CW00822157

Charlotte Fiell

HAIRSTYLES

Ancient to Present

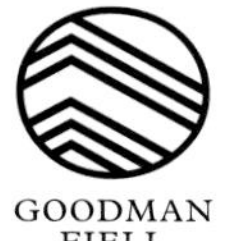

GOODMAN
FIELL

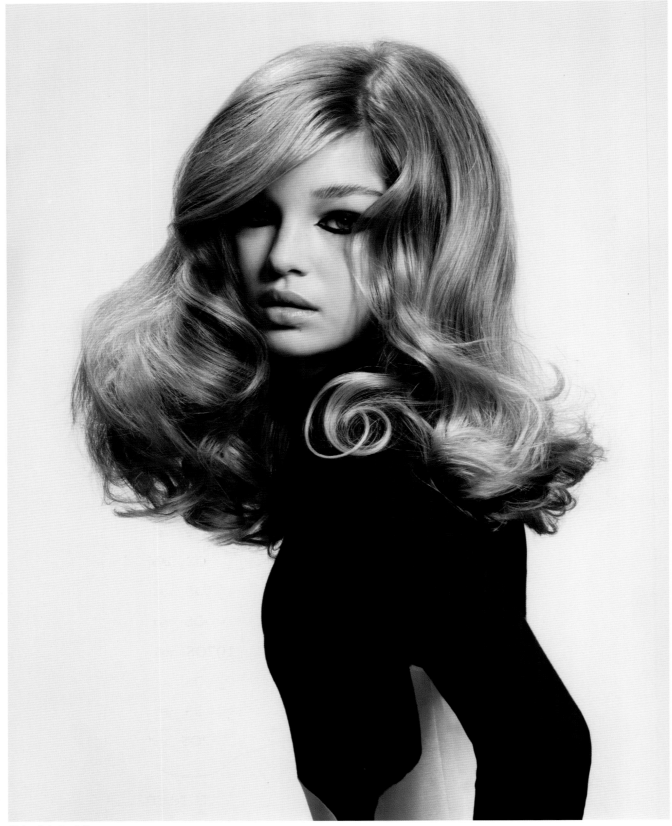

Hairstyle by Louis Byrne, 2009

Contents

Published in 2013 by Goodman Fiell
An imprint of the Carlton Publishing Group
20 Mortimer Street
London W1T 3JW

www.carltonbooks.co.uk

A CIP catalogue record for this book is available from the British Library.

ISBN 978-1-84796-040-5

Printed in China

FOREWORD

Hairdressers should never stop learning. To create a great hairstyle you have to have precision, symmetry and balance as well as an appreciation of the overall shape and style. Hairdressing is about rules and to perfect the craft takes years. Once you master the craft you can take your work that step further. It's at this point that you can commit random acts, disrupt the rules and let creativity take you to a new place, but, before you get there, you must learn how to cut technically. Then you can work towards artistry. Hair is like a canvas on which you can use your self-expression to create something unique and take that expression into many different areas such as photography and live shows. For me this involves sharing what I've done and what I know and giving purpose to everything I do. The medium of hair is an incredible way of artistic expression, like a temporary installation, an amazing image, or an ever-moving, kinetic sculpture and, like all great works of art, the art of hair is your own beholder.

Hairstyle: Ancient to Present is a wonderful testament to the enduring creativity of the hairdresser and also the discipline's unique cultural importance over the centuries. Hairdressing is a craft that needs a remarkable level of skill and this book demonstrates clearly and comprehensively, that the head is the perfect blank canvas for fabulous creations when practitioners have the necessary talents. I am very honoured to be a part of this wonderful book and trust that it will be a rich source of inspiration.

Anthony Mascolo

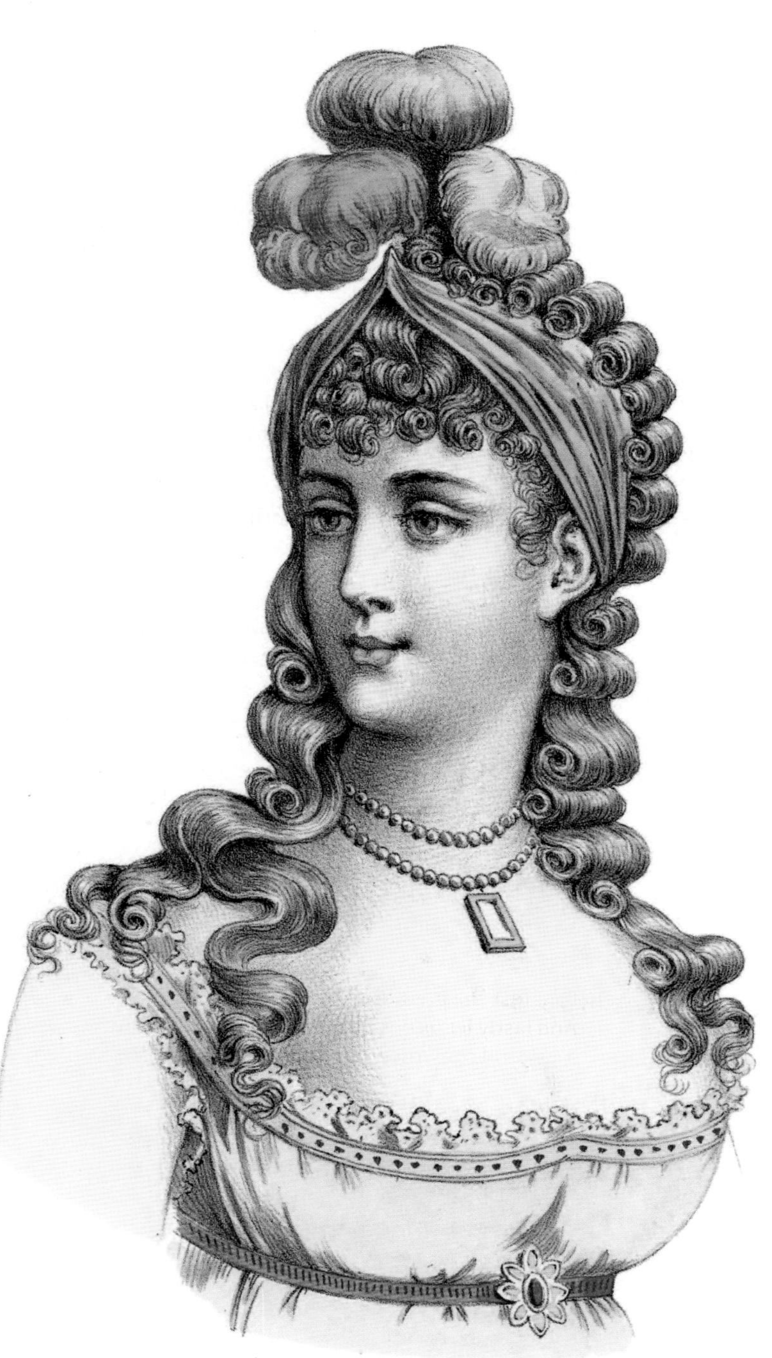

Coiffure Directoire, 1790s,
Album de Coiffures Historiques, E. Nissy

HAIRSTYLES: POWER & STATUS

Although hair and fashion are inextricably linked, hairstyling is often regarded as a vague afterthought in the fashion world, when it is actually an intrinsic part of it – the way a model's hair is styled is an integral element of a catwalk projection or a fashion marketing campaign, yet all too often the creators behind the coiffured creations are the unknown and unsung heroes of fashion image-making. This is not a new phenomenon; indeed the status of the hairdresser has always been slightly hazy, part-artisan, part-artist... the seemingly younger brother of the couturier or the milliner. In fact, hairstyling is itself a difficult discipline to pin down; it can be seen as an art form, a craft skill and even a design process. The transitory nature of a hairstyle – which can be blown away by a passing wind or washed away in a downpour – has also meant that it has been more difficult to record as a cultural phenomenon because it does not have the physical permanence of a garment or designed object. This inherent ephemerality has meant that hairstyling has largely been ignored as a significant research subject by cultural historians. This book sets out to readdress this, revealing the extraordinary skill and imagination of hairdressers down the ages, the majority of whom are long forgotten. With images that document an incredible variety of historic styles, this publication also surveys the work of today's leading hairstylists. It demonstrates that hairdressing is and has always been a vibrantly creative discipline, as well as a barometer of the wider cultural landscape in which it exists.

The story of hair is itself a winding and multi-stranded history that reflects the role of women in society. It traces their status and aspirations, while mirroring the wider economic, political and cultural contexts of the period in which specific haircuts were created. Every culture has hairstyles unique to it, and in Western society for centuries every season has had its own identifiable fashion, whether it's an elaborately structured and powdered wig of the 18th century, an elegant Victorian chignon, undulating Marcel waves of the Belle Époque era, or a late 1970s brightly dyed Punk crop. This lavish and sumptuously illustrated publication sets out to comprehensively trace this previously untold story and, in so doing, it is hoped that the social and cultural relevance of the hairdresser's art will finally be reappraised and given the status it so richly deserves. Moreover, this work is also intended to act as a visual celebration of this remarkably inventive cultural phenomenon.

Different hair types are linked to cultural identity, while various cultures have diverse notions of beauty. Indeed beauty shop culture can be seen as a magnifying lens on wider cultural norms; for example, in African-American culture the hair salon is an important gathering place that functions as a vital cultural institution almost on par with the church. While in earlier times, the act of going to a hair salon rather than "dressing" hair at home was an important step towards female emancipation. It is no surprise that the modish bob so beloved by flappers of the Art Deco period, which swept aside centuries of carefully constructed hairpieces, festoons of ribbons and elaborate pinning, coincided with a period of unprecedented economic and political liberation for young women. Indeed the history of hairdressing is ultimately the visualised account of women's changing role in society.

We should also remember, that human hair is itself a very human attribute, with the only other animal that has hair that continuously grows being the musk ox. We all face, through the hair growing on our bodies, our cultural and biological roots on a daily basis; indeed it defines what it is to be human – it is ultimately an ever-growing expression of the human condition. It is also a marker of ethnicity; for example, oriental hair has a round cross-sectional profile, while Afro hair has a flattened eliptical form and Caucasian hair an oval one. These differently formed cross sections cause the hair to grow in markedly different ways – to curl, frizz or hang dead straight. It emerges that hair is not only a remarkably durable part of the body, but it also stores and records our unique genetic material making it individual to every single person on the planet. Hair is also the stuff of stories; everybody has a hair story – and it is these anecdotal tales of bad hair, good hair, dyed hair, frizzy hair, thinning hair etc. that we can collectively identify with. Ultimately our hairstyles reflect our self-image as individuals set against the prevailing culture of our times.

And lastly let us not forget, that although the dressing of hair is a cultural construct that is a powerful signifier of creative individuality, personal identity, political views and socio-economic status, it is also explicitly linked to female sexuality. Indeed today there are still many cultures around the world where women's heads are covered to hide their supposedly suggestive locks. Certainly, throughout the ages, the dressing of hair has been an important female activity that has enriched the idea of femininity by beautifying its subjects. As Martin Luther noted, hair is indeed, "the richest ornament of women" and its rich visual history is waiting to be rediscovered on the following pages...

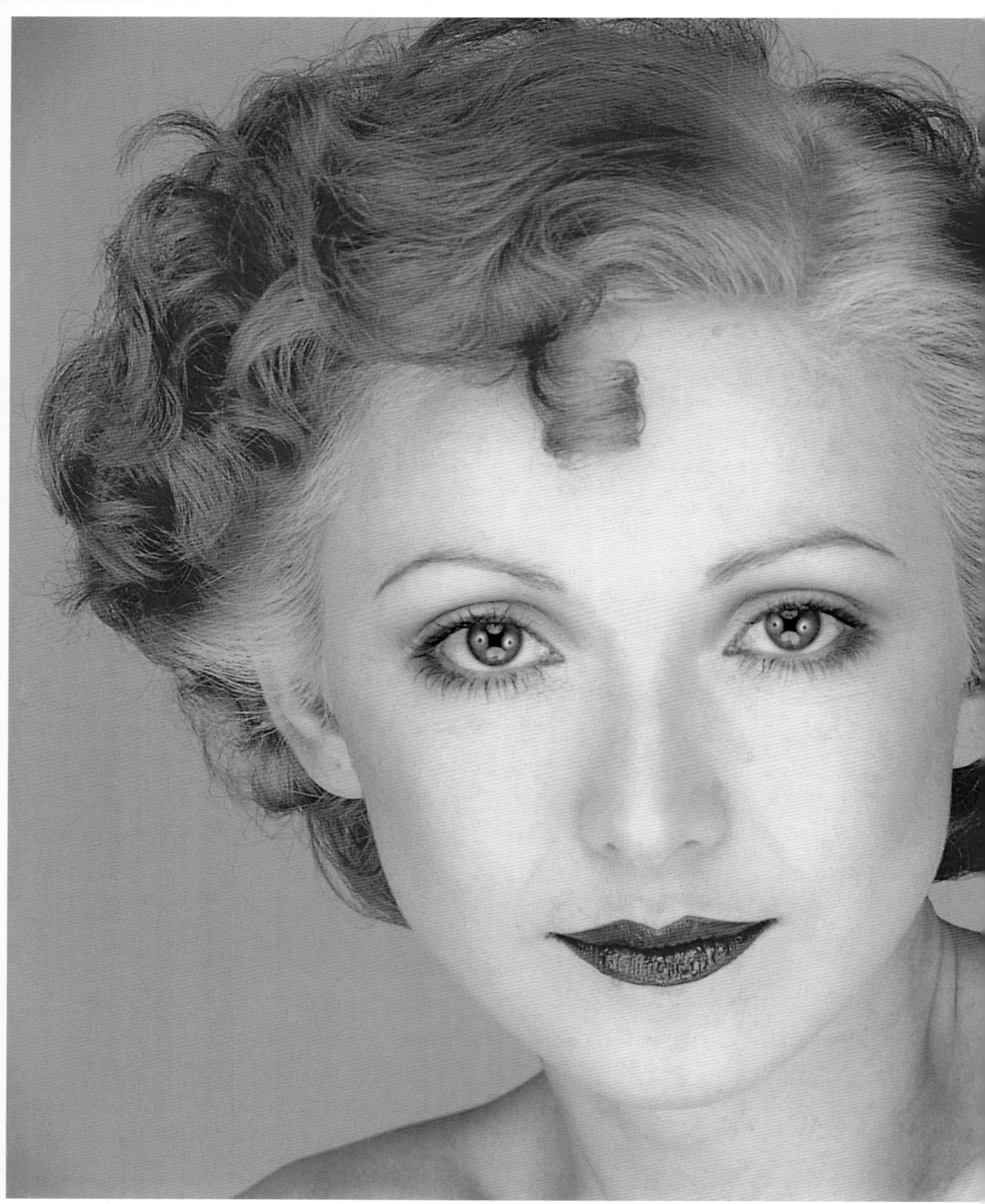

Hairstyle by Keith Wainwright of Smile, 1979–80

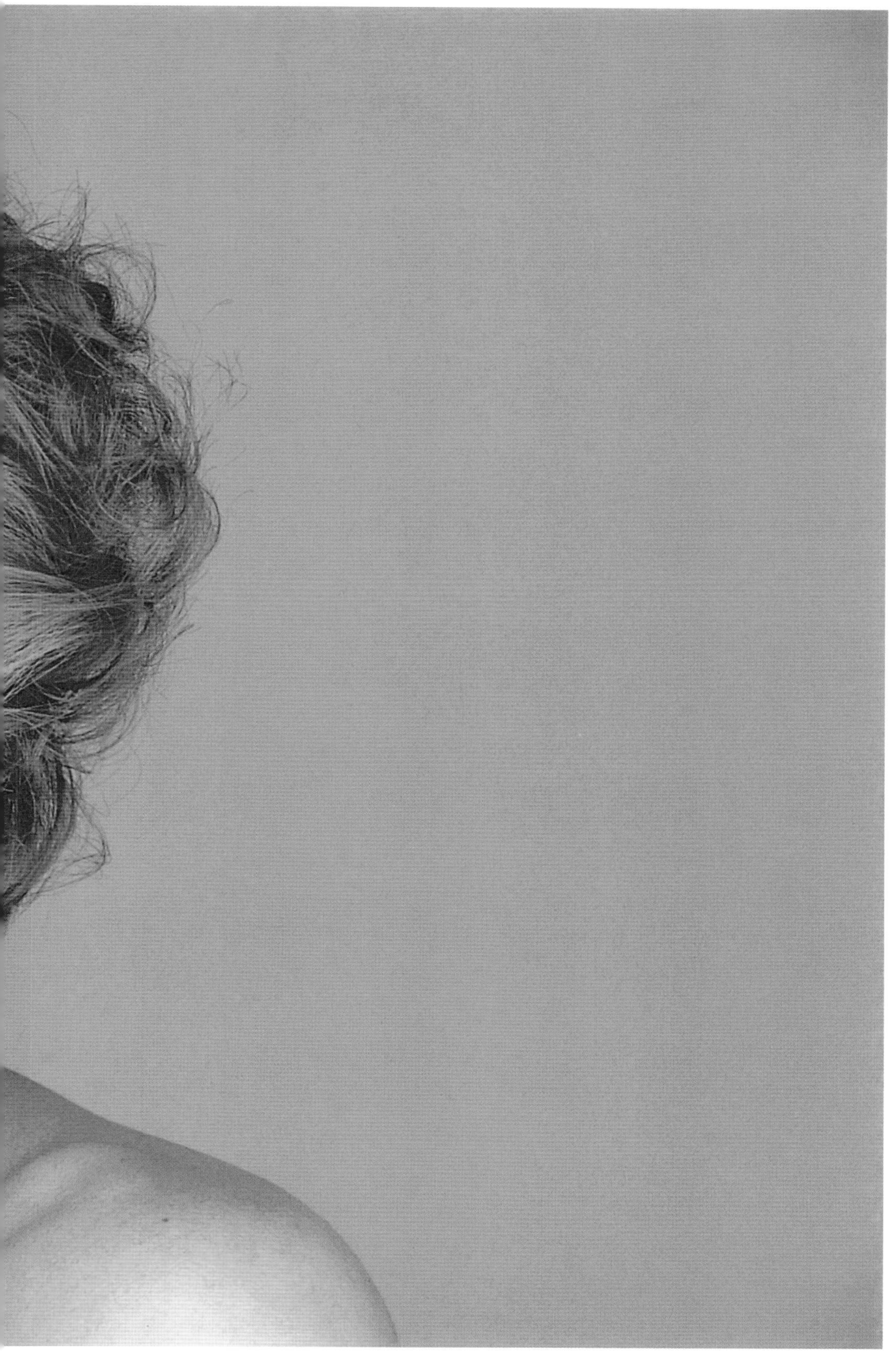

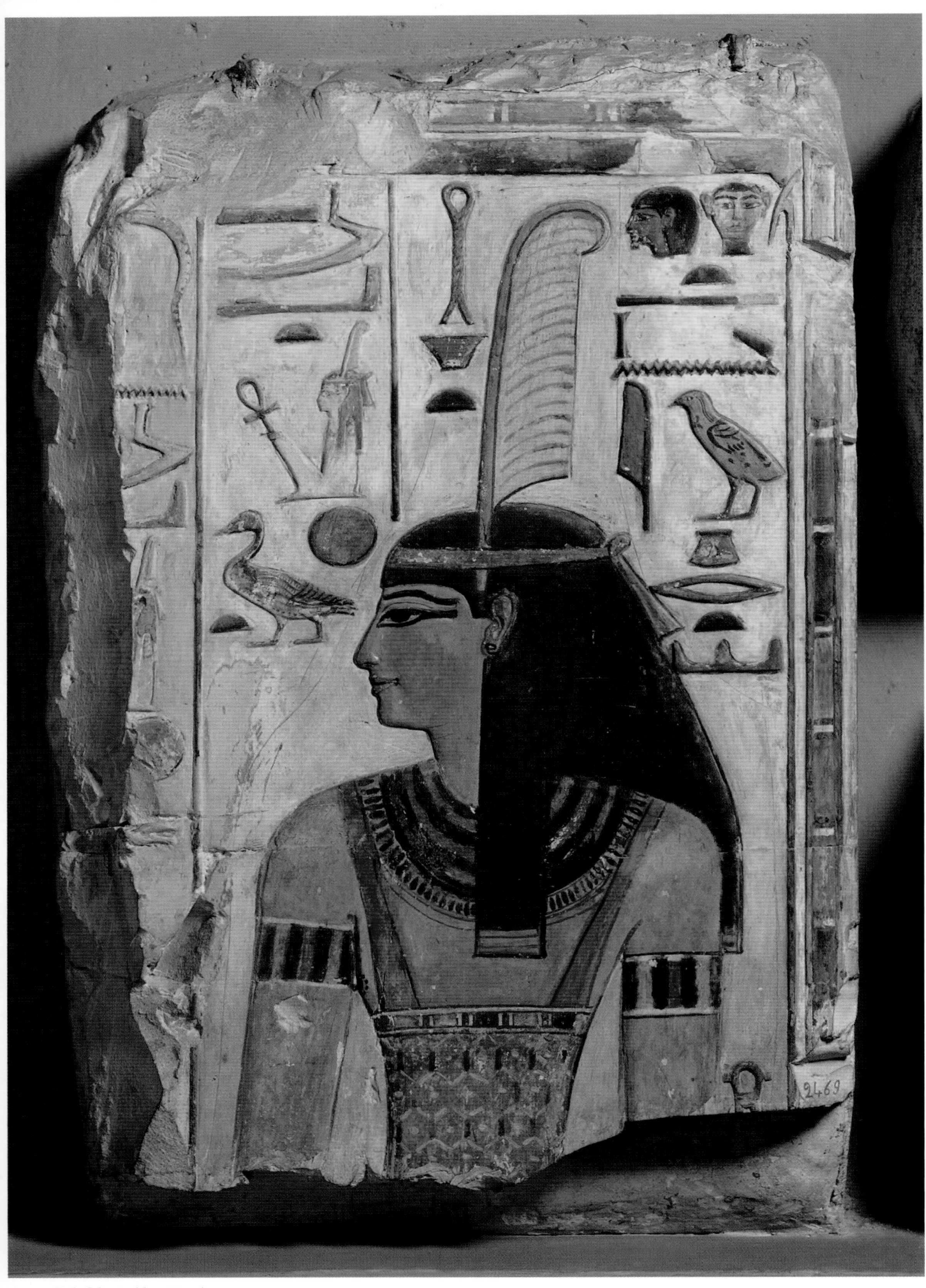

'Bas-relief of the Goddess Maat',
New Kingdom (XVIII–XXV dynasty)

ANCIENT

ANCIENT EGYPT From ancient times onwards women have devoted a huge amount of time and money to the dressing of their hair in order to embellish their beauty. As J. P. C. Bicknell noted, "Historical research has shown that your tonsorial artist is by no means a comparatively modern innovation, but that he plied his craft skillfully many thousands of years ago." (*Progress*, Summer Issue 1938, p.89). The study of ancient Egyptian monuments and sculptures certainly reveal a civilisation where women styled their hair with immense care. For women of high status, the elaborate adornment of their hair was the literal pinnacle of their overall attire. Wearing cleverly constructed wigs on their shaved heads, the women of ancient Egypt wore their hairpieces in styles that were artistically enriched with leaves, jewellery and carved combs, sometimes crafted to represent leopards or antelope. It was, however, only royal women that were allowed to wear hair jewellery that represented the asp – the sacred snake of the ancient Egyptians. It was also only women of high status that could afford wigs made from real hair, while poorer women made do with wigs made from wool. In Ancient Egypt, there appear to have been various dedicated hairdressing establishments that made wigs of plaited hair impregnated with a mixture of beeswax and resin to hold their shape. The British Museum has in its collection a number of wigs from this period, as well as several surviving wig-boxes that have come from various tomb excavations. Experts believe that because in Egyptian times the notion of sexual activity and the idea of reincarnation were so closely linked, that the presence of wigs in burial chambers is not just part of a cache of precious objects signifying the deceased's status, but may well also be an allusion to rebirth after death. And as such, hair in Ancient Egypt was not only a mark of wealth and rank, but also a signifier of sexual attraction – just as it still is today.

ANCIENT GREECE Unlike the Egyptians, Greek woman were blessed with a smoother hair texture that meant it was easier to style their locks. Instead of shaving their heads and wearing wigs, Grecian women allowed their hair to grow long, often curled on their forehead and at the sides of their heads, then drawn into a pony-tail or elaborate bun at the nape of the neck and held in place with diadem, hairbands, hair pins, strings, hairnets and ribbons. The elegant line and subtle adornment of Grecian hairstyles echoed the soft flowing lines of their diaphanous garments. One distinctive hairstyle especially favoured by young Greek woman was the so-called "Melon" which divided the hair into ribbed segments that ran from the forehead to the back of the neck. Curling irons and hairbrushes were used to create these types of elaborate hairstyles, while beeswax was used to set the curls and tresses in place. Greek maidens also used ash, henna and coloured waxes to change the tone of their hair, and because blonde hair was a rare but highly prized ideal within Greek culture, they even tried bleaching their hair. It is no surprise that Hesiod described Helen of Troy, the greatest beauty of Greek mythology, as "fair-haired". Indeed the poet Sappho also waxed lyrical about the beauty of golden hair, writing:

> My mother always said
> that in her youth she was
> exceedingly in fashion
> wearing a purple ribbon
> looped in her hair.
> But the girl whose hair is yellower
> than torchlight need wear no
> colorful ribbons from Sardis -
> but a garland of fresh flowers.

In Greek mythology, hair was inexplicably linked to the idea of sexuality and power. The Greek poets Homer and Anacreon both saw hairstyles as not only an essential ornament of women but also a corrective against the forces of uncivilised nature. Indeed there was a plethora of recognisable hair ornaments with which unruly tresses were subdued including, according to William Smith's *Dictionary of Greek and Roman Antiquities* (1875), "the Sling", which was a broad band worn across the forehead made of metal or leather; the "Kekryfalos" – a fine hair net sometimes made of gold; the "Bag" that was used to cover the majority of the head and was manufactured from silk or wool, and lastly the "Miter" which was a turban-like band of coloured cloth that was wound around the hair and worn in various styles. According to J. P. C. Bicknell, "In the Ancient Greek civilisation the fashionable courtesans wore their hair dressed in many wonderful fashions and tinted blue, red, green and every conceivable colour of the rainbow." Significantly the Greek hairstyles depicted in the fine arts of the time show a remarkable level of craft. It is not surprising that, according to A. Mallemont, the author of *L'Art de la Coiffure Française* (1900), the patricians of Ancient Rome imported young Greeks taught by the great masters of Athenian hairdressing, "but if they failed to satisfy them, woe betide them!"

ANCIENT ROME In his famous instructional elegy, the *Ars Amatoria* (The Art of Love), the Roman poet, Ovid advised women to, "Arrange your hair with art, all its charm will depend on how much or how little care you bestow on it." In this ancient guide to dating, Ovid also gives us an insightful glimpse into the plethora of styles that were fashionable in Ancient Rome, noting, "There are a thousand styles of hairdressing. Each woman must know how to choose that which suits her best, and as to this matter, her mirror will be her wisest councilor... A loose and curly arrangement is most becoming to one, while an artistic gathering up of locks is better suited to another's features. Some ladies even seek to dress their hair in waves or wider twists whose rhythmic lines recall the undulations of the sea. The careless-looking style of hairdressing is admirably suited to many kinds of beauty; but nothing requires a greater amount of art than this apparently unstudied manner of wearing the hair."

During the earliest Roman period, women adopted Greek hairdressing practices and wore their hair relatively simply, often with their hair twisted up in a loop above their foreheads and then bound with a narrow band, sometimes made of gold or silver. This band provided a convenient fixing for the crown-like headdress worn during feasts or sacrifices. As time went on, however, more elaborate styles became fashionable. During this period there were numerous recognisably distinctive styles: the "Miter", the "Tholia", the "Strophe", the "Anademia", the "Vesica", the "Reticulum", the "Influa", the "Vittae", the "Corymbion", the "Calanthic", the "Calyptric" and the "Flammeum" – with their names often referring to the various things that were used to create them, from silk ribbons and finely woven gold hairnets studded with precious stones or pearls to strips of woollen cloth and veils.

As the Roman Empire expanded, its victories, conquests and triumphal processions gave women an increasing excuse for more elaborate hairstyles – intricate coiffures that were the embodiment of Roman refinement. In particular, the Roman conquest of the Germanic Tribes on the banks of the River Rhine had a huge influence on the hairstyles of the day. The German tribes favoured blonde or red hair and used "spuma batava" (Batavian foam) made from beechwood ash to lighten hair. This hair-bleaching dye, also known as Savon de Hesse, became extremely popular in Ancient Rome. Certainly by 300 BC Roman hairdressers were using numerous concoctions to produce the desired blonde look, and women who could afford it would wear wigs made from natural blonde imported hair. History recalls that during the so-called "Blonde Epidemic" in Rome, shops were opened that traded blonde and red hair imported from Germany for exorbitant sums of money. And if they couldn't afford this, then Roman women also used henna to give their naturally dark locks an attractive reddish tone.

The Flavian Period saw a marked change in hairstyles, with the earlier looped tresses above the forehead and the simple gathered buns falling from fashion. Instead the high-ranking women of Imperial Rome adopted something altogether more sophisticated, with tower-like constructions of tightly curled loops that incorporated hairpieces and wiring to achieve the desire effect. The Roman satiric poet, Juvenal, gives us a description of a patrician lady at her toilette and attended by her slave who adopts this so-called "Flavian Nest" style: "Finally the slave builds up on her lady's head a many-storied edifice, which makes her look like Andromache from the front; whereas, seen from behind, the effect produced is of another order. There are locks of curly hair, cushions that swell the proportions of the structure, little side curls that fringe the forehead and the ears. These mysteries of the toilette, this anxious care of the tresses, constitute the chief occupation of the Roman ladies."

As fashions moved on, during the second century, Roman hairstyles became simpler again with the hair plaited and then formed into a bun at the back of the head or a coronet on top of the head, which was then frequently secured with a large decorative pin. Hairdressing in the third century revealed the fashion for deeply waved hair, while the fourth century saw Roman women wearing their hair in large flattened buns often entwined with ribbons. During the Roman period there were numerous hairdressing establishments where women would go to get their hair styled into the latest and ever-changing fashions of the day. Many Roman women also owned slaves who were trained to attend to their elaborate coiffures in the comfort and privacy of their own homes. Certainly the time and money merited on these fabulously coiffed constructions, reveals that the styling of hair was seen as an important cultural occupation that ultimately expressed the urbane civilisation of Imperial Rome, and the high status of many of its citizens.

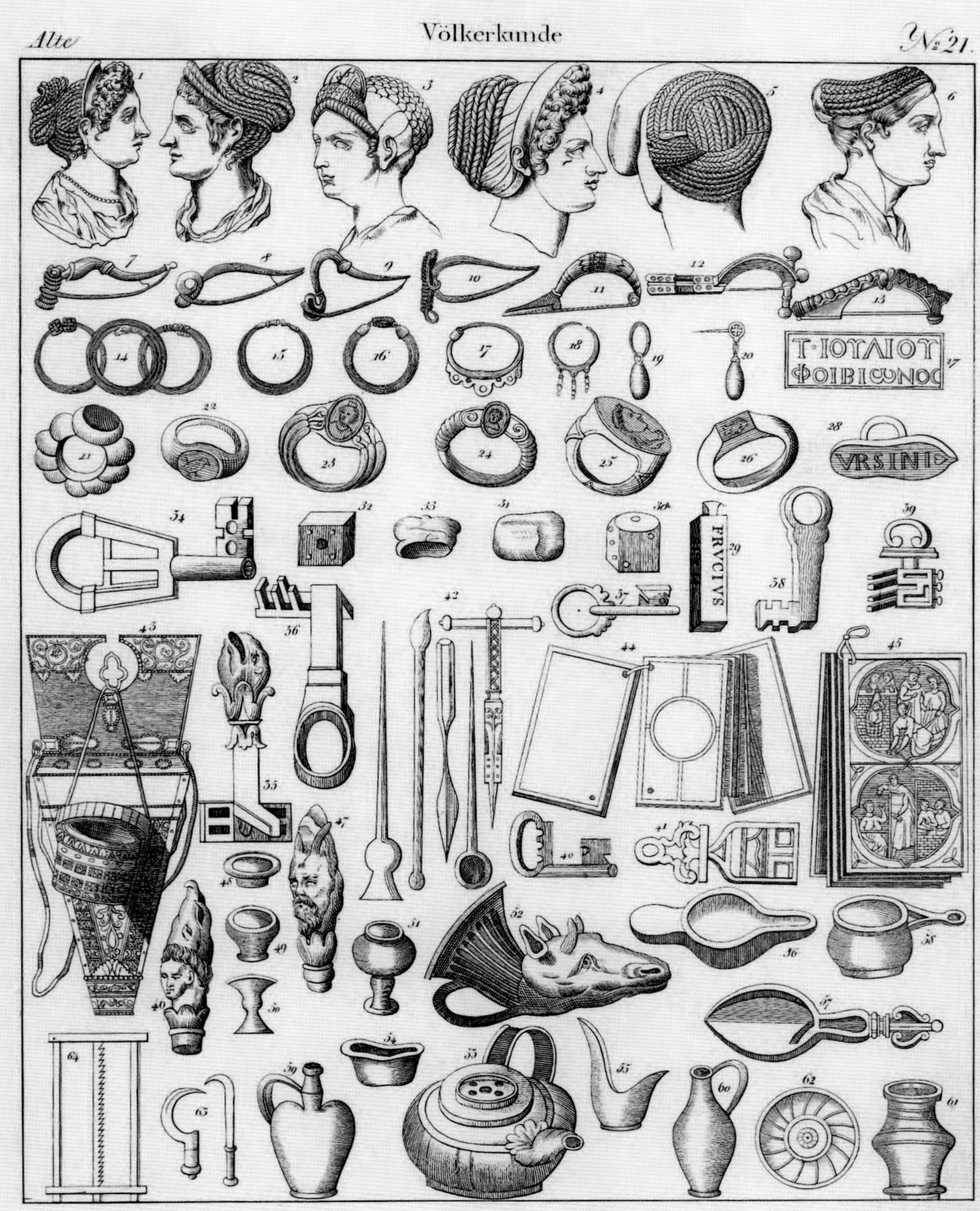

Roman hairstyles and artifacts *Systematische Bilder-Galerie zur Allg. Dt. Real-Encyclopädie*

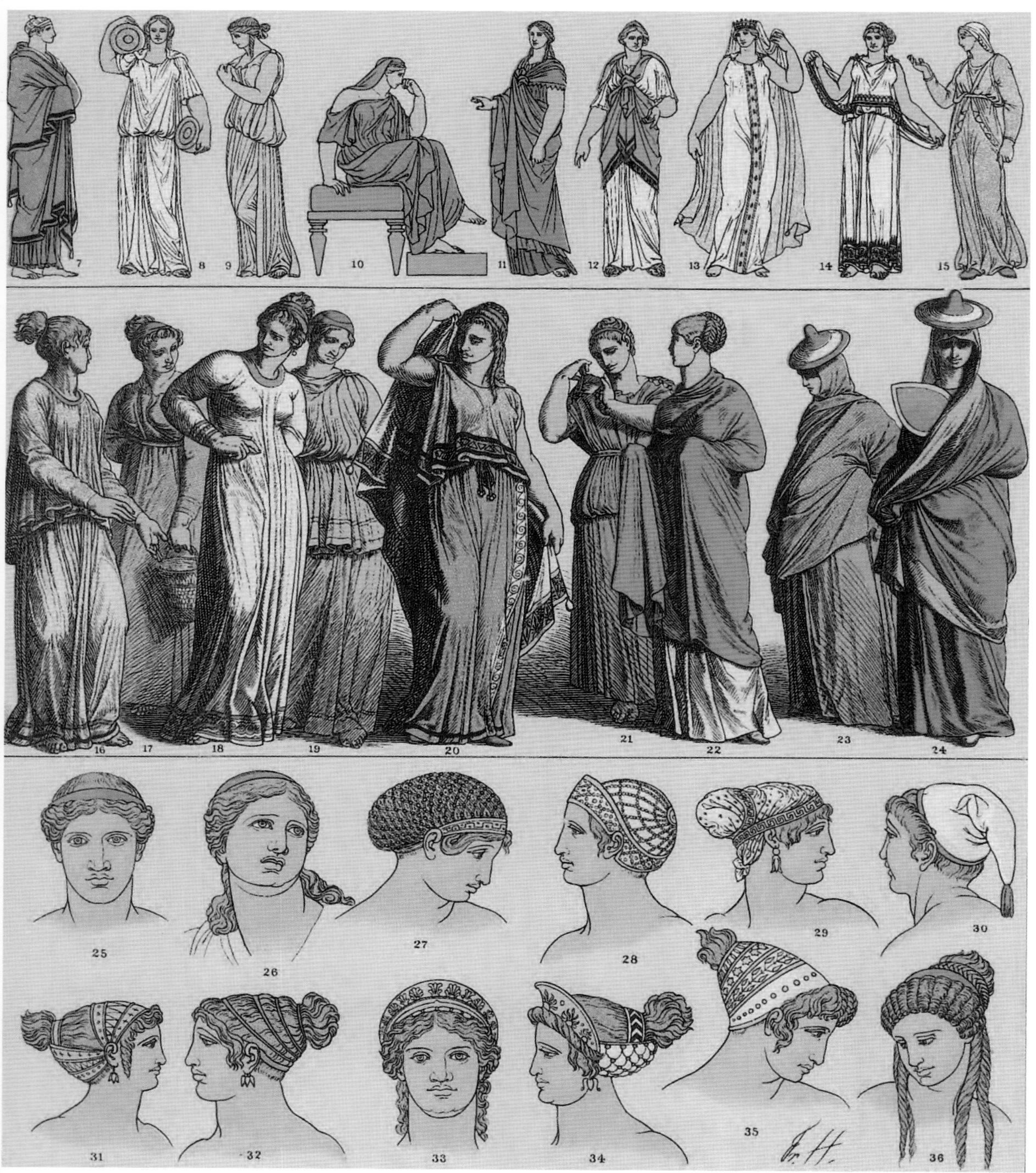

Ancient Greek hairstyles

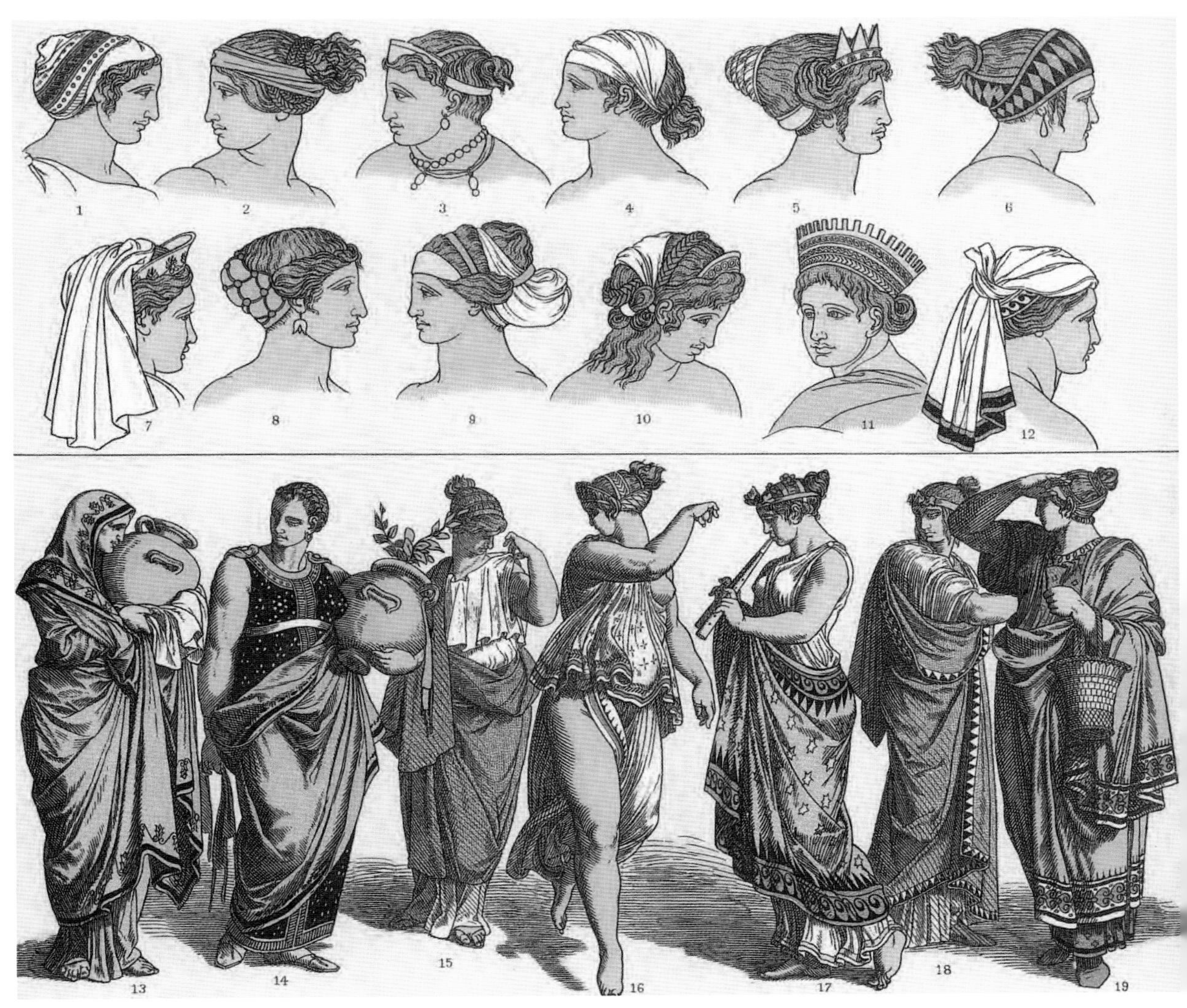

Ancient Greek hairstyles

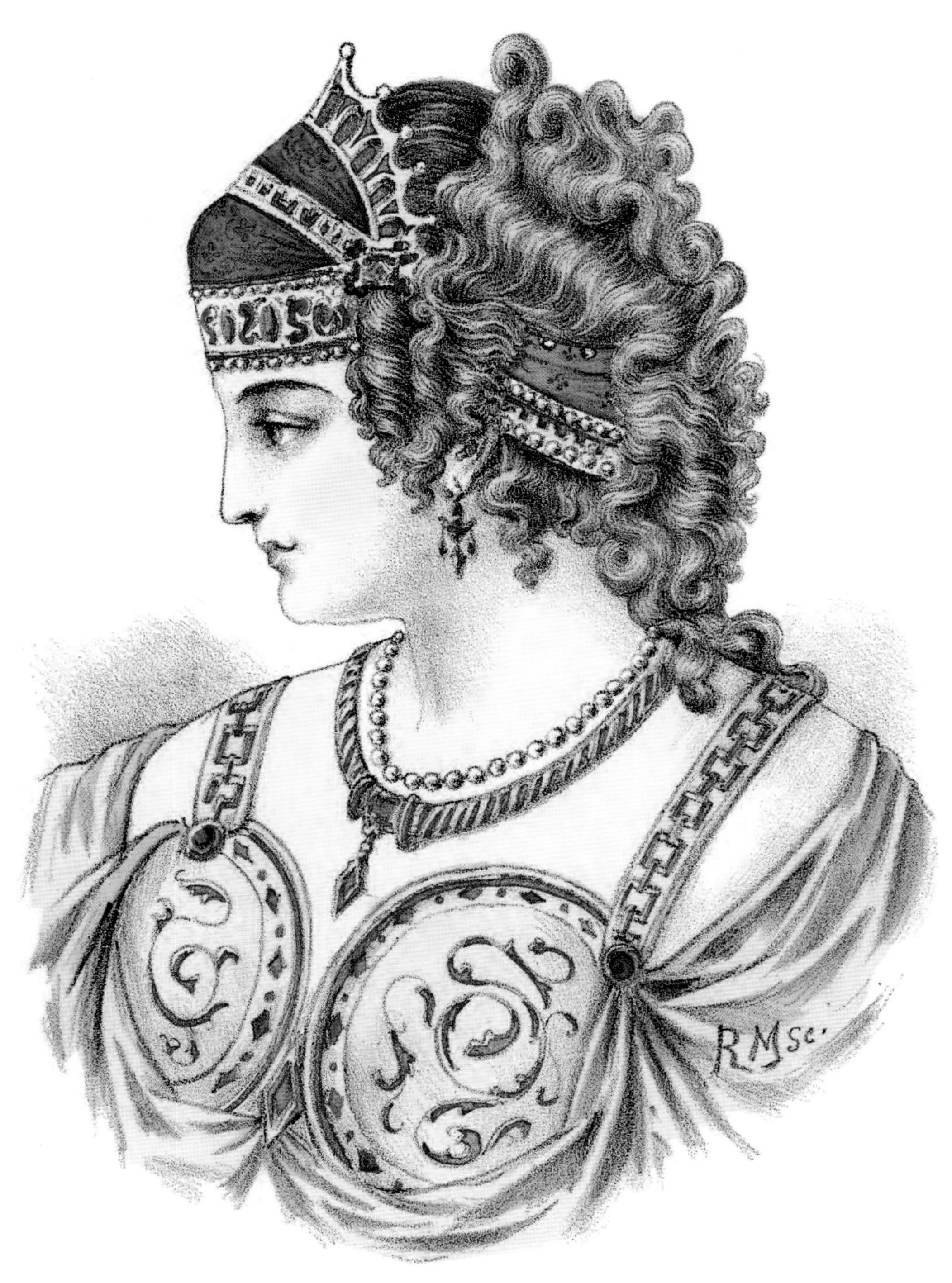

Greek hairstyle, *Album de Coiffures Historiques*, E. Nissy

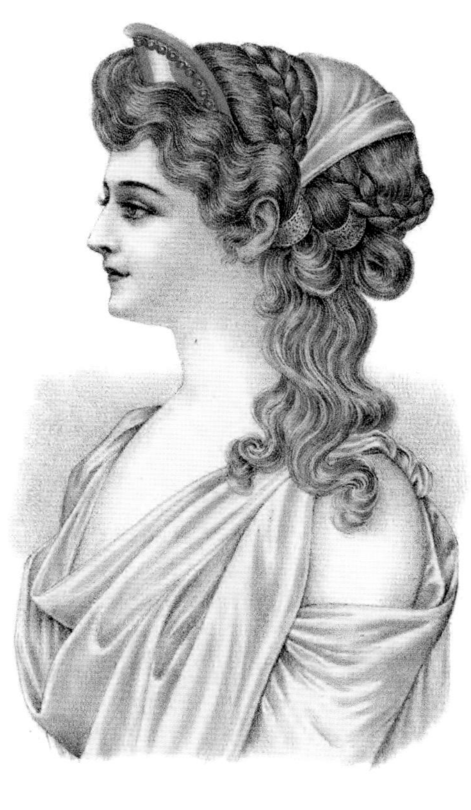

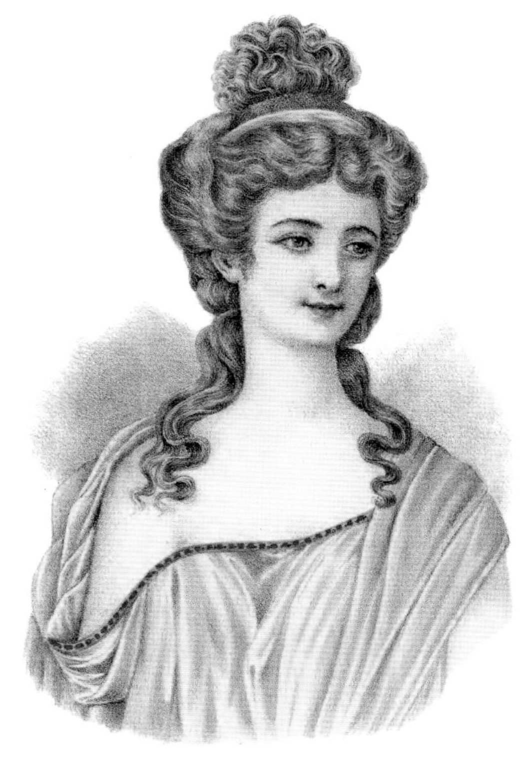

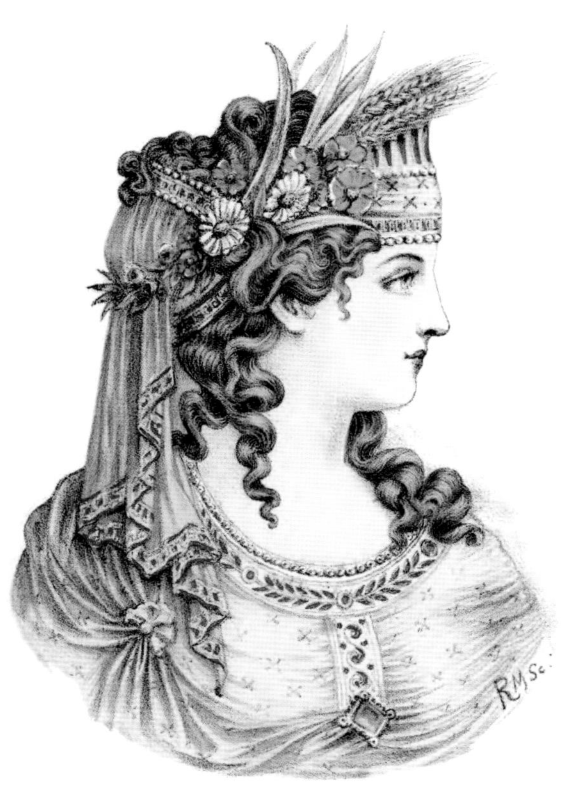

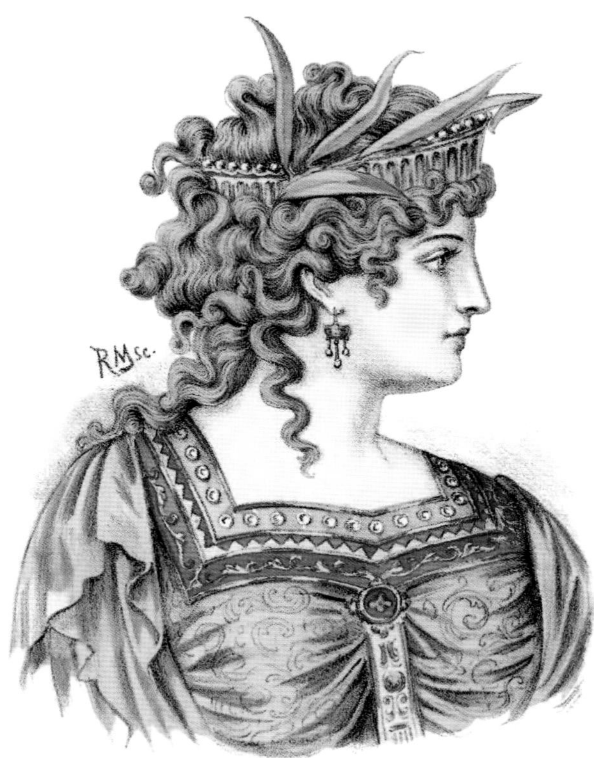

Greek hairstyles, *Album de Coiffures Historiques*, E. Nissy

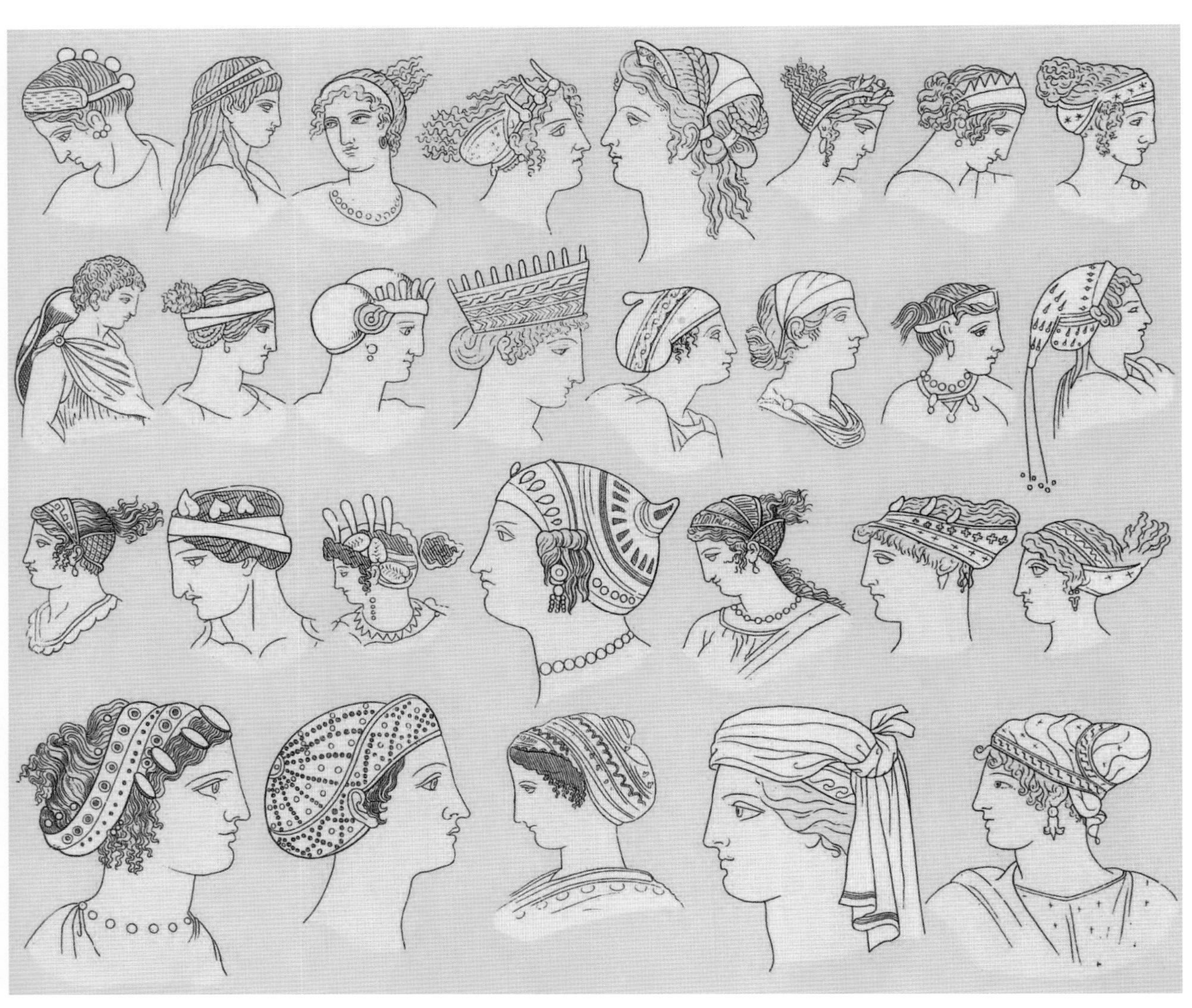

Ancient Greek hairstyles,
Le Costume Historique, A. Racinet

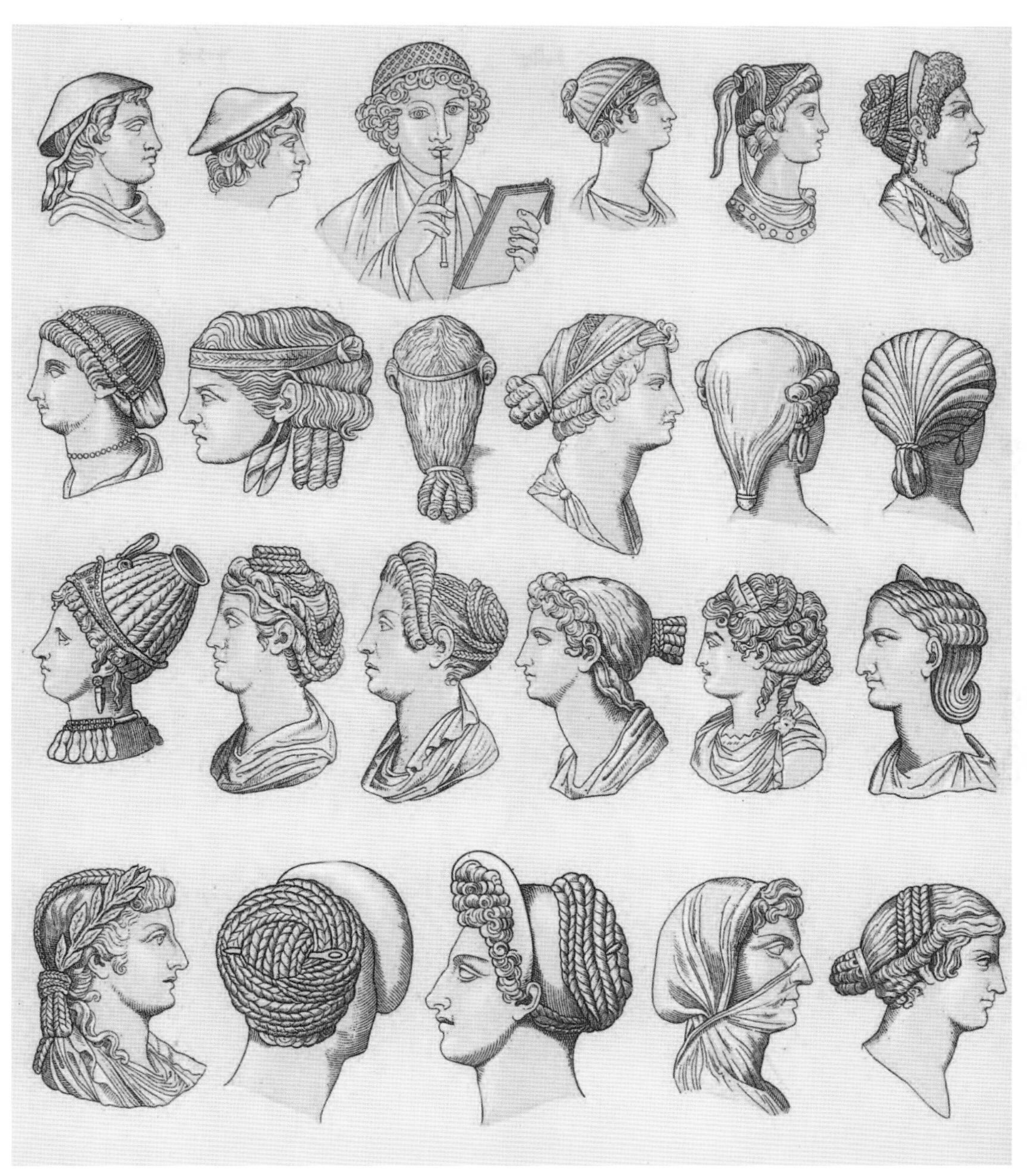

Roman hairstyles, *Le Costume Historique*, A. Racinet

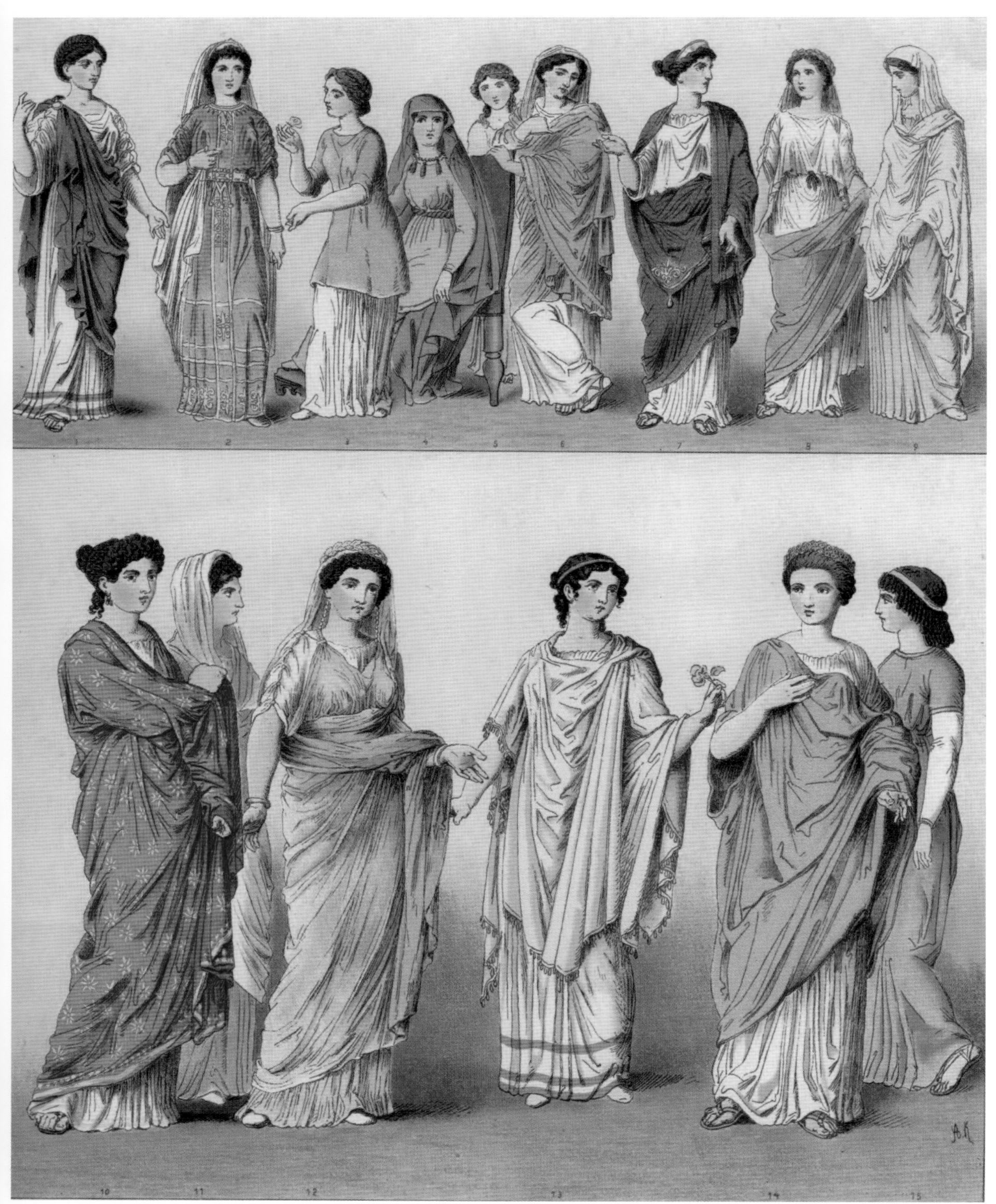

Roman female costumes, showing different hairstyles, lithograph by Eugen Köhler

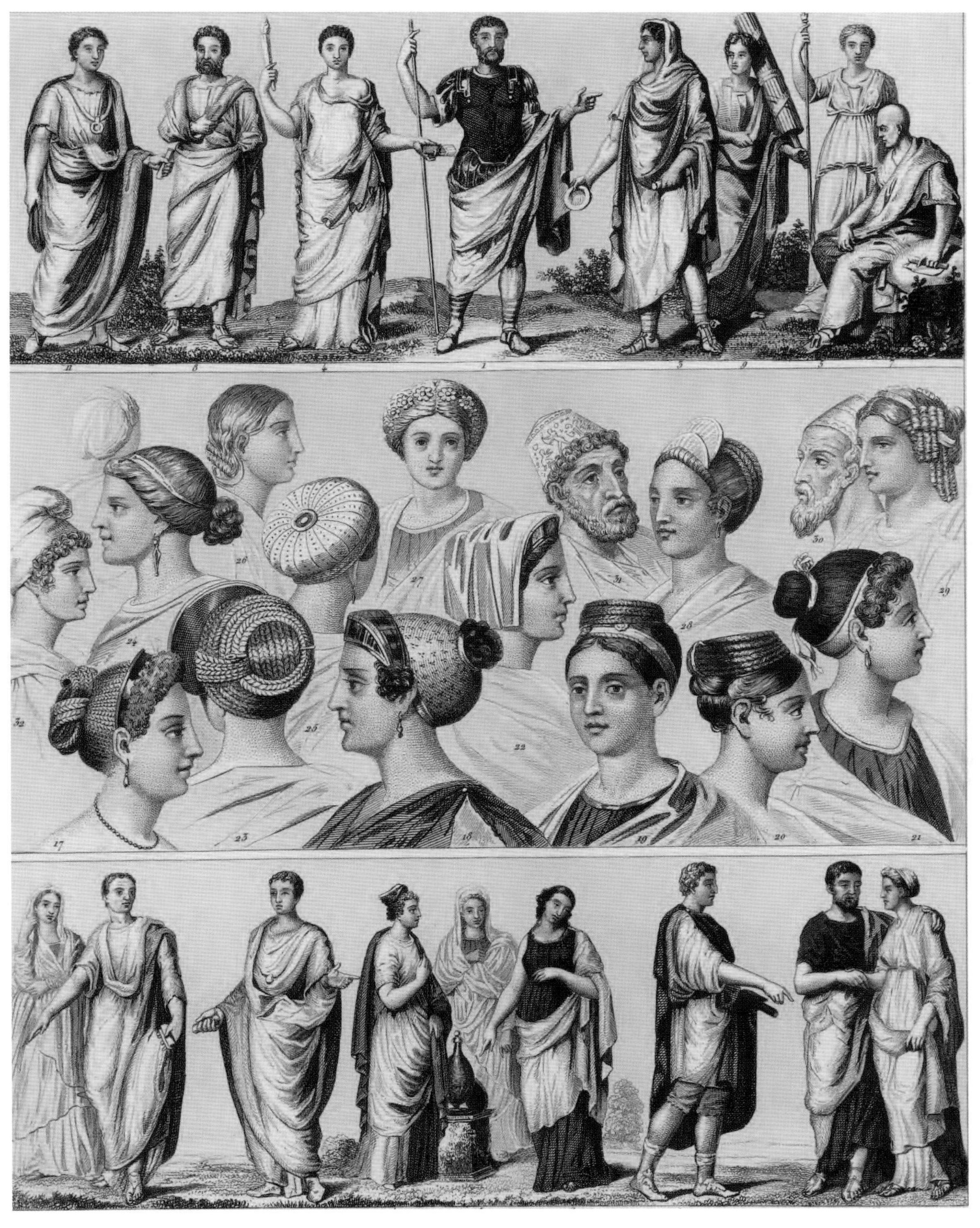

Roman hairstyles, lithograph
by Henry Winkles

'Portrait of Girl' fresco, from Pompeii

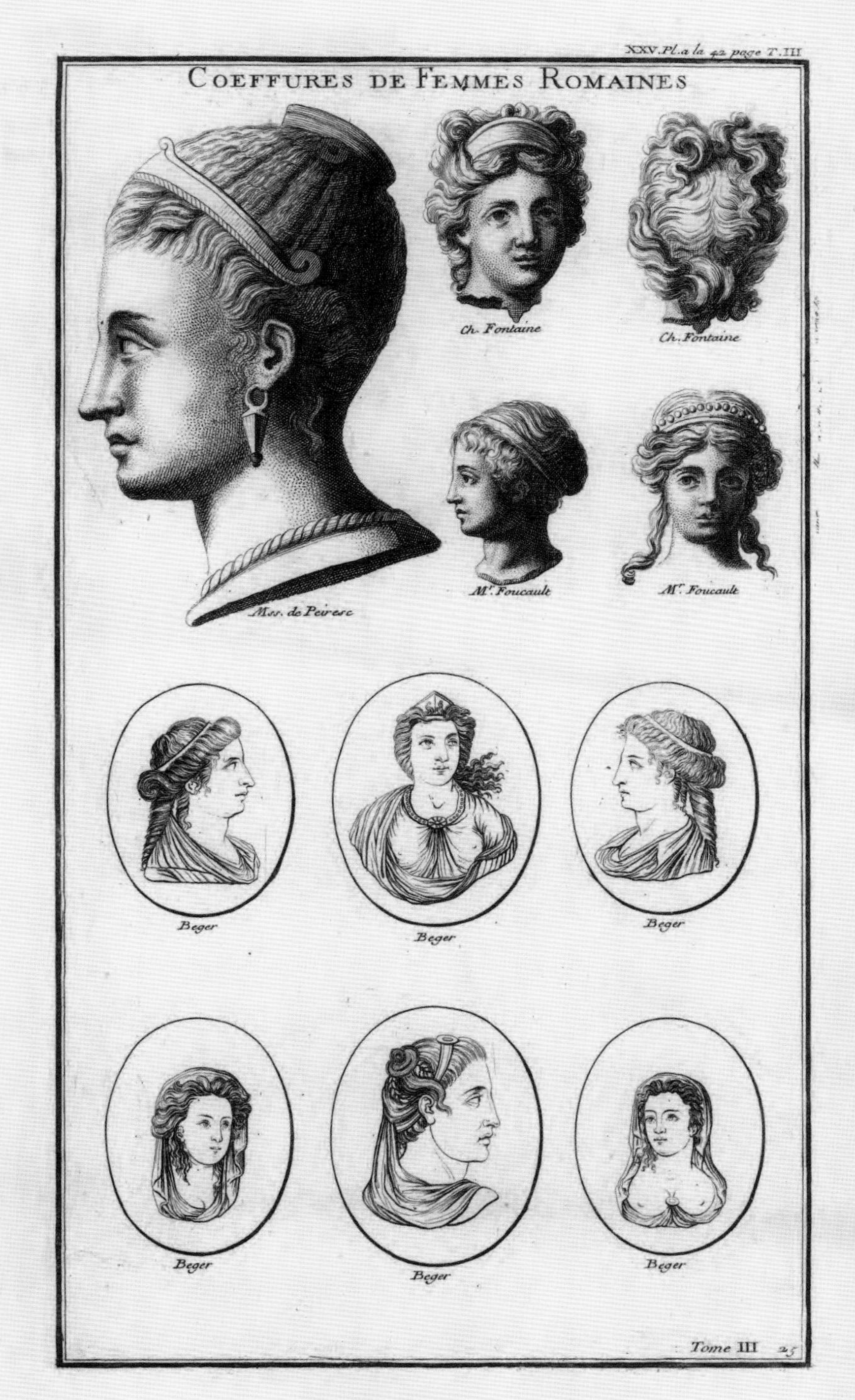

Roman hairstyles, *L'Antiquité Expliquée, et Representée en Figures*, Bernard de Montfaucon

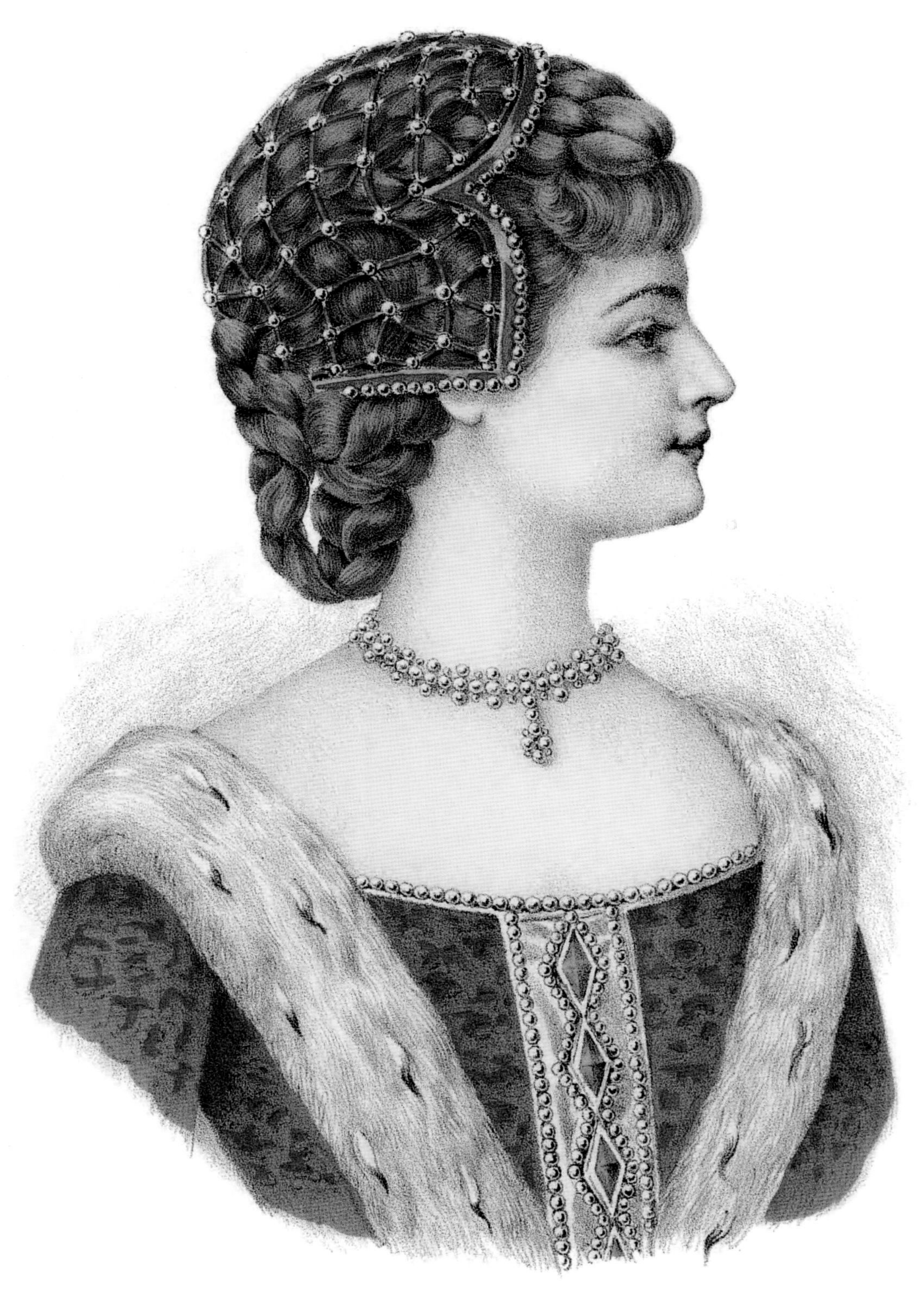

Middle Ages hairstyle, *Album de Coiffures Historiques*, E. Nissy

MIDDLE AGES

Spanning the fifth century to the 15th century, the Middle Ages, also known as the Medieval Period or the Dark Ages, saw a distinctive stylistic shift in the way women's hair was styled. The elaborate coiffures of the ancient world were initially replaced with a fashion for simpler styles and the wearing of veils that often hid much of the head. The more austere hairstyles of this early Medieval era mirrored the rise of Christianity and its emphasis on modesty, especially for women. Often young women wore their hair loosely and held in place down their backs with a circlet, while older women appear to have preferred wearing their hair in either a coil or a bun. Often it was only the hair on the forehead that was visible underneath the veils, and this was simply parted down the centre and then gently waved on the temples.

During this period, however, Byzantine-inspired styles imported from the Orient, thanks to the Crusades, also became popular. And by the 12th century, it had become fashionable for women to wear their hair in braids that were loosely plaited, and which were sometimes so long they almost touched the ground. Often ribbons were used to bind these braids so as to give a fashionable cross-gartered look. Ribbons were also twisted into tapering points as a way of creating the illusion of longer plaits. In the late 12th century, the length of braids became shorter and often they were looped and pinned across the forehead to create a headband of plaited hair. Another fashionable hair ornament in the 14th century was a wide band of material known as a "Barbette" that was worn under the chin and then pinned upwards onto a circlet worn on the head, thereby leaving only a small amount of hair showing. During this period there was also a fashion for "Ram's Horn" plaits – braids that were coiled onto the sides on the head and then pinned into place.

During the 15th century, more elaborate styles began to take hold, which often enclosed the hair in bag-like nets set with jewels or into tapering steeple-like cones, known as "Hennin" onto which transparent veils were attached. Padded wirework "Templers" that were worn on the sides of the head also became fashionable, as were turban-like headdresses that often took the form of a fabric-covered padded roll. As the French journalist and man of letters, Octave Uzanne noted, "During the 14th century ladies wore feathers in their hair. Some built up their tresses in the shape of bushel measures, more or less high. Others imprisoned their locks in a sort of net called 'crestine', 'crépine' or 'crépinette'. The tufts at the sides of the head formed horn-like excrescences... Never were splendour and extravagance in head-covering carried to such an excess as during the first half of the 15th century. The hair itself was but a trifling item in the luxury of decoration lavished on the female head."

One of the most elaborate of these head-covering decorations was a two-coned headdress known as the "Butterfly" that enjoyed a short-lived popularity in the 1470s. Despite the fact that for the most part women's hair was covered with veils during the Medieval period, fair-coloured tresses were especially favoured and women often dyed their hair to acquire a lighter shade than nature intended; indeed in France during this period the process of bleaching hair became known as "se blondoyer". During this time, ladies also extensively plucked their hairlines in order to attain fashionably high foreheads, which were seen as a sign of noble beauty and wealth. Of course, the elaborate hairstyles of the Middle Ages were solely the preserve of noblewomen, and women of the serf class wore far simpler hairstyles; older women usually had short or shoulder-length hair covered with a linen bag or a plain barbette, while most unmarried girls wore their hair loosely down their backs with a simple circlet or fillet holding it in place. The late 15th century, however, saw the full blossoming of the Renaissance period, which freed women from the cumbersome veils of the previous feudal era and gave rise to hairstyles that mirrored the seismic social changes that were occurring in the different countries across Europe.

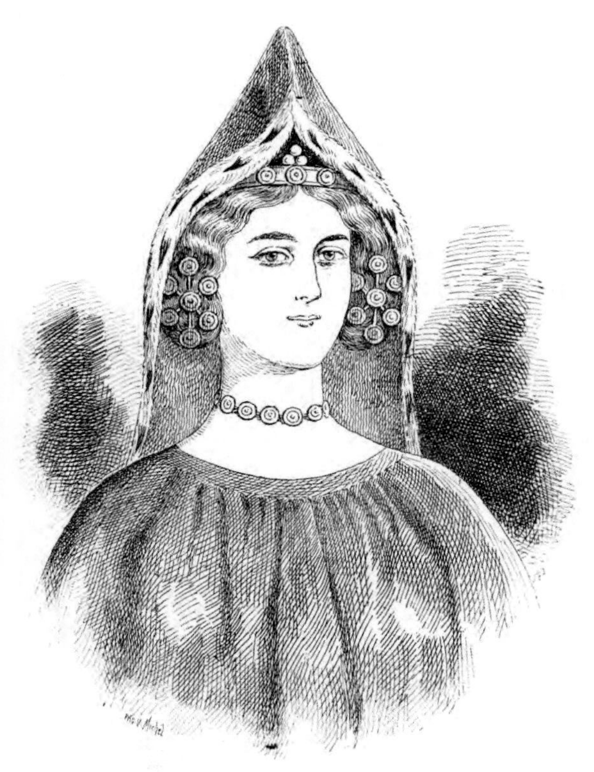

‘L’Aumusse’ hairstyle, c.1200, *L’Art de la Coiffure Française*, A. Mallemont

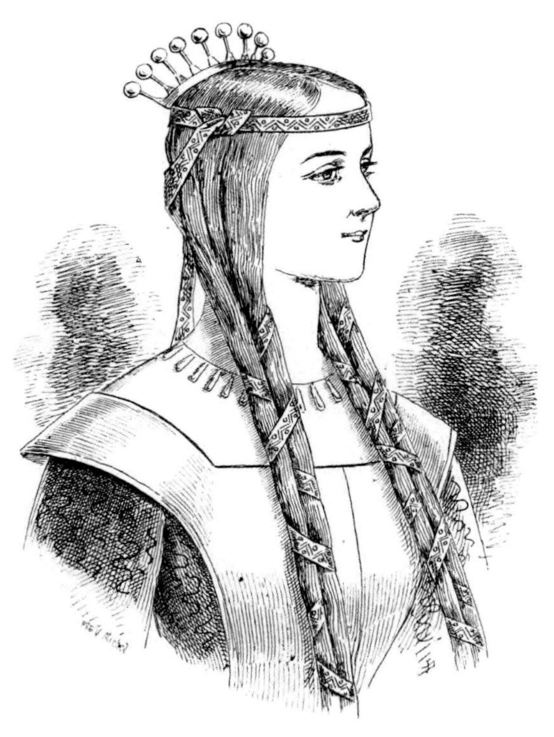

‘Le Fréseau’ hairstyle, Middle Ages, *L’Art de la Coiffure Française*, A. Mallemont

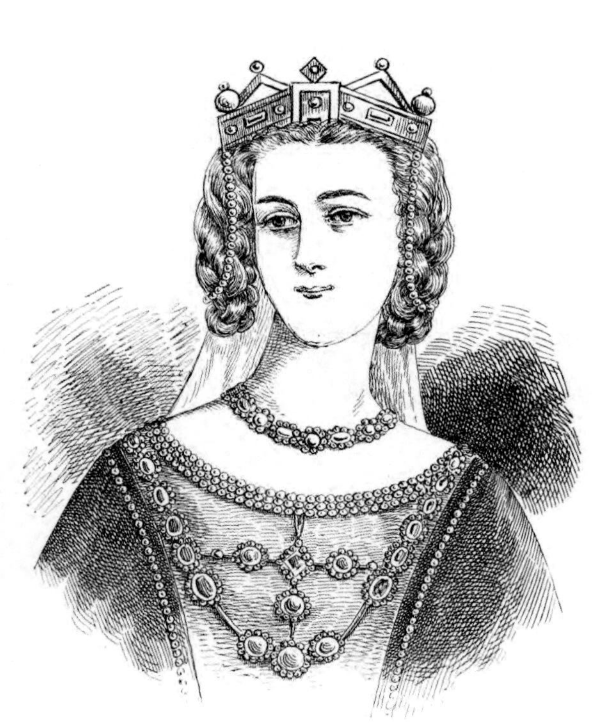

Queen Mérovée, Middle Ages, *L’Art de la Coiffure Française*, A. Mallemont

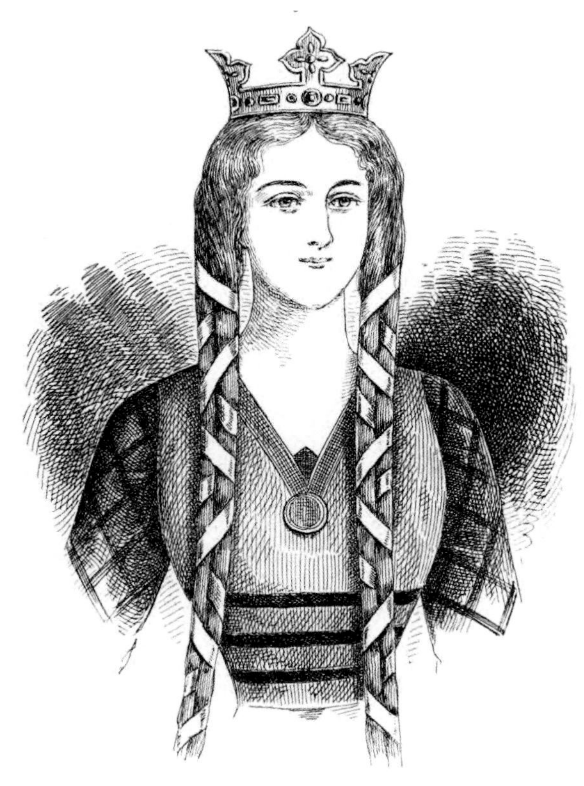

Queen Clotilde, Middle Ages, *L’Art de la Coiffure Française*, A. Mallemont

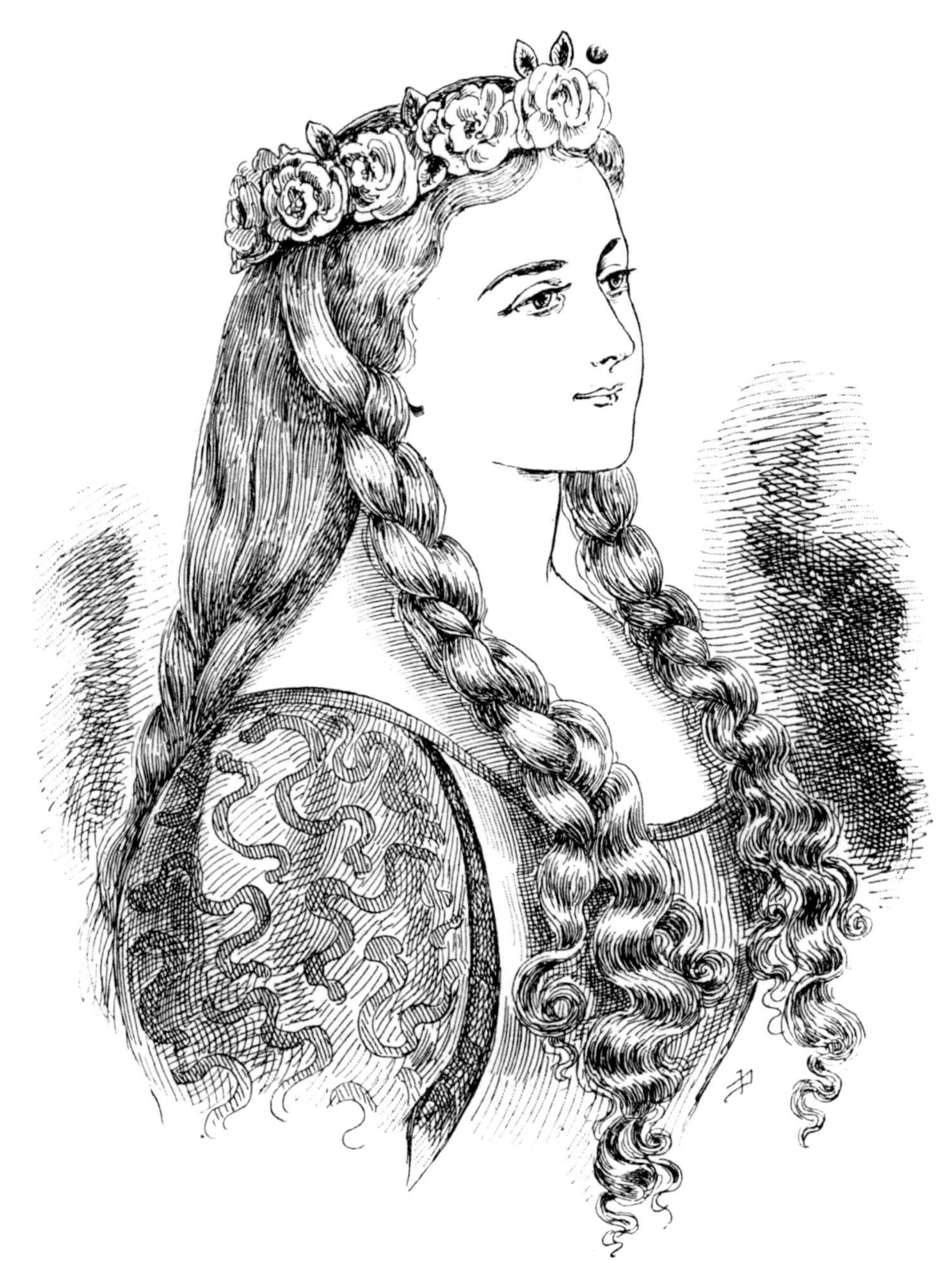

'Le Chapel' hairstyle, Middle Ages, *L'Art de la Coiffure Française*, A. Mallemont

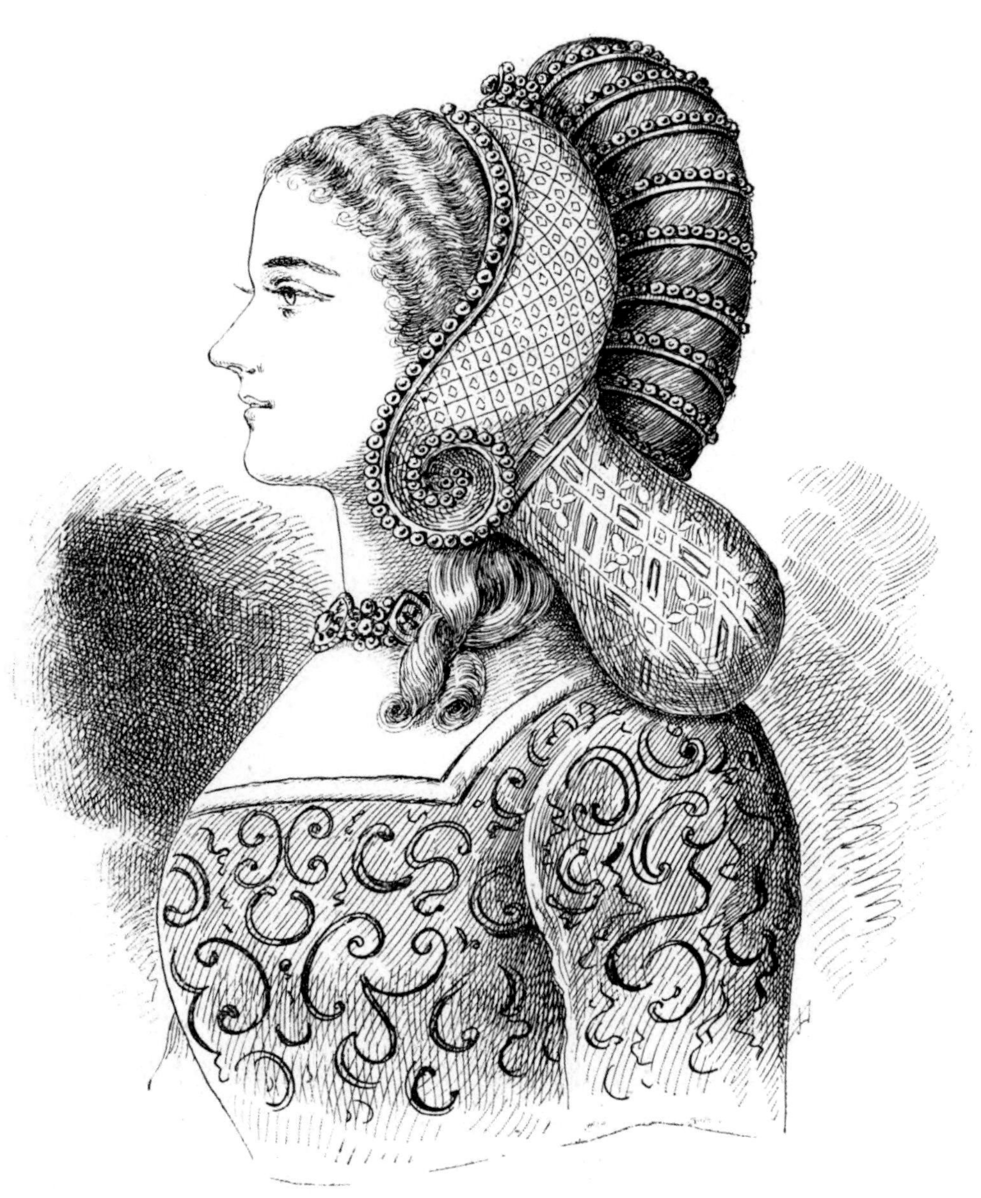

Hairstyle, Middle Ages, *L'Art de la Coiffure Française*, A. Mallemont

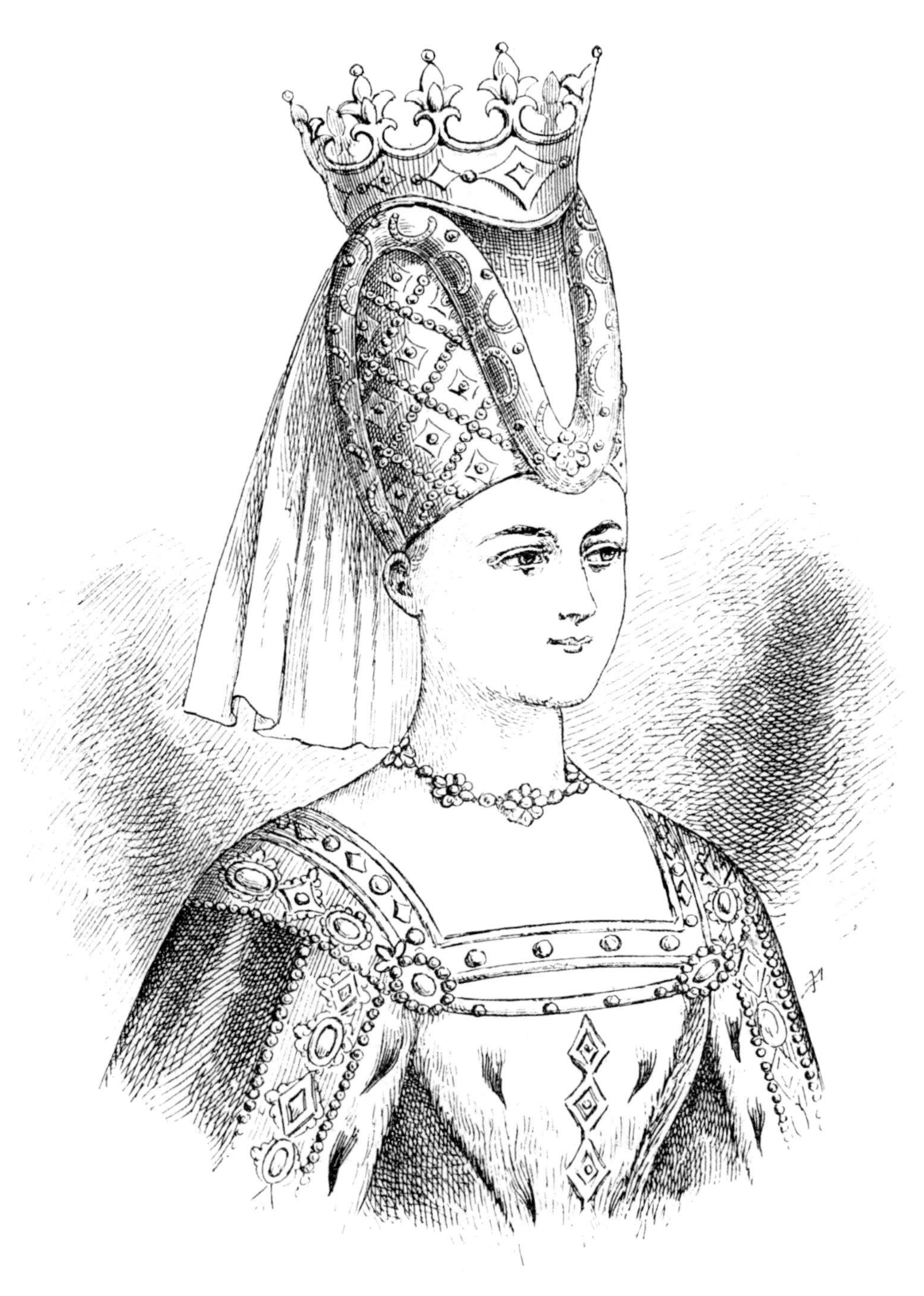

Isabeau of Bavaria, Queen consort of France, late Middle Ages/ Renaissance, *L'Art de la Coiffure Française*, A. Mallemont

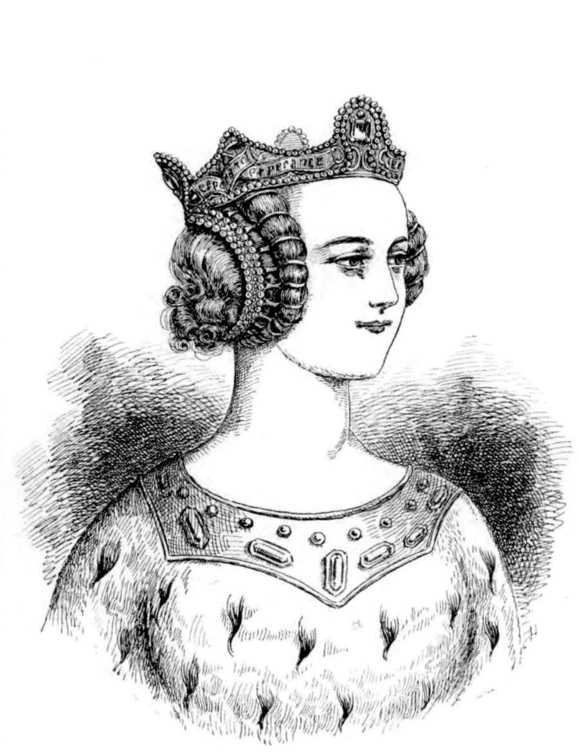

Hairstyle, Middle Ages, *L'Art de la Coiffure Française*, A. Mallemont

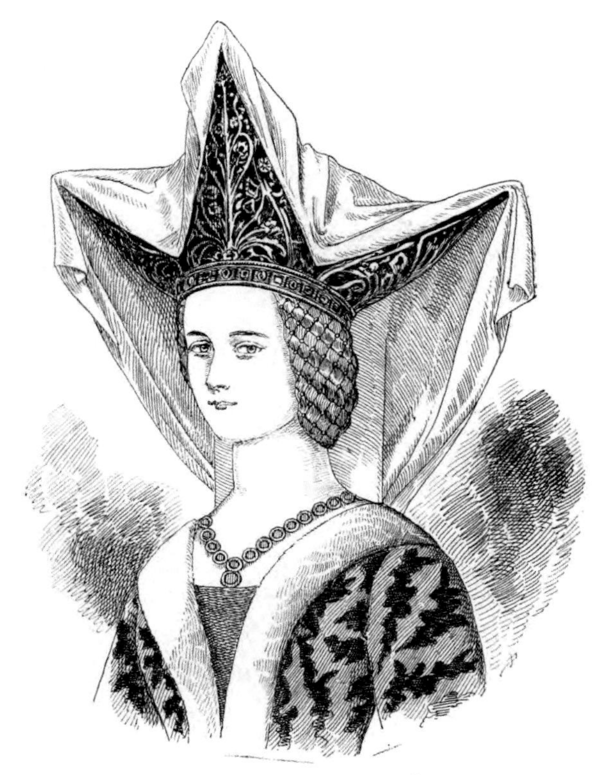

Three-pointed star hairstyle, 15th century, *L'Art de la Coiffure Française*, A. Mallemont

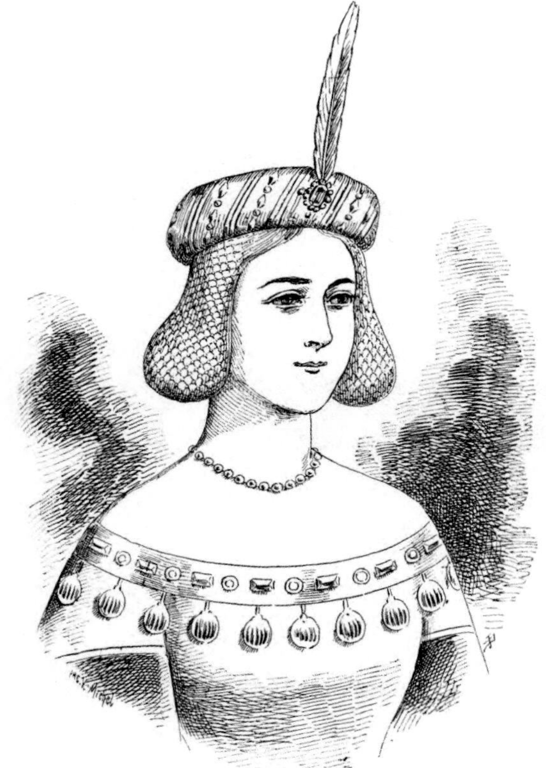

'Crespine with birette', c.1200, *L'Art de la Coiffure Française*, A. Mallemont

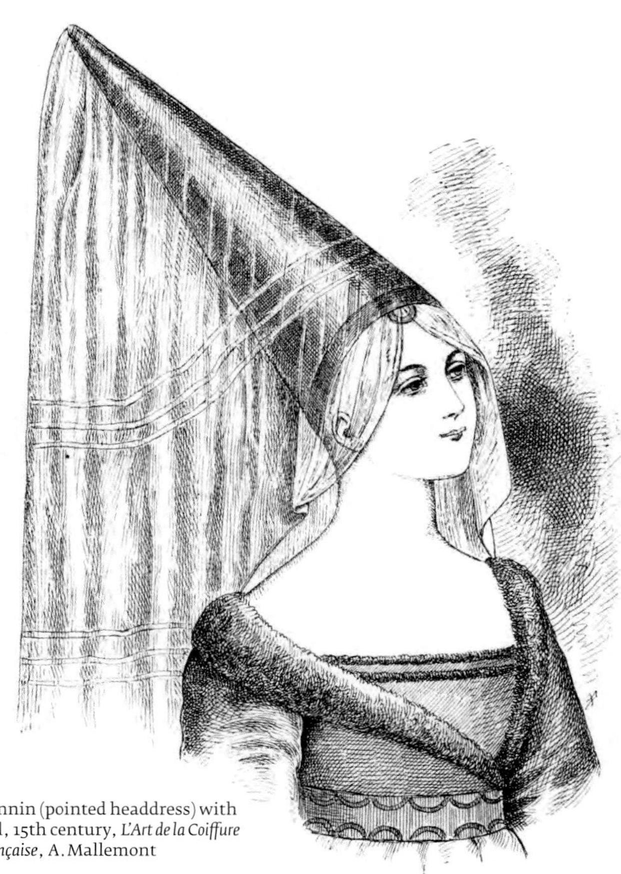

Hennin (pointed headdress) with veil, 15th century, *L'Art de la Coiffure Française*, A. Mallemont

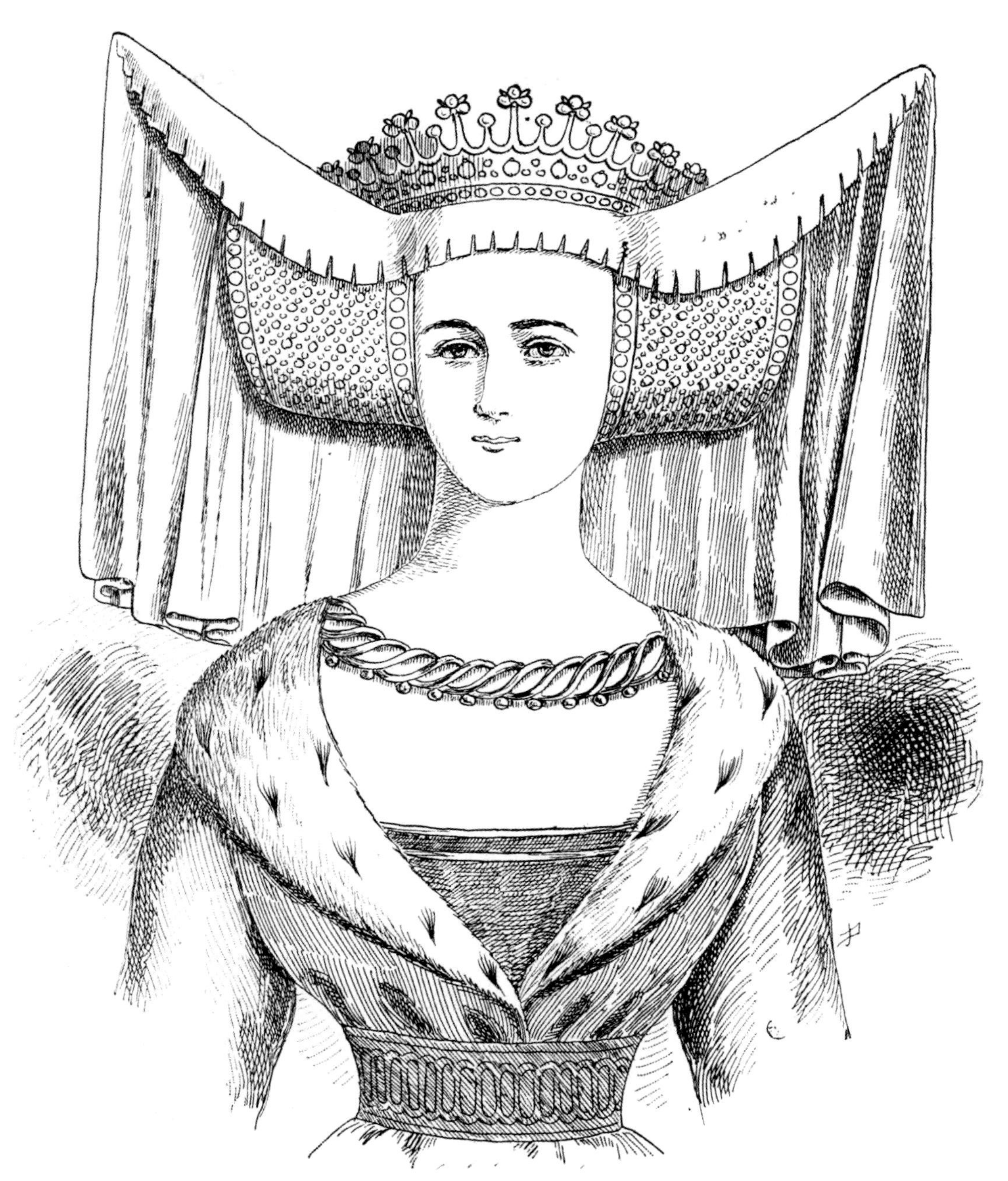

'Coiffure Cornue' (Horned Hairstyle), arranged upon a crown, 15th century, *L'Art de la Coiffure Française*, A. Mallemont

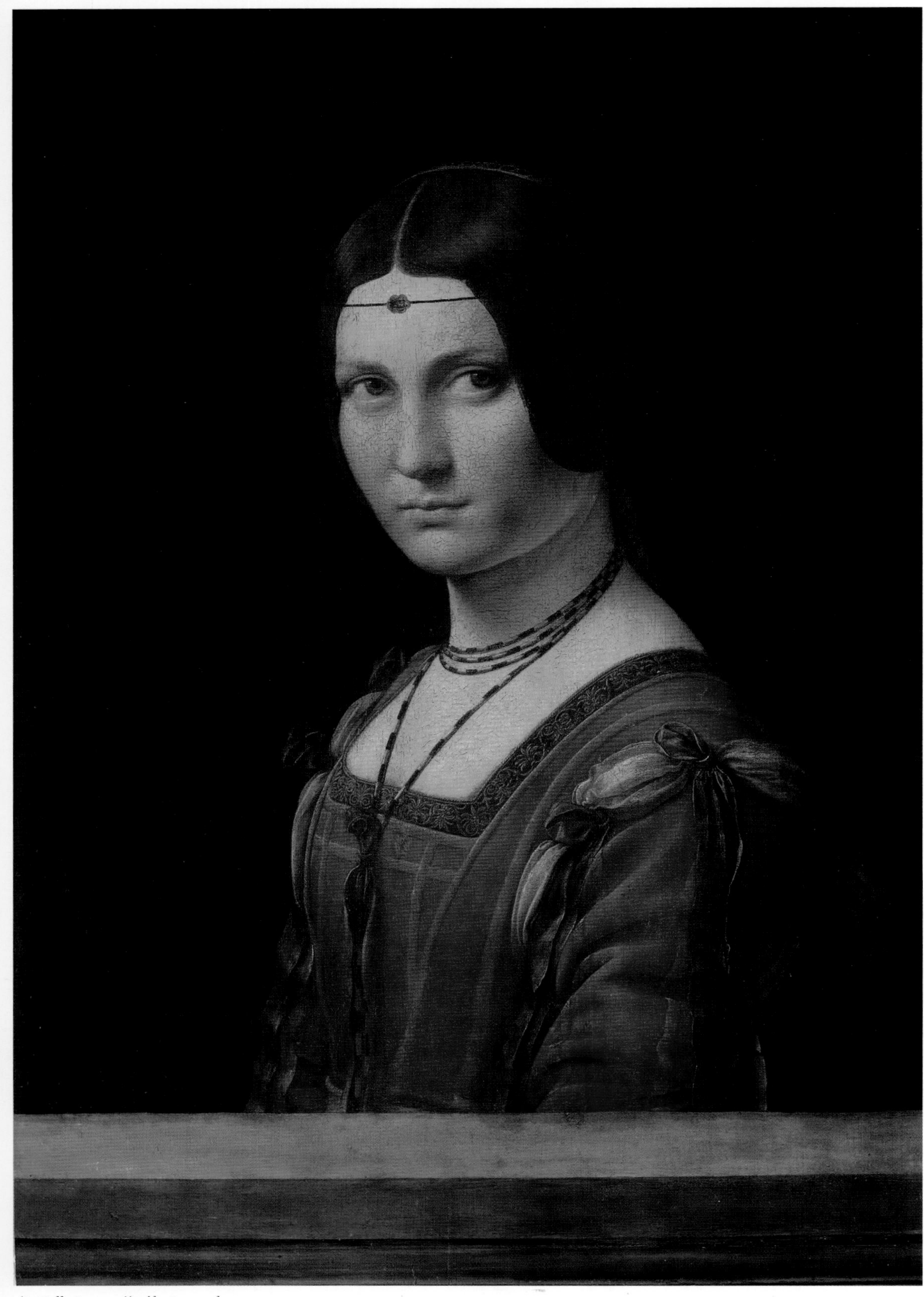

'La Belle Ferronnière' by Leonardo da Vinci, 1490–96

RENAISSANCE

Emerging from the long shadows cast by the Dark Ages, the Renaissance marked a period of rapid economic growth as European countries moved from a feudal system to a trade-based society that saw the rise of the merchant classes. This led to a blossoming of cultural activity, encompassing not only politics and the sciences but also the arts, and this in turn altered the concept of female beauty. Looking back to the elegant classicism of Ancient Greece and Rome, the Renaissance era rejected the overwhelming God-fearing religiosity of the Middle Ages, and instead adopted a more secular outlook based on classical humanist philosophy – and this cultural transition had a huge bearing on the role of women in society and, of course, what they did with their hair.

The 16th century saw the demise of the veil, which was to be fashionably replaced by the small cap, a vogue initially imported into France, Italy and England from Spain. This new form of headdress allowed more of the hair to be shown. In Tuscany, for example, it was popular to wear a long plait with just the crown of the head covered by a tight-fitting cap or simple diadem, while in Spain the hair was swept upwards with a jewelled and feathered cap placed atop and set at a jaunty angle. Another headdress that was popular in Italy during the Renaissance period is known as "la Belle Ferronnière" after a portrait of an unknown woman in the Louvre, which is attributed to Leonardo da Vinci. This simple but dramatic embellishment consisted of a thin gold chain or rope of pearls with a jewel or large pearl (known as a "Ferronniére") set at its centre, which was worn across the forehead and then fastened at the back of the head, allowing the hair to flow naturally beneath it. The effortless simplicity of this hair ornament reflected the Italian Renaissance's sensual glorification of female beauty and, by enhancing hair that was worn naturally, this elegant circlet also helped to enforce its seductive charms.

Another fashion popular in the 1560s and 1570s was a heart-shaped coiffure that had initially originated from Venice. For this modish hairstyle of the Tudor period, the hair was centre-parted and then dressed on either side over crescent-shaped pads, with the hair at the back of the head coiled and pinned at the nape of the neck. During the late Renaissance period, another new form of headdress became *de rigeur*: a stiffened, wide band of satin or velvet that was often bejewelled or trimmed with fur, such as ermine. This elegant headdress framed the face and allowed the wearer's hair to flow naturally behind it. As Octave Uzanne noted, it "made a very harmonious setting for their faces. The hair was curled and allowed to fall on the neck. Certain court ladies, following a fashion set by Margaret of Navarre, curled the hair over the temples and dressed it high over the forehead. The first metal hairpins were invented in England in 1545. Prior to this invention, the hair was held in place by means of pins and very fine and flexible skewers, all made of wood." These new hairpins meant that it was easier to secure more elaborate headdresses, such as the exquisite jewel-encrusted ones worn by Elizabeth I of England.

Indeed "Good Queen Bess" reputedly owned over a hundred different wigs and her striking red hairpieces subsequently sparked a trend among fashion-conscious women of the time, who attempted to dye their own hair the same eye-catching golden hue. During Elizabeth's reign, according to J. P. C. Bicknell, "Women of all classes spent as much money as they (or their unfortunate husbands) could possibly afford on ornament to decorate their coiffure, frequently chains of rich jewels, silver and even gold; it seems that the most beautiful ladies wore their hair so loaded with heavy ornaments of every kind that they could scarcely move." The hairdressers of the day were also highly skilled in using false hairpieces known as "postiches" to create these elaborately coiffured confections. It would seem that most noble women supplemented their own locks with natural hairpieces, including the ill-fated Mary Queen of Scots who reportedly possessed a number of wigs and who wore a lace-edged headdress that dipped at the forehead, which was briefly fashionable among her female sympathisers until she fell from grace.

By the 1580s a new "Pompadour" style had also started to gain popular currency, which incorporated pads and wire frames to heighten the overall coiffure. The Renaissance had freed women from the medieval veil and all its suppressive associations, and instead its poets and artists celebrated the beauty of hair in all its guises. As the distinguished Neo-Platonic poet, Francesco Petrarch – who is sometimes referred to as the "Father of Humanism" – wrote in his *Il Canzoniere* (Song Book) at the very start of the Renaissance period: "She let her gold hair scatter in the breeze. A new young angel carried by her wings." And certainly by this remarkable era's close, women were enriching the natural beauty of their locks through the use of intricate ornamentation, rather than hiding their tresses under a cloaking veil of religious modesty.

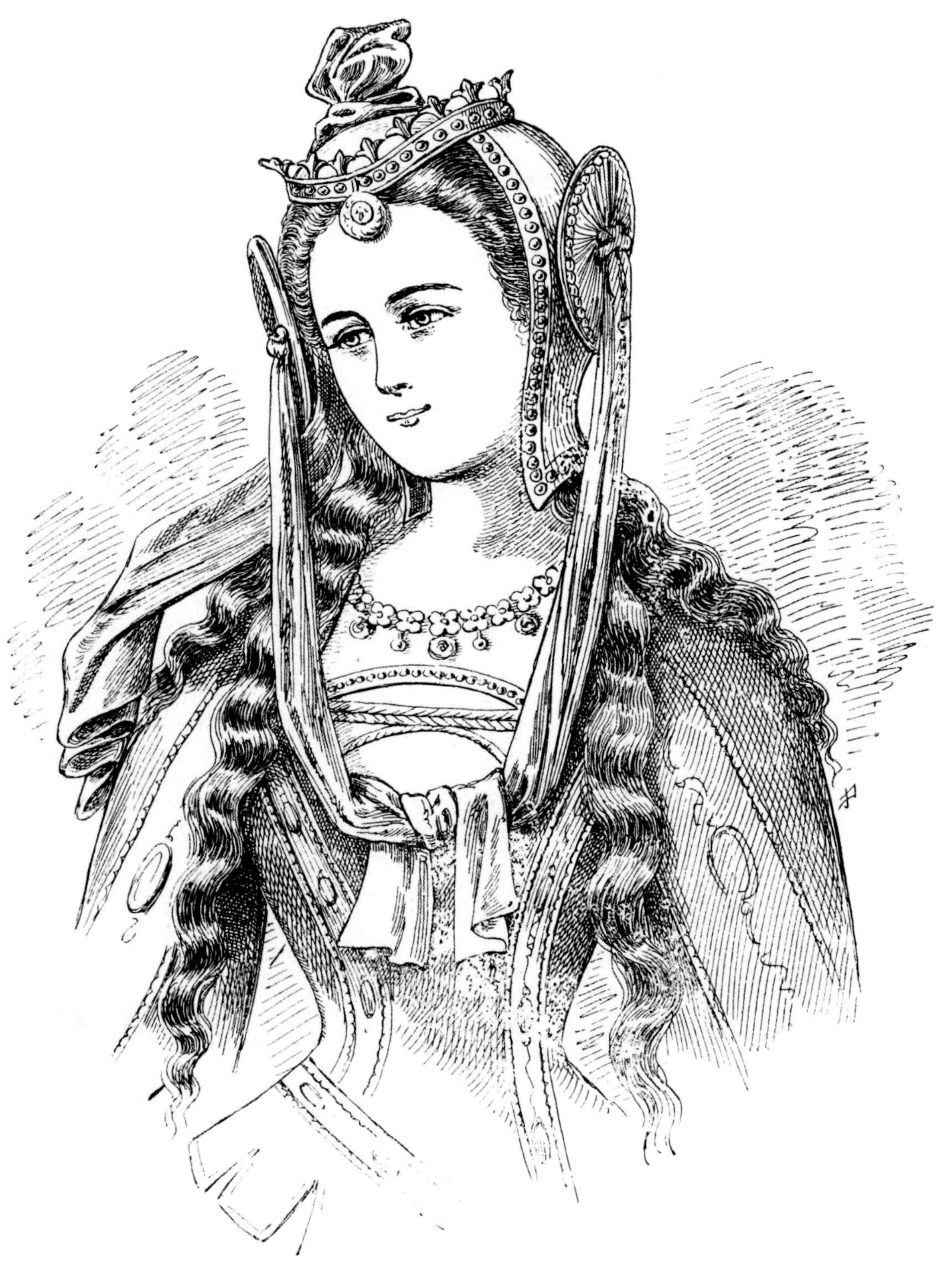

Renaissance hairstyle, end of 15th century, *L'Art de la Coiffure Française*, A. Mallemont

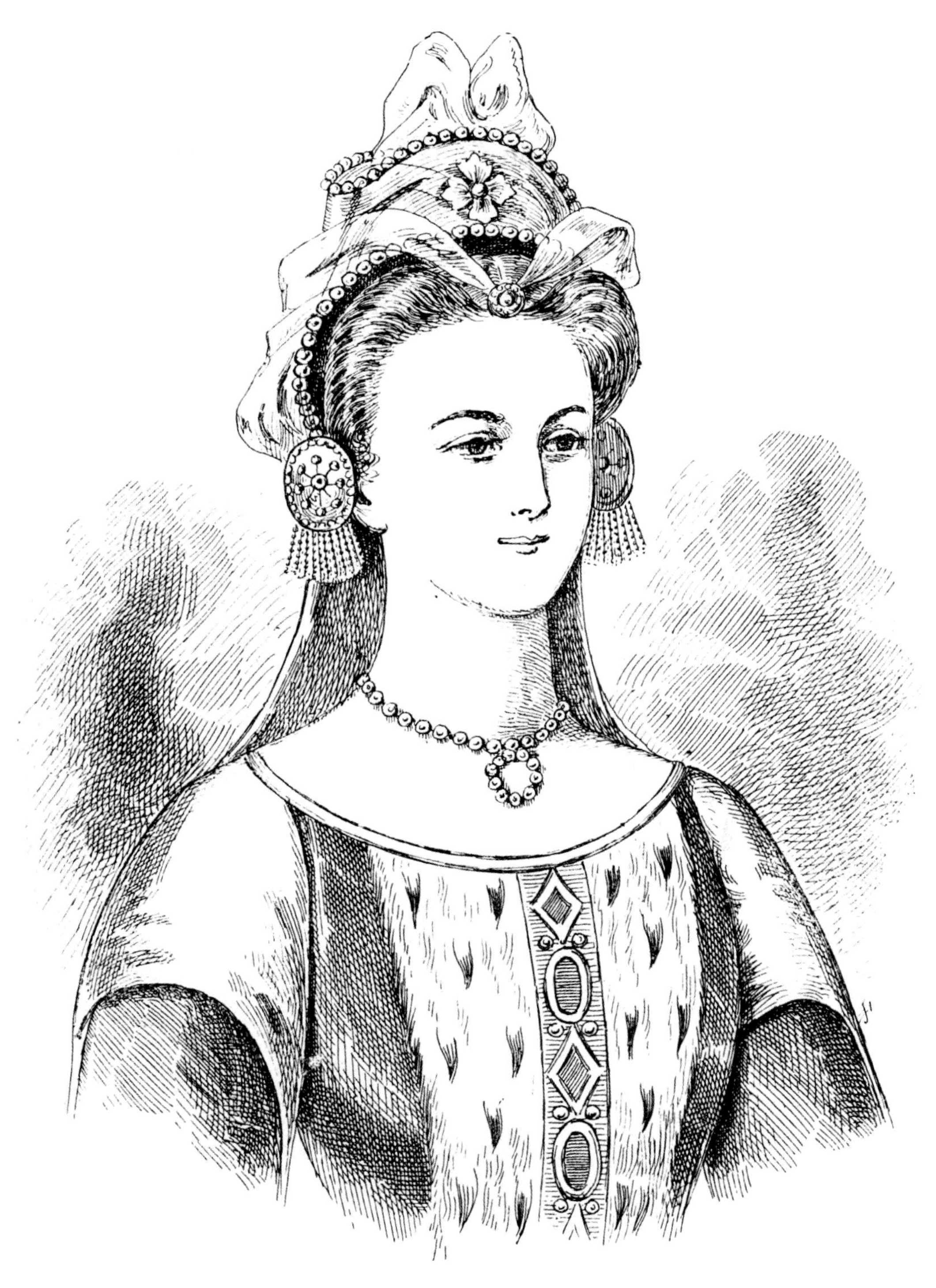

Young girl's hairstyle, 15th century,
L'Art de la Coiffure Française, A. Mallemont

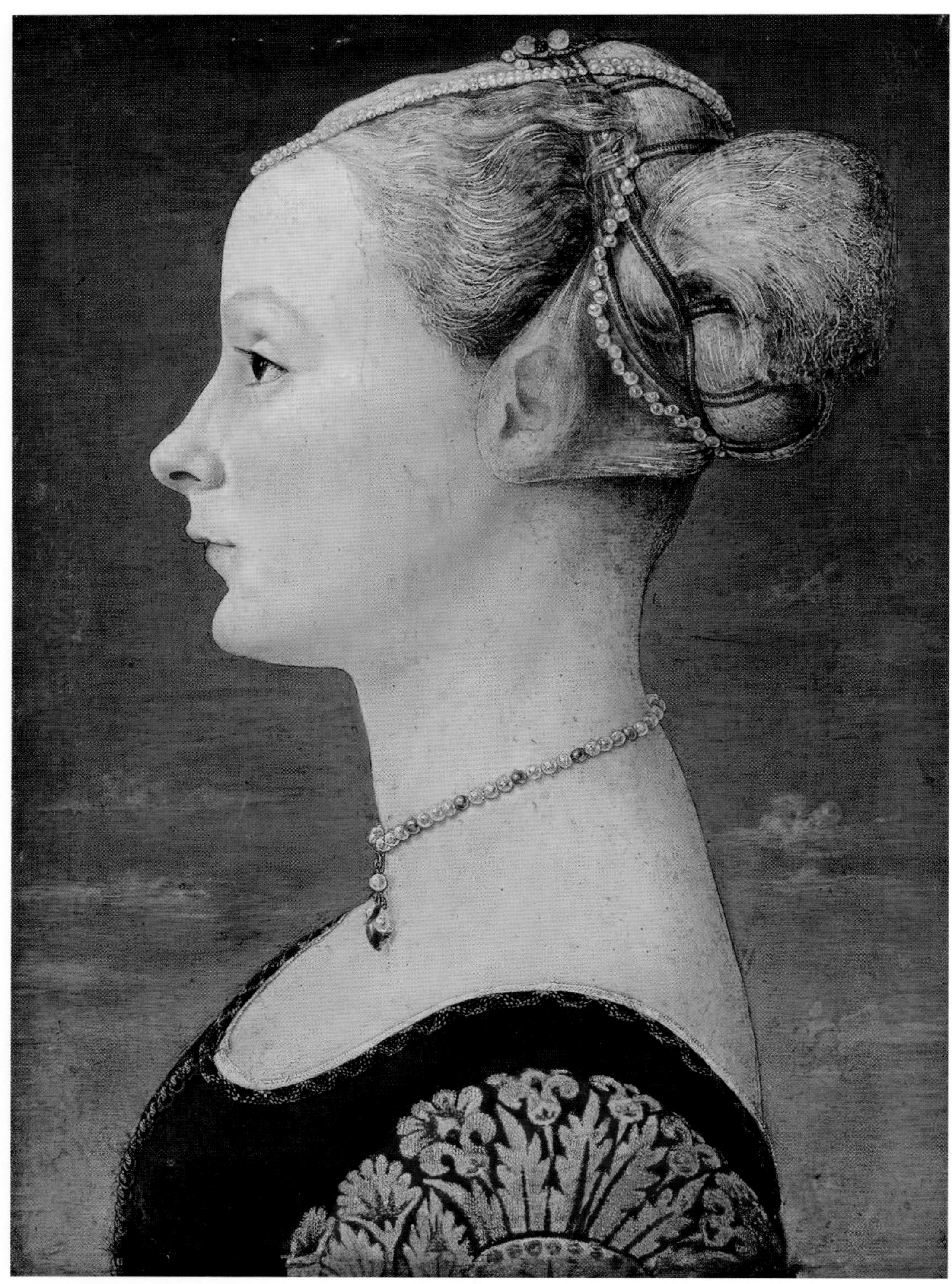

'Portrait of a Woman', attributed to Piero Pollaiuolo, c. 1470s

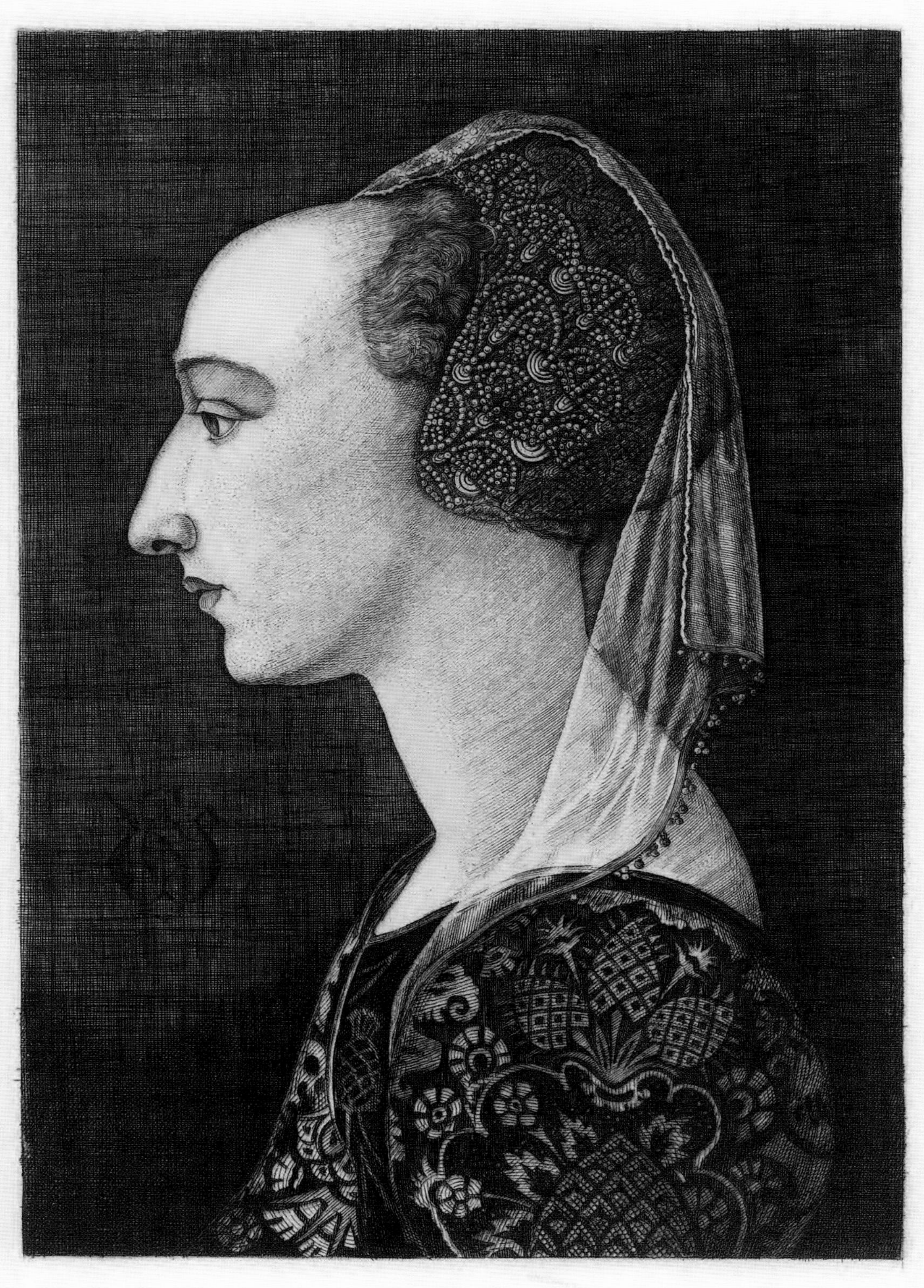

Engraving of 'Portrait of a Lady in Red', painting by Florentine artist, acquired as a portrait of Isotta da Rimini by Piero della Francesca, c.1460–70

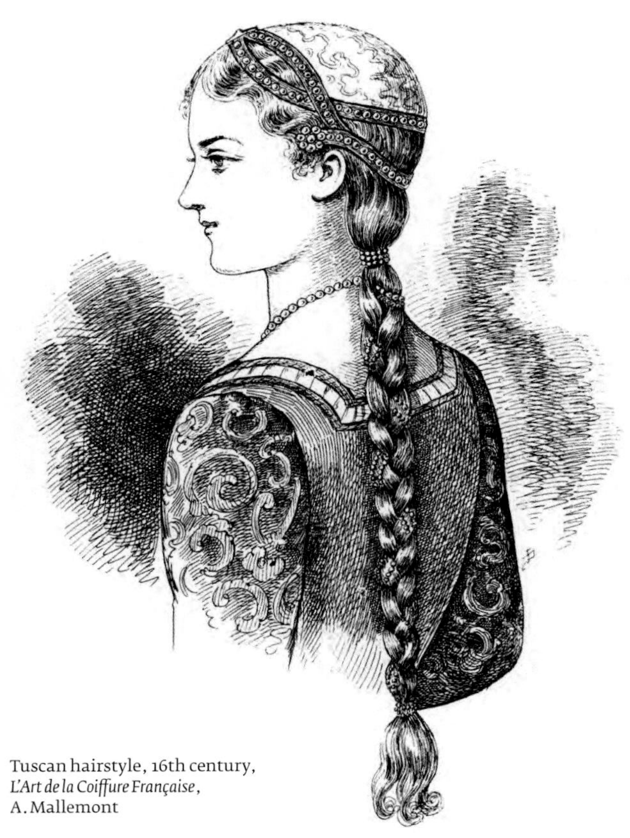

Tuscan hairstyle, 16th century,
L'Art de la Coiffure Française,
A. Mallemont

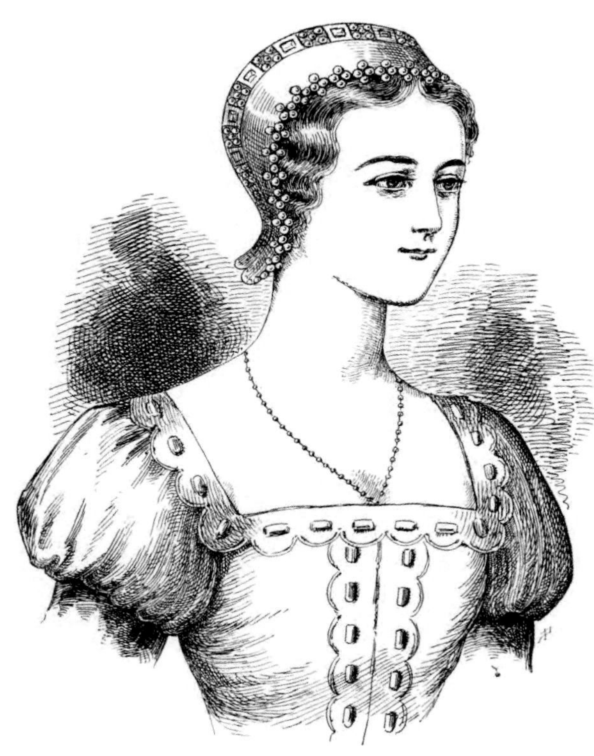

French hairstyle, Renaissance,
L'Art de la Coiffure Française,
A. Mallemont

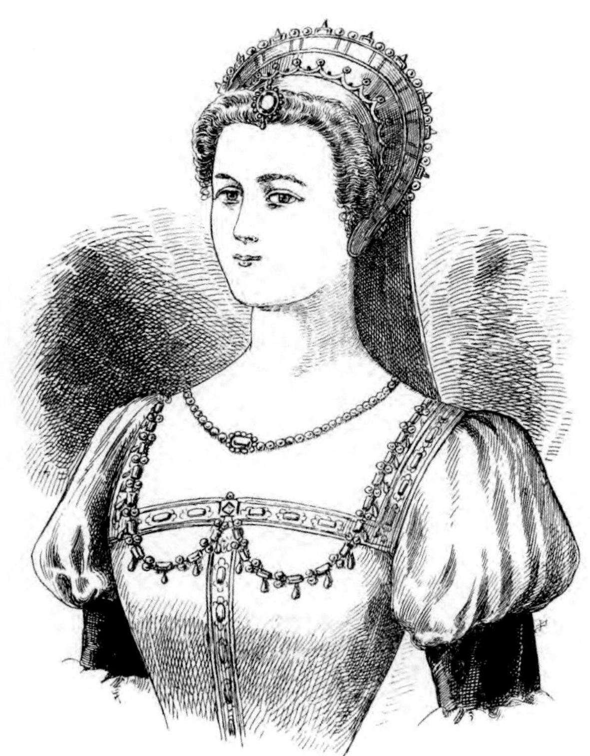

Italian hairstyle, Renaissance,
L'Art de la Coiffure Française,
A. Mallemont

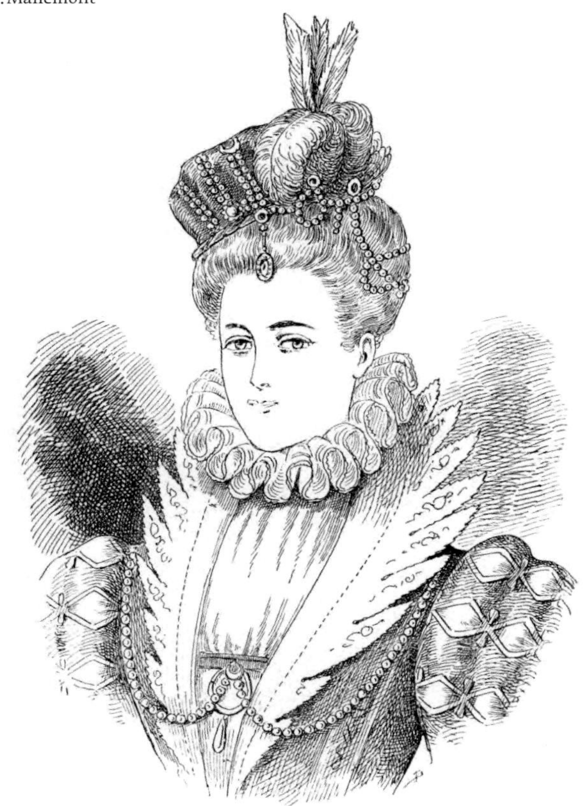

Spanish hairstyle, Renaissance,
L'Art de la Coiffure Française,
A. Mallemont

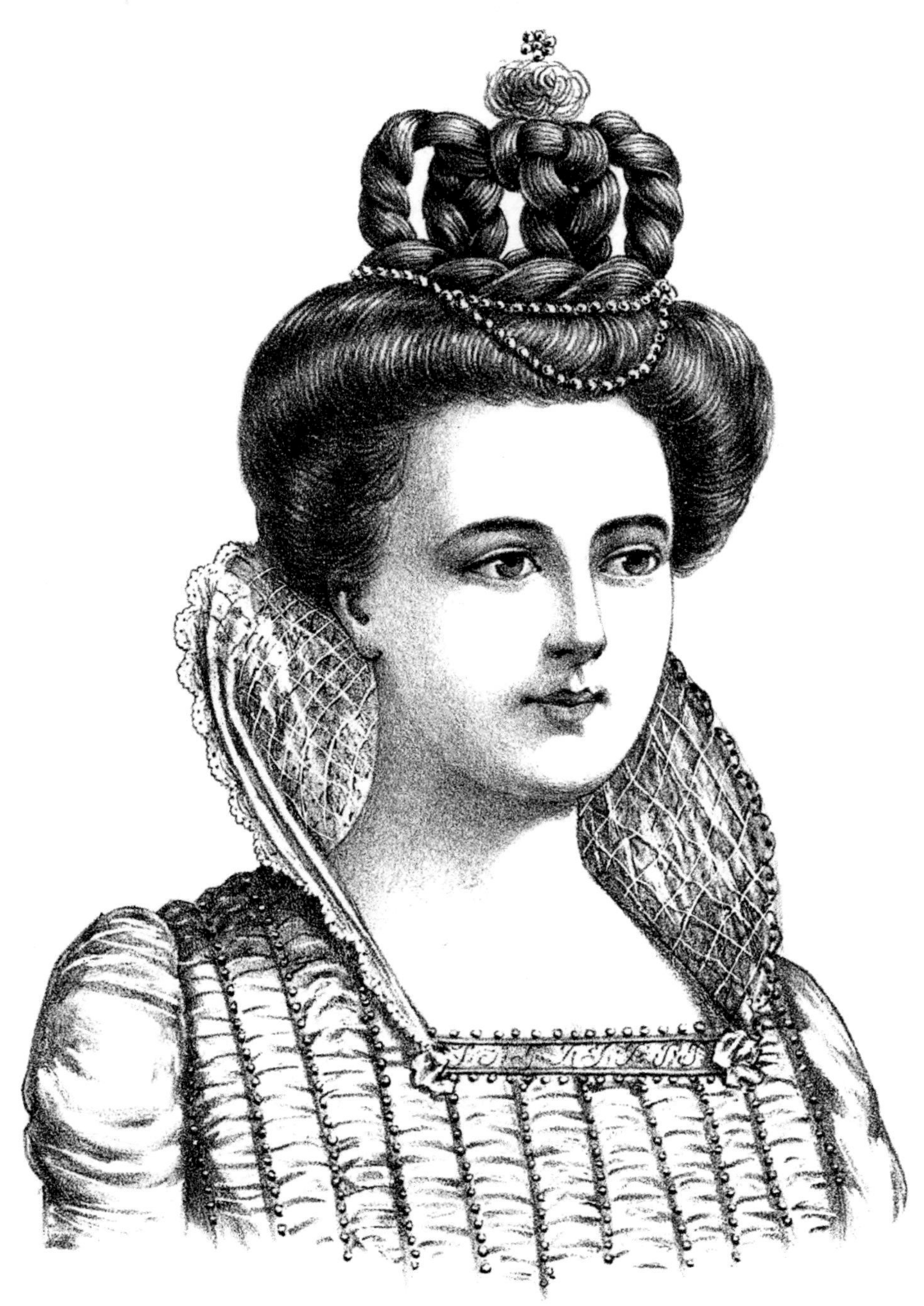

Crown-like hairstyle in the style of Mary Stuart entwined with pearls, *Album Historischer und Phantasie-Frisuren*, Heinrich Moritz

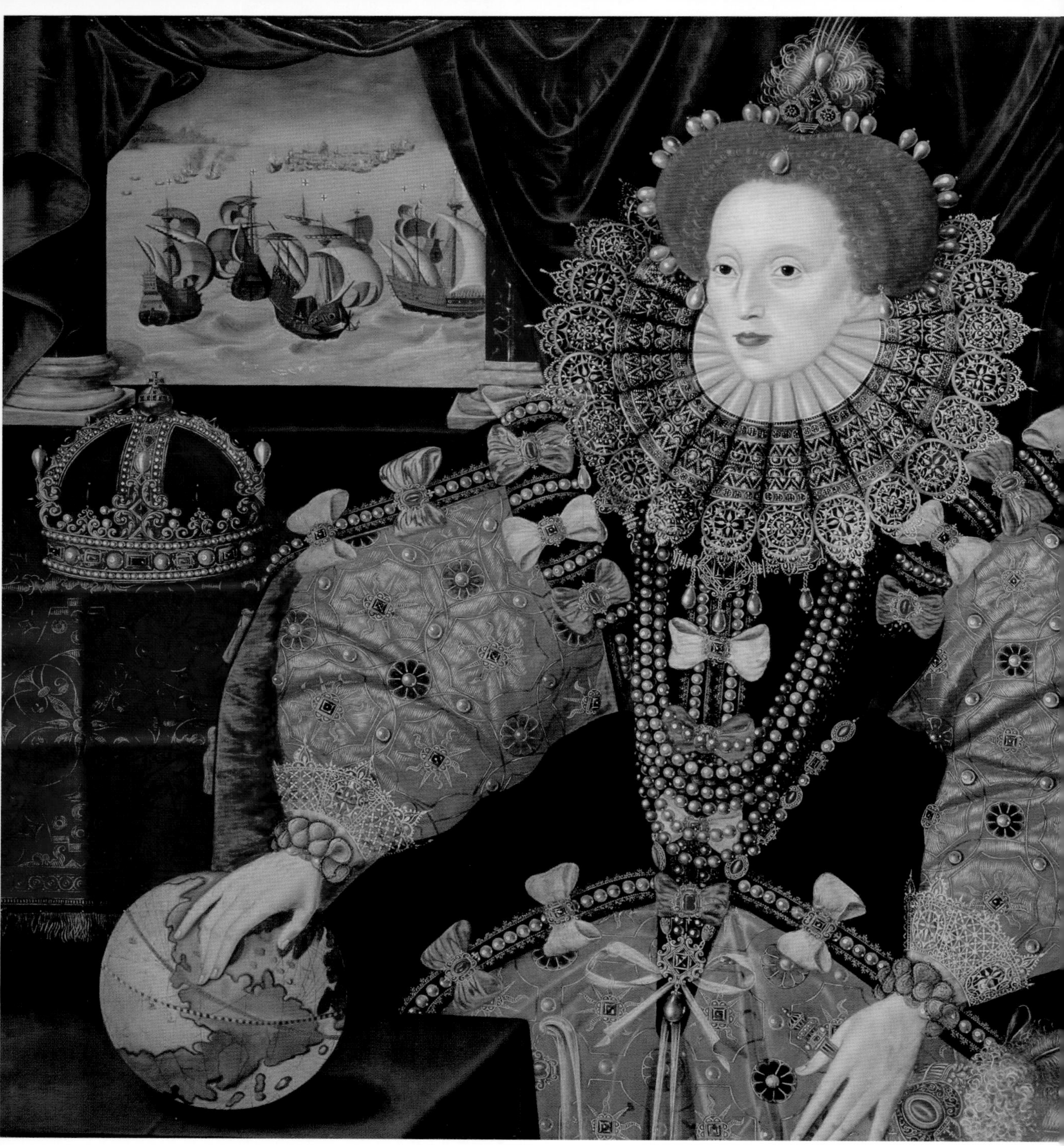

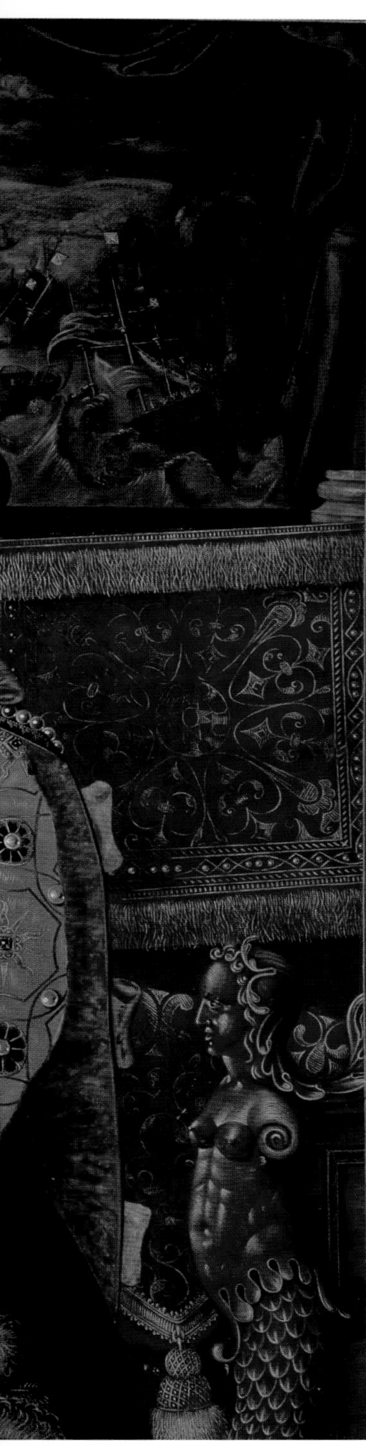

'Portrait of Queen Elizabeth I' by Marcus Gheeraerts the Younger, 1590s

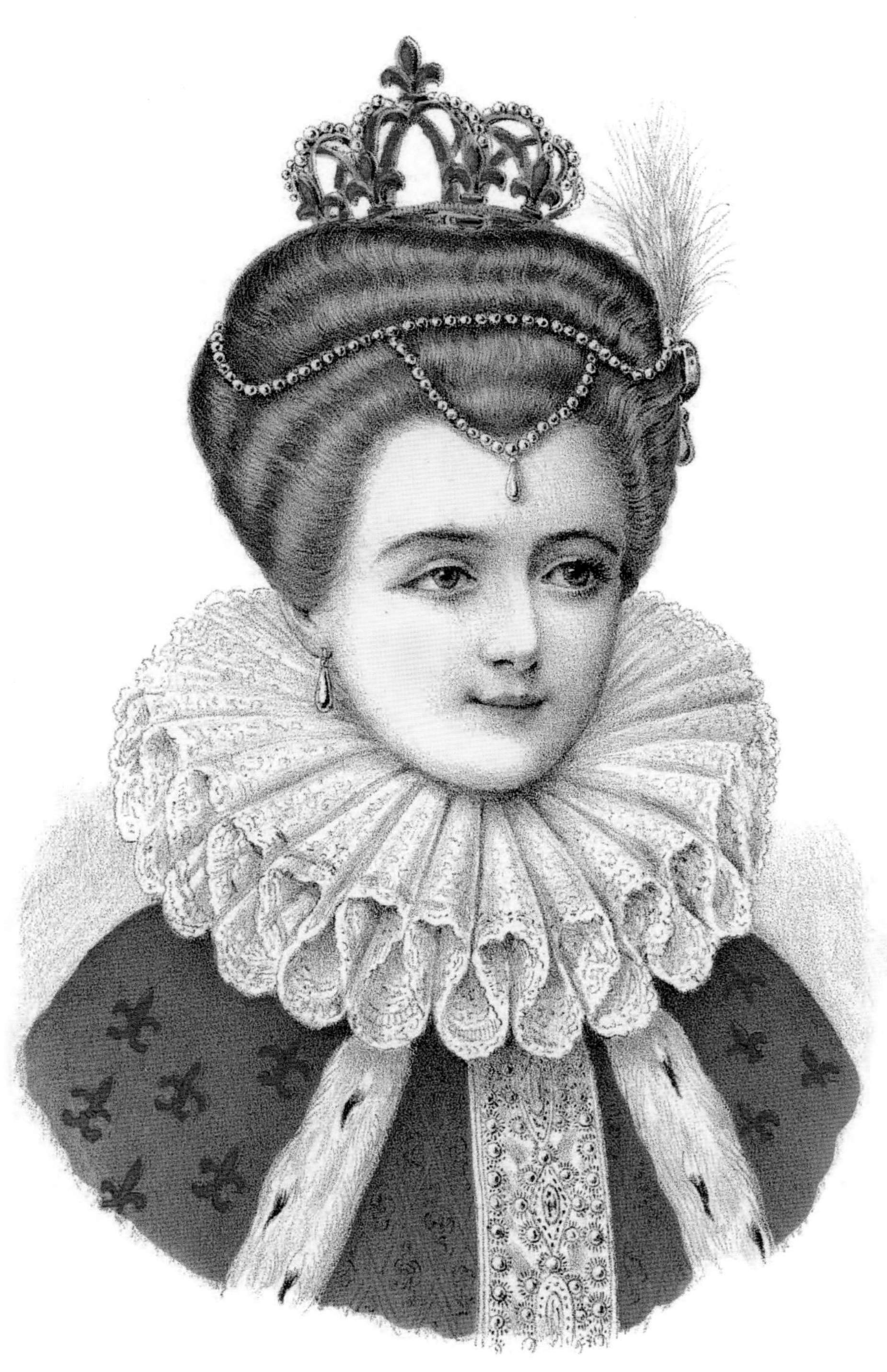

Henri III hairstyle, *Album de Coiffures Historiques*, E. Nissy

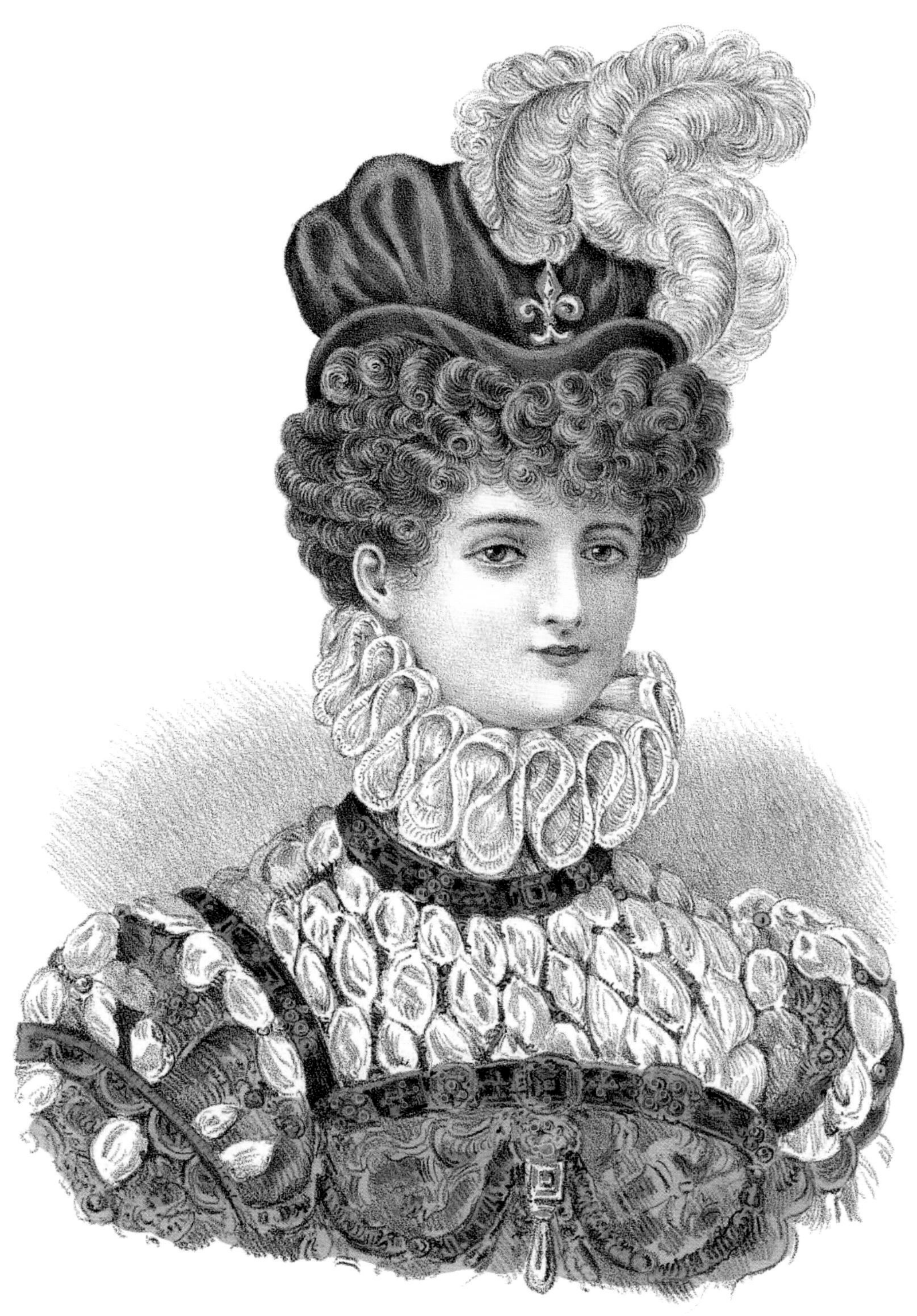

Elizabethan hairstyle (1558–1603),
Album de Coiffures Historiques, E. Nissy

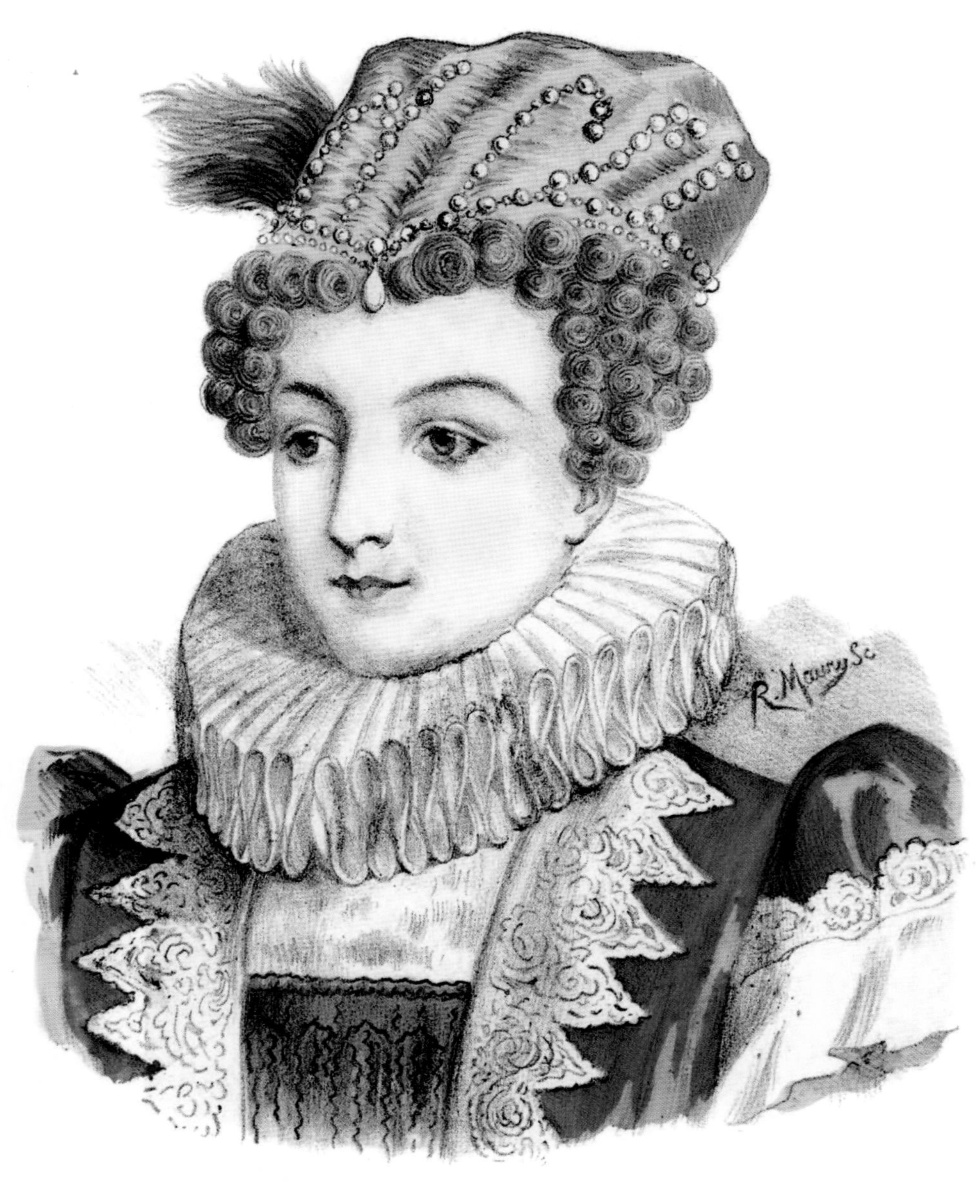

Henry IV hairstyle, Marguerite of Navarre,
Album de Coiffures Historiques, E. Nissy

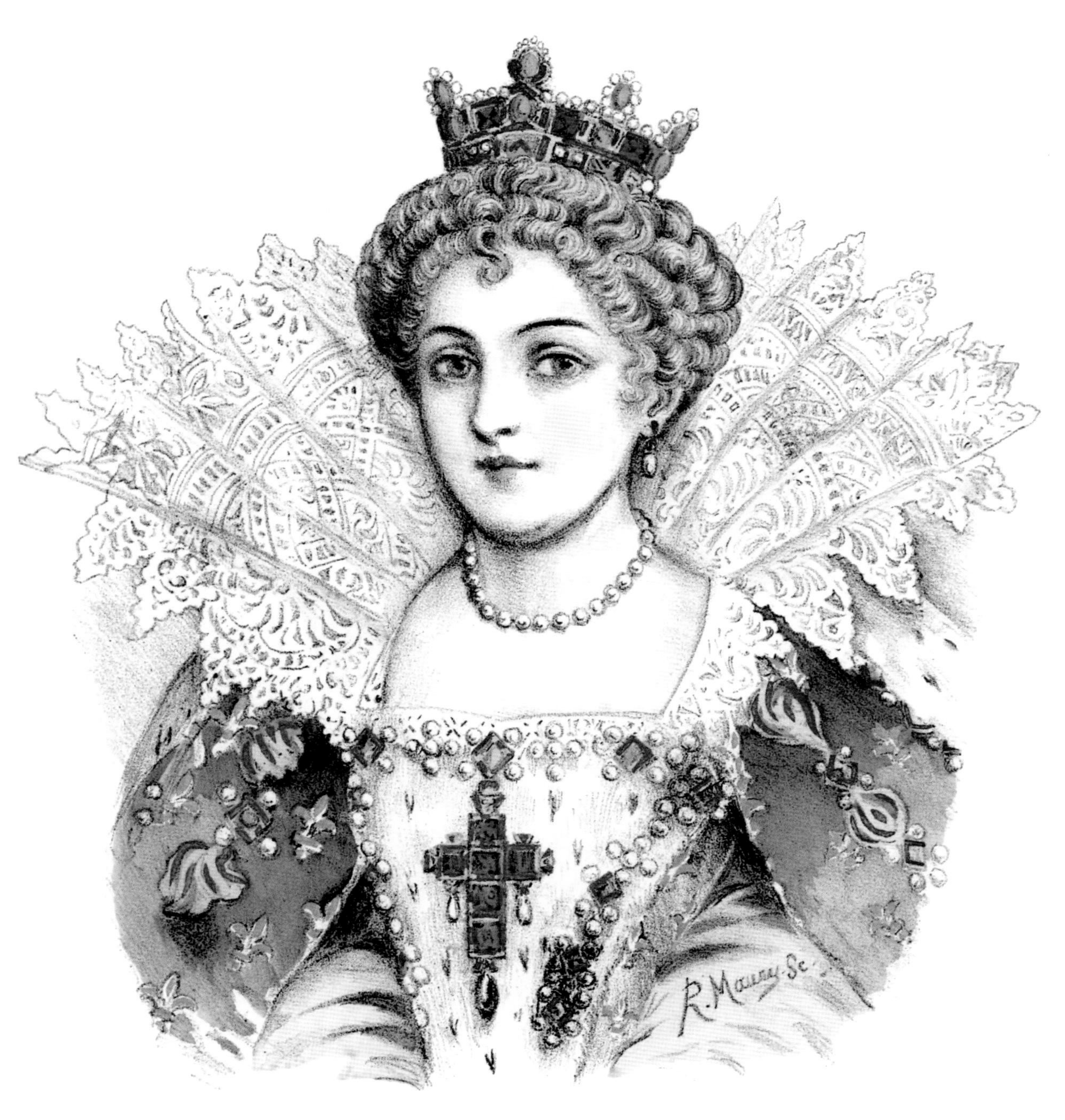

Henry IV hairstyle, Marie de Médici,
Album de Coiffures Historiques, E. Nissy

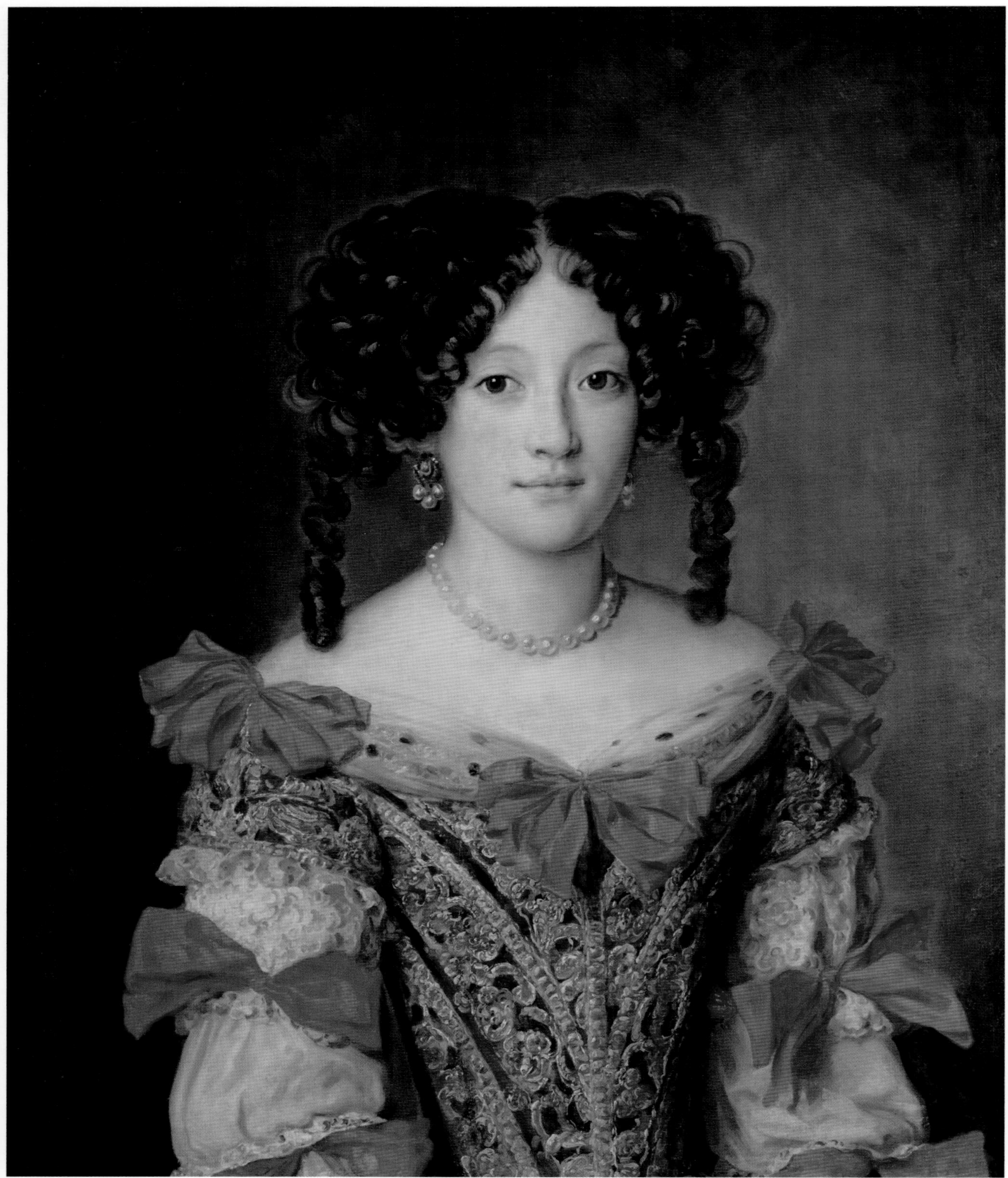

'Portrait of a Woman' by Jacob Ferdinand Voet, c.1670s

17TH CENTURY

Fashions in hairstyling changed very gradually during the first quarter of the 17th century, with the Spanish-influenced style that had been so favoured in the Elizabethan court still remaining *à la mode* until around 1620. Around this time a new fashion influenced by the French court began to emerge in which a small fringe was worn and a few loose curls, known as "Bouffants", were allowed to prettily frame the sides of the visage. In 1625, Charles I of England married Henrietta Maria of France and subsequently the hair fashions emanating from France became even more popular, with men and women wearing their hair or wigs loosely curled and at a shoulder-length in the Royalist "Cavalier" style. Another fashionable import from France was "Cadenettes", tiny plaits of hair that were tied with ribbons known as "Gallants". It was also during this era that ladies, who had previously relied on the hairstyling services of other womenfolk, began to employ male hairdressers to attend to the increasingly technical demands of their fashionable coiffures.

In England, the Civil War (1642–1651) brought in its wake a less ebullient style, with the Parliamentarian "Roundheads" and their supporters preferring a more modest style of hairdressing that accorded with their Puritan religious beliefs – to this end, women wore their hair short and straight, or brushed back and covered with an unadorned white close-fitting cap. During this Commonwealth period, another less austere style was also worn by less fanatical Puritan ladies that comprised of shoulder-length hair that was curled into ringlets and then simply beribboned. This soberness in personal grooming, however, did not last for long and when the English monarchy was eventually restored to the throne in 1660, the subsequent reign of the opulently bewigged Charles II marked a renewal of interest in the lavish dressing of hair.

During this period, it would appear that both sexes became highly "hair-conscious" and spent large amounts of time and money on their luxuriant coiffures – with expensive wigs made of horse hair, yak hair and human hair being worn by those who could afford them. These periwigs appear to have needed constant attention – cleaning, curling and powdering, and probably frequent delousing too. As the famous diarist and wig-wearer Samuel Pepys wrote in an entry on January 23 1660, "Thence to my office and there did nothing but make up my balance. Came home and found my wife dressing of the girl's head, by which she was made to look very pretty."

Certainly in France in the latter half of the 17th century, there was a multitude of fashionable styles to choose from – including the long-forgotten "Bretaudié" introduced by a hairdresser called "La Vienne" (the Viennese) and the mane-like "Hurlupée" that was made fashionable by the Duchesse de Nevers in the 1670s. Madame de Sévigné wrote in a letter dated March 18 1671: "Madame the Duchesse de Nevers came in with her hair dressed in the most ludicrous fashion, though you know that as a rule I like uncommon hairstyles. La Martin had the fancy to create a new coiffure and had cropped her! Her hair had been cut and rolled on paper curlers, which had made her suffer death and agony a whole night long. Her head was like a little round cabbage – nothing at the sides. My dear, it is the most ridiculous sight you can imagine."

Also known as the "à la Maintenon" after Madame de Maintenon (who later became the second wife of King Louis XIV of France), this fashionable hairstyle involved frizzing the hair into something resembling a woolly lamb's fleece and then allowing an abundance of "rogue" curls to charmingly frame the face. In England during this period, women tended to wear their hair centre-parted and then styled their fringes into flat curls on their foreheads, while the hair on the sides of their heads was curled into soft ringlets and the hair at the back of their heads was drawn up into a bun. By the 1670s, there was an increasing fashion for even tighter ringlets that cascaded into a mass of clustered curls around the sides of the face, while the hair at the back of the head was left long so that it could fall seductively onto a women's bare shoulders.

In 1680, the Marquise de Fontange inadvertently sparked another hairdressing trend while out hunting. With her hair blowing annoyingly in her face as she rode, the Marquise gathered her loose locks up with a ribbon and tied them into a knot over her forehead. This new "Coiffure à la Fontange" became immediately fashionable at the Court of Versailles, where it was taken to exaggerated voguish extremes with a mass of curls surging above the forehead and a large bun protruding from the back of the head, which was known as a "Chou" (cabbage). Often these so-called "Fontanges" worn by the aristocratic ladies of the day were crowned with a curious cap-like fan, normally made of tightly pleated muslin supported on a wire frame that was worn almost like a cockscomb on top of the head and often embellished with bowed ribbons and gauffered lace.

Around the end of the century, "Fontange" headdresses reached their fashionable zenith with many featuring long lace or linen lappets that either hung down the sides of the face or were looped up and pinned. There were a great number of different ways to style hair under these striking headdresses, and the way that the hair was set and curled was given different names. "Favourites", for example, were curls positioned on the temples; "Confidants" were smaller curls sited by the ears; "Crève-coeurs" (heartbreakers) were the small curls that were located at the nape of the neck and "Bergers" (shepherds) were curls that were looped high into a puff-like confection. On top of this abundance of curls, the highly stacked "Fontange" headdresses were kept in place using various types of pins, known as "Firmaments" (constellations), "Guêpes" (wasps) and "Papillons" (butterflies). However, if ladies' hairstyles of the 17th century had seemed somewhat excessive, it was nothing

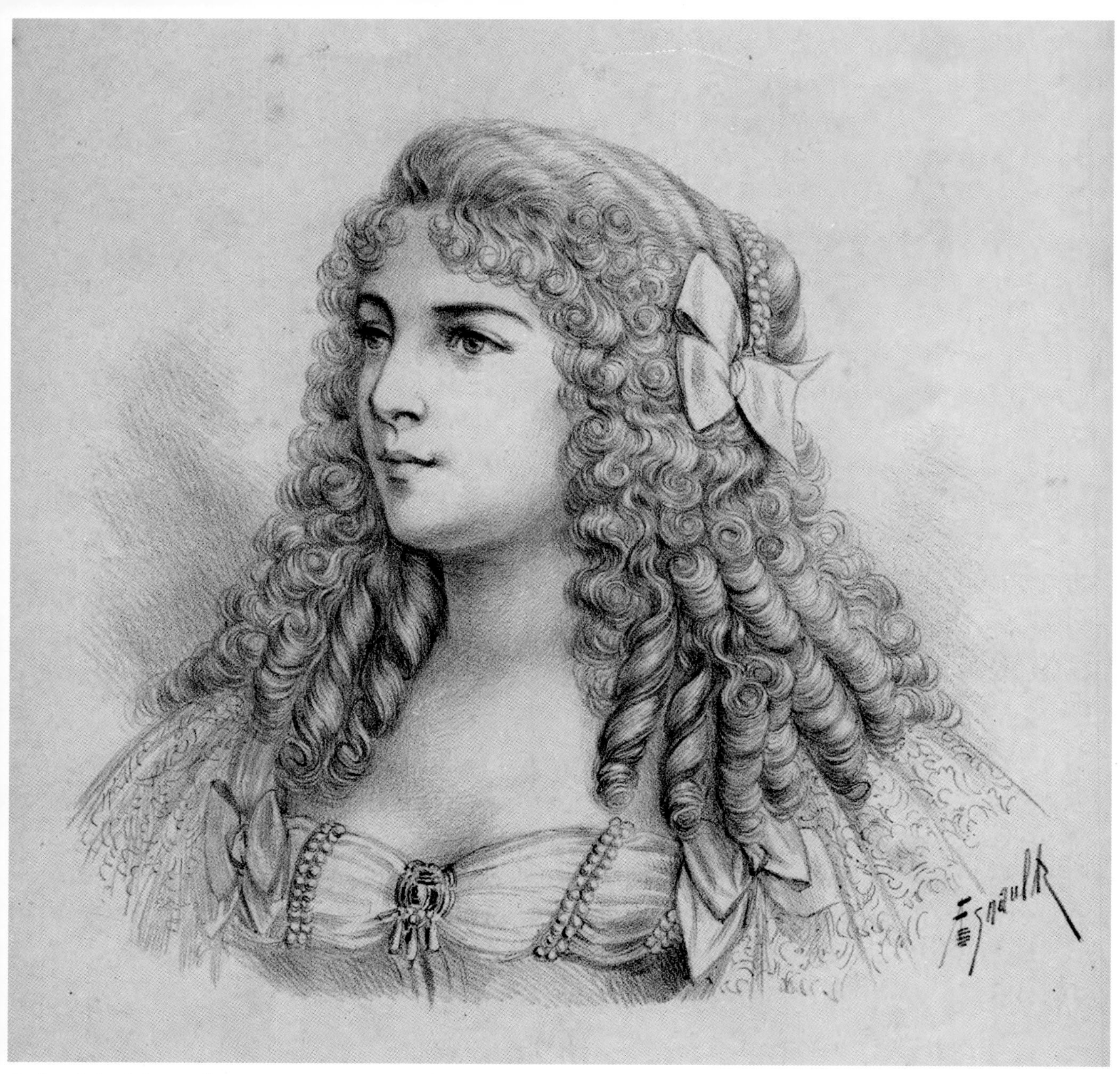

Louis XIII hairstyle (recreated by Auguste Chaplin of la Comédie Française)

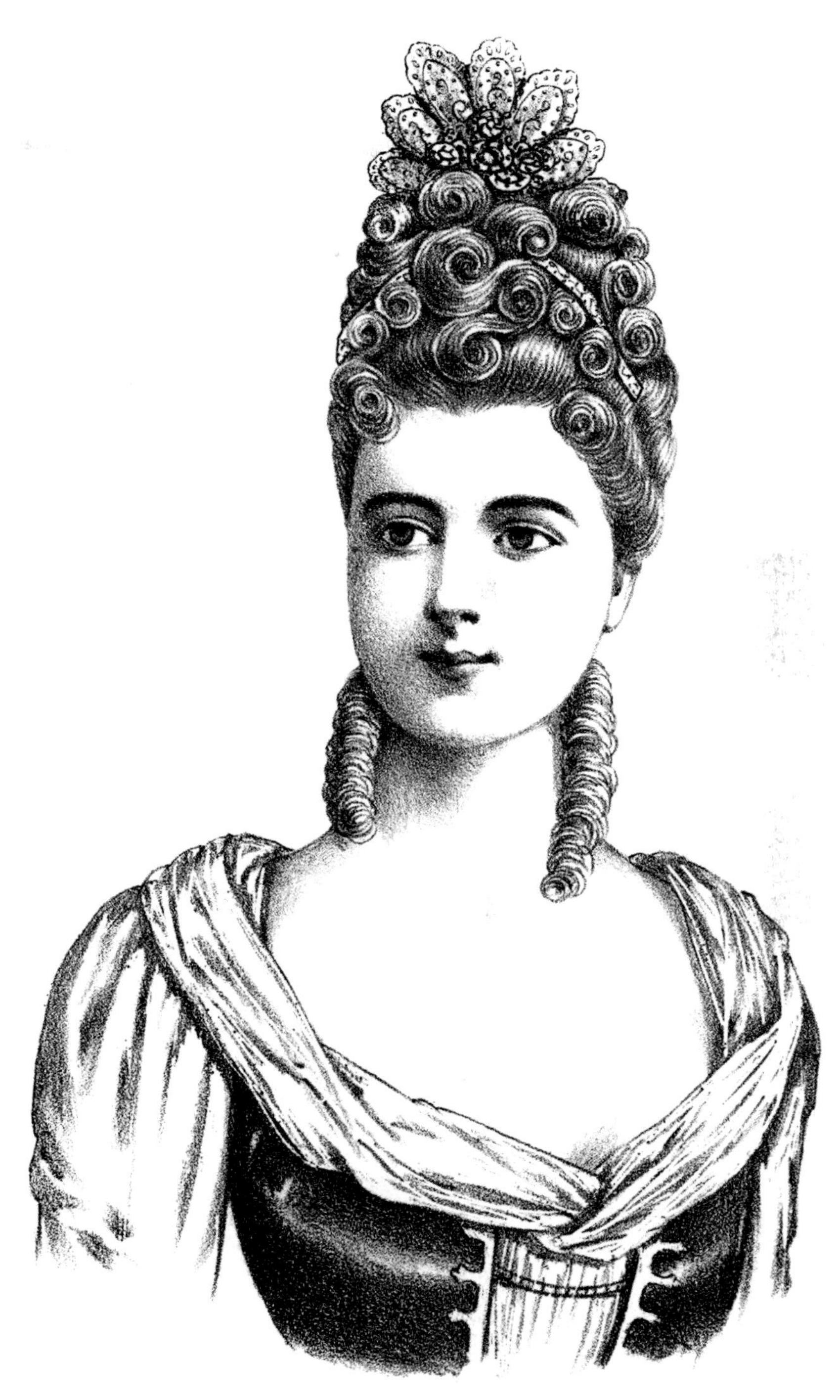

Louis XIV hairstyle, c.1690, *Album Historischer und Phantasie-Frisuren*, Heinrich Moritz

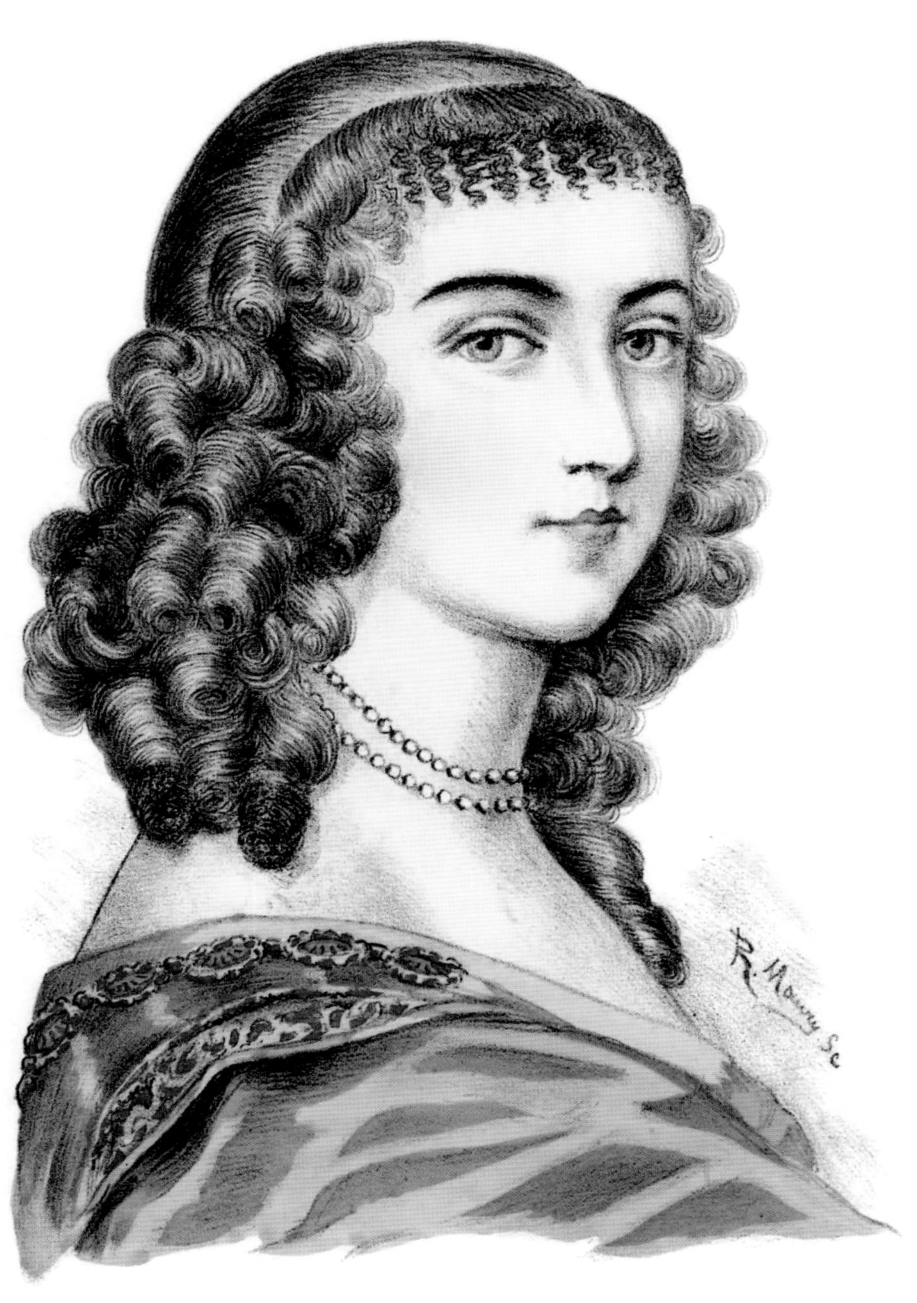

Louis XIII hairstyle, Ninon of Lenclos, *Album de Coiffures Historiques*, E. Nissy

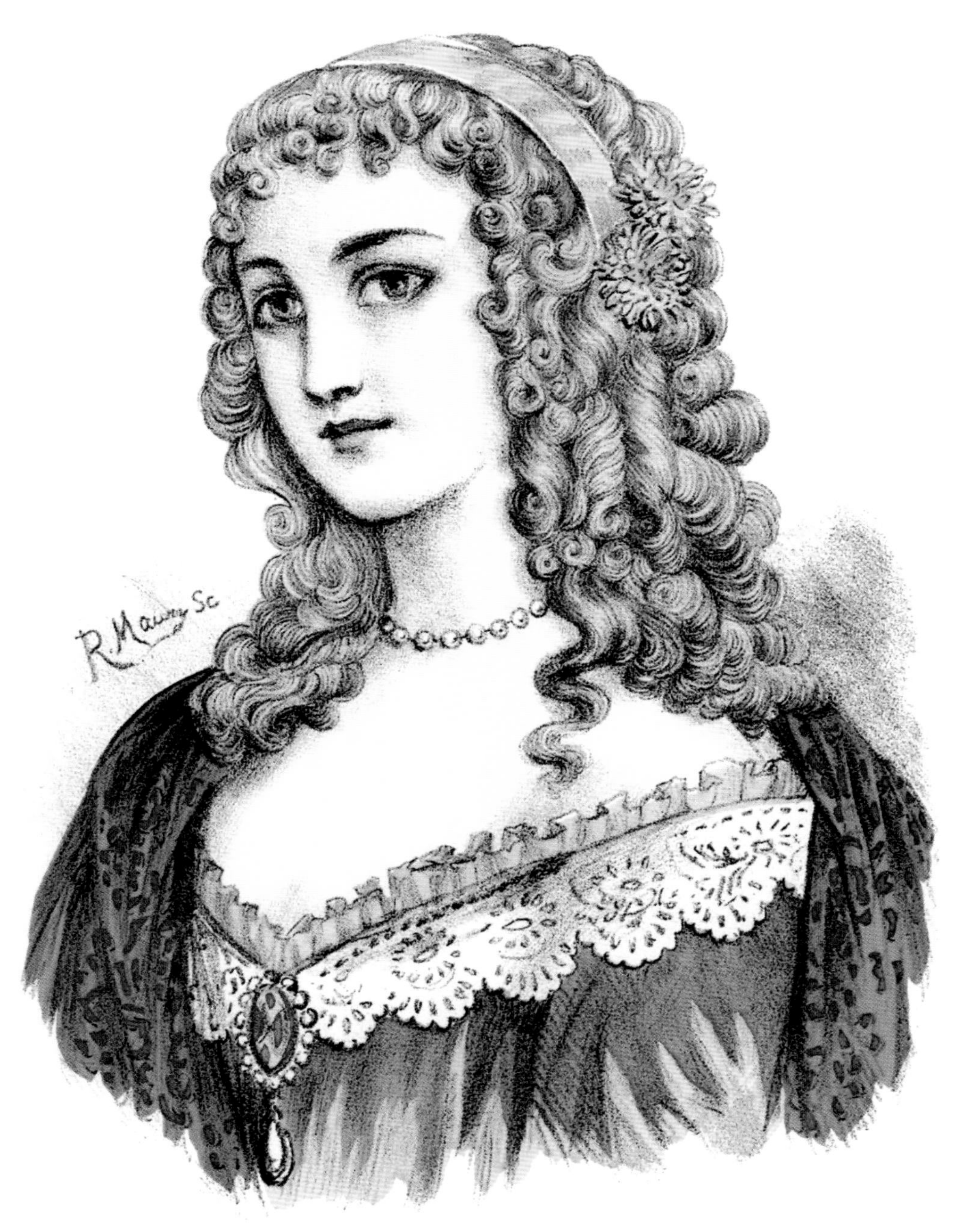

Louis XIII hairstyle, *Album de Coiffures Historiques*, E. Nissy

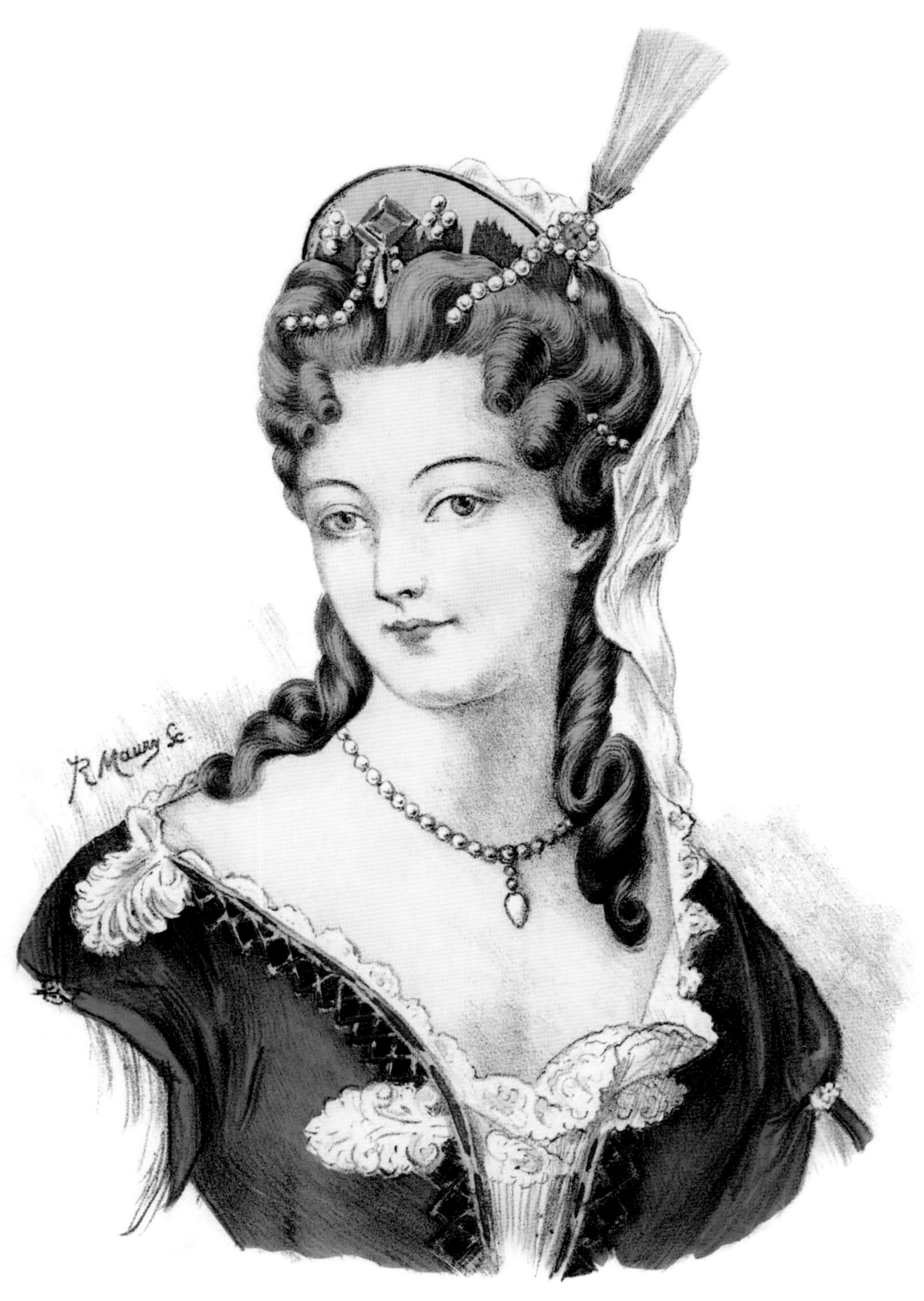

Louis XIV hairstyle, Duchesse of Maine,
Album de Coiffures Historiques, E. Nissy

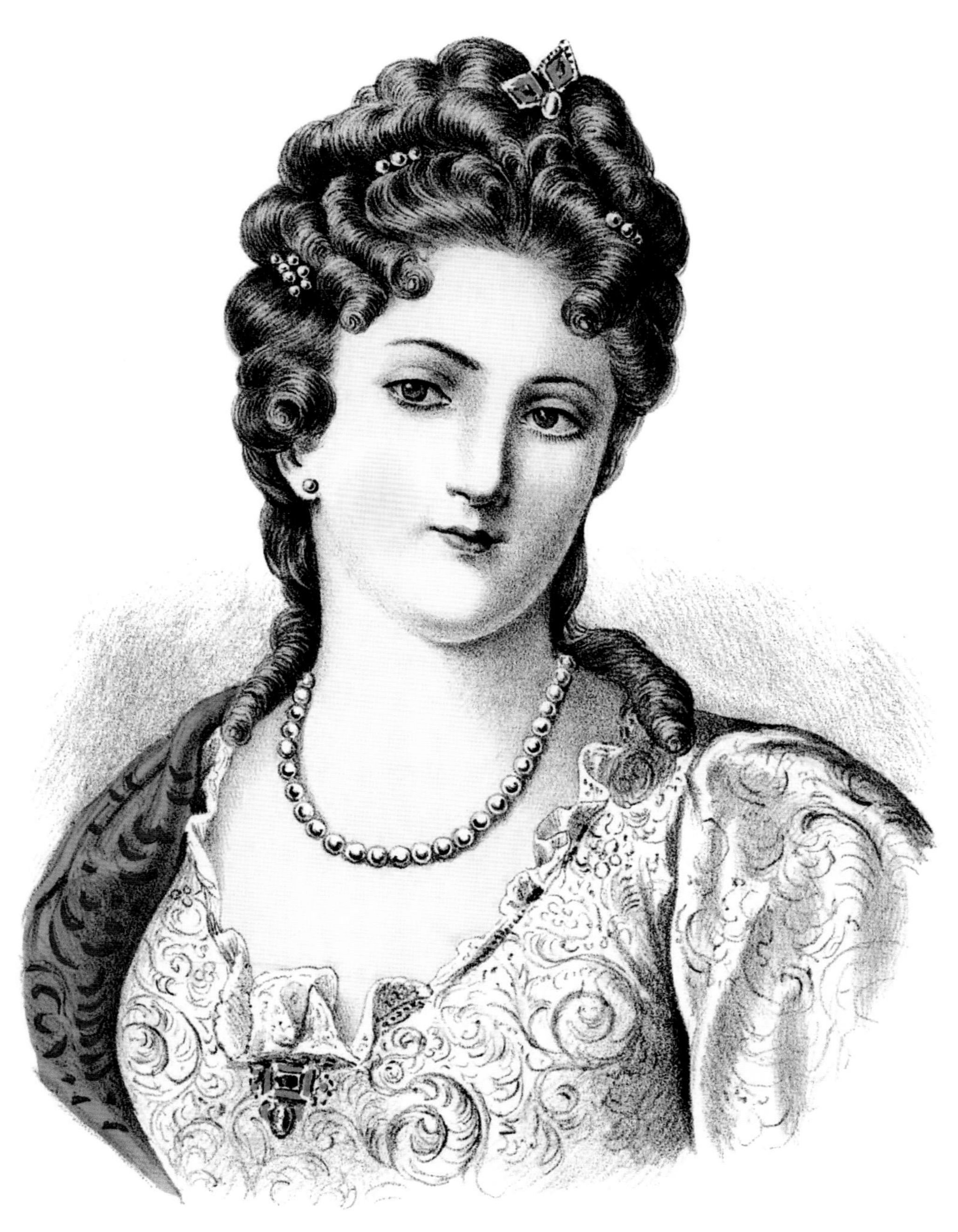

Louis XIV hairstyle, Duchesse of Bourgogne,
Album de Coiffures Historiques, E. Nissy

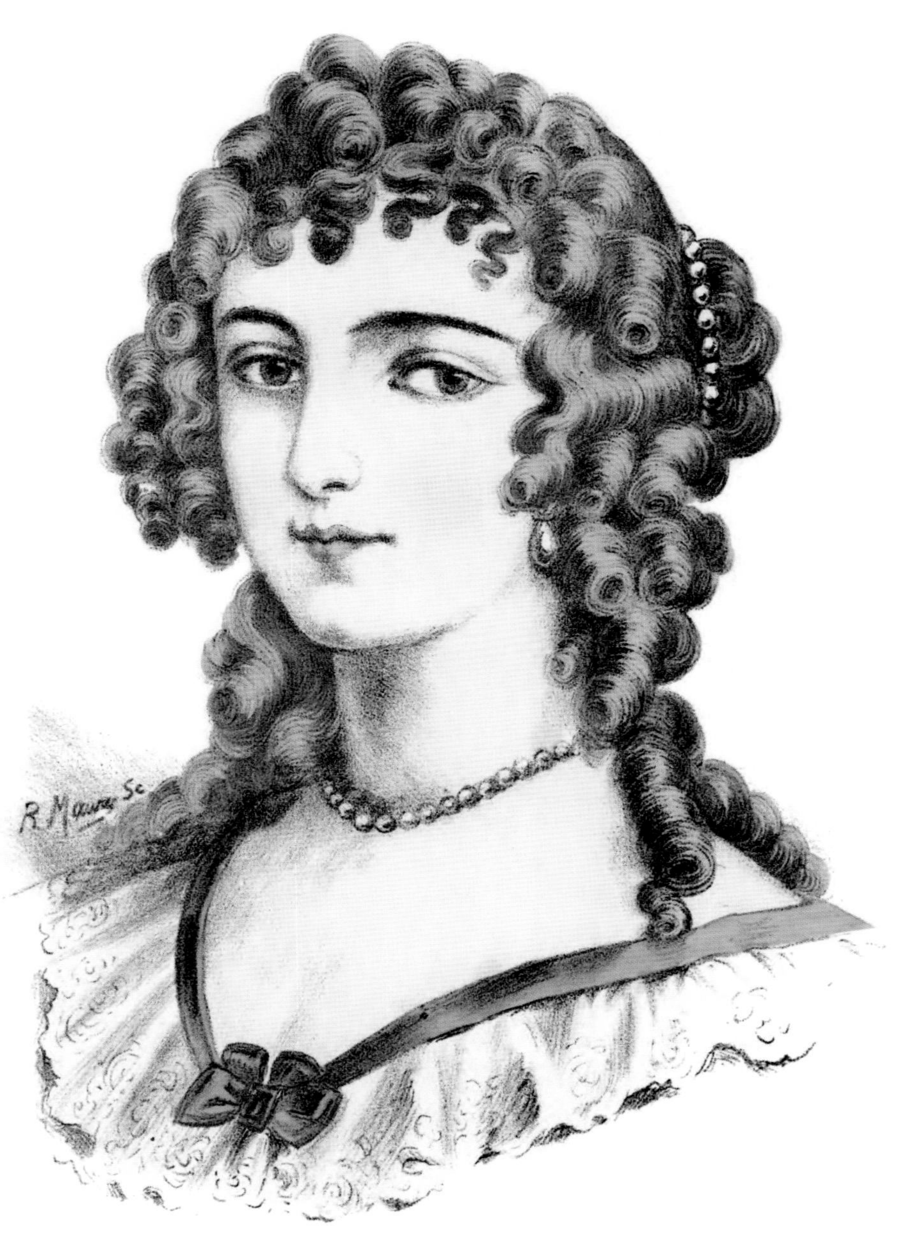

Louis XIV hairstyle, Madame de Maintenon,
Album de Coiffures Historiques, E. Nissy

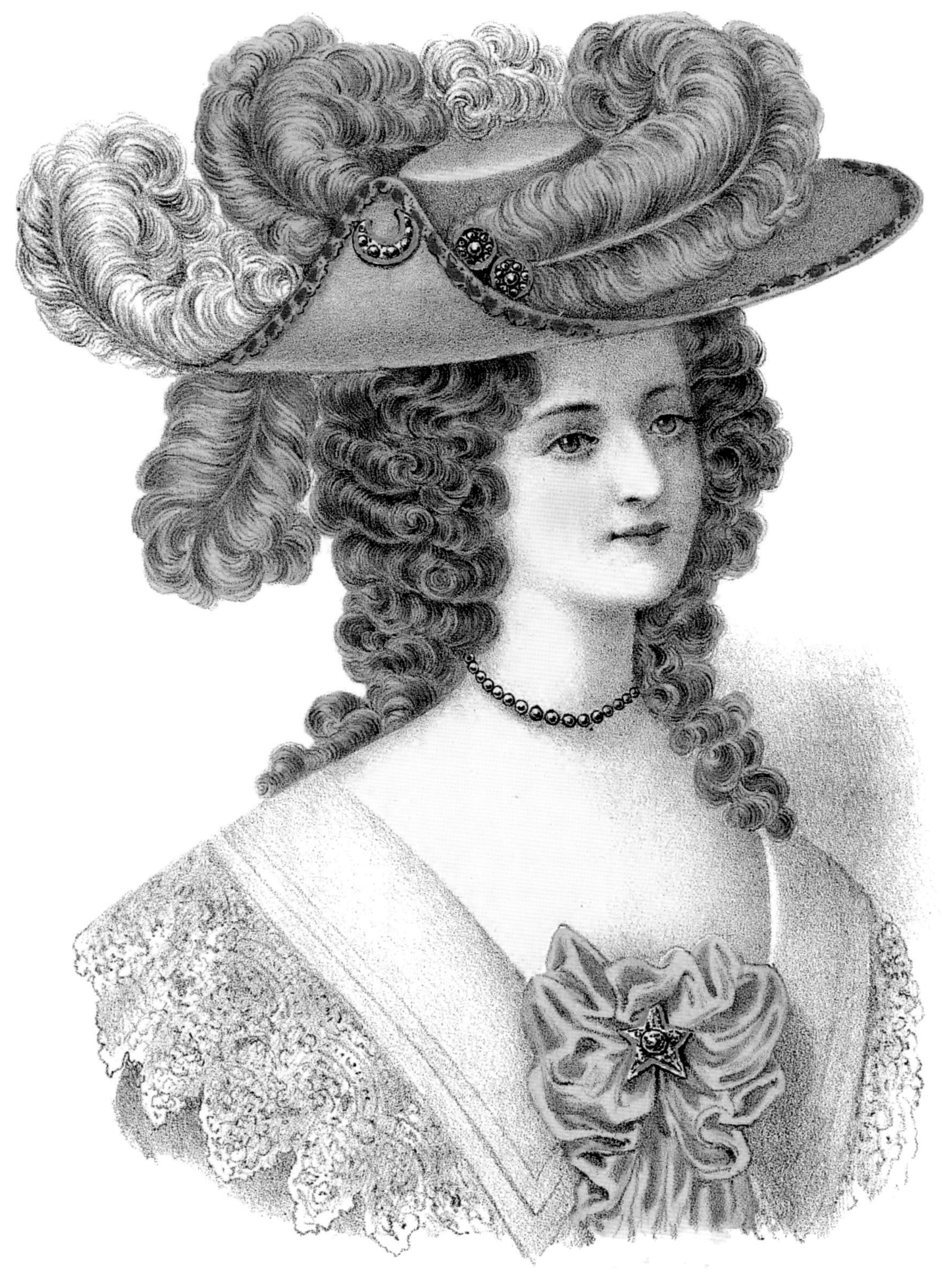

Louis XIV hairstyle, *Album de Coiffures Historiques*, E. Nissy

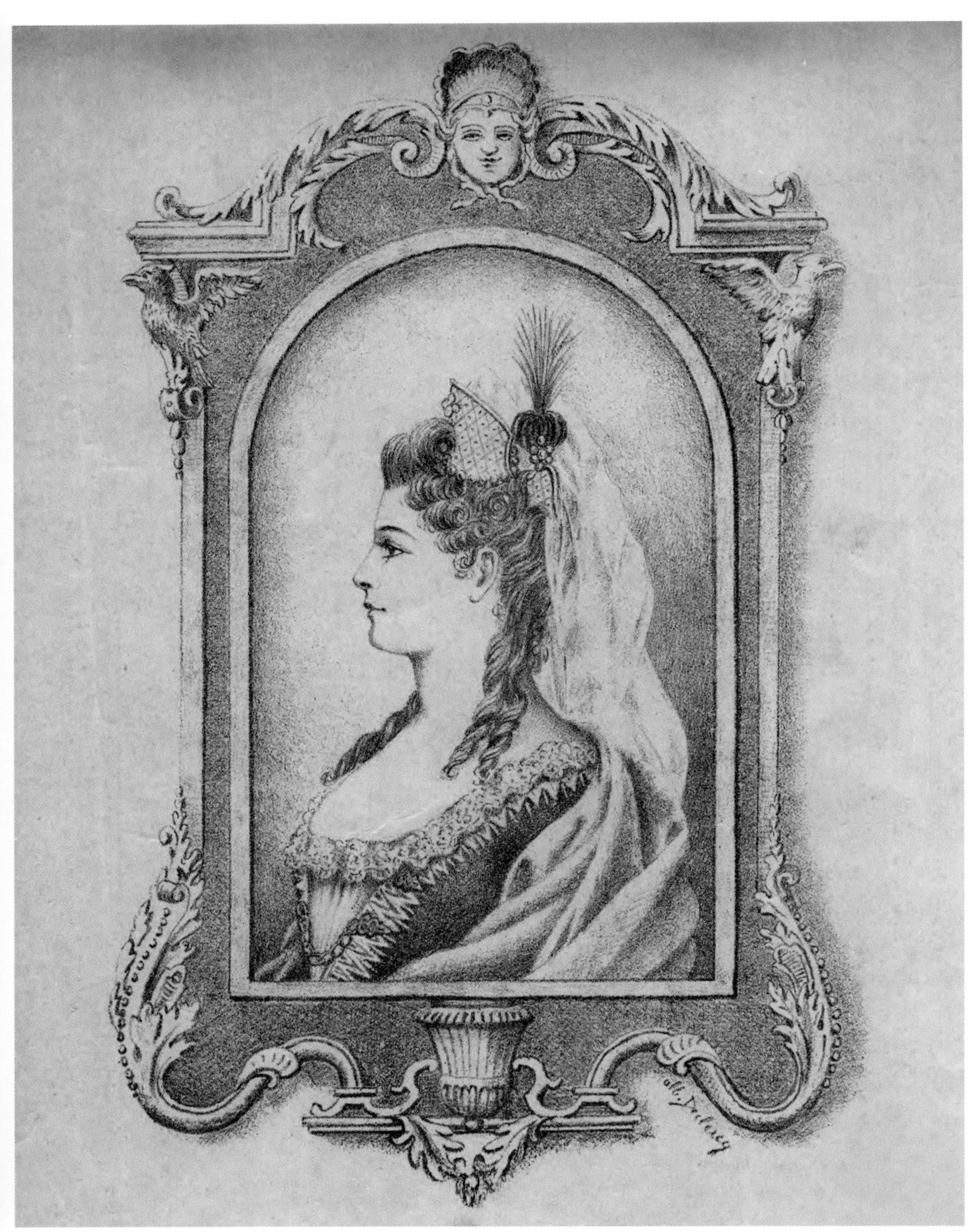

Hairstyle of the Duchesse du Maine,
c.1692, *Paris-Coiffeur*, J.Caumont

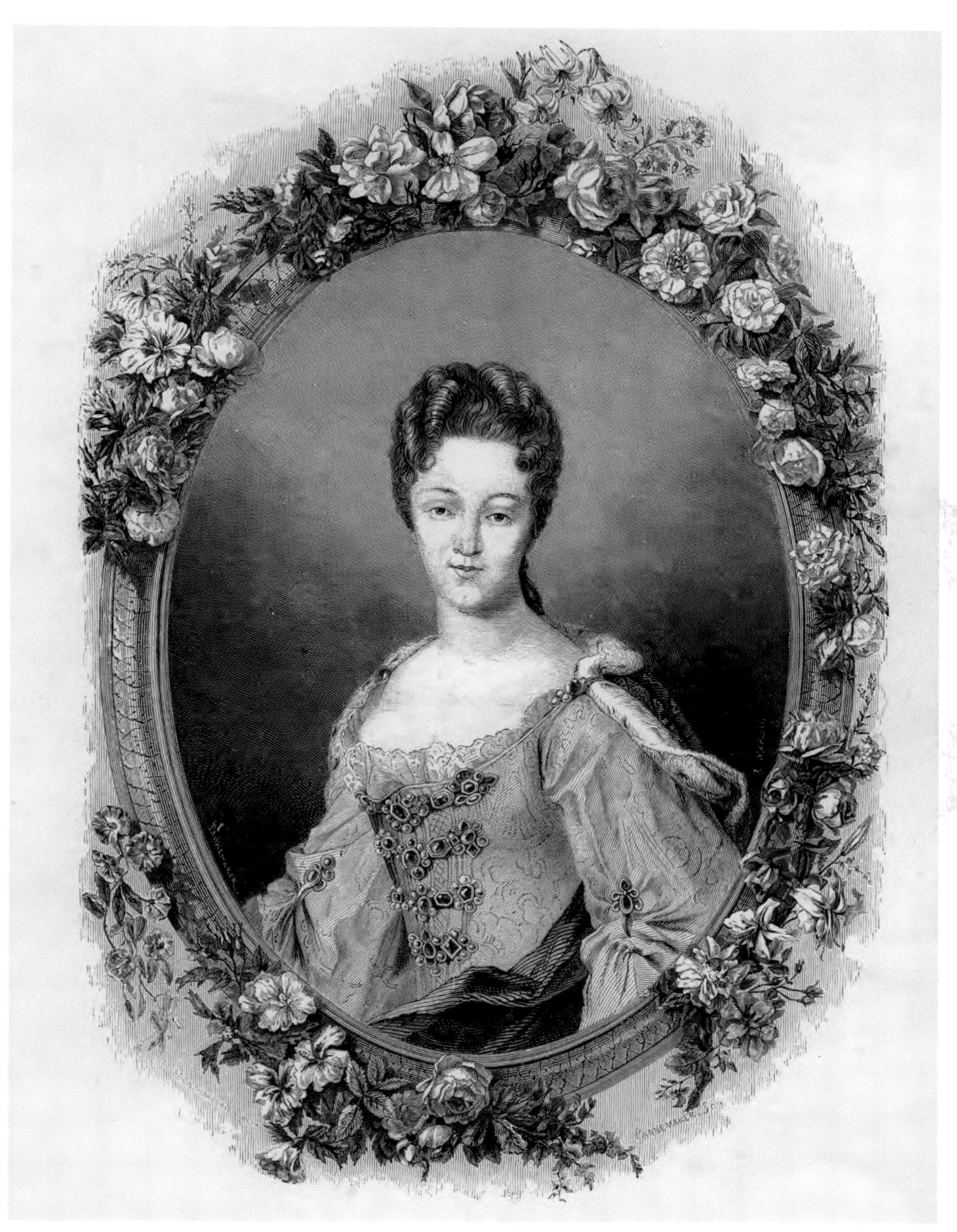

Coiffure of Princess Adelaide de Savoie, Louis XIV,
L'Art dans le Coiffure, J. Caumont

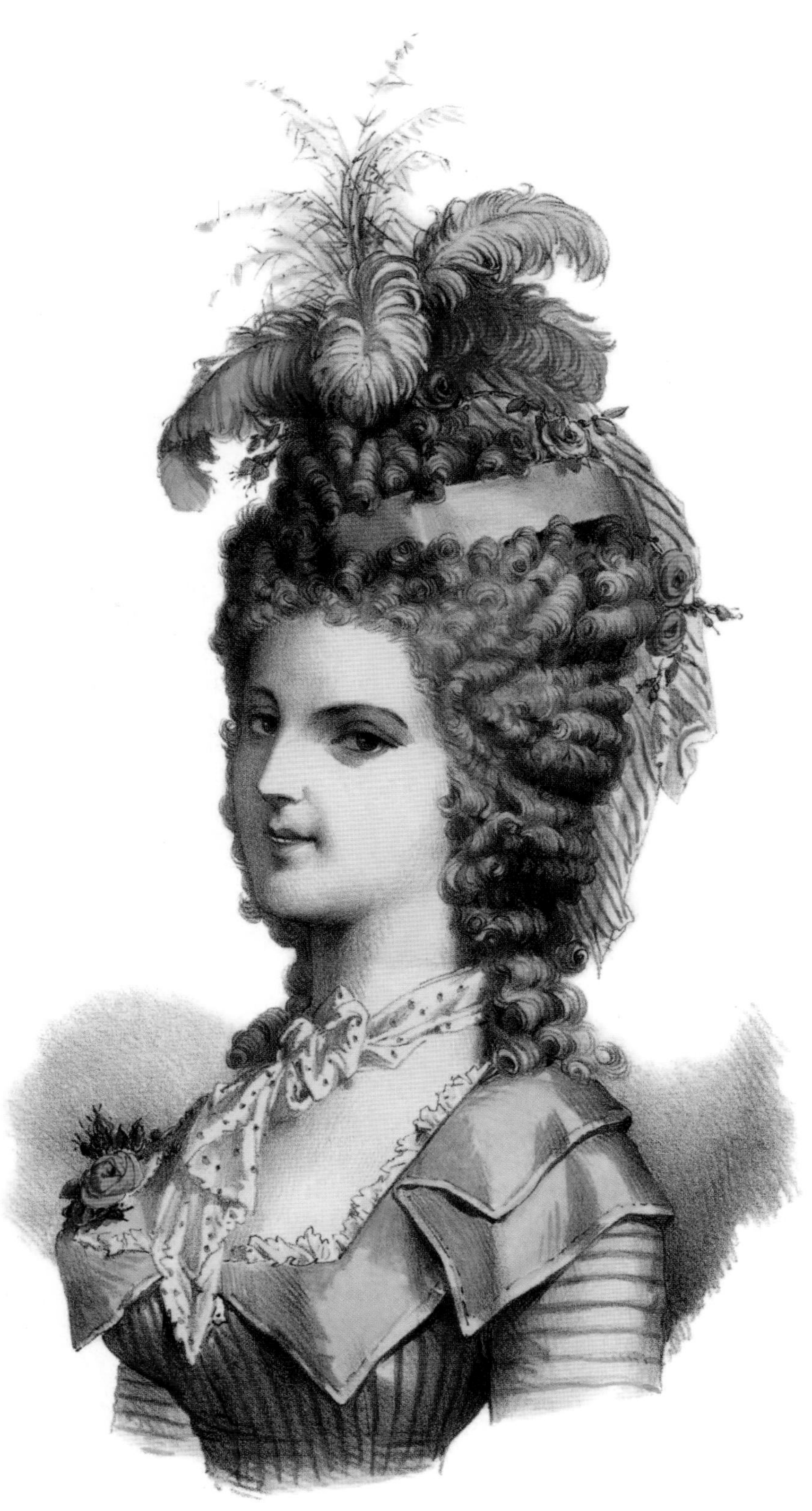

Hairstyle taken from a fashion journal published in 1789, *Le Moniteur de la Coiffure*

18TH CENTURY

At the start of the 1700s the high fan-like "Fontange" headdress was still a popular feature of ladies' coiffures, but by the 1710s it was reducing in size and height, and often women wore their hair without any form of headdress and hanging loosely curled upon their shoulders. For courtly occasions, however, women began wearing decorative caps, trimmed with bows, frills or even made entirely of lace with their hair worn up in buns beneath them, thereby enhancing the line of the neck. During the 1720s, it became increasingly fashionable for women to wear their locks in rolls or waves beneath these decorative "Cornette" caps. As time progressed, these shepherdess-style mop-caps became increasingly fancy with large bows attached to their backs and, from the 1730s to the 1750s, a coiffure known as the "Tête de Mouton" (The sheep's head), which consisted of a profusion of small curls and tight ringlets, became exceedingly popular to wear under these fetching headdresses.

Another hairstyle that became popular during the period between the 1740s and the 1760s was a simple "top-knot" which was embellished with bunches of ribbons, as well as artificial flowers, decorative hairpins, strands of looped pearls or semi-precious jewels. This was also the era of the "Pom-Pom" which was a confection of feathers, flowers, lace, jewels and even butterflies, which was attached just above the hairline with the wearer's tresses piled up beneath it. As the century progressed so did the size and height of the wigs; around 1760 the new "Taupe" (mole) style arrived that consisted of the hair on the back of the head being drawn up into a helmet-like hill and the front locks tightly curled in a coronet-like fashion. In 1763, the hairdresser and wig-maker Frison established the first ladies' hairdressers guild. This enterprising hairdresser also invented the new "Greek style" which quickly became all the rage among the fashionable women of the day. Around this time, ladies when wearing morning dress or in a state of *negligé* wore their hair in nets or bags – but when they went out in the afternoons or evenings they spent a large amount of time skillfully dressing their hair into these elaborate and classical styled arrangements.

It was, however, the 1770s that saw towering wigs become quite literally the height of fashion. In around 1772, the soaring "Full Headdress" or "Opera-Box" made a dramatic appearance with the hair greased and powdered into dizzying constructions, at times measuring an astonishing four feet from the tip of the chin to the top of the head. A contemporary journalist wrote of the fashionable "Cabriolet" style: "Conceive two great wings on either side of the face, sticking out seven or eight inches, and three or four beyond the biggest noses in the kingdom, the said wings fastened at the back to a full linen bag containing the voluminous collection of hair which ladies, at this moment, regard as their most precious ornament. Above all this is piled a sort of framework of ribbon puffings, which looks as if it were tied together with a rosette of the same ribbon near the back of the skull." This coiffure was soon replaced by the even more outrageous powdered "Pouf" which was fashioned from yards of gauze material into a mountainous construction onto which were attached an overabundance of decorative ornaments, including flowers, fruit, vegetables, feathers, stuffed birds, dolls, miniature figurines of shepherdesses and shepherds as well as mythical allegories. As Auguste Racinet noted in his comprehensive *Le Costume Historique*: "The 'Pouf' was sometimes a rustic poem, an English park where we saw a windmill, groves, streams, sheep, or it was a setting for an opera, the development of a panorama."

After the vogue for the "Pouf" faded, "Hérissons" (hedgehogs) became extremely common, which according to Octave Uzanne were "like huge sapper's busbies, hoar-frosted with powder" and which were described in the *Gentleman's and London Magazine* in 1777 as, "Hair carried one storey higher and projects with a high peak over the forehead... and is quite new from Versailles." The trend-setting wife of Louis XVI, Marie Antoinette, frequently changed her hairstyle, and all the fashionable ladies of the French court quickly copied her ever-increasingly elaborated coiffures – or even concocted styles of their own. Among the most notable coiffures of the day were the "Désir de Plaire" (desire to please), the "Chien Couchant" (hound), the "Parc Anglais" (English park), the "Sentiments Repliés" (returned feelings), "la Plume d'Amour" (the feather of love) and the "Vol d'amour" (flight of love). Other hairstyles harked back to ancient times and were inspired by Greek mythology, such as the coiffures "à la Vénus", "à la Junon" (Juno) or "à la Driade" (Dryad). In 1772, the 39-volume *L'Eloge des coiffures adressé aux Dames* (In Praise of Women's Hairstyles), was published in Paris. This staggeringly comprehensive celebration of the coiffeuse's art not only outlined 96 different hairdressing methods but also illustrated a staggering 3,744 models of hairstyles, some of which necessitated the hairdresser having to climb a small ladder in order to ply his craft.

Perhaps the most notable hairstyle of the period, however,

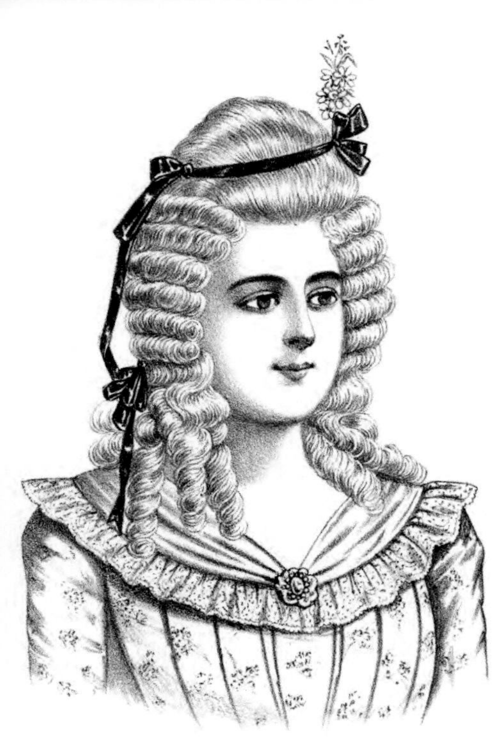

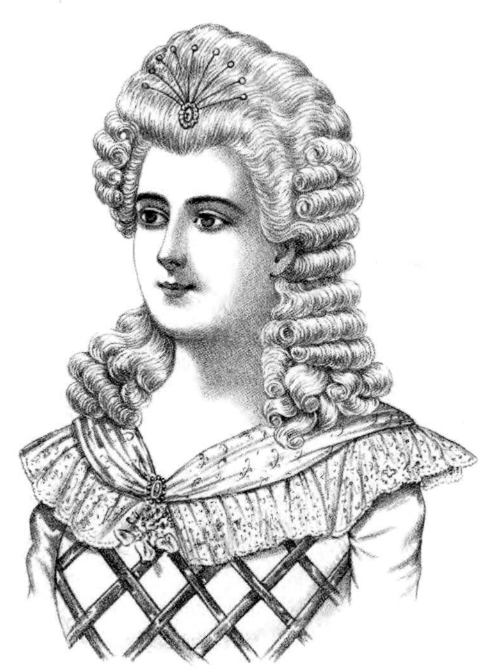

was "à la Frégate" (also known as "à la Belle Poule") that incorporated a model "man o' war" ship riding on waves of rippling hair – celebrating the supposed victory in 1778 of the French Belle Poule frigate against the HMS Arethusa (which had been previously captured from the French by the British). As an early example of a highly patriotic and thereby political hair statement, this nautical hairstyle also came to be known as the "Frégate de Junon" – commemorating another sea battle the following year, in which the 32-gun Junon frigate captained by Vicomte de Beaumont and another French frigate known as the Gentille heroically captured the Royal Navy's much larger 64-gun HMS Ardent. Another well-known hairstyle of this period was known as "à la Minerve" and consisted of a high wig dressed with up to ten ostrich feathers, which was made fashionable by Marie Antoinette. Of course, the satirical cartoonists of the day, in both France and England, took enormous pleasure in poking fun at the ridiculous excesses of hair fashions worn by ladies of the upper echelons of a society that was so starkly divided by class privilege, but often their depictions were a grotesque exaggeration of reality.

A truer representation of these elaborate hairstyles can, however, be found on the pages of James Stewart's seminal treatise, *Plocacosmos: or the Whole Art of Hair Dressing; wherein is contained, ample rules for the young artizan, more particularly for ladies, women, valets, etc. as well as directions for persons to dress their own hair*, which he self-published in 1782. Apart from being illustrated with beautiful engravings of the then-fashionable coiffures of the day, this landmark publication also gave practical advice on wig wearing and the time-consuming preparation of perukes, as well as more general haircare tips for the fashionable lady. For example: "All that is required at night is to take the cap or toke off, as any other ornament, and as you put them on, you can easily know how to take them off: with regard to the hair, nothing need be touched but the curls; you may take the pins out of them, and, with a little soft pomatum in your hands, stroke the hairs that may have started; do them with nice long rollers, wind them up to the roots, and turn the end of each roller firmly in to keep them tight, remembering at the same time the hair should never be combed at night, having always so bad an effect as to give a violent headache next day. After the curls are rolled up, touch them with your pomatumy hands, and stroke the hair behind; after that take a very large net fillet, which must be big enough to cover the head and hair, and put it on, and drawing the strings to a proper tightness behind, till it closes all round the face and neck like a purse, bring the strings round the front and back again to the neck, where they must be tied; this, with the finest lawn handkerchief, is night covering sufficient for the head." Around this time, English ladies, most notably Georgiana, Duchess of Devonshire, sported fashionable powdered padded wigs with loose curls falling around the shoulders, on which they wore large-brimmed hats with huge feathers set at a jaunty angle.

The immense weight of the lofty wigs so fashionable in the 1780s and the extraordinary amount of time it took to precisely dress them meant that they were in vogue for only a relatively short, if highly memorable, period of time. In

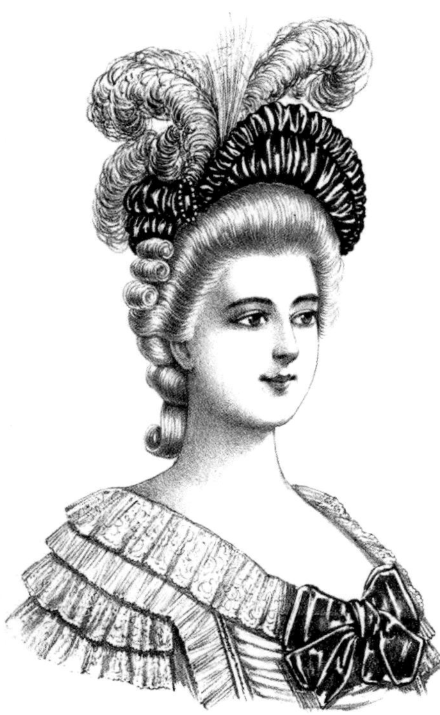

Left: Louis XVI hairstyle with ribbon and flowers
Right and middle: Louis XVI hairstyles, *Album Historischer und Phantasie-Frisuren*, Heinrich Moritz

fact, the fashion for towering wigs collapsed almost overnight when Marie Antoinette's hair began to fall out following the birth of her son, Louis Charles (the Dauphin of France), in 1785, and she took to wearing caps and had her hair styled into the less formal "Coiffure à l'Enfant". The adoption of this simpler style was also no doubt a recognition of the growing revolutionary sentiment stirring among the French populace – to put it plainly, the follies of excessive tall-wigged coiffures were not politically expedient during this period of increasing social unrest. After the Storming of the Bastille in Paris on July 14 1789, there was a marked change in hairstyles. The French Revolution heralded in its own distinctive fashions, which were in accord with the Republic's democratising motto: "Liberté, égalité, fraternité".

To mark the changing times, many women wore their hair curled at the front and then allowed the rest of their locks to fall naturally to their shoulders, while Parisiennes also wore their hair "à la Nation" or "aux Charmes de la Liberté" – the latter seemingly to involve the wearing of a small posy of myrtle interspersed with tricolor ribbons that conveyed support for the Revolution. Two other French hairstyles that were popular during the Revolutionary period were known as "à la Titus" – a short cut of curled hair bound with a circlet – and the "Porc-epic" (Porcupine) – a spiky dishevelled style that was boyishly becoming.

Just as Samson lost his strength when the treacherous Delilah cut his hair, so too did the power of the French aristocracy disappear as their hair was brutally shorn in preparation for the guillotine. Somewhat morbidly after the death of Robespierre, however, there was a trend for what can only be described as guillotine chic – with women wearing their hair extremely short "à la Victime" in imitation of the way condemned women's hair was cut so it would not interfere with the blade of the guillotine. Around 1798 also saw the rise of "Les Merveilleuses" (The Marvellous Ones), ladies of a Post-Revolutionary elite who copied the fashions of ancient Athens. These elegant women frequently sported the classically inspired "Merveilleuse" style comprising a profusion of curls drawn together on top of the head with ringlets at the sides and back, and then smaller curls at the front. This hairstyle was an act of defiance against the revolutionary austerity of the French Revolution's "Reign of Terror" and a coiffured celebration of the despised Robespierre's eventual fall from grace. Among the "Les Merveilleuses" set there was also a vogue for wearing fair wigs during the day and dark-haired wigs at night, with fashionable ladies changing their wigs frequently throughout the day. Reputedly Madame Tallien and Madame Barras, two renowned socialites of the Directoire period, owned thirty such wigs each, in an array of different colours that they wore in the "Merveilleuse" style or other Greco-mania-inspired styles – giving them a suitably fashionable and winsome Neo-Classical look. Two leading hairdressers of the day, Rey and Duplan, reportedly made a fortune from the sale and dressing of such classically inspired wigs.

Although during the Directoire period in France (1795–1799) there was a predilection for Neo-Classical hairstyles, there was also a vogue for loosely curled, somewhat fluffy wigs that were embellished with Turkish-inspired "Mameluke Turbans" adorned with feathers, which were elegantly exotic. This fashion also became hugely popular in England with fashionable Georgian ladies wearing these semi-turbans with huge ostrich feathers dyed in various shades or adorned with black heron plumes. Sometimes the ostrich feathers were reputedly three times the height of the wearer's head, which meant that women had to contort themselves in carriages and the like. This style was notably documented in James Gillray's cartoons of the period, revealing the functional shortcomings of this rather glamorous if short-lived form of headdress. Although the hairstyles at the close of the century were a little more subdued than the dazzlingly structured and ornament-embellished follies created during the reign of Louis XVI, they still revealed that the dressing of hair was an important pastime for the fashionable elite, and that the idea of female attractiveness remained inextricably bound to the idea of beautiful hair.

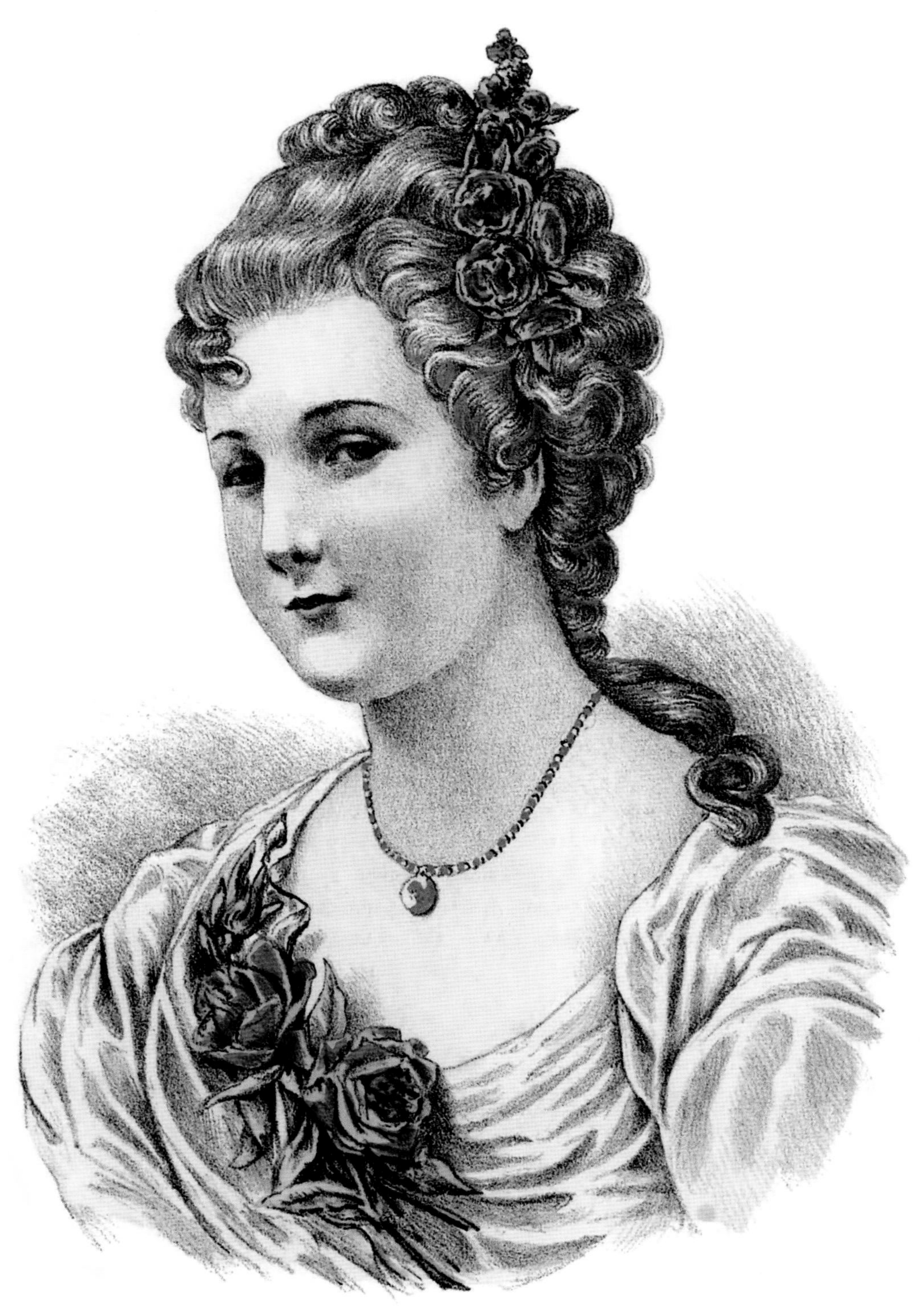

Madame de Parabère, Louis xv hairstyle,
Album de Coiffures Historiques, E. Nissy

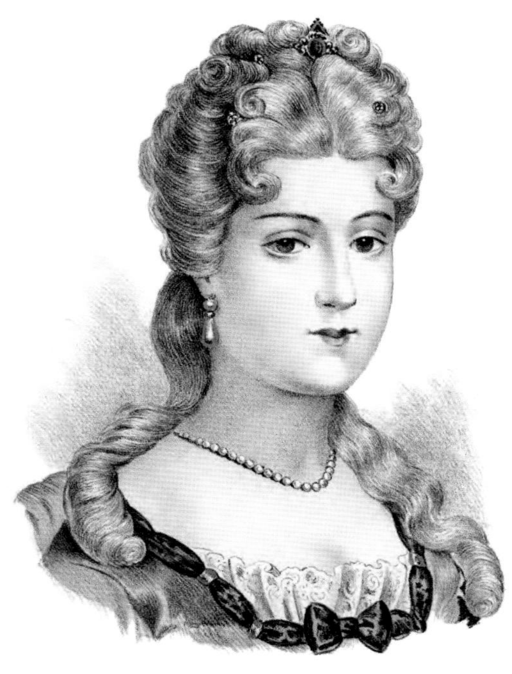

Louis XV Hairstyle, Elisabeth of Orléans, *Album de Coiffures Historiques*, E. Nissy

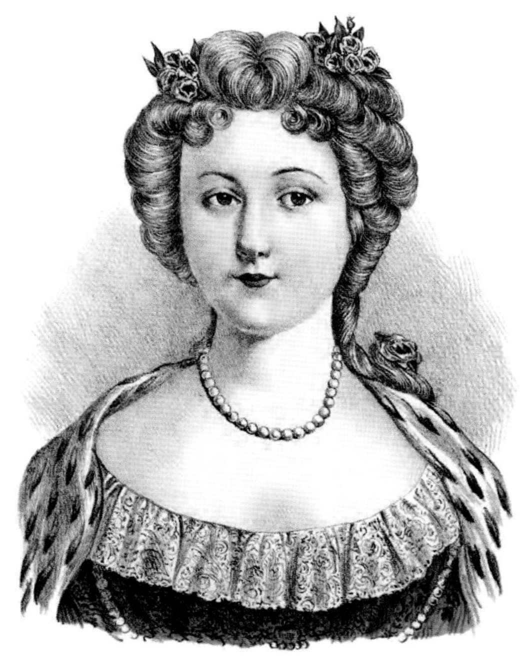

Marie Leczinska, Louis XV hairstyle, *Album de Coiffures Historiques*, E. Nissy

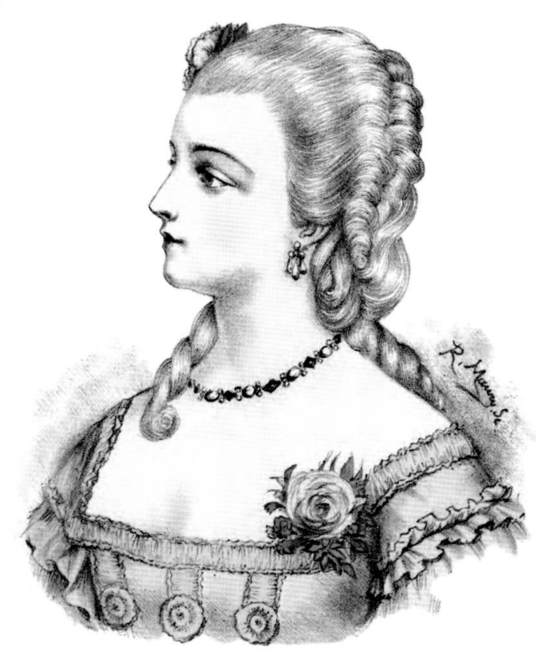

Madame Du Barry, Louis XV hairstyle, *Album de Coiffures Historiques*, E. Nissy

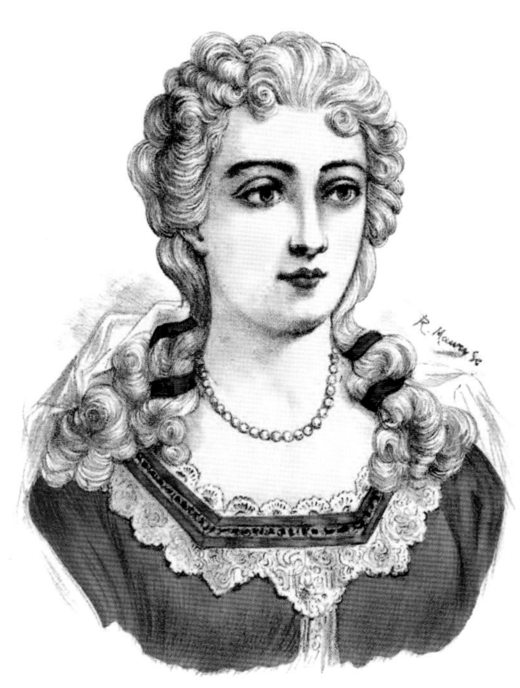

Adrienne Lecouvreur, Louis XV hairstyle, *Album de Coiffures Historiques*, E. Nissy

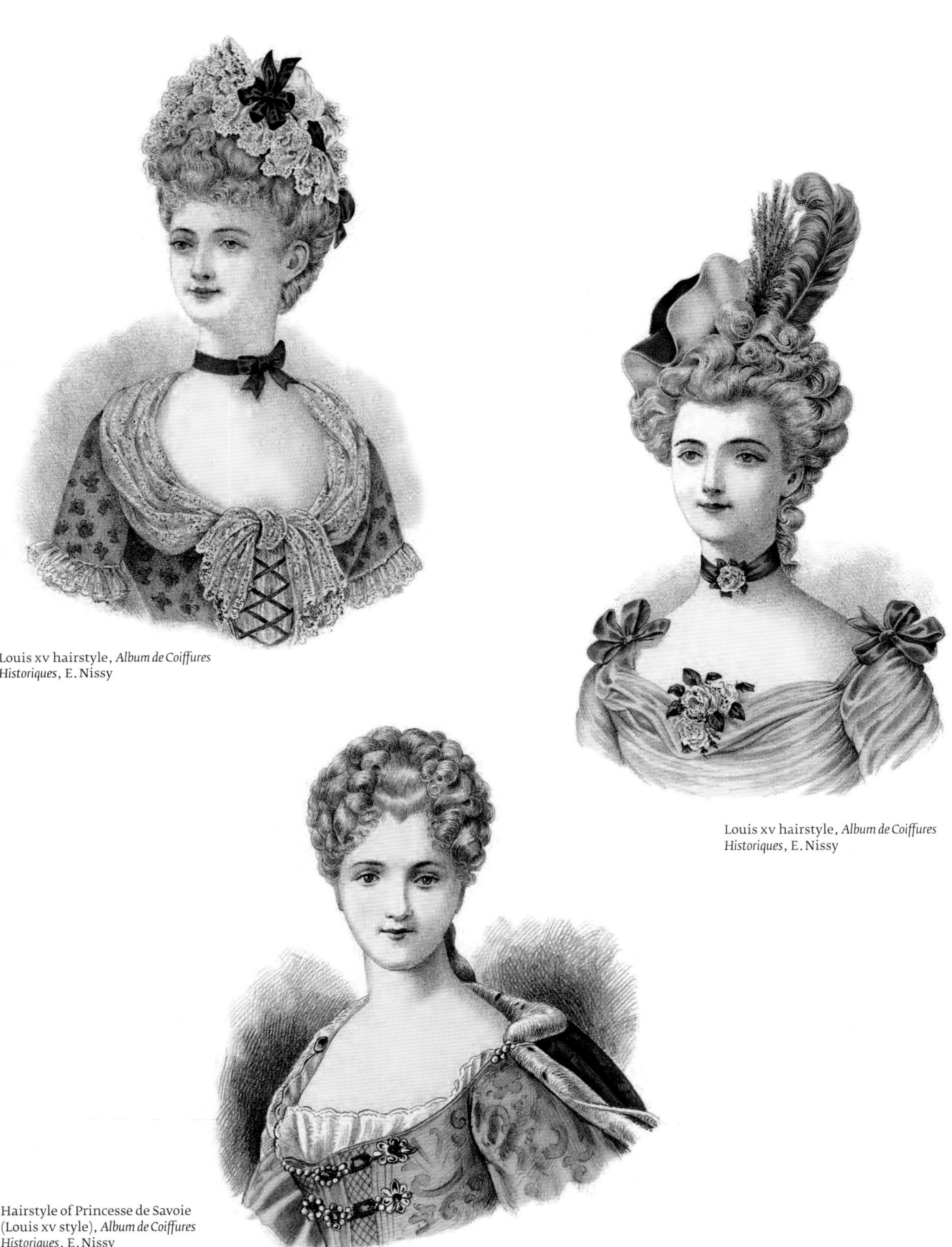

Louis xv hairstyle, *Album de Coiffures Historiques*, E. Nissy

Louis xv hairstyle, *Album de Coiffures Historiques*, E. Nissy

Hairstyle of Princesse de Savoie (Louis xv style), *Album de Coiffures Historiques*, E. Nissy

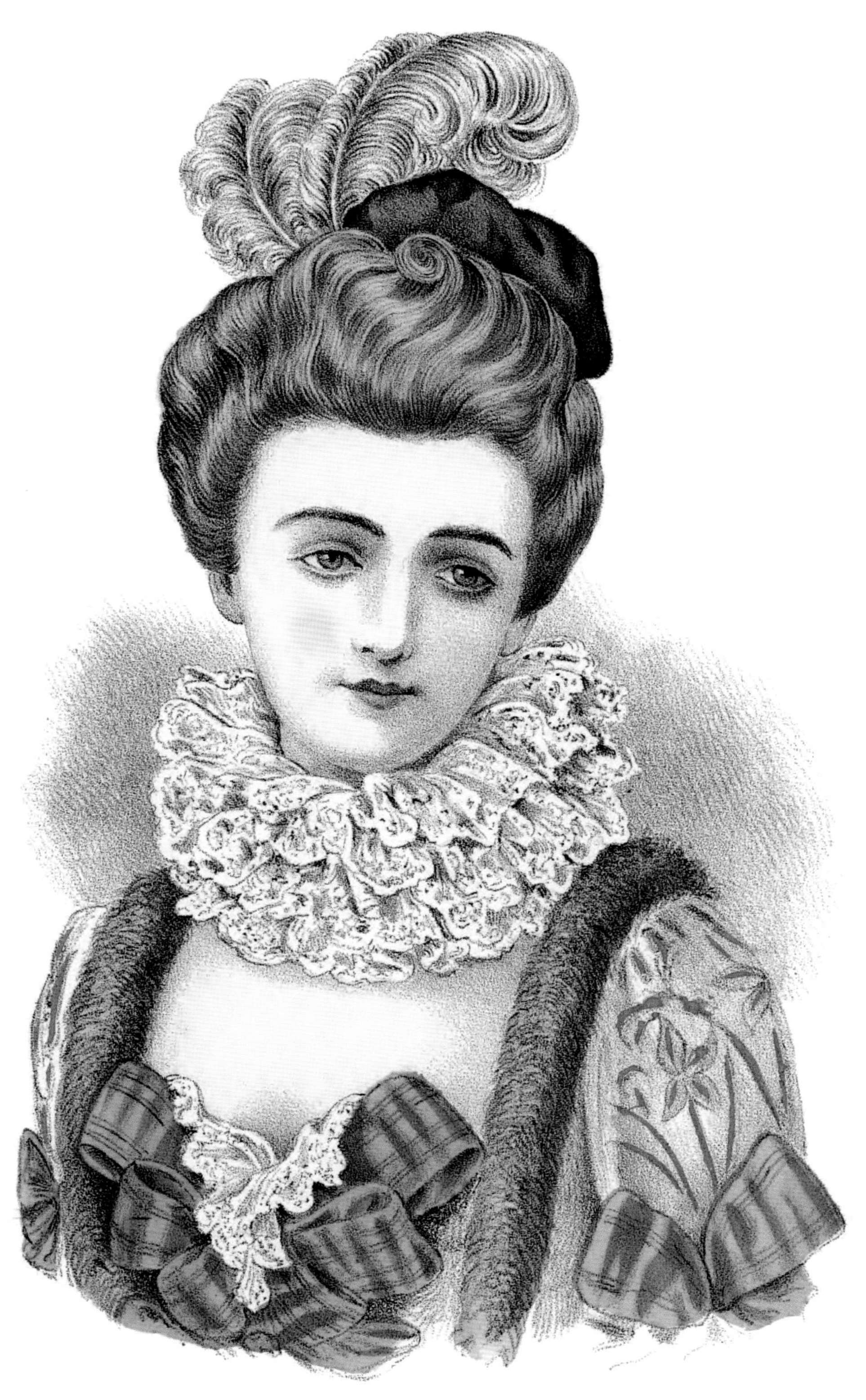

Louis xv hairstyle, *Album de Coiffures Historiques*, E. Nissy

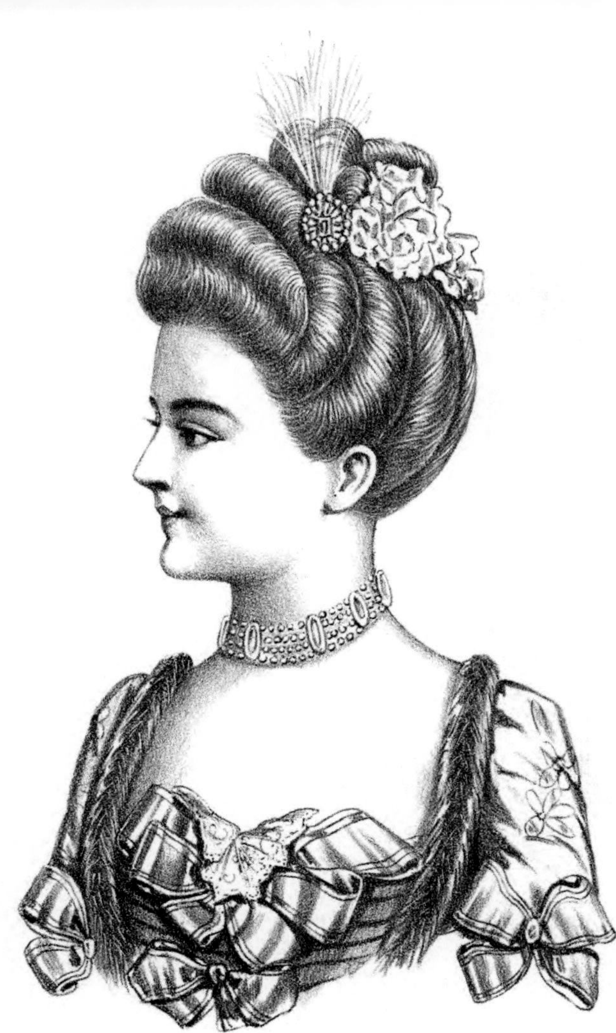

Louis xv hairstyle, *Album Historischer und Phantasie-Frisuren*, Heinrich Moritz

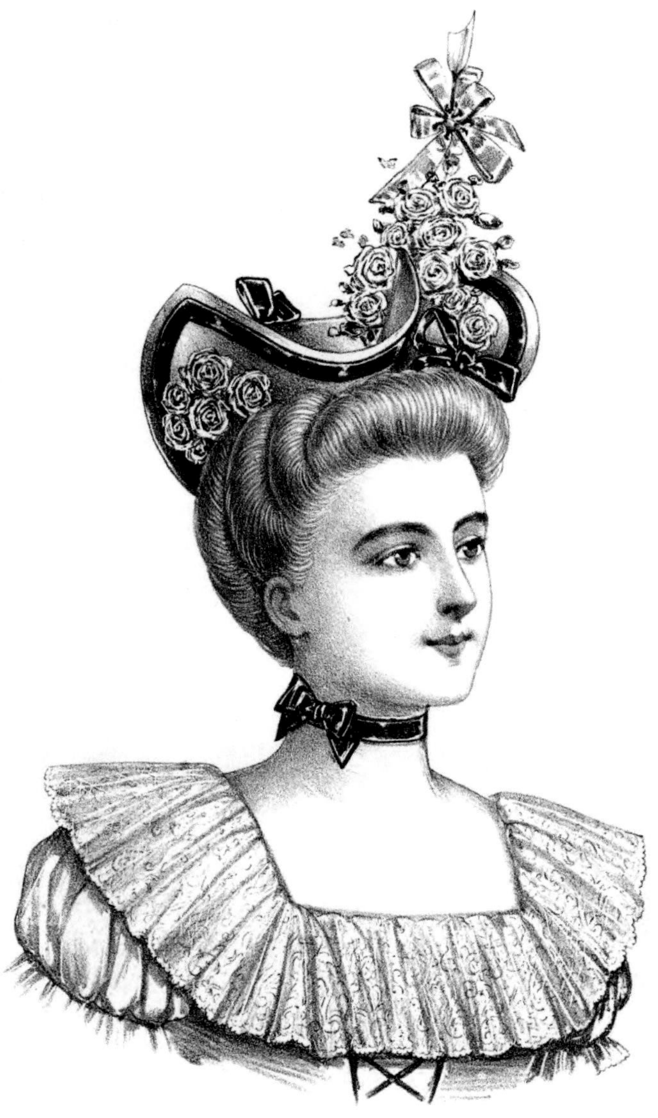

Louis xv hairstyle with hat, *Album Historischer und Phantasie-Frisuren*, Heinrich Moritz

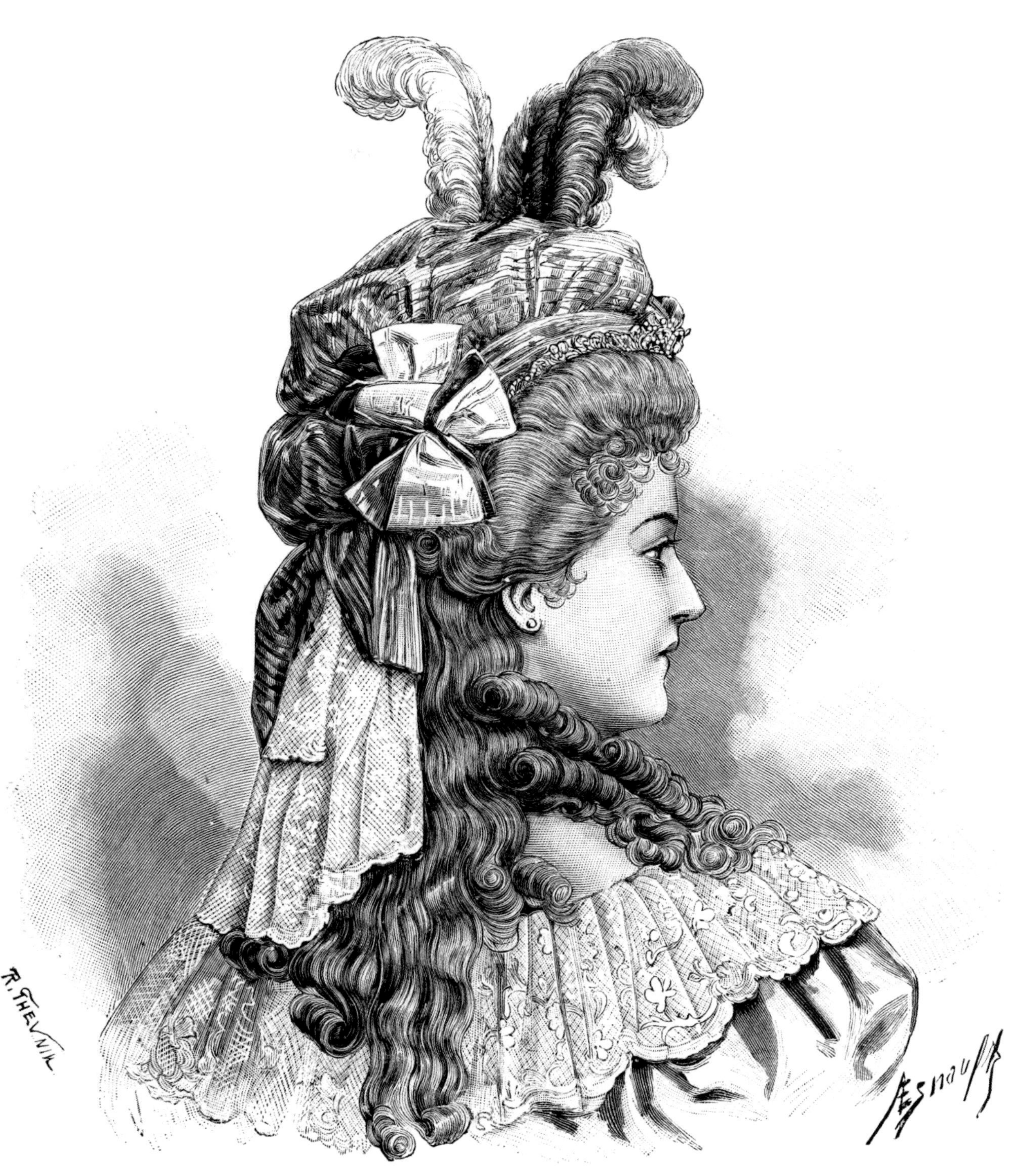

Louis xvi coiffure, *L'Art dans la Coiffure*, J. Caumont

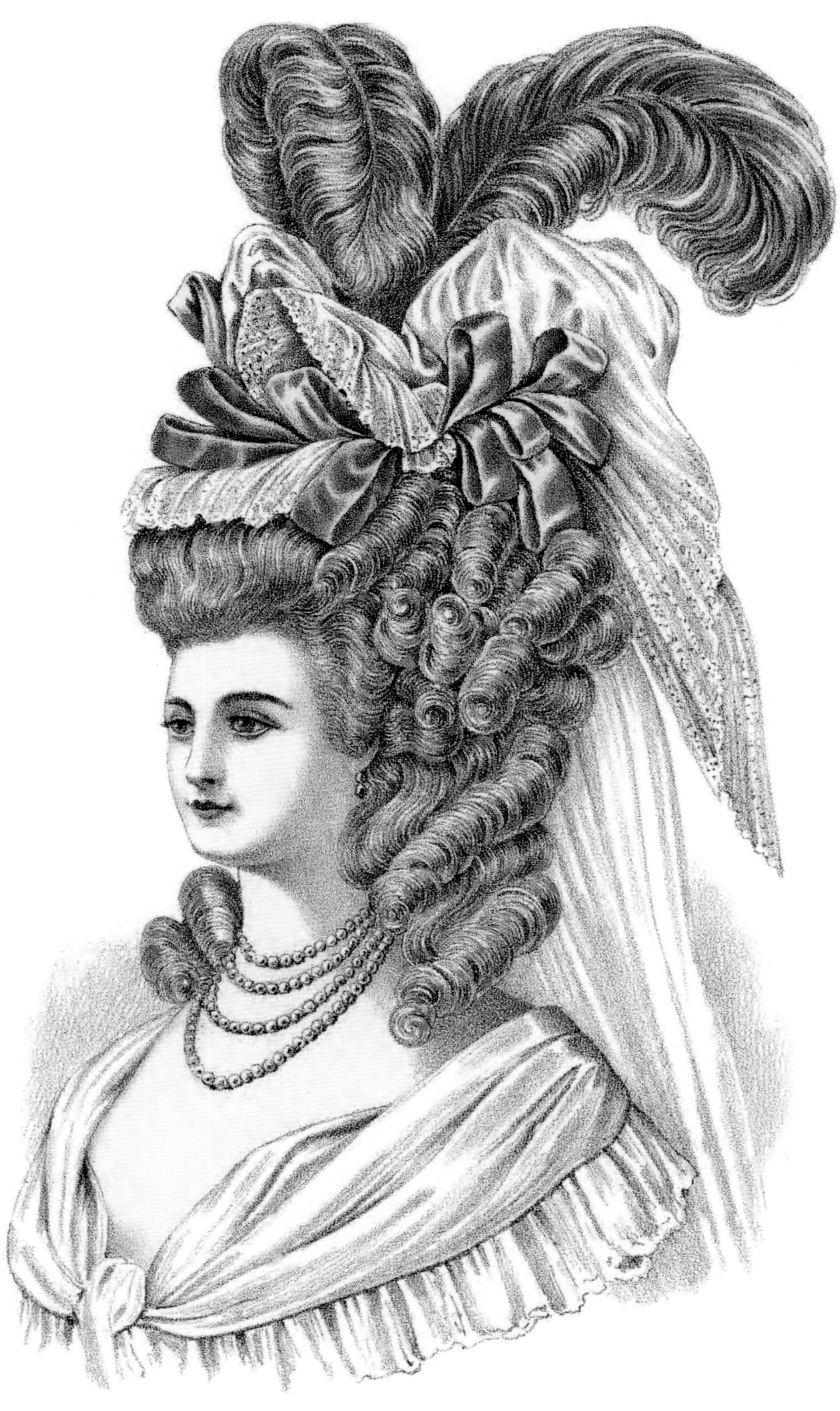

Louis xvi hairstyle, *Album de Coiffures Historiques*, E. Nissy

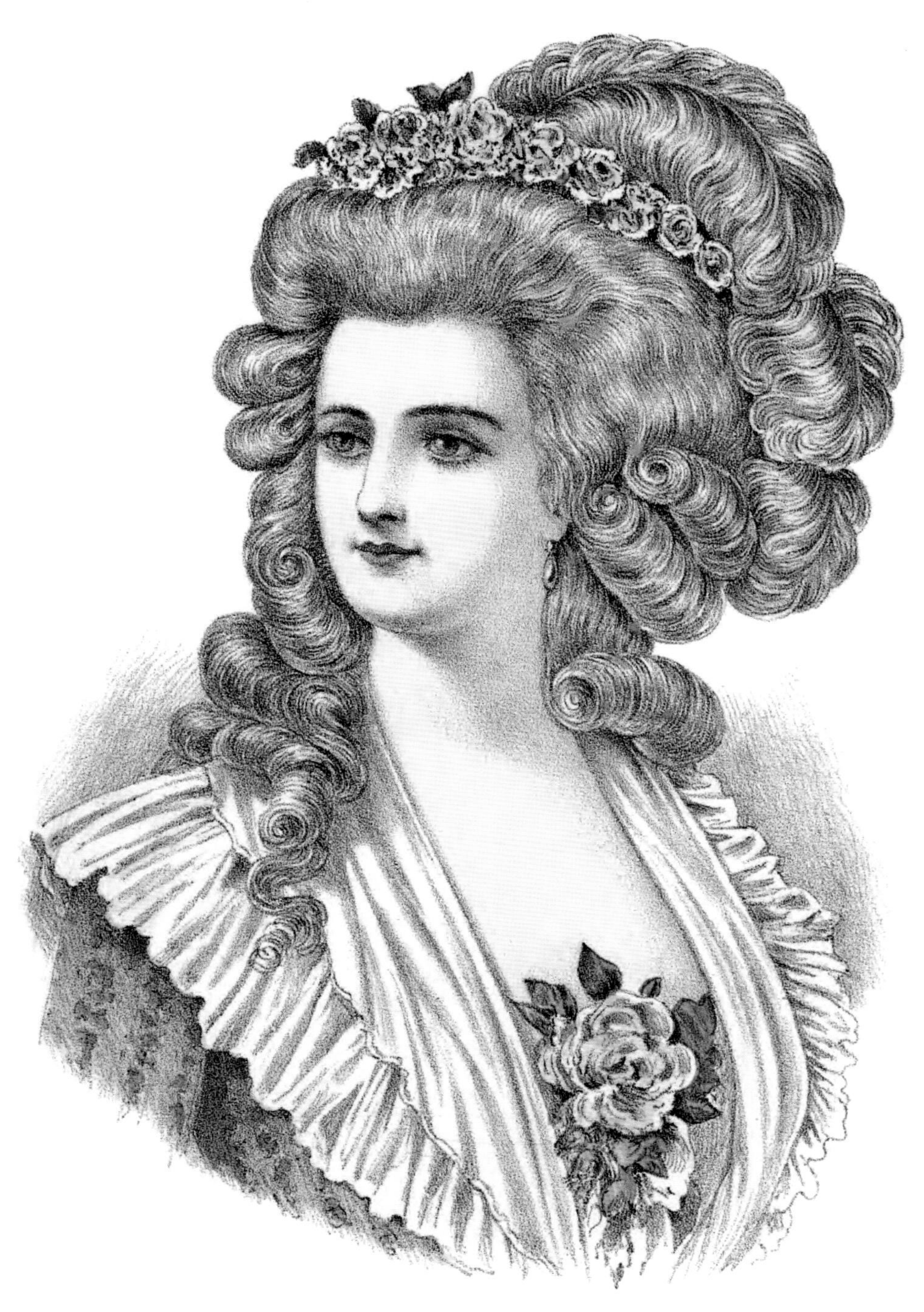

Louis XVI hairstyle, *Album de Coiffures Historiques*, E. Nissy

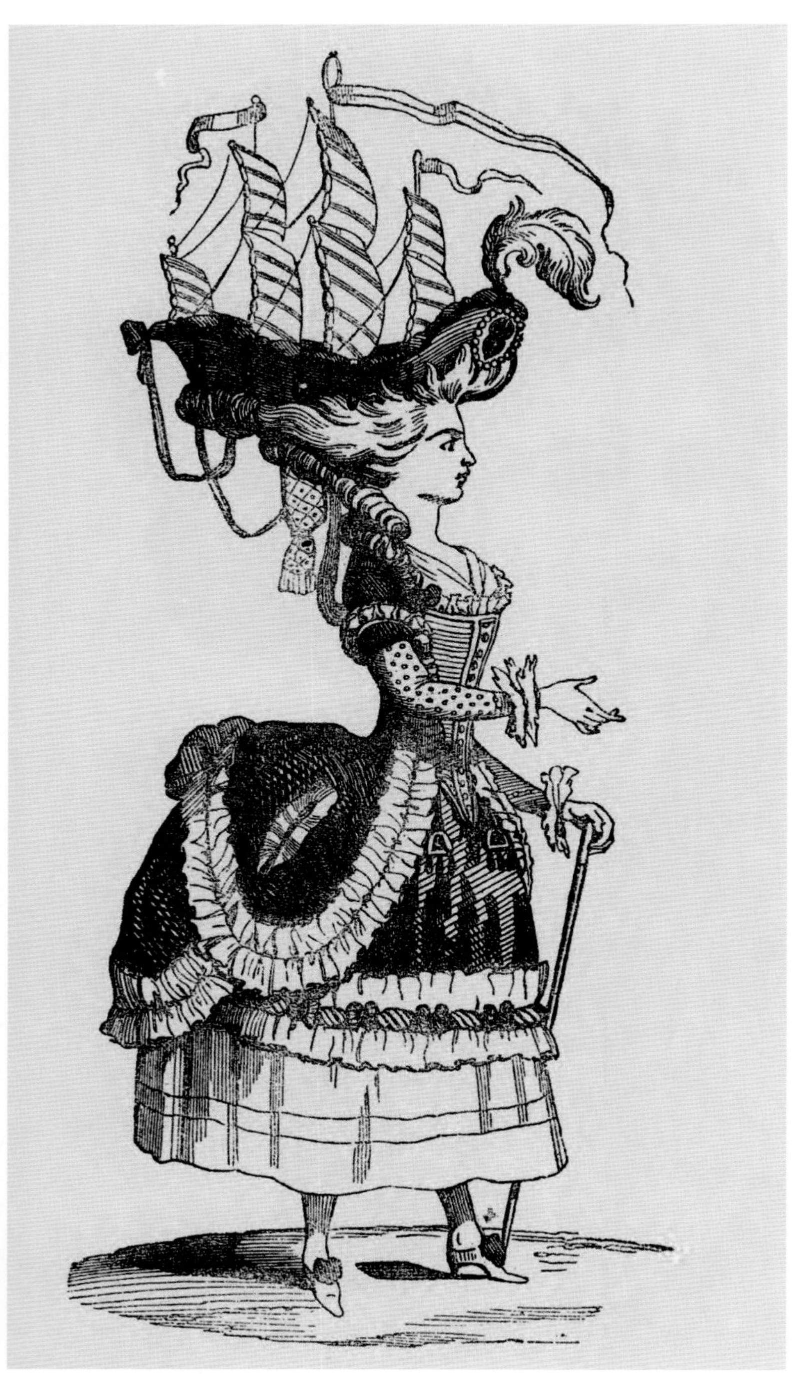

'Coiffure à la Belle Poule', France,
Louis XVI

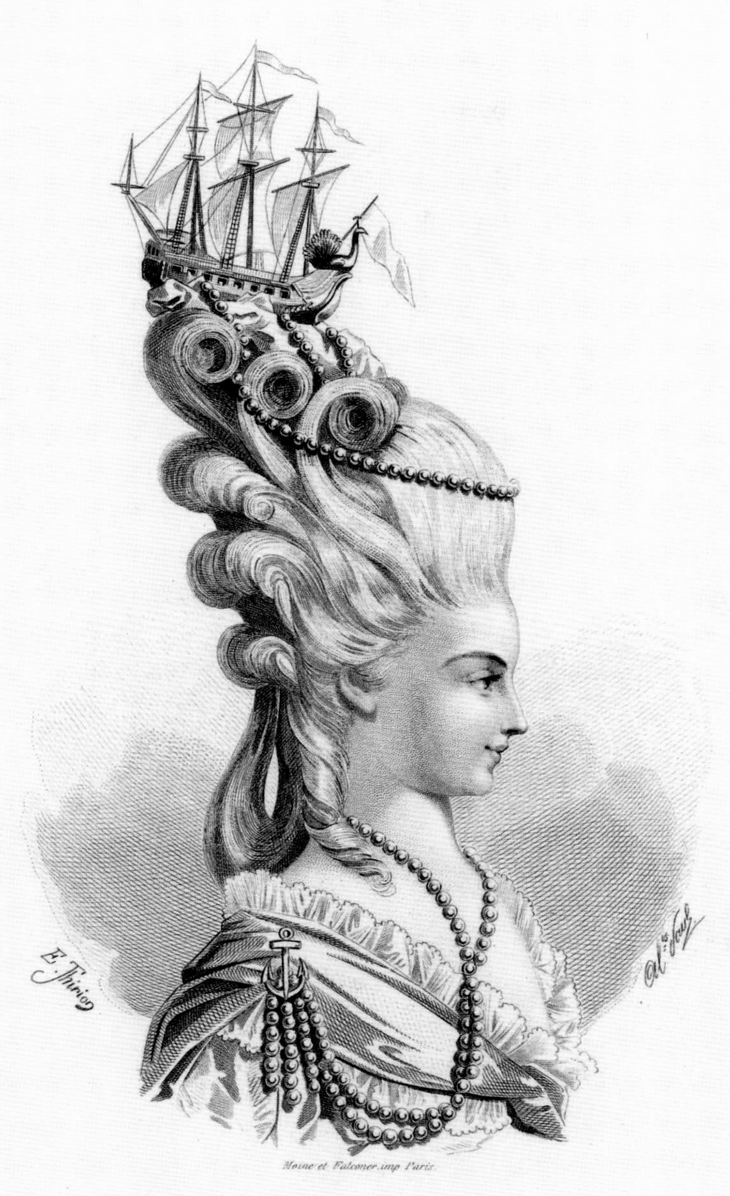

'La Frégate La Junon' hairstyle,
Louis XVI, engraving by E. Thirion

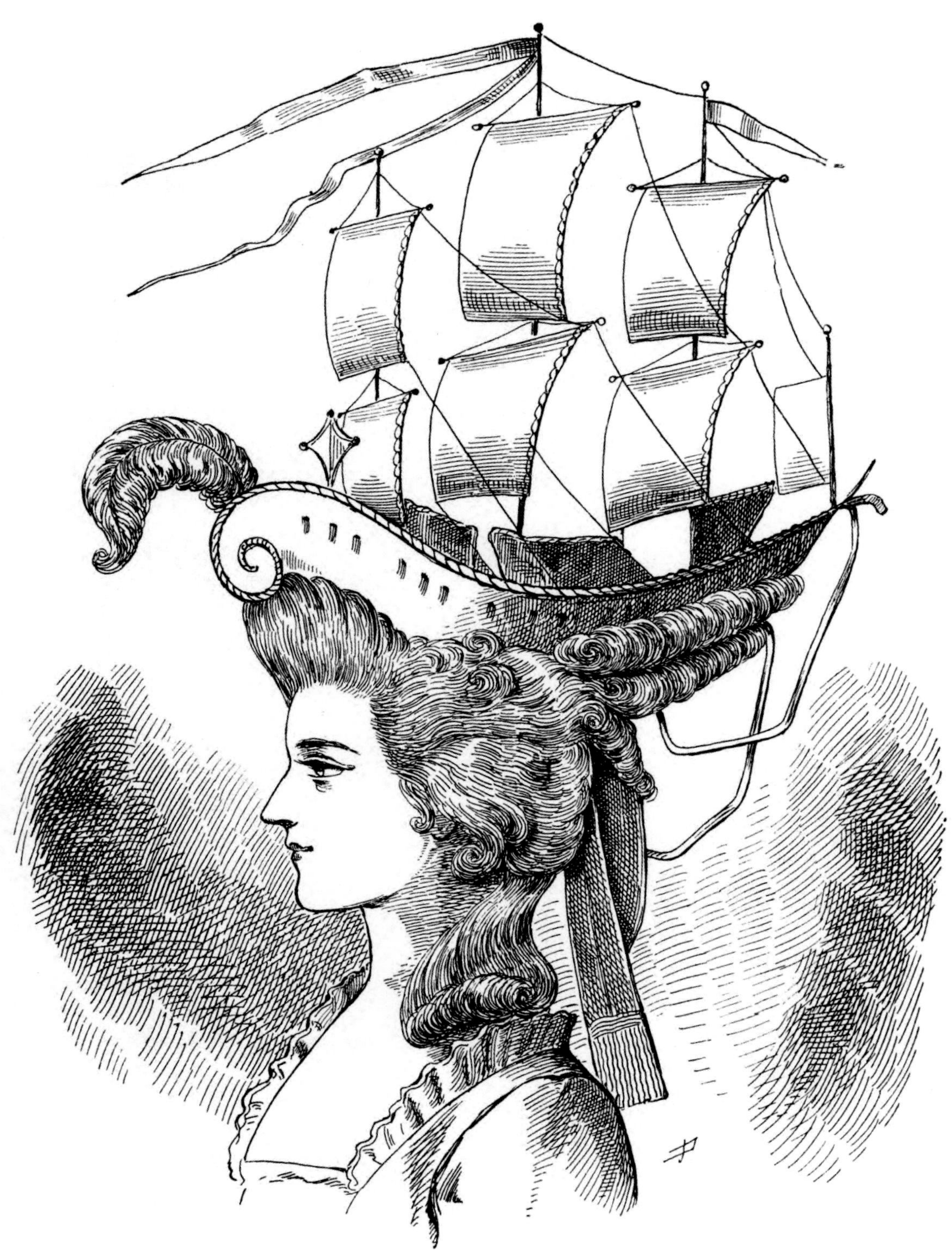

'Coiffure à la Belle-Poule', Louis XVI,
L'Art de la Coiffure Française, A. Mallemont

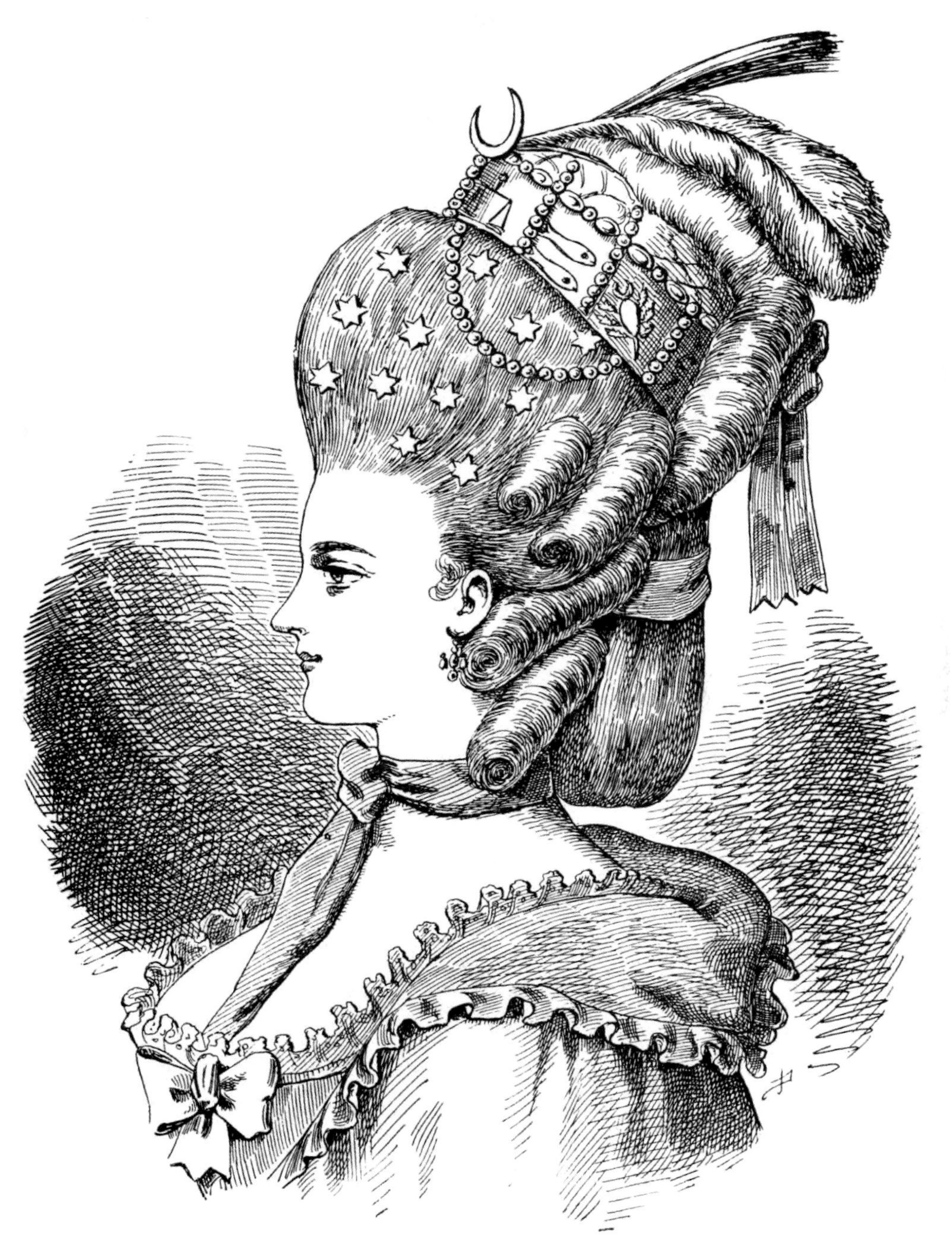

'Zodiac' hairstyle, Louis XVI, *L'Art de la Coiffure Française*, A. Mallemont

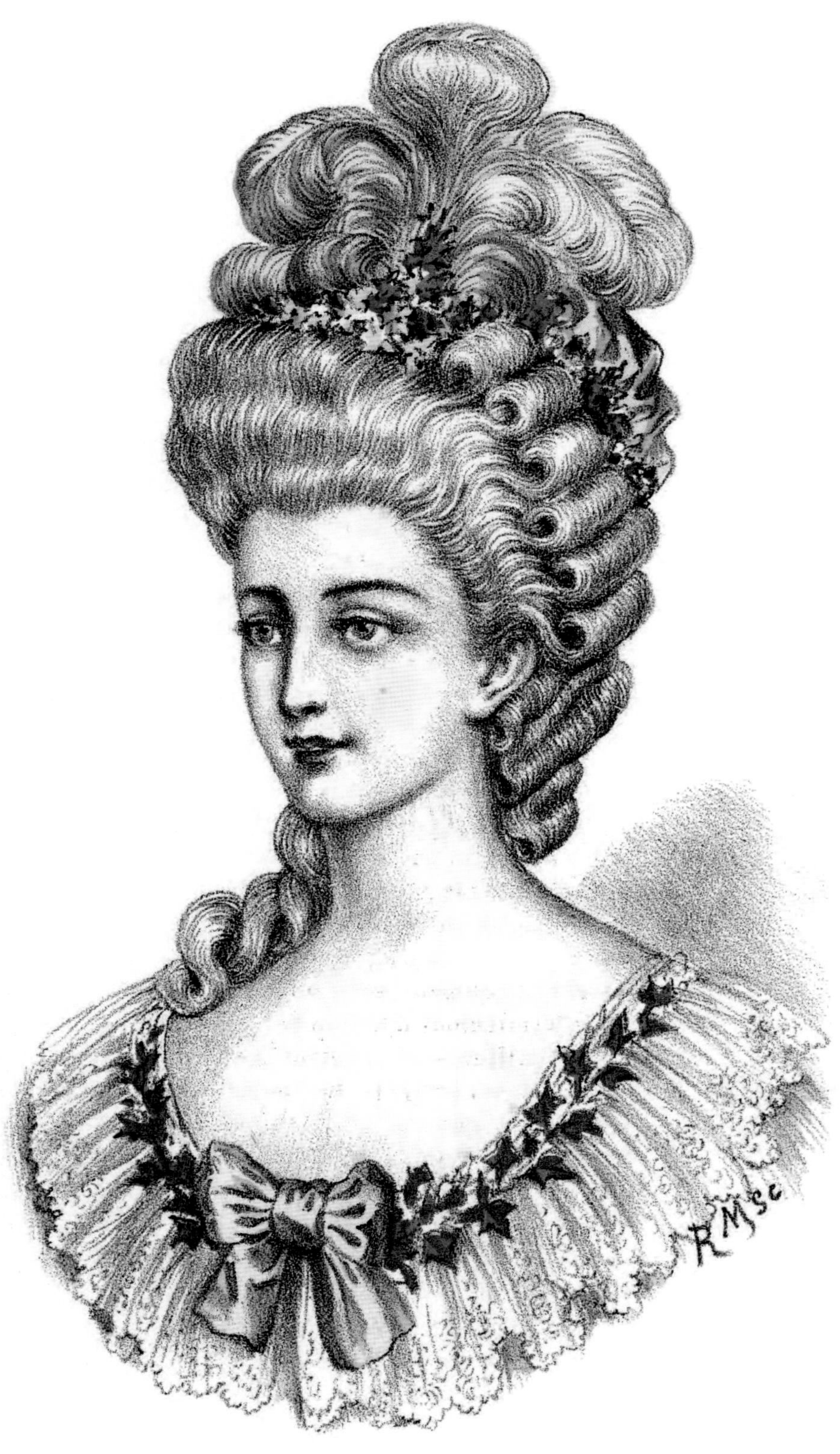

Louis xvi hairstyle, *Album de Coiffures Historiques*, E. Nissy

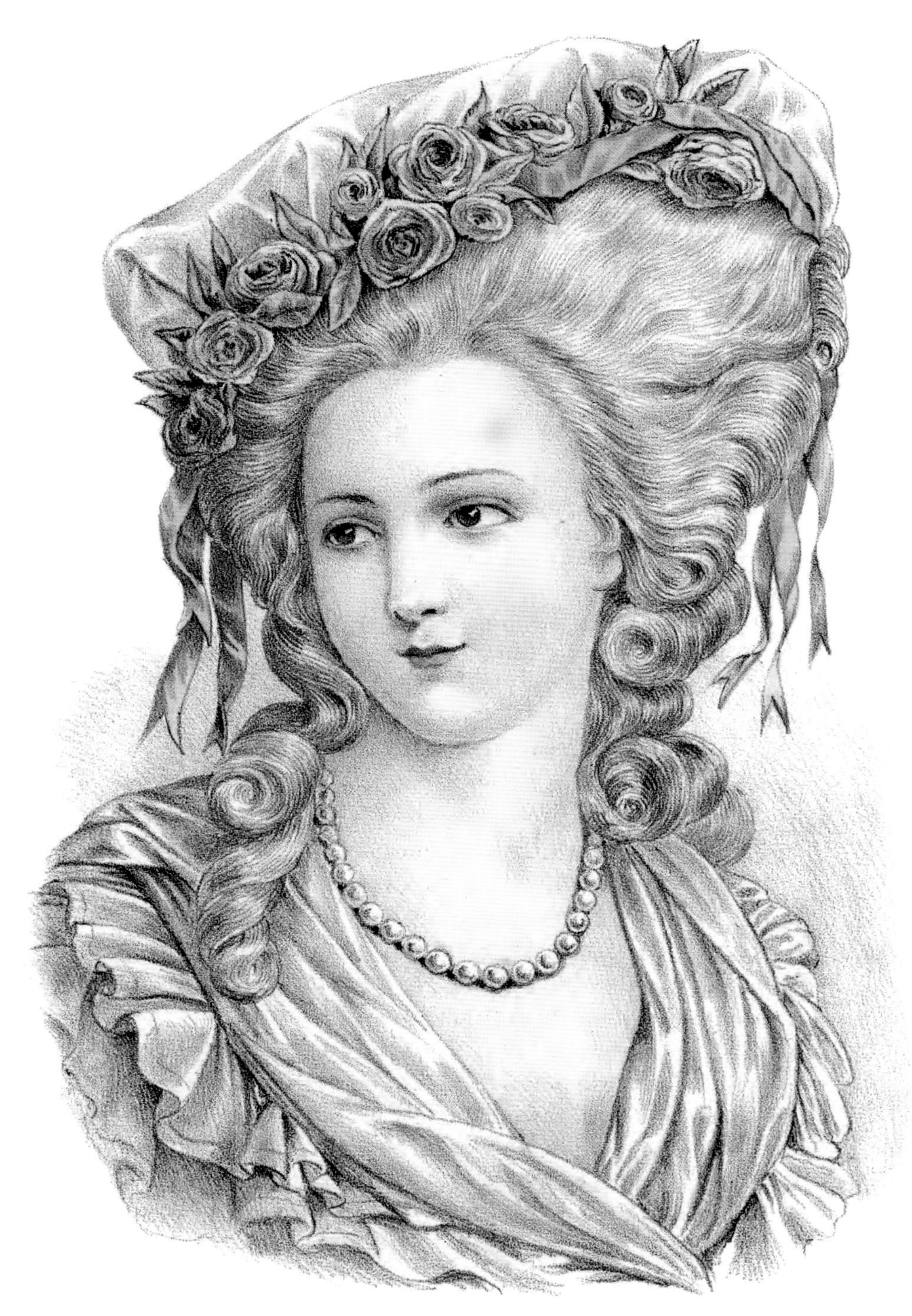

Princess de Lamballe, Louis xvi hairstyle,
Album de Coiffures Historiques, E. Nissy

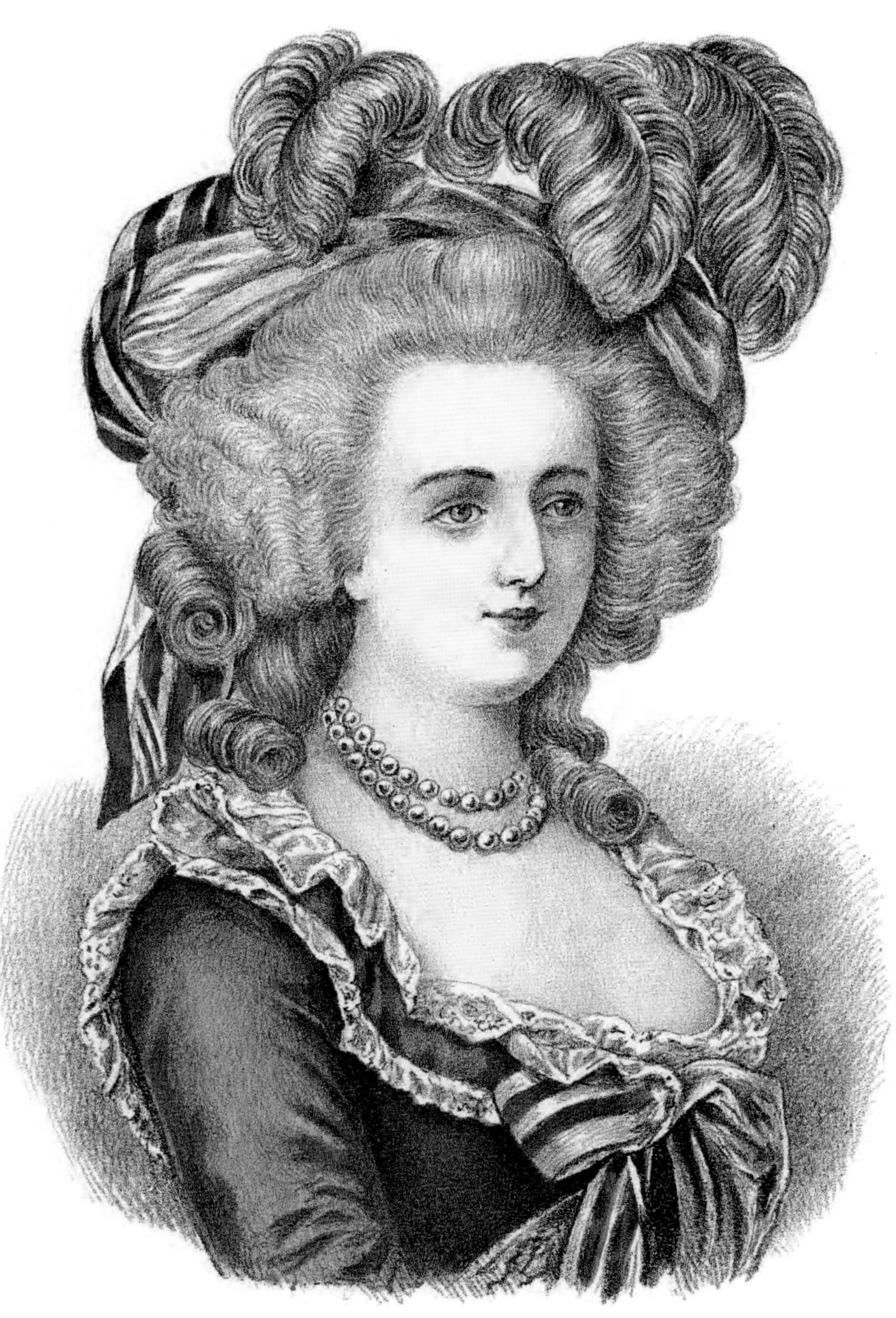

Marie Antoinette, Louis XVI hairstyle,
Album de Coiffures Historiques, E. Nissy

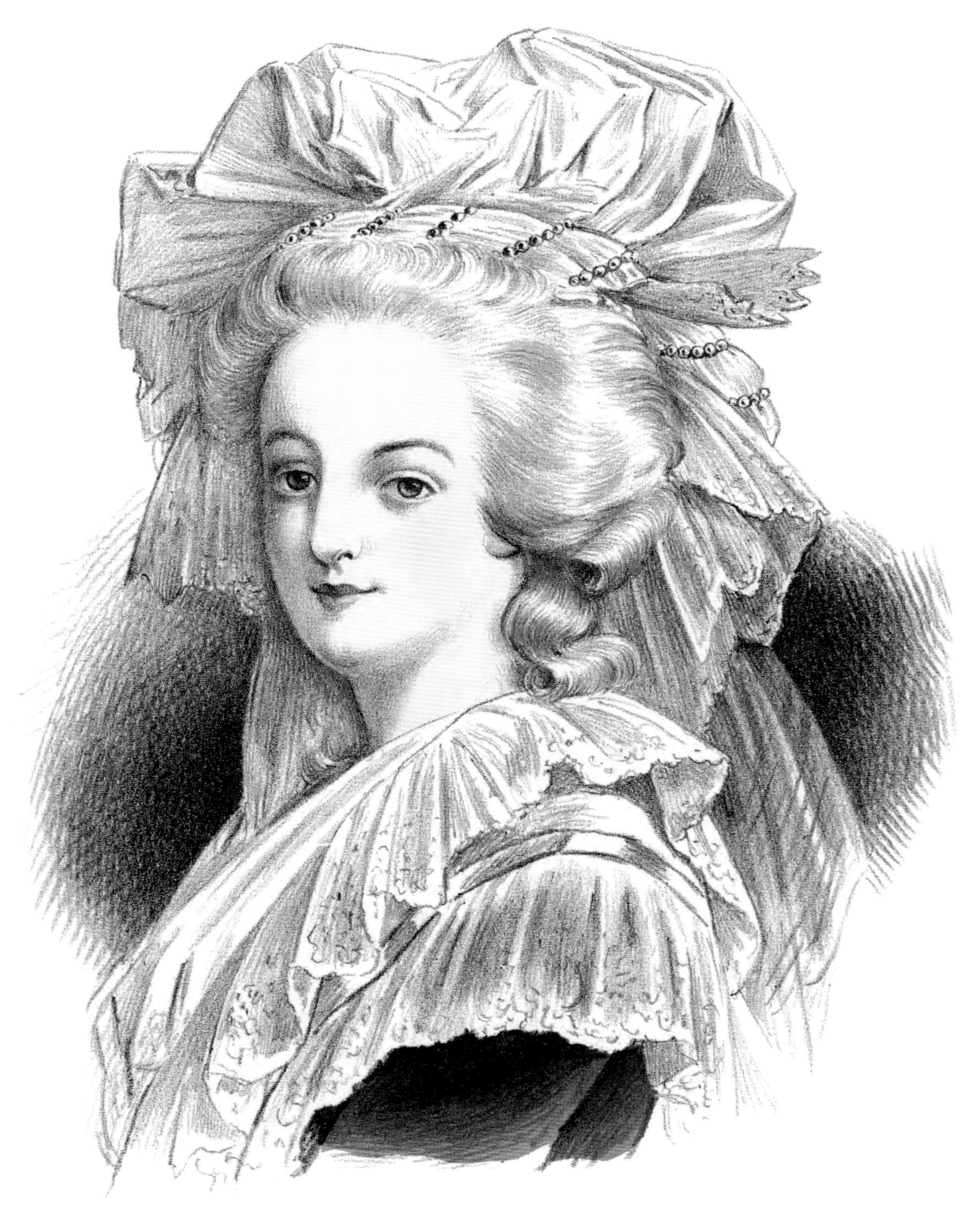

'Coiffure de Gala', Marie Antoinette,
Album de Coiffures Historiques, E. Nissy

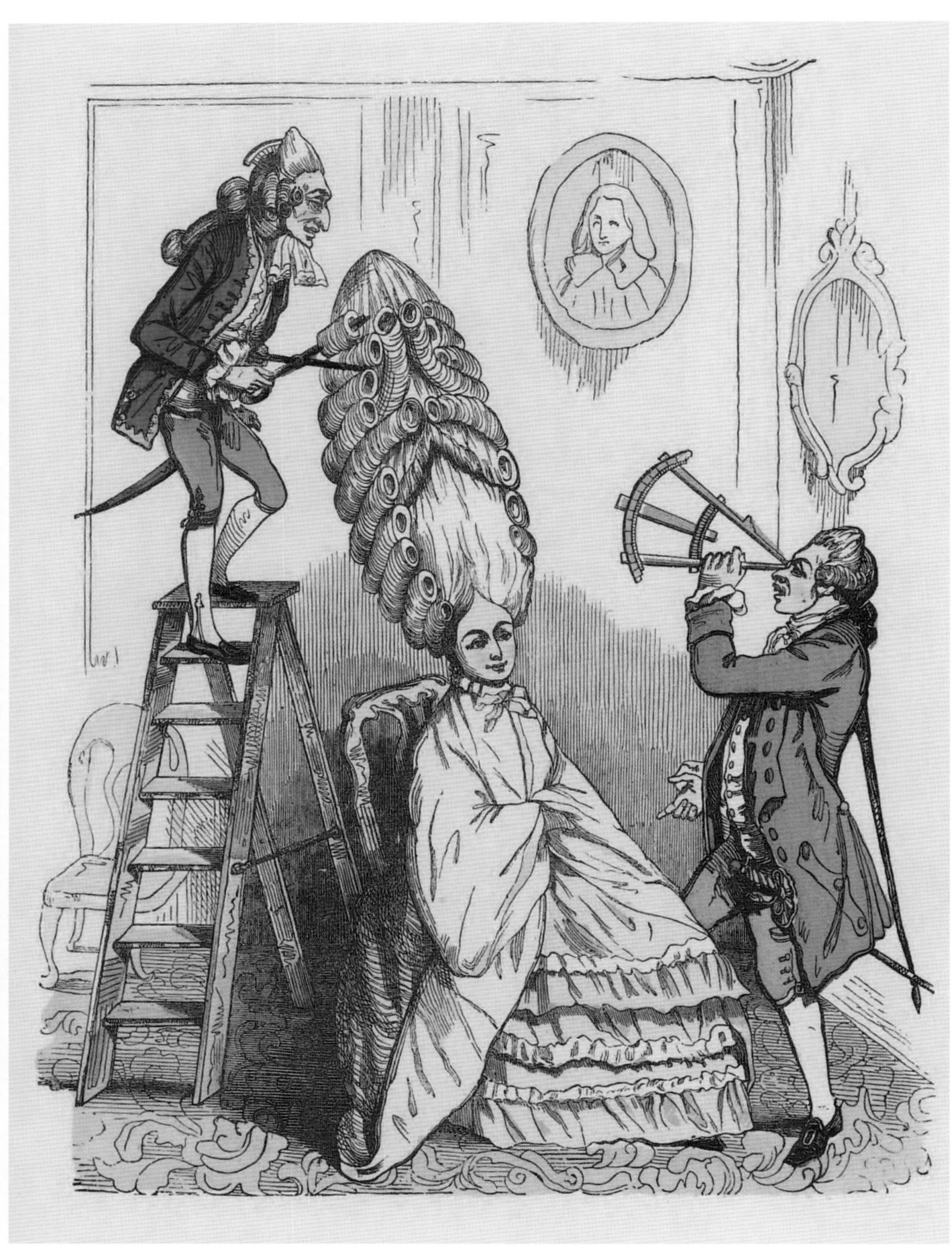

'Hair styled from upon a ladder' caricature from the 18th Century, after M. Darly

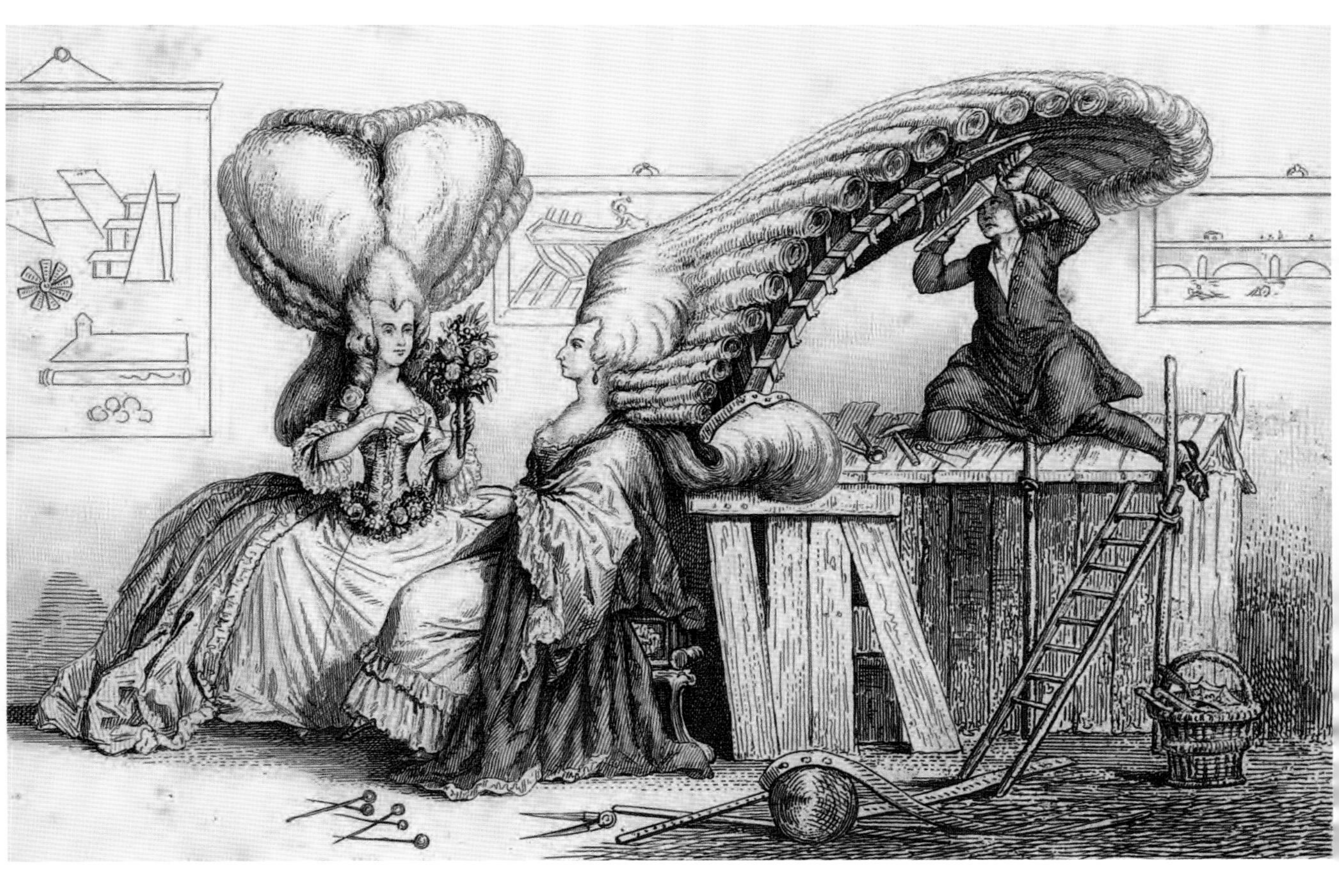

'Academie de Coiffures' cartoon,
Modes Des Grandes Coiffures, 1788

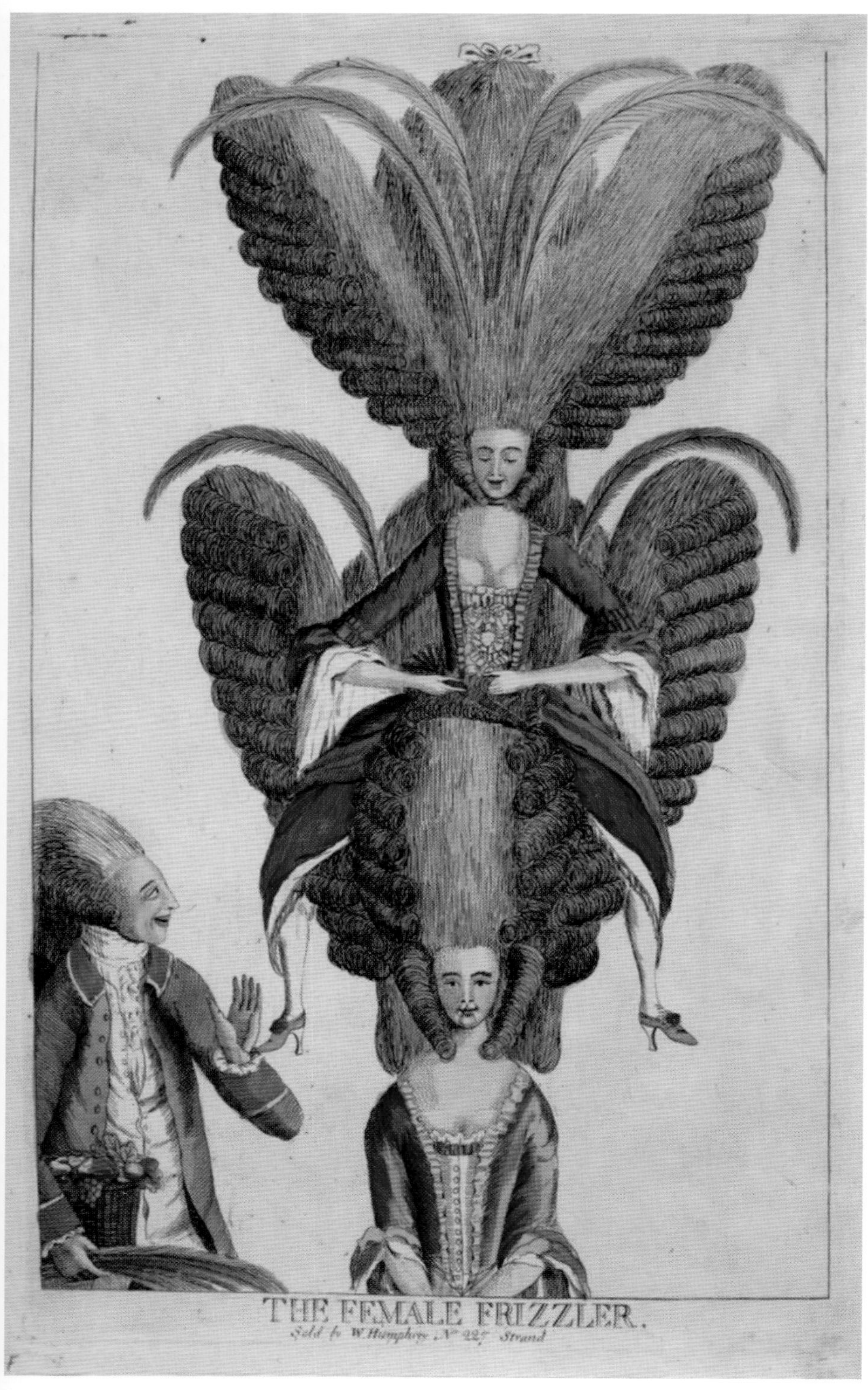

'The Female Frizzler', British cartoon, c.1775–1800

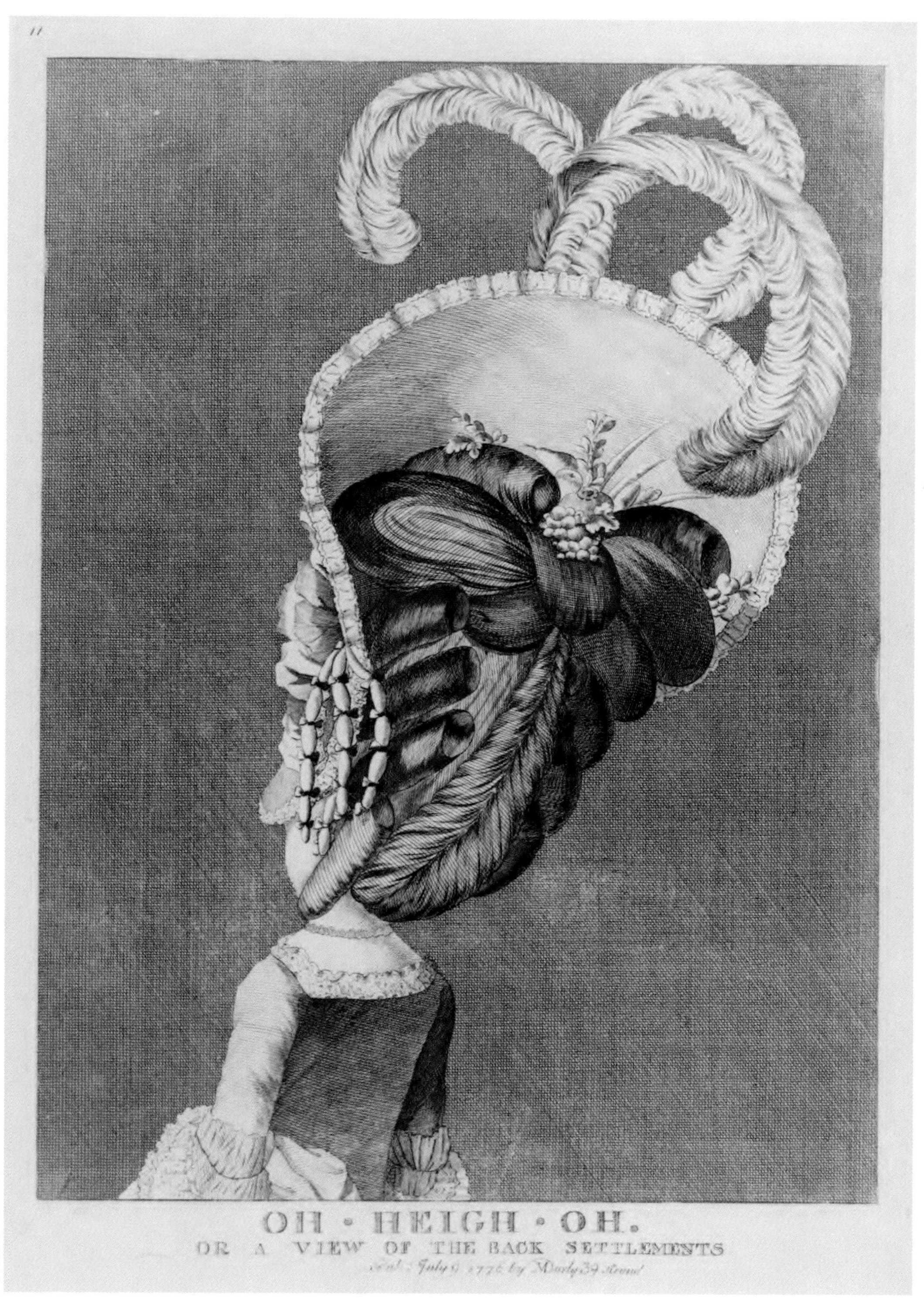

'Oh Heigh Oh, or, A View of the Back Settlements', published by M. Darly, 1776

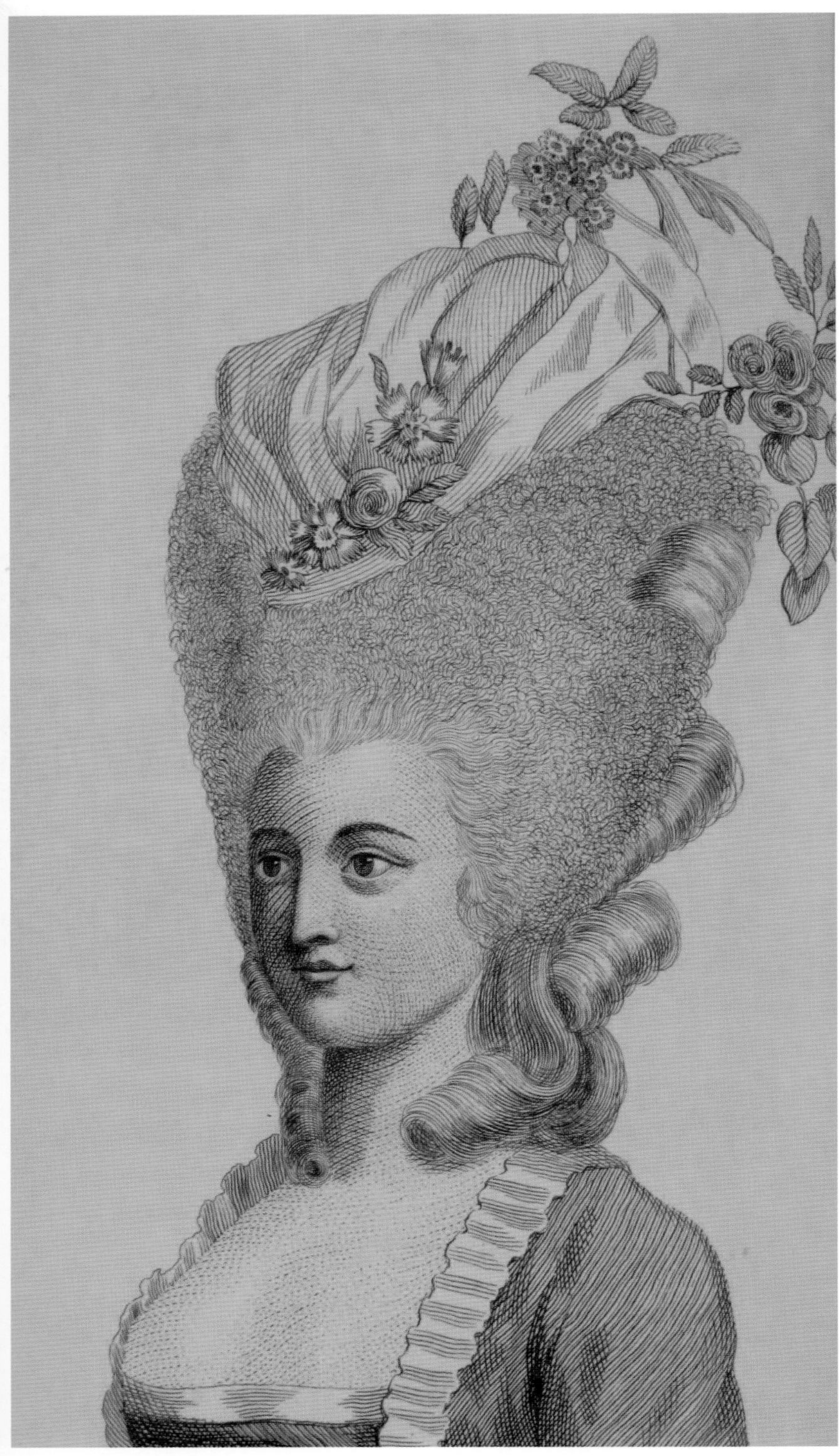

Louis xvi hairstyle, *Plocacosmos*,
James Stewart, 1782

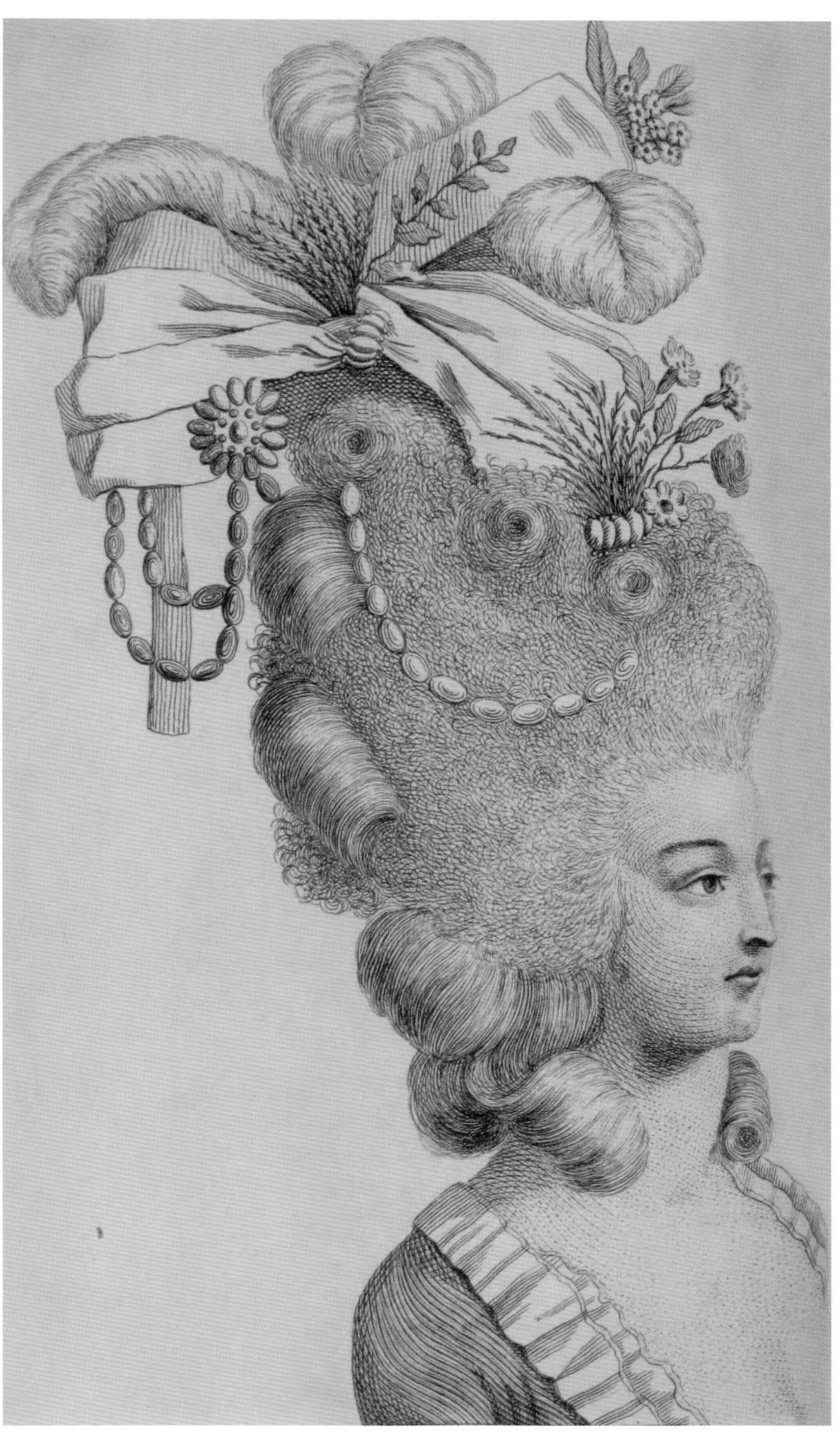

Louis xvi hairstyle, *Plocacosmos*,
James Stewart, 1782

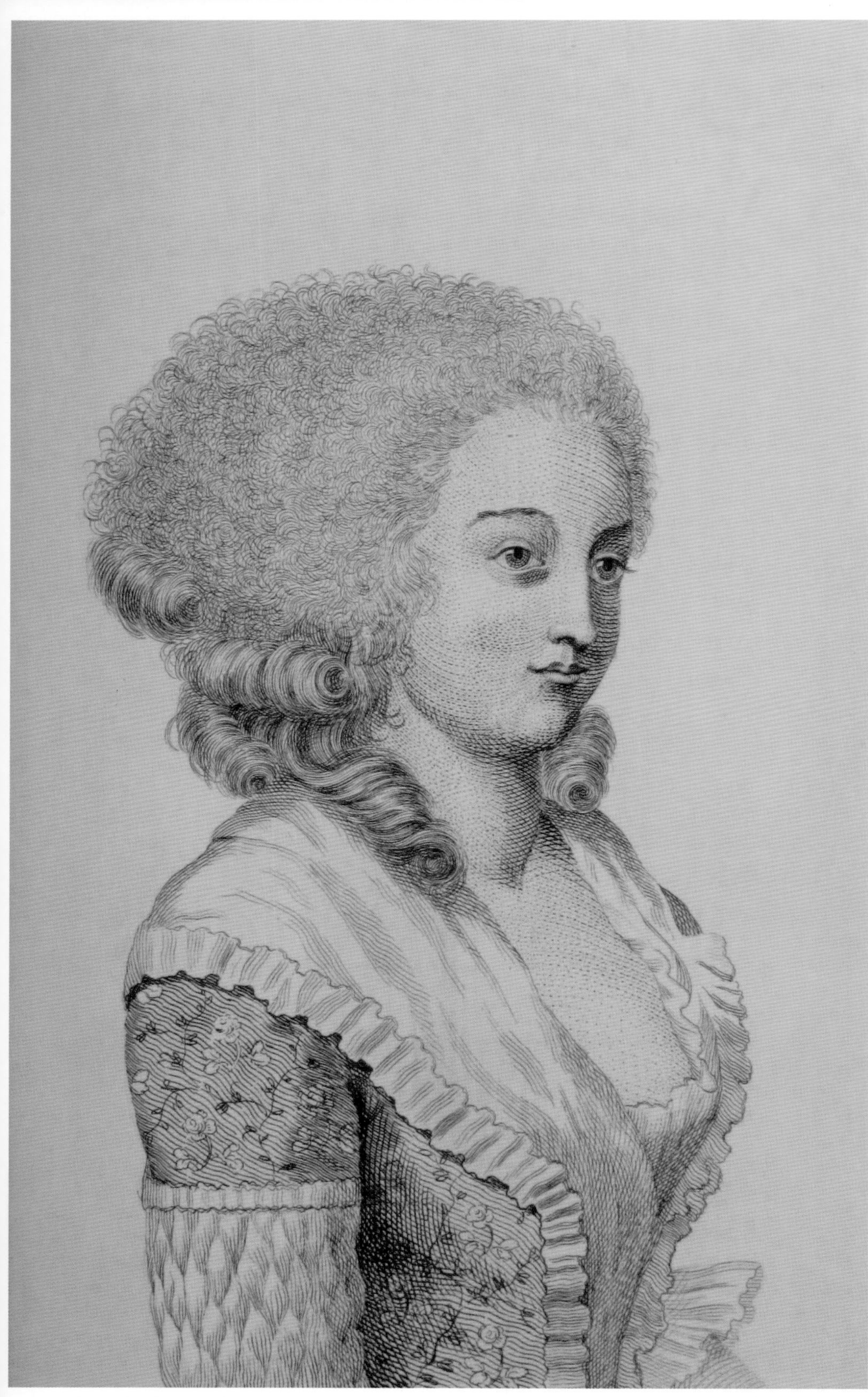

Louis XVI hairstyle, *Plocacosmos*,
James Stewart, 1782

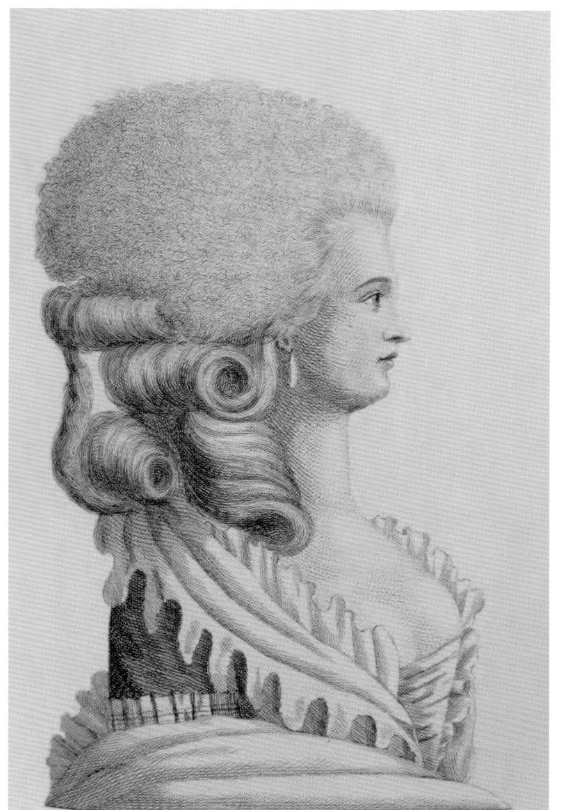
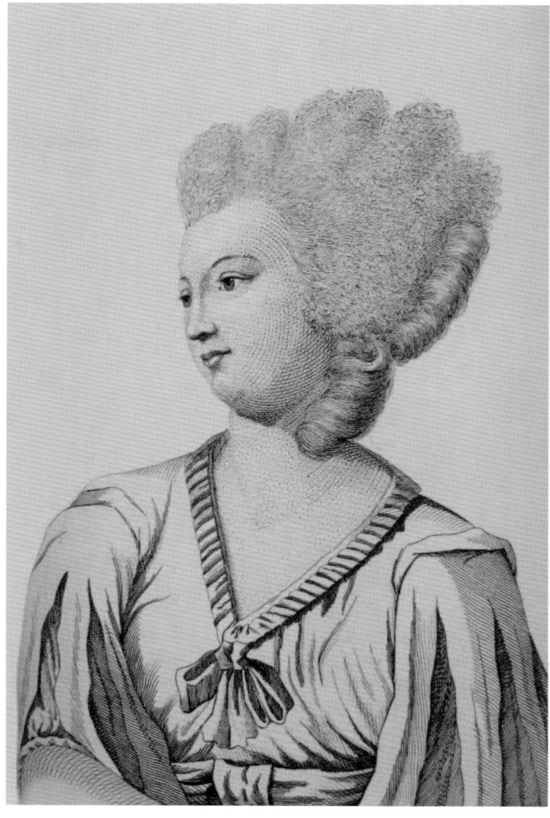
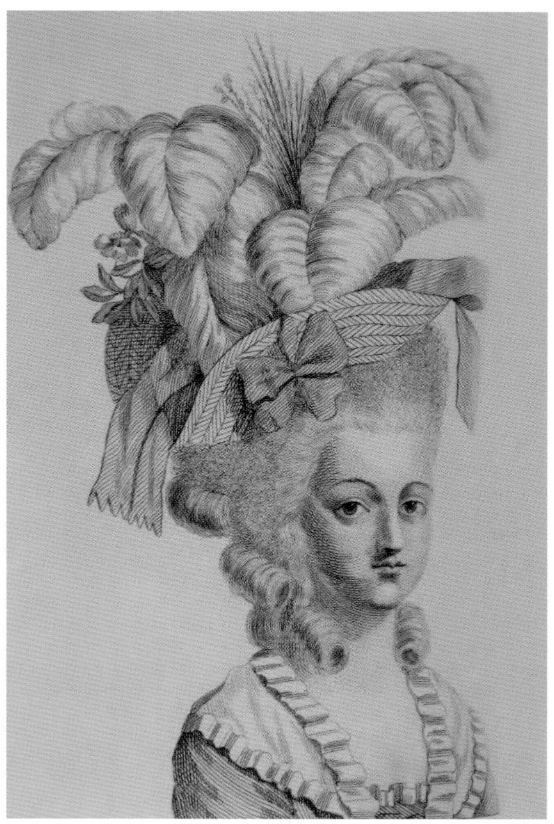
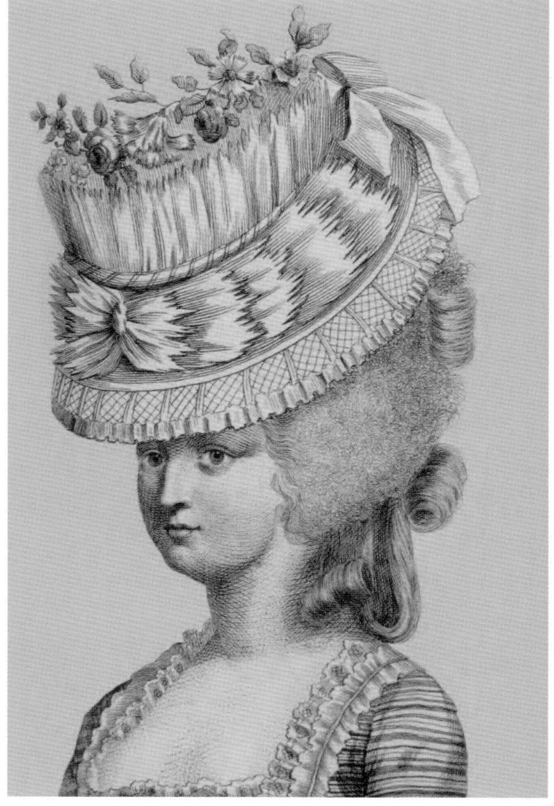

Louis xvi hairstyles, *Plocacosmos*,
James Stewart, 1782

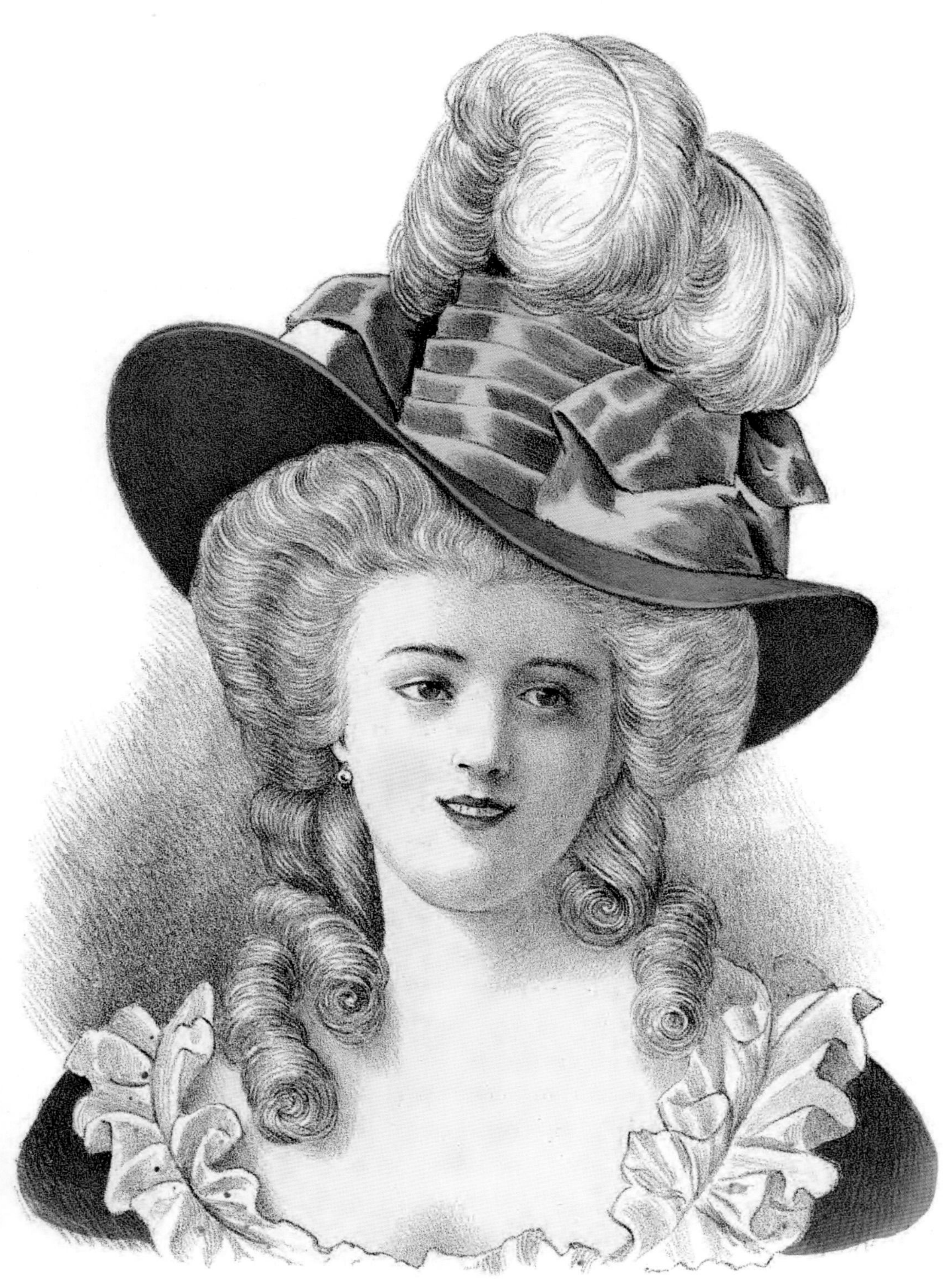

Louis XVI hairstyle, *Album de Coiffures Historiques*, E. Nissy

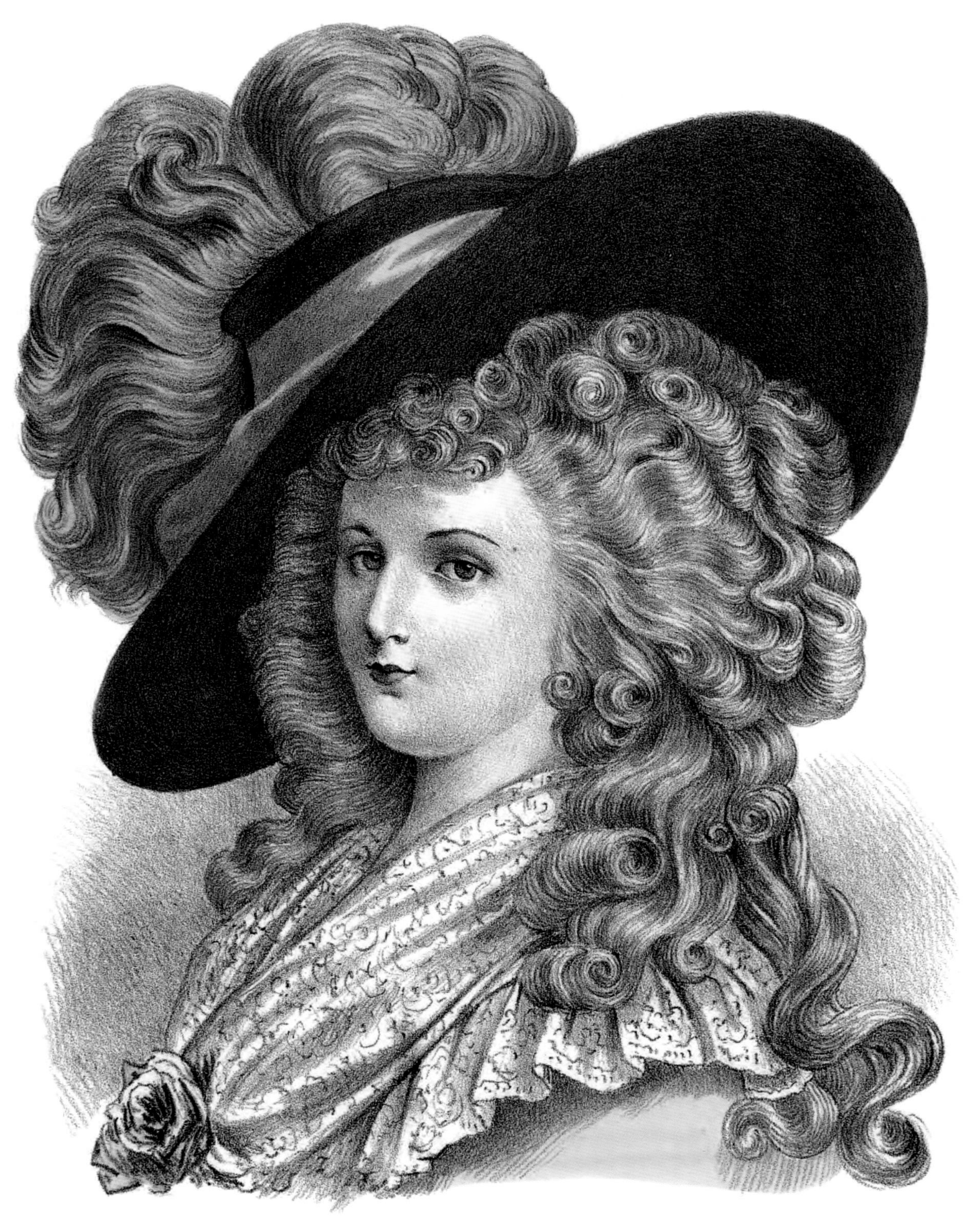

Louis XVI hairstyle, after the Duchess of Devonshire, *Album de Coiffures Historiques*, E. Nissy

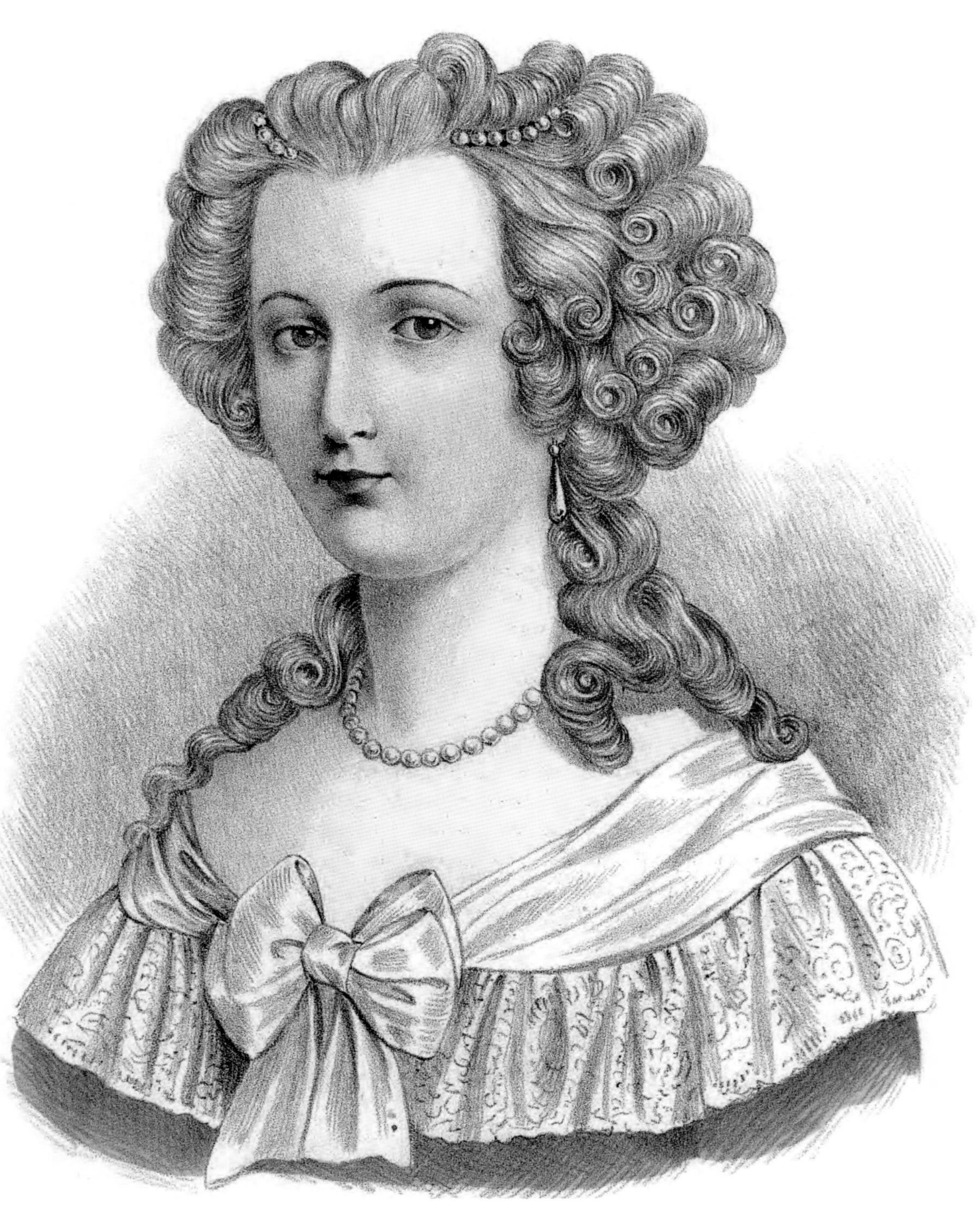

Marie Antoinette, Louis XVI hairstyle, *Album de Coiffures Historiques*, E. Nissy

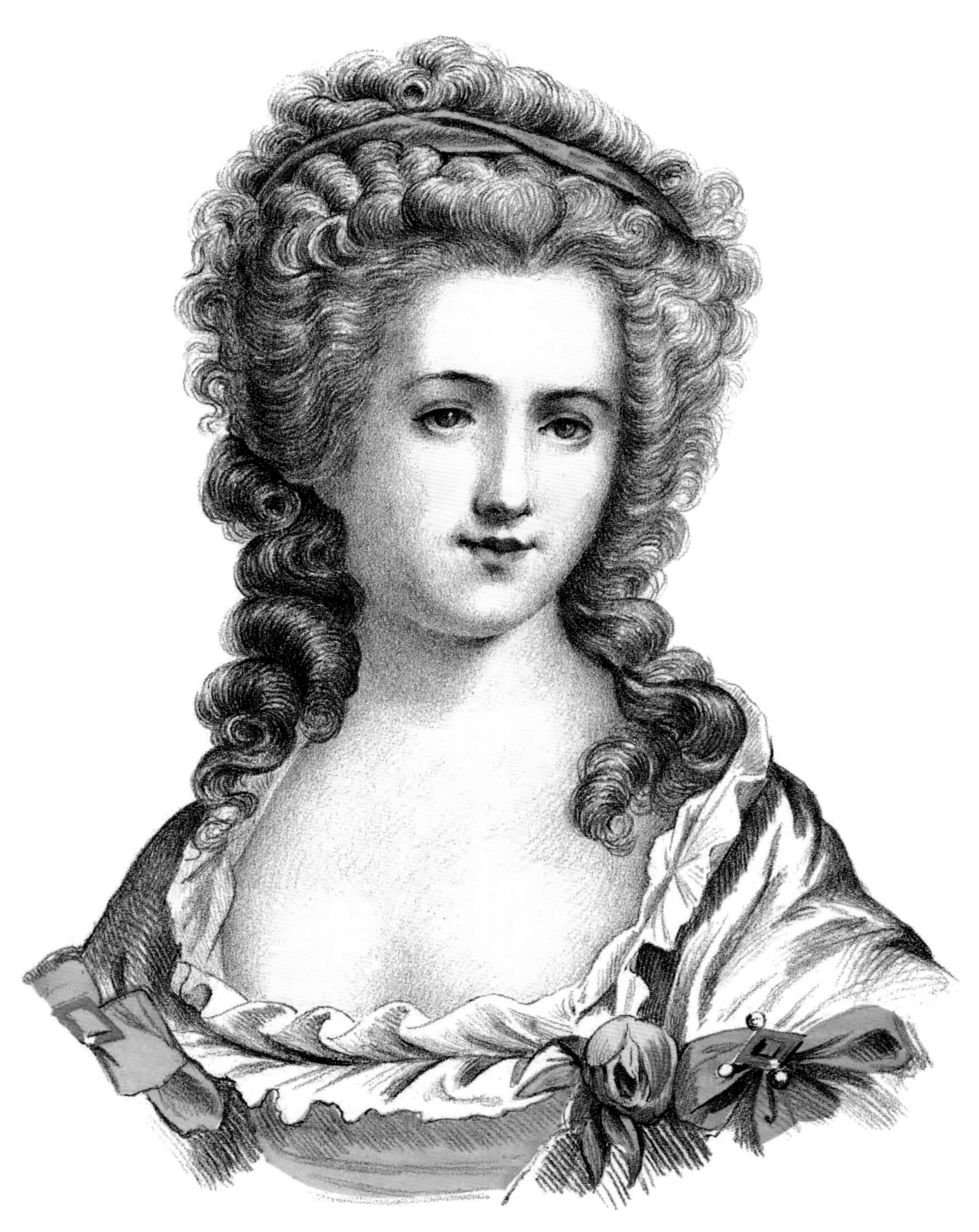

Madame de Montesson, Louis xvi hairstyle,
Album de Coiffures Historiques, E. Nissy

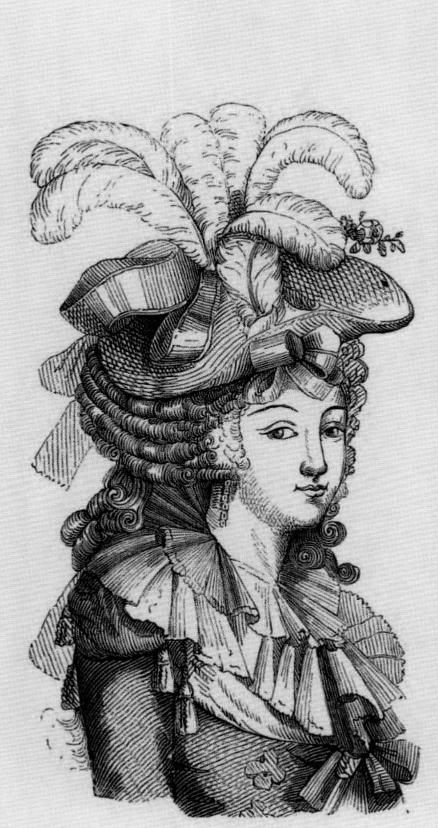

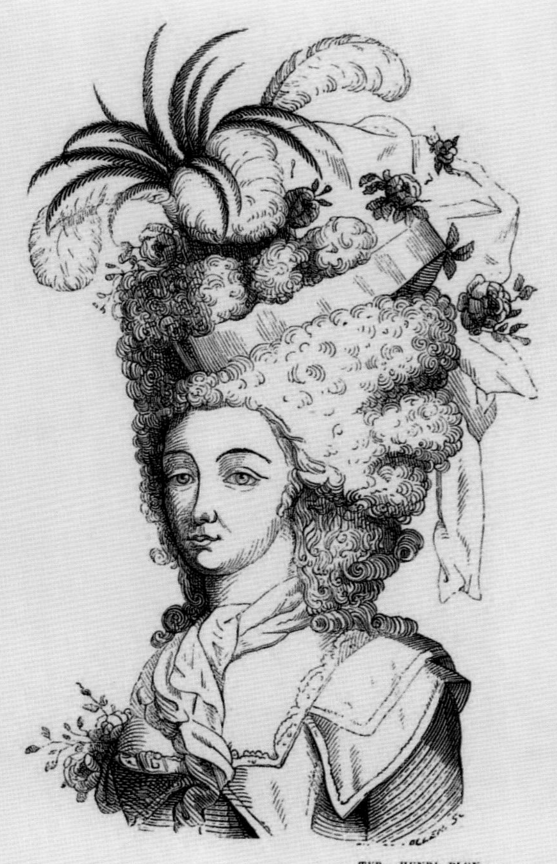

TYP. HENRI PLON.

COIFFURE A LA NATION

COIFFURE AUX CHARMES DE LA LIBERTÉ

« Se trouve à Paris, chez DEPAIN, coiffeur de dames et auteur de ces coiffures. – Le sieur Depain continue toujours d'enseigner l'Art de Coiffer. »

'Hairstyle for the Nation and Hairstyle for the Charms of Freedom', fashion plate etching, 1790s

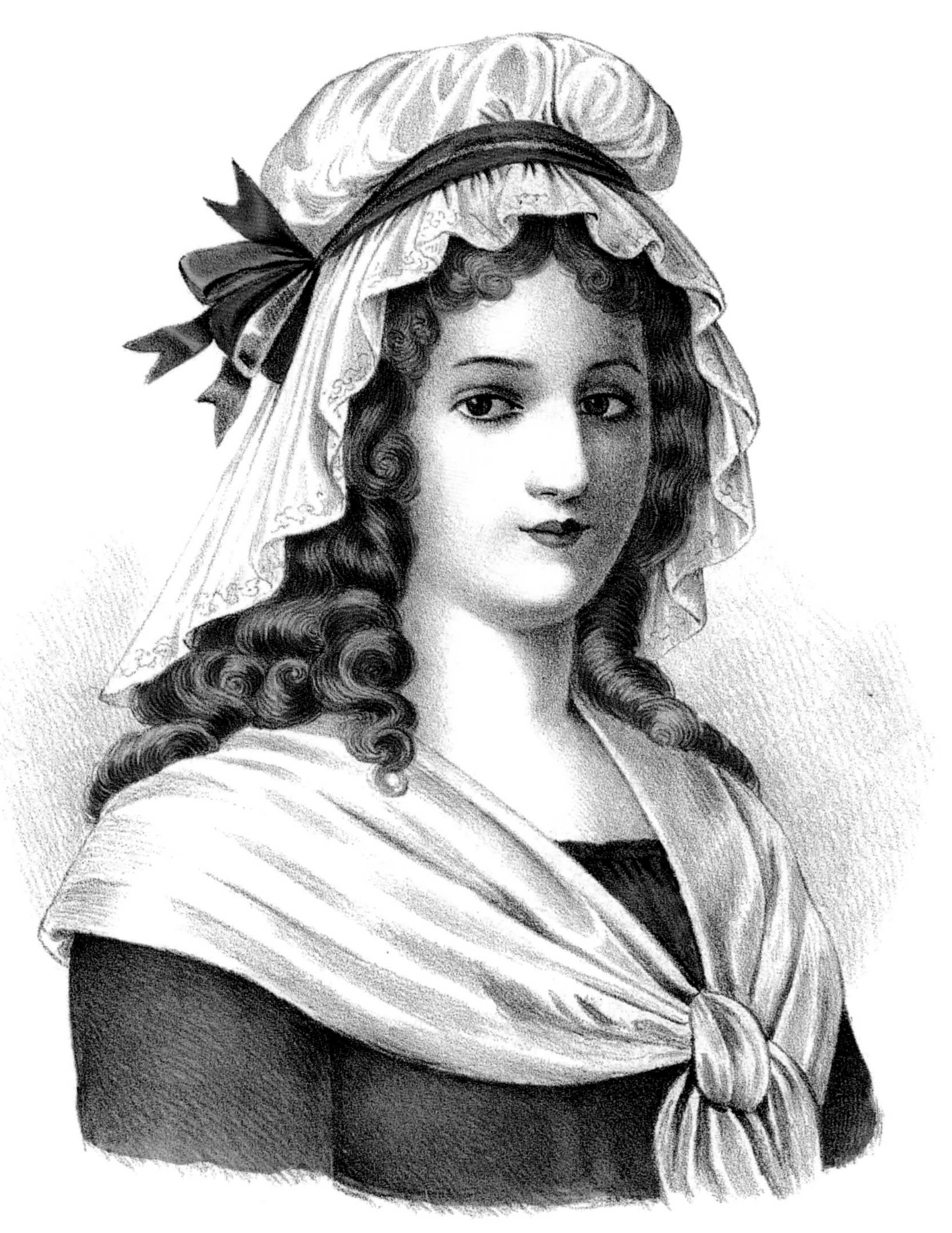

Charlotte Corday, First Republic hairstyle, *Album de Coiffures Historiques*, E. Nissy

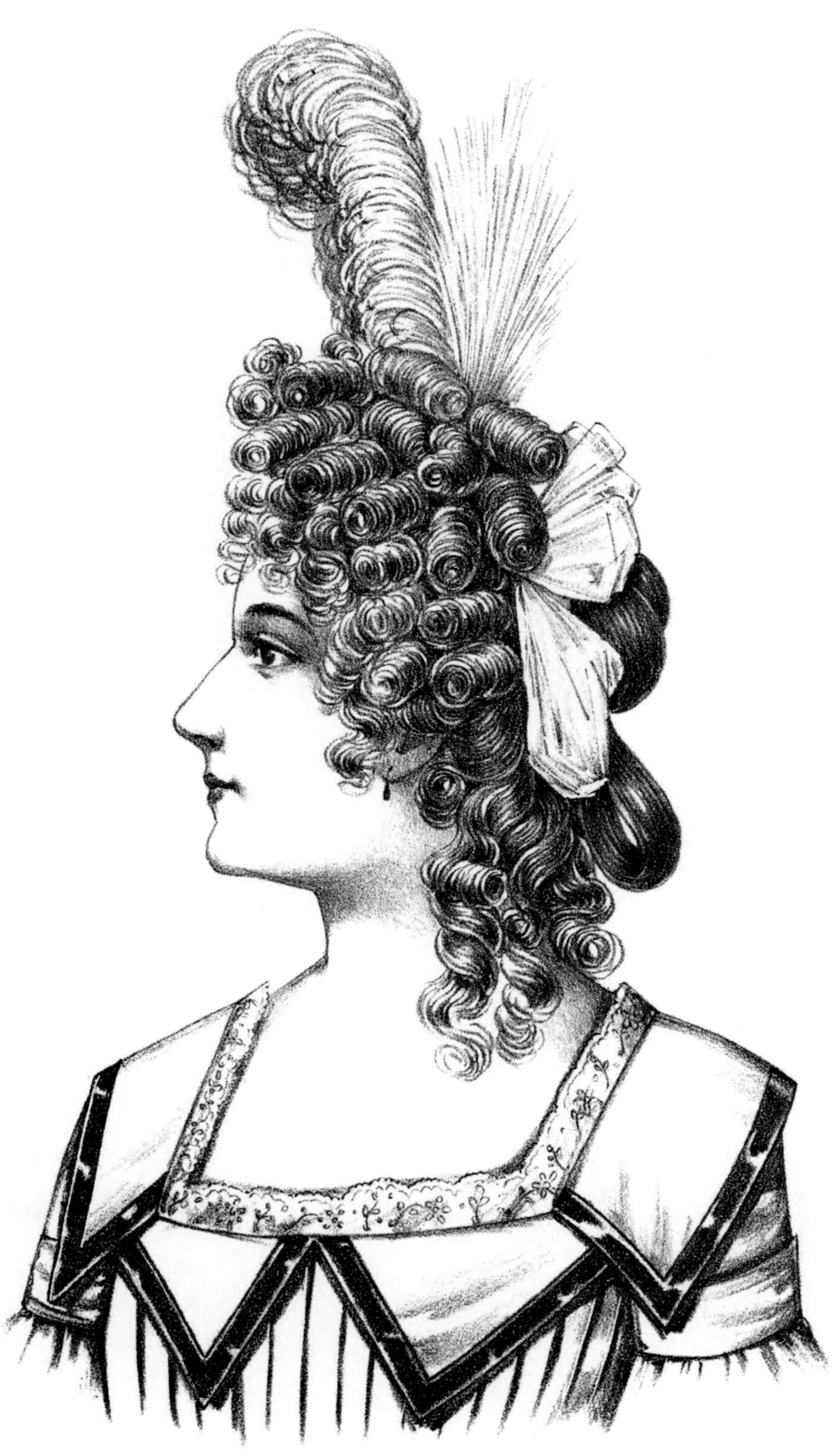

Revolution hairstyle, *Album Historischer und Phantasie-Frisuren*, Heinrich Moritz

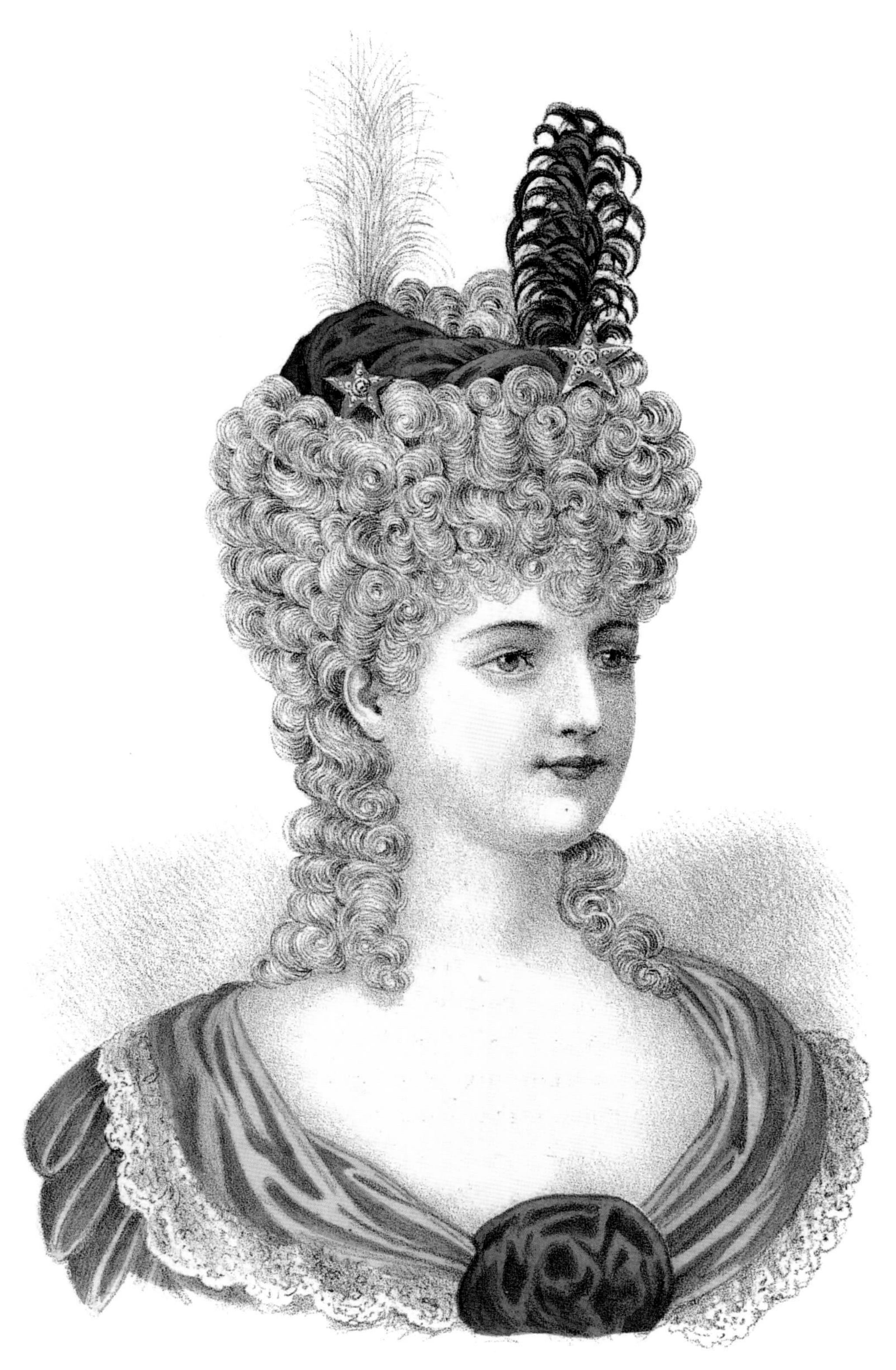

Hairstyle of a 'Merveilleuse', *Album de Coiffures Historiques*, E. Nissy

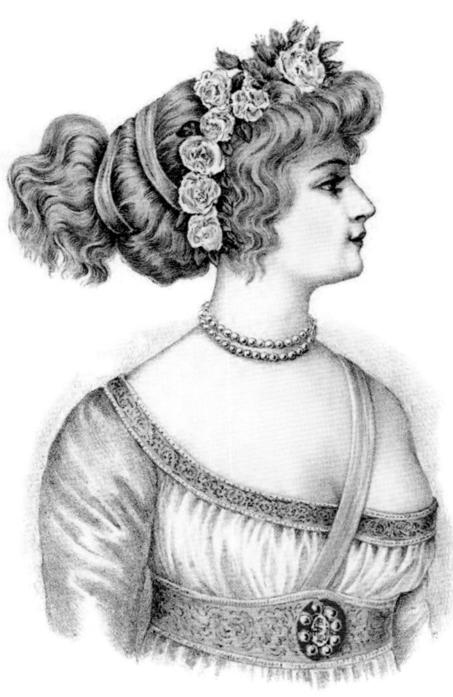

Coiffure Directoire, 1790s, *Album de Coiffures Historiques*, E. Nissy

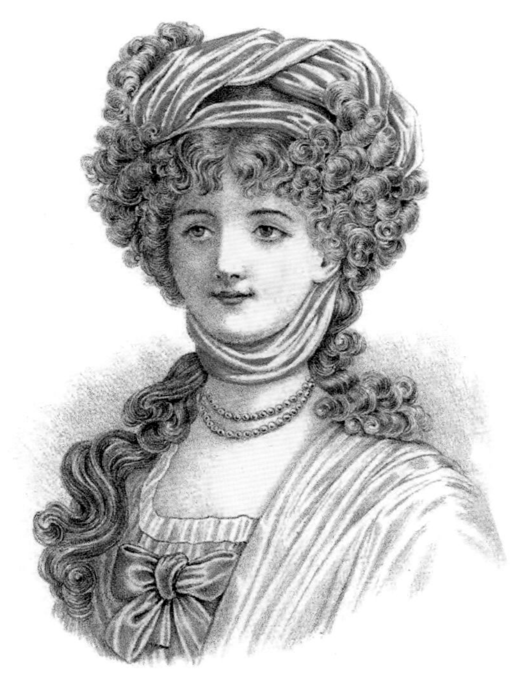

Coiffure Directoire, 1790s, *Album de Coiffures Historiques*, E. Nissy

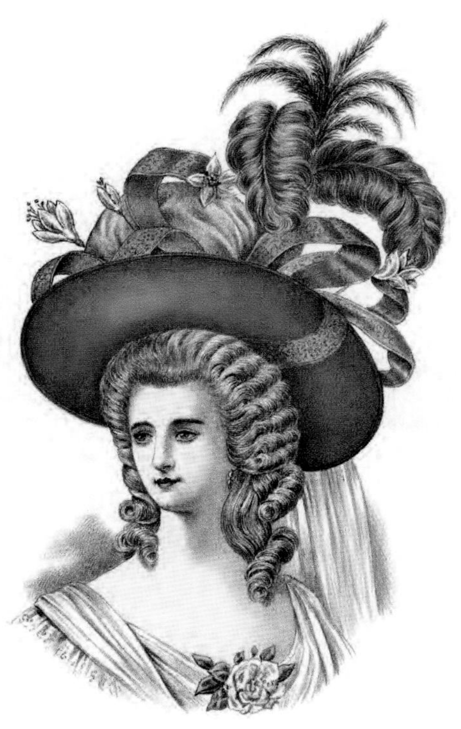

Coiffure Directoire, 1790s, *Album de Coiffures Historiques*, E. Nissy

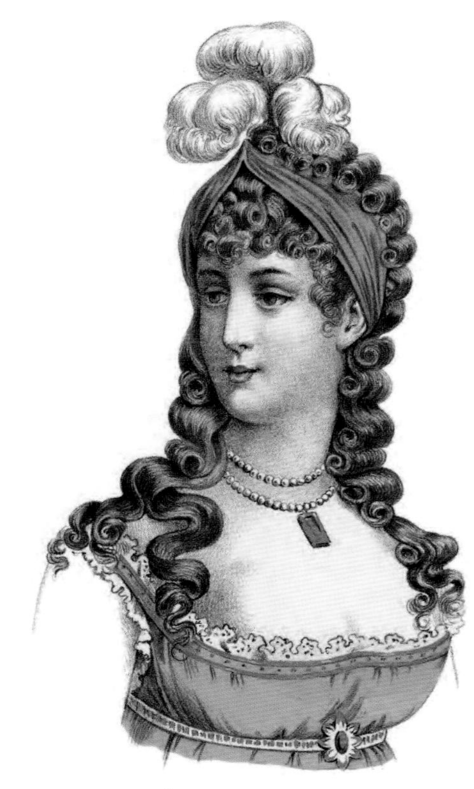

Coiffure Directoire, 1790s, *Album de Coiffures Historiques*, E. Nissy

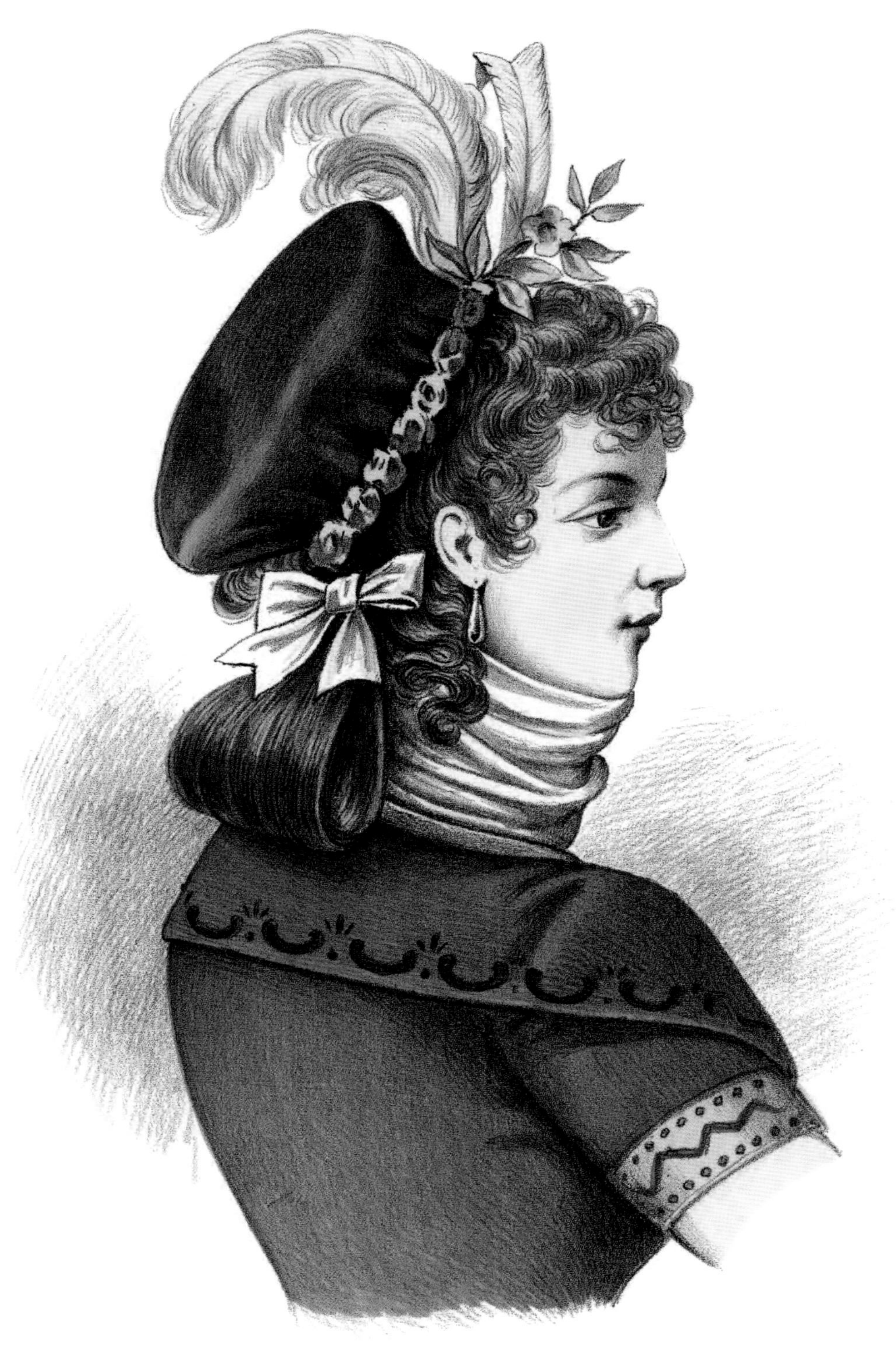

Dame Galante, Coiffure Merveilleuse, 1792, *Album de Coiffures Historiques*, E. Nissy

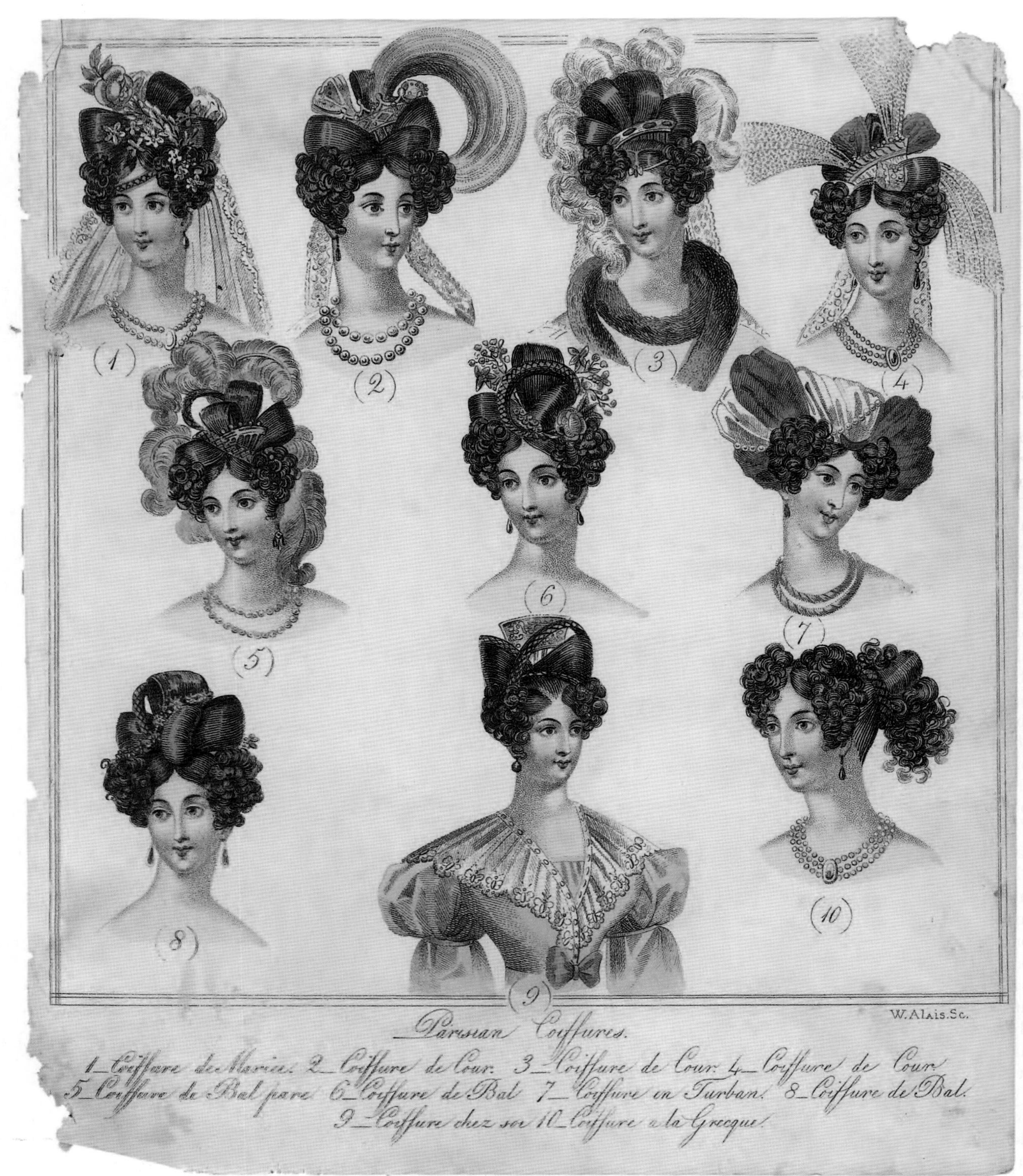

Parisian Coiffures: 1. Bride's hairstyle; 2. Court hairstyle; 3. Court hairstyle; 4. Court hairstyle; 5. Hairstyle of Bal paré; 6. Ball hairstyle; 7. Turban hairstyle; 8. Ball hairstyle; 9. At home hairstyle; 10. Greek hairstyle, engraving by W. Alais, c. 1730

19TH CENTURY

The early years of the 19th century saw the continuing influence of Neo-Classicism within hair design. During the Consulate Period in France (1799–1804) it was quite common for ladies to wear their hair short during the day and then don elaborate wigs for the evening. While the majority of hairstyles of the period drew inspiration from ancient Greece, bonnets, turbans and curious duck-billed caps also became popular headdresses that were worn over short hairstyles. Other hairstyles such as "à la Cornelie", "à la Hollandaise" and "en Lantin" were also popular choices; the latter being a short crop of very tight curls worn close to the head that was inspired by a statue of Mercury in the Vatican.

The French Empire (1804–1814/5) saw Napoleon Bonaparte become "L'Empereur des Français" and this heralded in various other neo-classical hairstyles that were less austere, many made fashionable by his first wife, Josephine. As Octave Uzanne noted, "The smart coquettes of the Empire, after having cut their locks short like Titus and Caracalla, began to dispose their curls in imitation of the heads they saw on antique cameos and medals. The Empress Josephine, whose childish taste for gems is common knowledge, never appeared without the most splendid jewels in her hair." Later Napoleon's second wife, Marie-Louise, Archduchess of Austria, also became a trendsetter and wore her hair in large curls and drawn up into a large bun on the top of her head with a coronet or flowers pinned at its front. According to A. Mallemont, it was during this period that Duplessis established a hairdressing school where he taught students how to put hair into such buns or raise hair into a Minerva band. Another hairdresser of the time known as Palette also offered hairdressing courses and published a hairdressing journal.

In Regency England (1811–1820) ladies followed the French fashion for centre-partings and ringlets worn over the ears. The contemporary guide to etiquette titled *The Mirror of Graces* (1811) that was penned "By a Lady of Distinction" gave the following hairstyling advice: "Now, easy tresses, the shining braid, the flowing ringlet confined by the antique comb, or bodkin, give graceful specimens of the simple taste of modern beauty. Nothing can correspond more elegantly with the untrammelled drapery of our newly-adopted classic raiment than this undecorated coiffure of nature." Around 1815, longer hair became popular and gradually the unruly curls of the Greek styles gave way to a sleeker look, with often the hair drawn into a coil on the top of the head and then small corkscrew ringlets or loops of hair allowed to cover the ears. In the 1820s and 1830s, there was also a vogue for puffy clouds of soft ringlets worn at the sides and on the top of the head, with the front hair either centre-parted or drawn over the forehead, and the back hair formed into a chignon. Towards 1826, the "Apollo Knot" became a firm favourite for evening attire. This extraordinary style involved attaching plain, coiled or plaited false hair onto wires to create eye-catching loops that were worn vertically on top of the head. This amazing coiffure remained extremely fashionable until around 1836, and in later historic surveys of hairstyles it is often just referred to as "Coiffure 1830" having become so synonymous with the era in which it enjoyed its greatest popularity.

A number of other hairstyles that similarly incorporated loops of hair drawn up into various intriguing shapes also materialised in the 1830s. The young Queen Victoria (having ascended the British throne in 1837) wore some of these looped styles, however, by the late 1830s and throughout the 1840s a more natural and demure look became stylish, with hair drawn into a bun or coil and curls allowed to fall loosely at the sides of the head. Another coiffure that was extremely becoming on younger women was when the hair was clipped high at the sides and then allowed to tumble as fat ringlets. Of course, the hairstyles mirrored the aspirations and social changes occurring within society during this era. With rapid industrialisation and growing urbanisation, the Victorian age saw unprecedented economic expansion that gave rise to the development of the middle classes, and with this came new fashions for both clothes and hair. Throughout the 1850s and 1860s women wore their hair in a multitude of styles that often incorporated hairpieces, which were often bought in the new department stores of the day. During this period it was also common for ladies to grow their hair exceedingly long so it could then be dressed upwards onto the head to give a sense of volume and mass.

The early 1870s saw sweeps of hair drawn up into combs and enormous chignons, while many also opted for the Parisian style of flowing loose curls cascading down the back. There was also a passing craze for shorter, mannish styles, and the hairdresser Marcel Grateau found that frequently his customers with naturally straight hair would asked for it to be curled.

Marcel realised that if he could wave rather than curl the hair a more natural look could be obtained and, as his *New York Times* obituary later explained, "It was at this point in his life that his adoration for his mother and the happy chance that had given her a wonderful head of curly hair together served to make his fortune and elevate his whole profession. Setting himself to the task of finding a way of artificially producing waves like those in his mother's hair, after months of experiment he attained success. He found that by holding the curling tongs reversed he could produce his mother's coiffure on nearly every woman's head. The women in his quarter, not recognising genius, called his new style "poodle fashion". For months he had to beg each woman customer to permit him to use his new "ondulation". At last one woman consented to his doing so. Her wave lasted five weeks. Hearing of the new style, an actress called on Marcel

Left: Hairstyle of Queen Luise, the consort of King Friedrich Wilhelm of Prussia, 1800s
Right: 'Consulate' hairstyle, *Album Historischer und Phantasie-Frisuren*, Heinrich Moritz

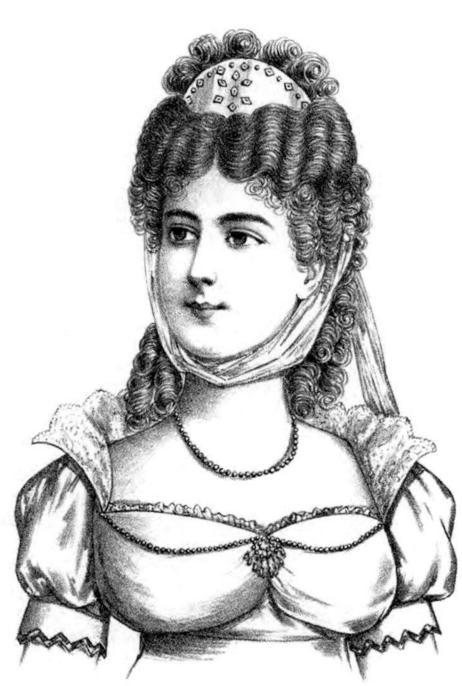

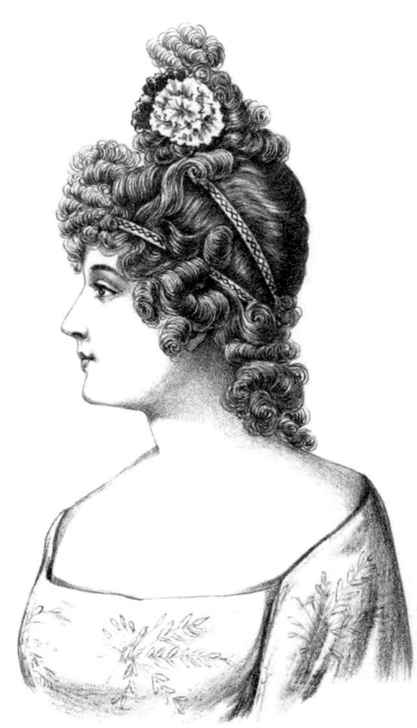

one day, and had her hair waved. She played in a music hall, and Marcel's fame was made in a night. The wave was taken up immediately by the theatrical world and professional beauties, the leaders of the social world following."

When Marcel first began to wave hair in 1872 using his specially designed heated tongs in his small hairdressing establishment in Montmartre, he charged just a few centimes a time. Within three years, however, so great was the demand for the "Marcel Undulation" he was charging anything up to five francs a head, and in 1882 he opened a magnificent salon in the heart of Paris, where he charged from 200 to 300 francs for 25 minutes of his precious time. By the mid 1880s Marcel's distinctive waved look had become all the rage and Marcel had amassed an enormous fortune thanks to his invention. Interestingly, although the fashion for hairpieces was increasingly waning during this period, Parisian hairdressers found that they could compensate for the lost revenue from the declining sales and dressing of wigs, by offering the fashionable "Marcel Wave" with its deep, regular and long-lasting rippled effect. From a commercial point of view the "Marcel Wave" was a godsend for hairdressers because it necessitated regular monthly trips to their salons. Certainly Marcel himself was under no illusion of his invention's impact, declaring: "The secret? Simply a knack in the turn of the wrist and a series of movements of the irons that makes the 'wave' lasting. I realised at once I was a benefactor to all womankind." He was also quoted as saying, "Fashions may come and go, but every woman in her heart yearns for wavy hair." Indeed, Marcel's invention of his wave-making curling tongs was not only a commercial boon for hairdressers in the closing years of the 19th century, but it was also an important impetus to the growth of the hair profession during the early decades of the 20th century.

During the late 1880s and 1890s the fashion was for less complex styles, which often incorporated small false "Martineau" hairpieces that were fashionably waved or curled using Marcel's heated irons. In the early 1890s many women wore a light fringe of loose curls and then the rest of their hair was gathered in a chignon, which sometimes was padded to give the illusion of greater volume. There was also a short-lived fashion for the curious "Teapot Handle" whereby hair was coiled at the back and then fashioned into a loop that rose at right angles to the crown of the head. By the turn of the century, pads were also being used at the front of the head to give a raised pompadour style, while the rest of the hair was drawn into a high bun, which was frequently supplemented in the evening with an aigrette – an ornamental tuft of plumes often made from the tail feathers of an egret. Certainly in the last quarter of the 19th century there were a large number of hairdressing journals being published, such as *The Hairdressers' Chronicle*, *La Coiffure Française Illustrée* and *Deutsche Allgemeine Friseur Zeitung* that helped to accelerate the seasonal fashion changes that occurred in hairstyling. The ensuing number of distinctly different coiffures that were seen on the pages of these magazines during this period is quite staggering, and demonstrates the hands-on skill and creative powers of the hairdressers. Certainly hairdressing was a significant cultural and commercial pursuit during the Victorian era, but hair also possessed a strong symbolic status within Victorian society. Many women wore lockets or other hair-incorporating mourning jewellery, thereby revealing the continuing and potent association of hair with life and love.

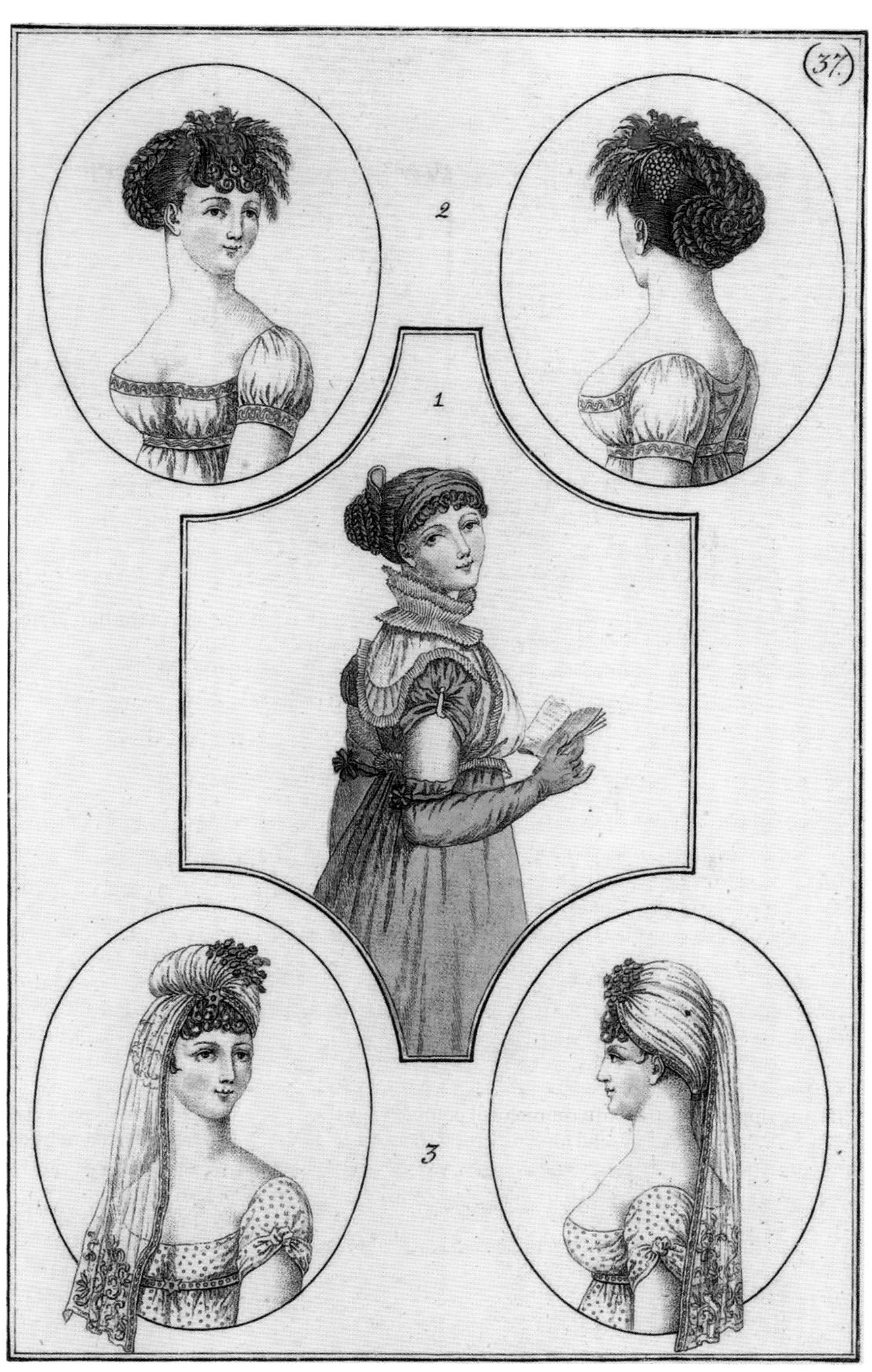

Parisian hairstyles, 1804, *Le Journal des Dames et des Modes Frankfurt*

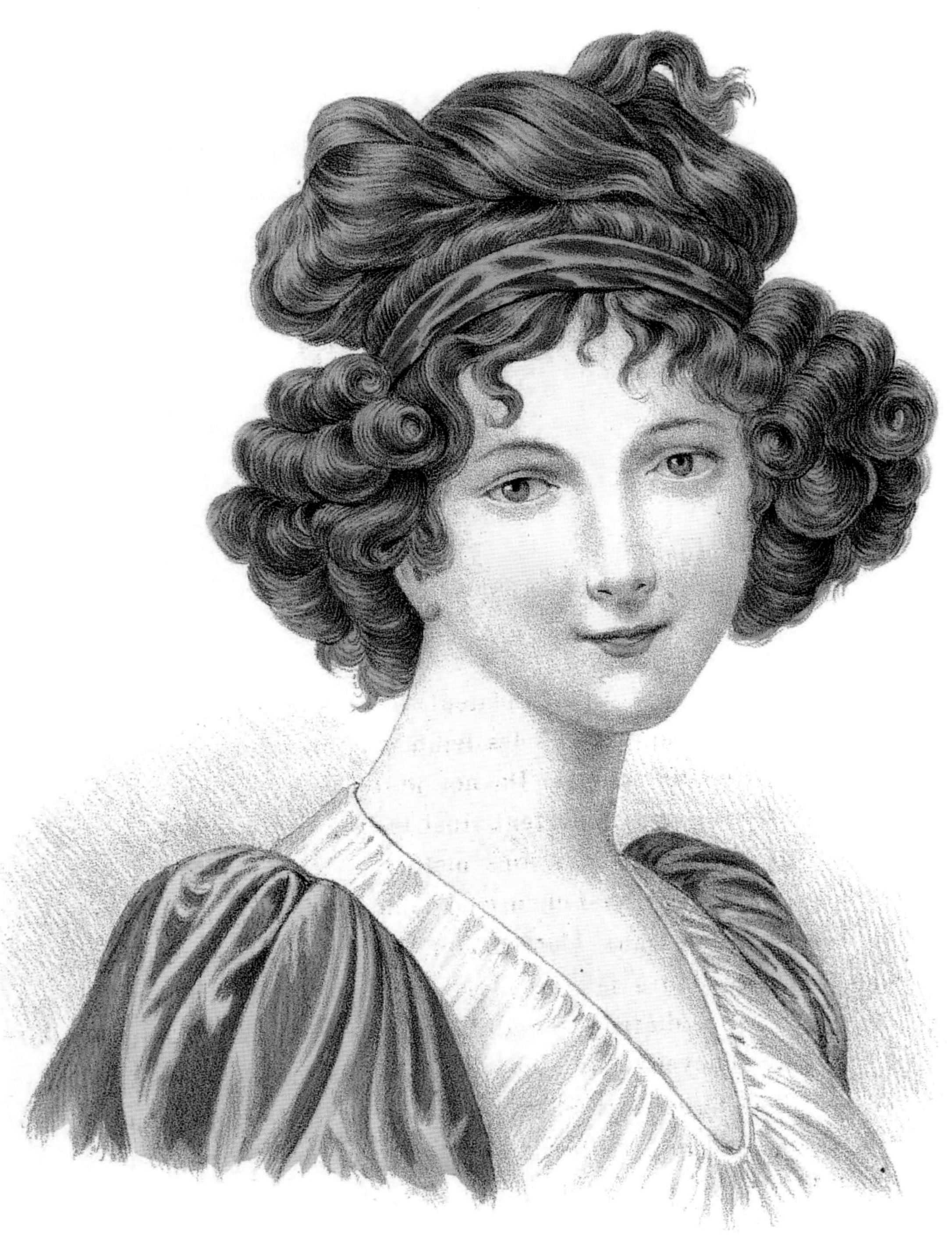

'Coiffure Fantaisie Empire' (Madame Le Brun), *Album de Coiffures Historiques*, E. Nissy

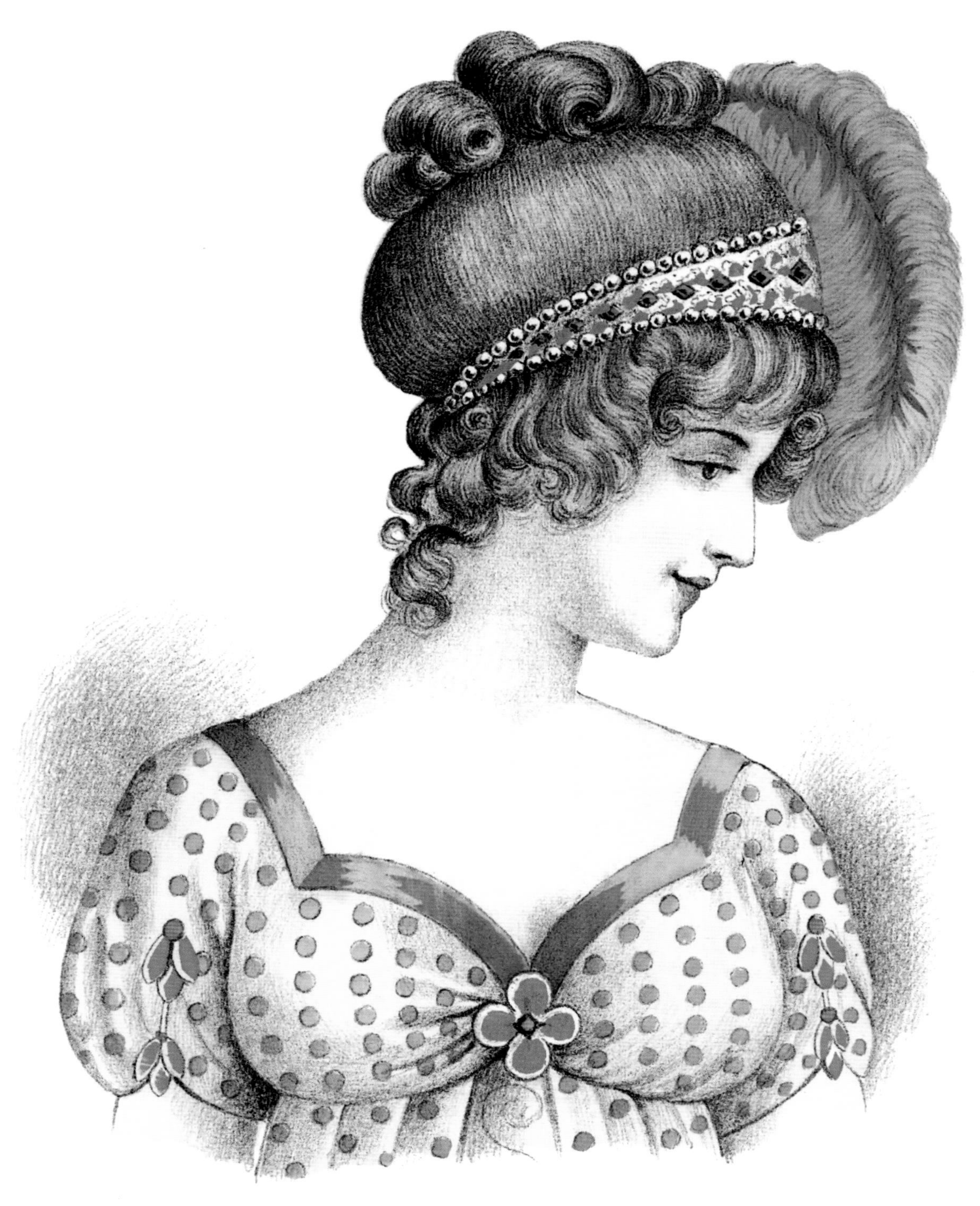

First Empire hairstyle, c. 1800–1810, *Album de Coiffures Historiques*, E. Nissy

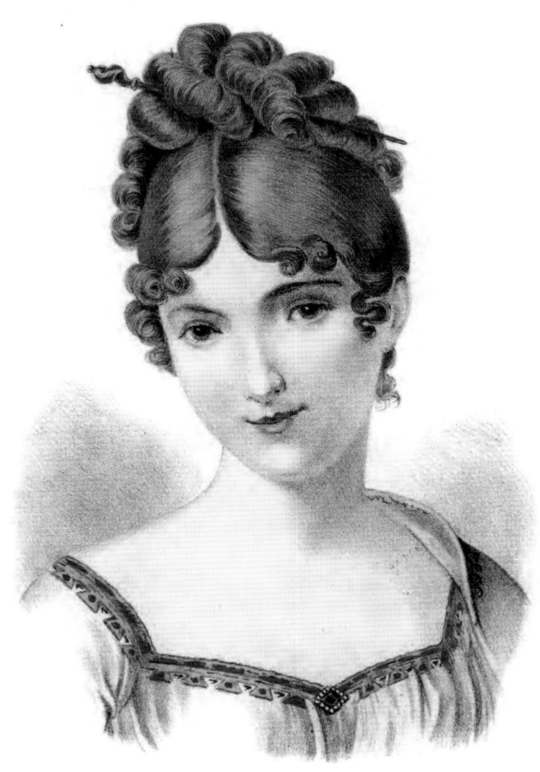
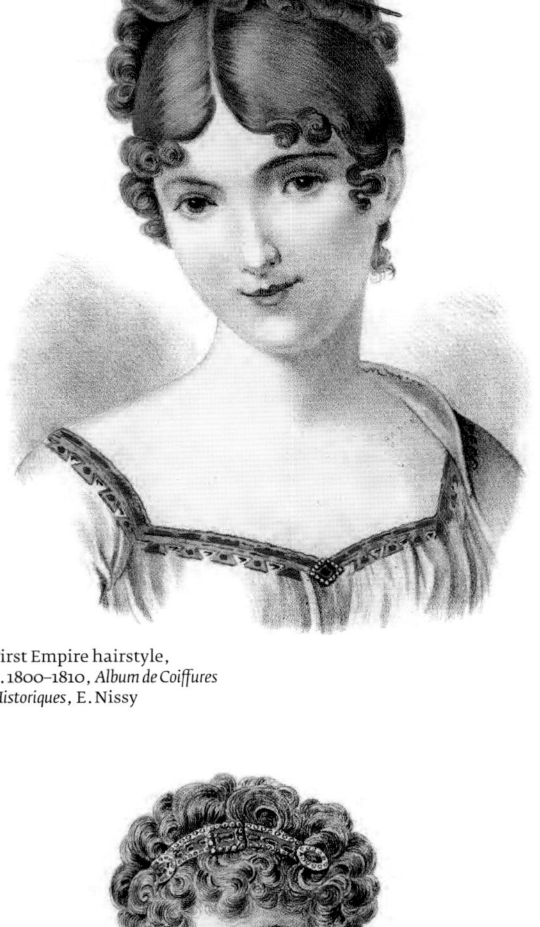

First Empire hairstyle, c.1800–1810, *Album de Coiffures Historiques*, E. Nissy

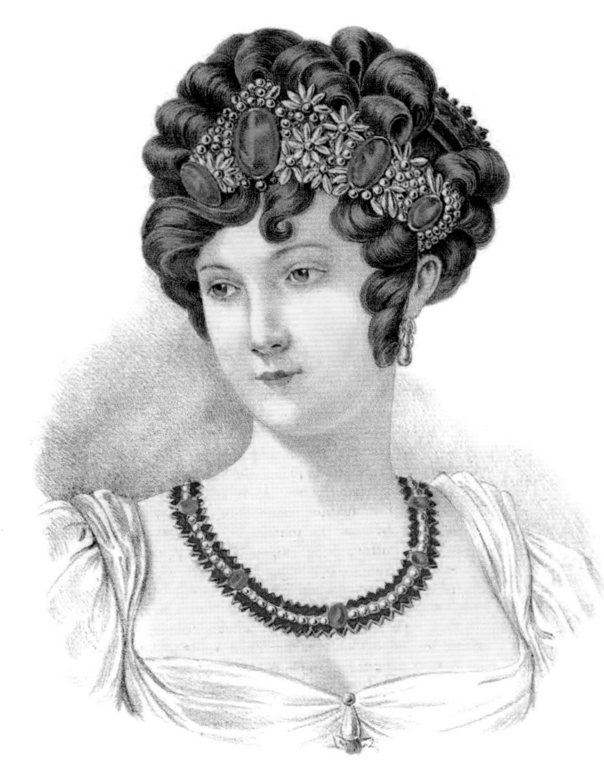

First Empire hairstyle, 1804–1814, *Album de Coiffures Historiques*, E. Nissy

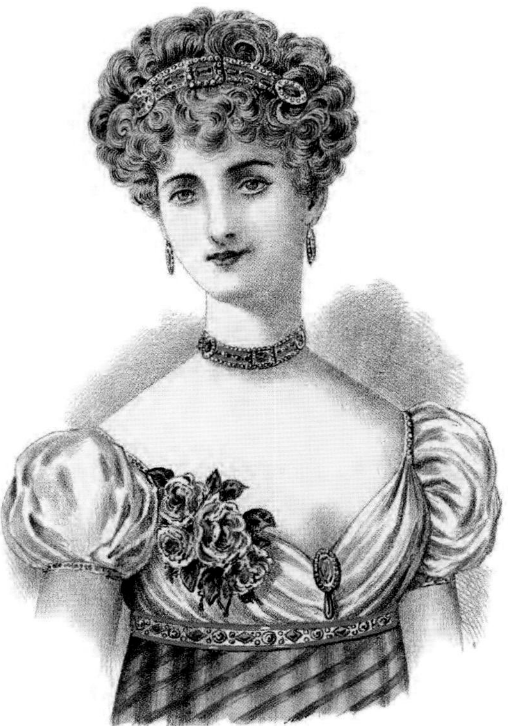

Empire hairstyle, 1810s, *Album de Coiffures Historiques*, E. Nissy

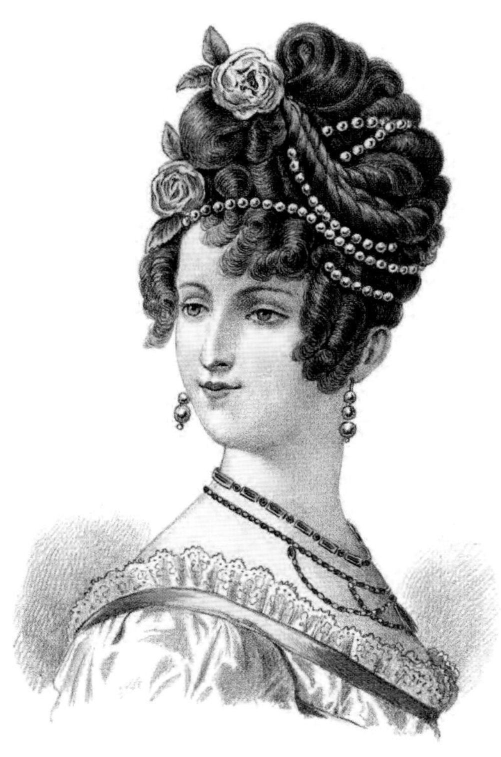

Restauration hairstyle, *Album de Coiffures Historiques*, E. Nissy

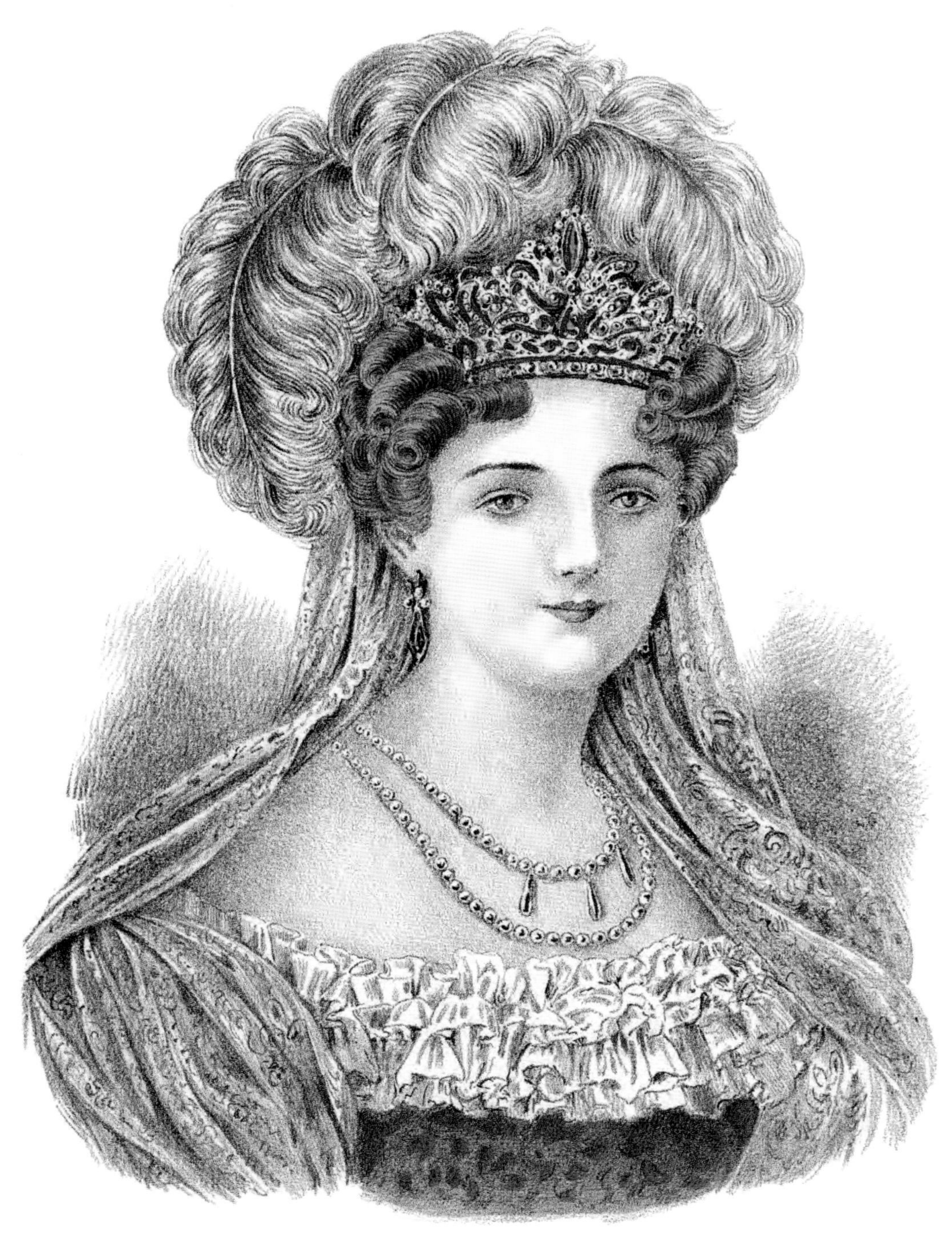

Restauration hairstyle, *Album de Coiffures Historiques*, E. Nissy

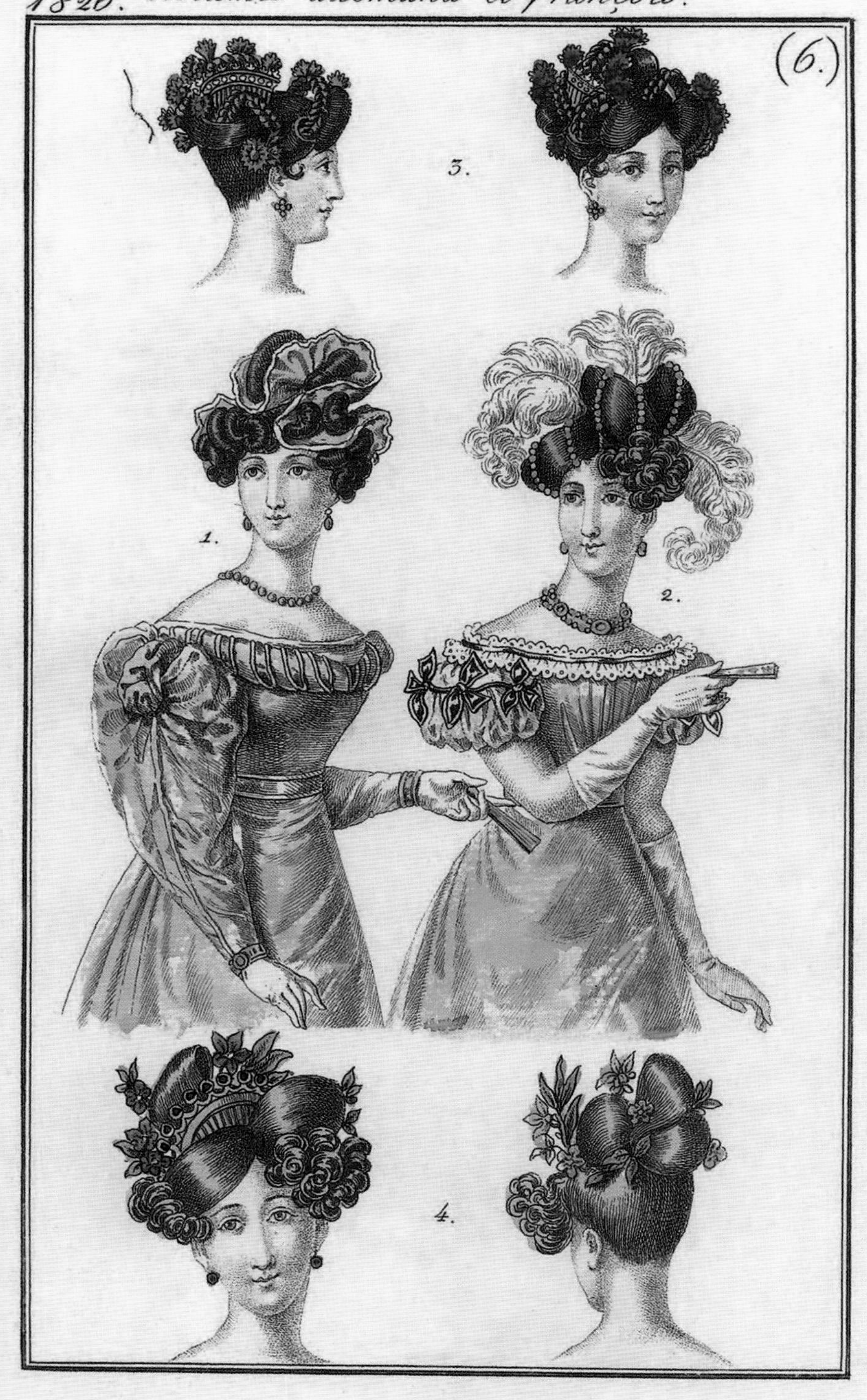

German and French hairstyles, 1826, *Le Journal des Dames et des Modes Frankfurt*

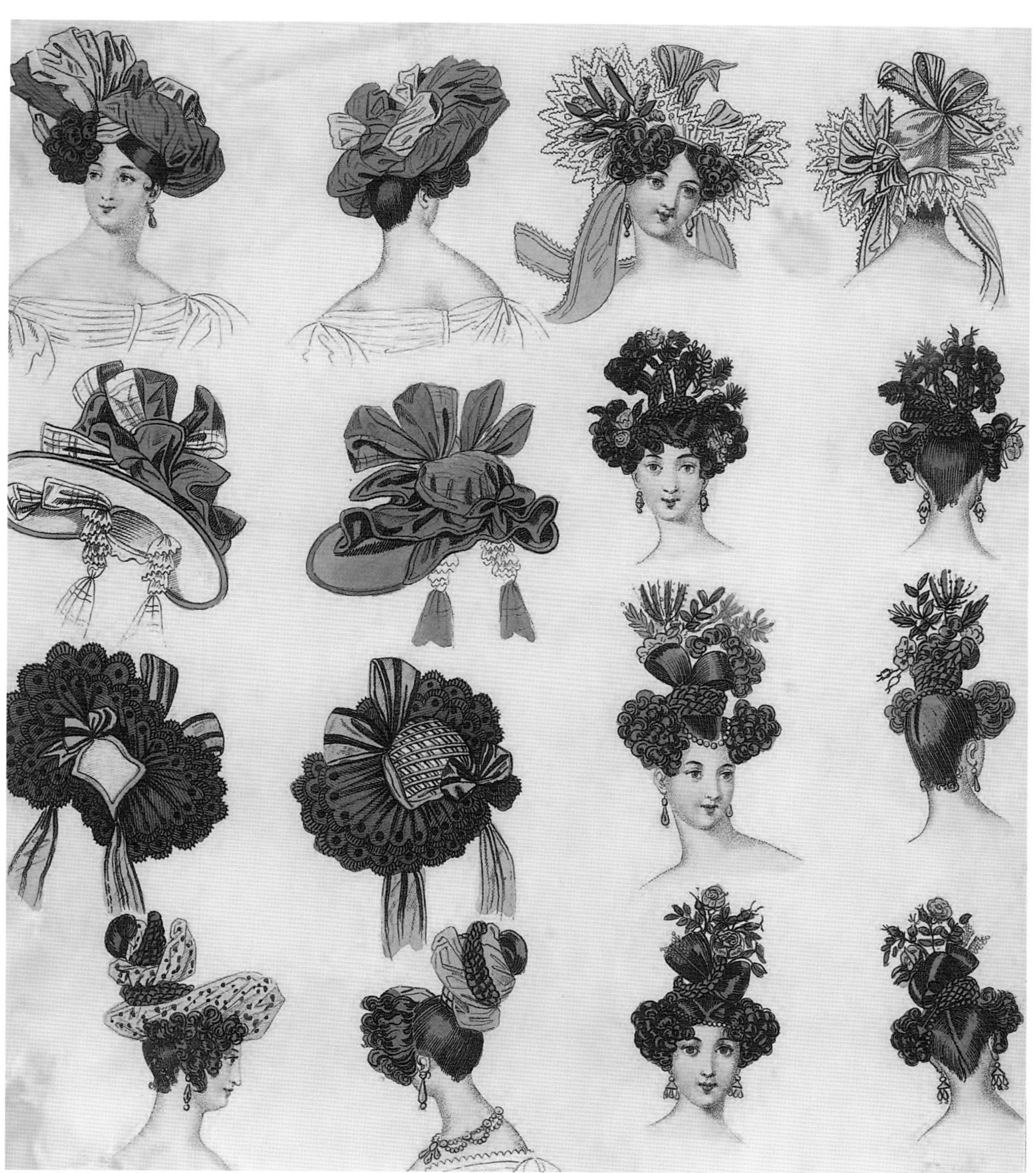

'Newest Fashions for April 1829, Fashionable Head Dresses', engraving by W. Alais

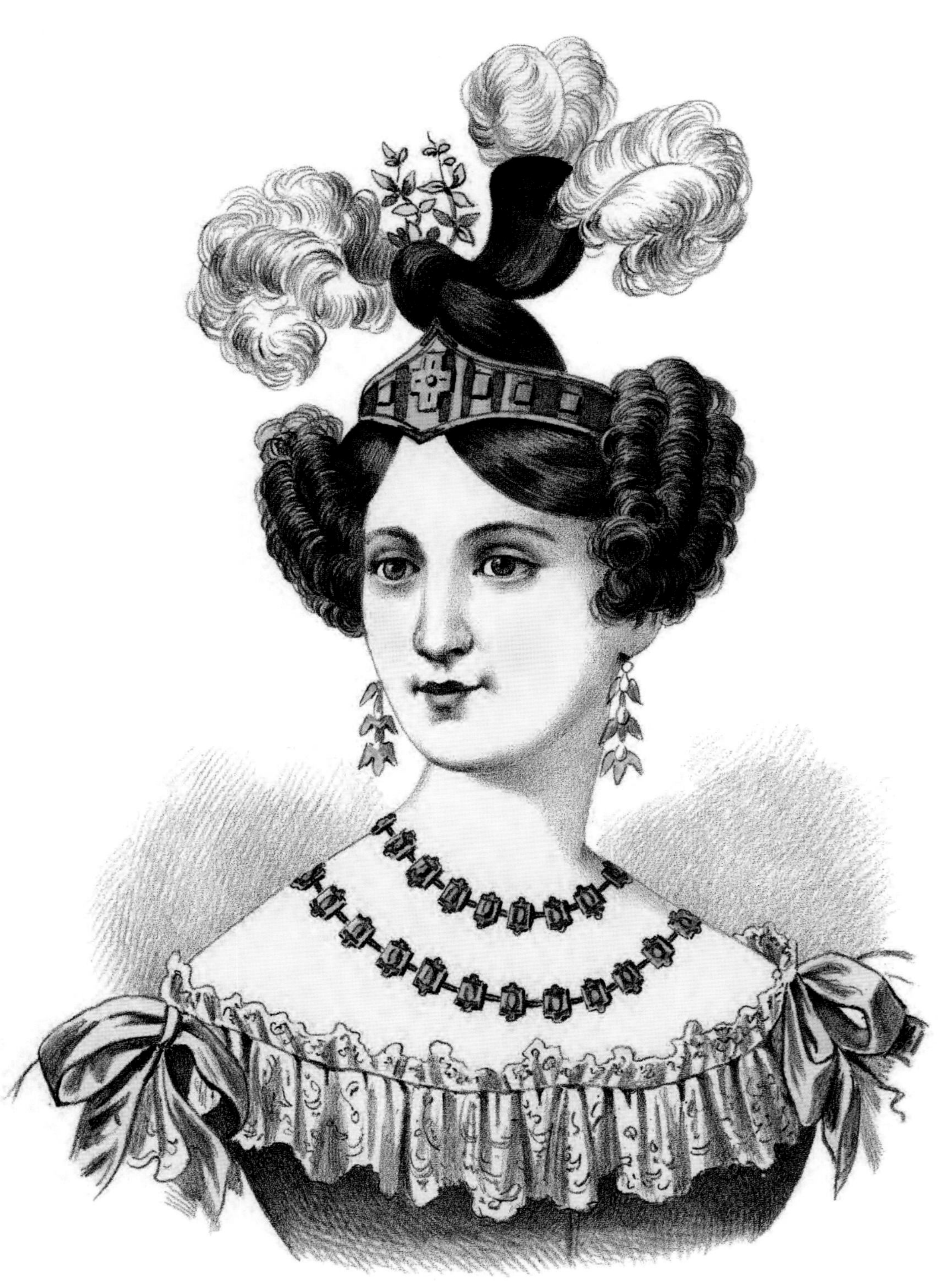

'Coiffure à la Girafe' (The Giraffe hairstyle), 1830s , *Album de Coiffures Historiques*, E. Nissy

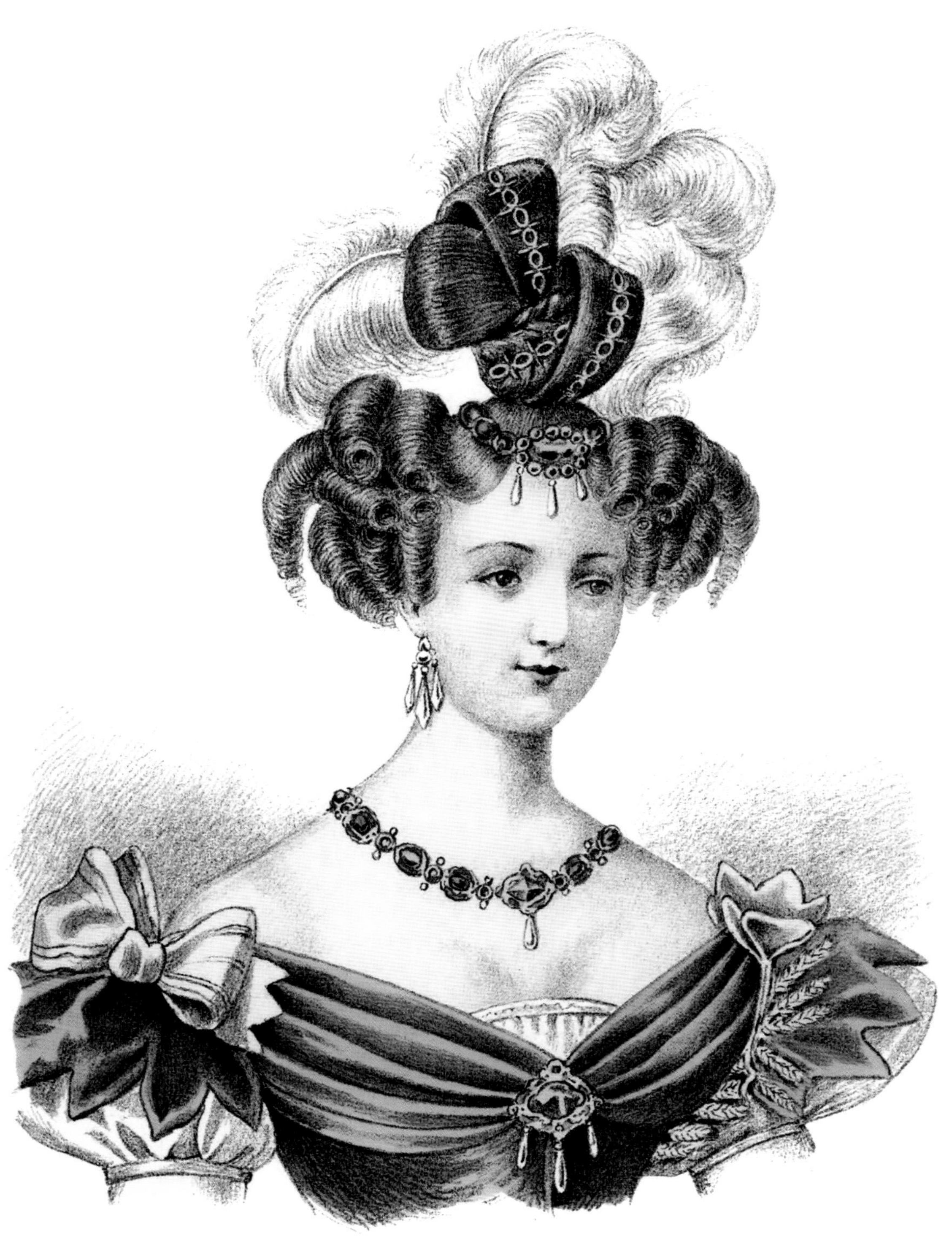

'Coiffure 1830', *Album de Coiffures Historiques*, E. Nissy

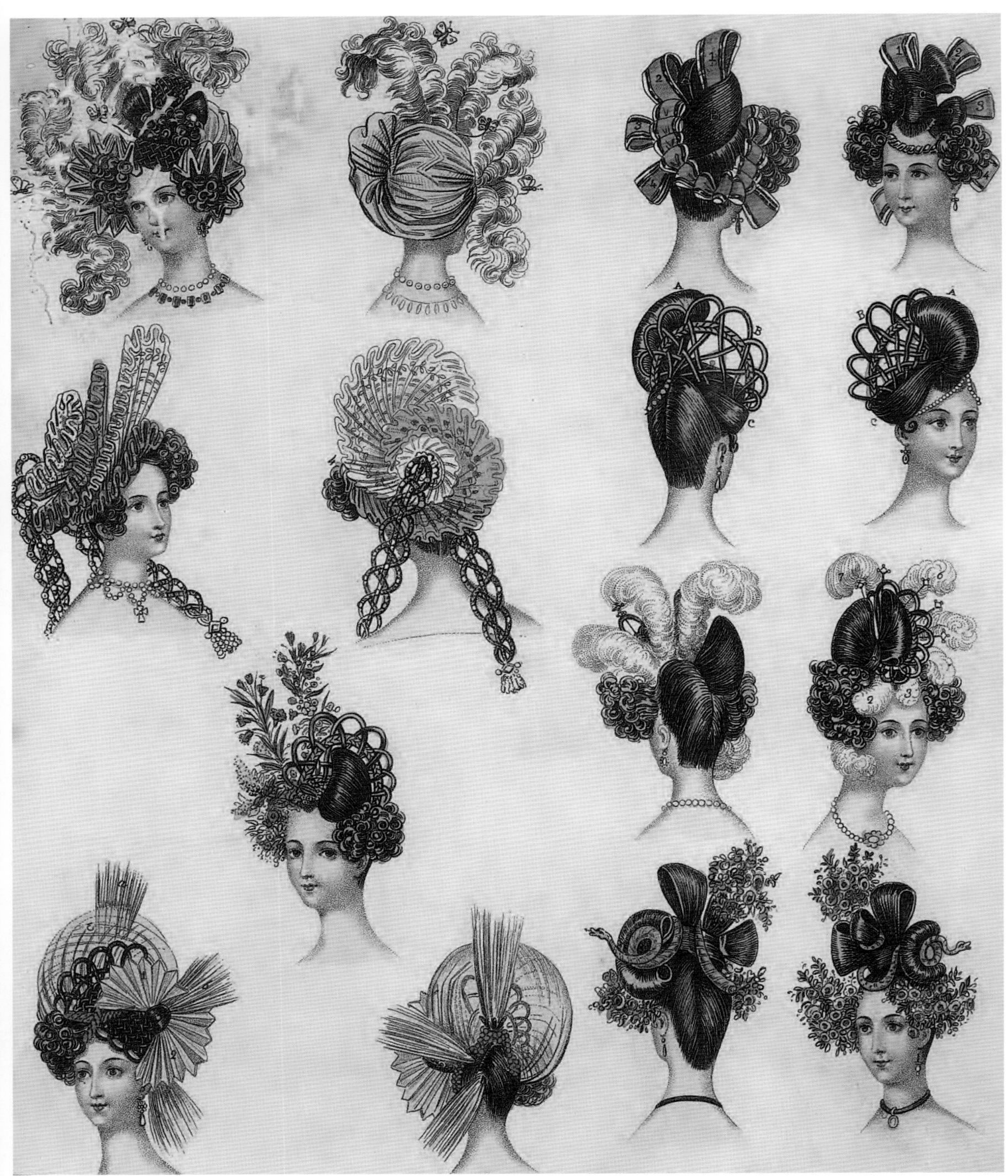

'Hairstyles by Mr. Ball, Oxford Street, Fashionable Head Dresses for June', 1830

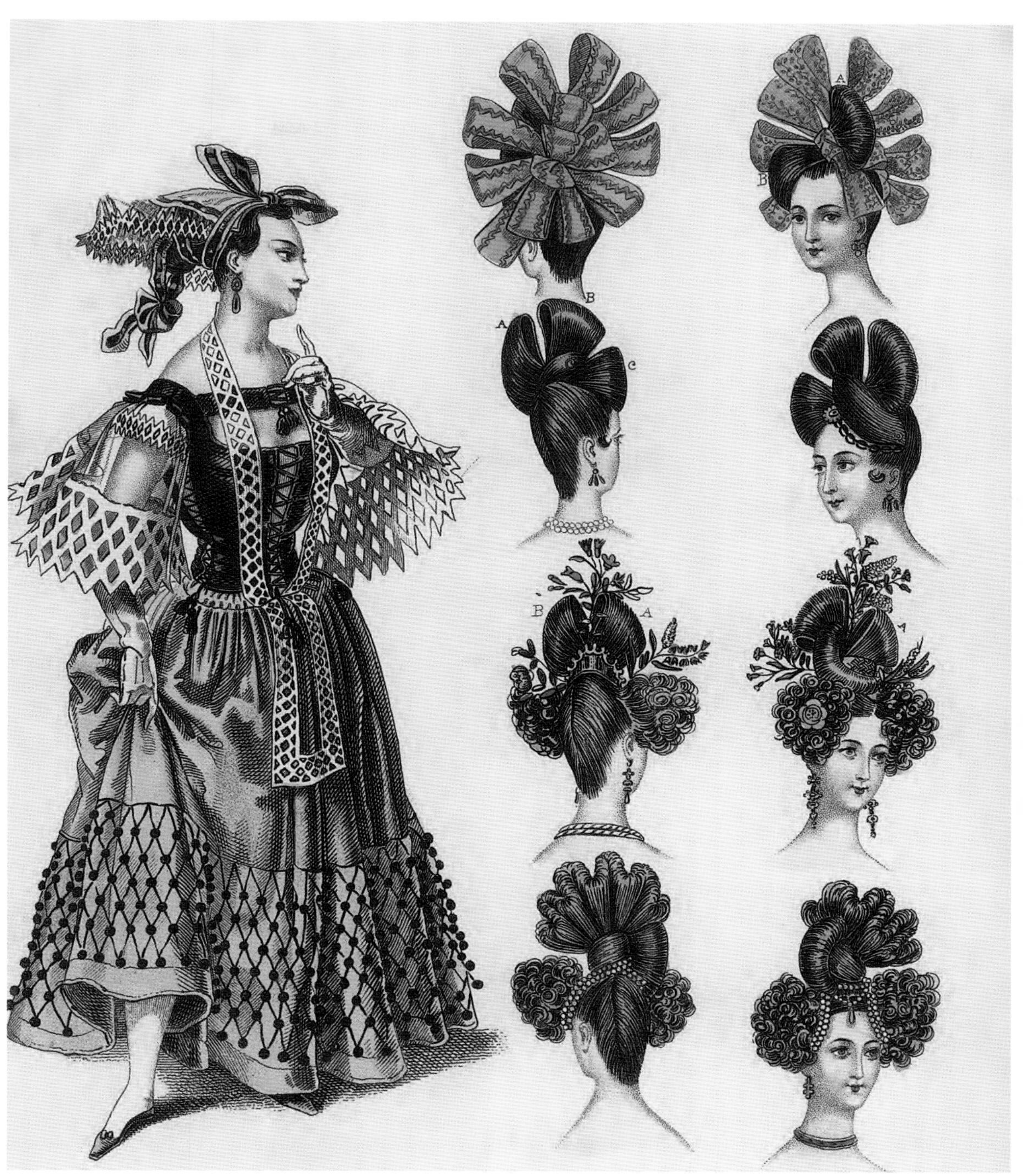

'Newest Fashions for July 1830, Fashionable Coiffures, Costumes of all Nations No. 50 – Spanish'

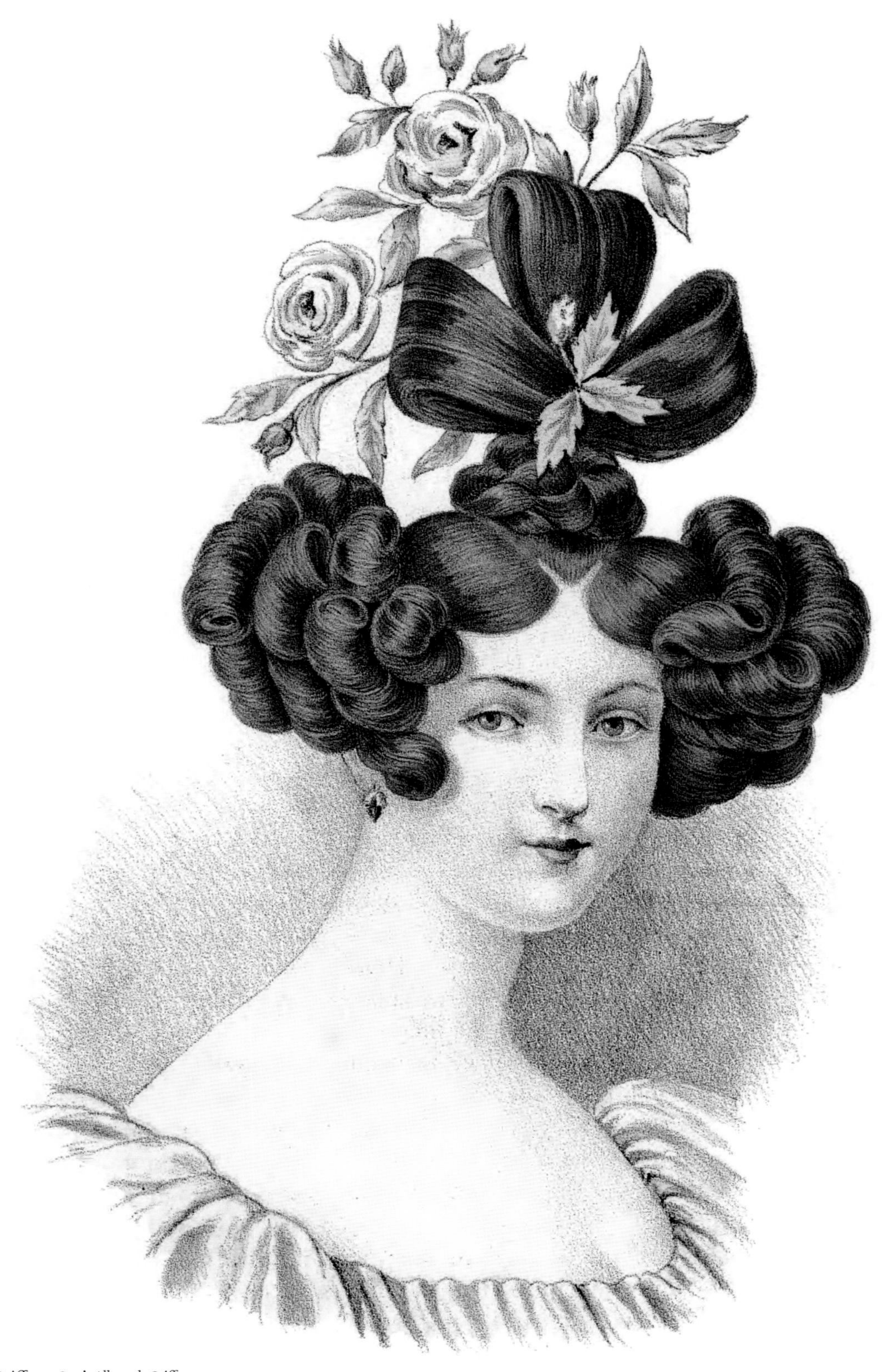

'Coiffure 1830', *Album de Coiffures Historiques*, E. Nissy

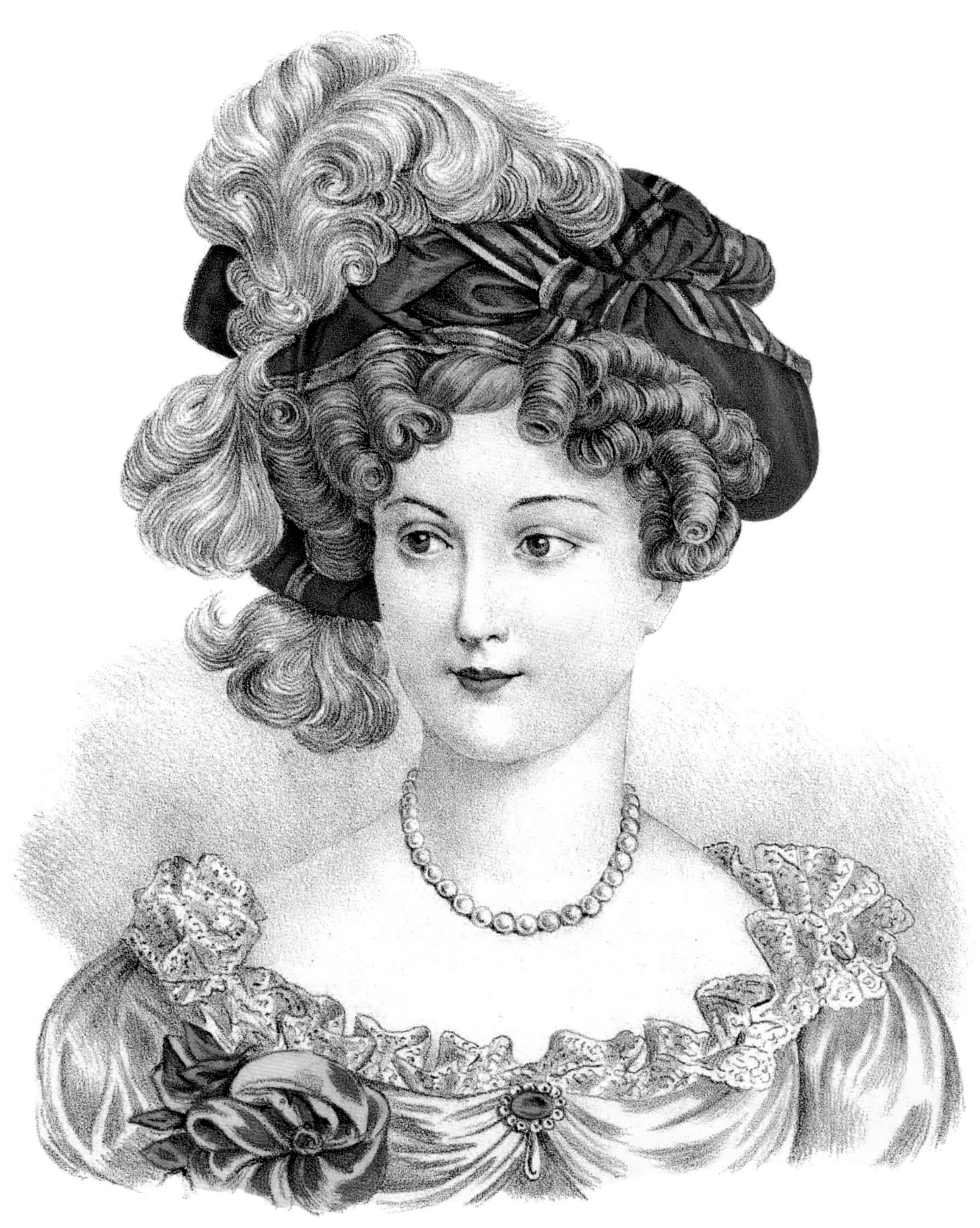

Coiffure of the Duchesse de Berry, 1830,
Album de Coiffures Historiques, E. Nissy

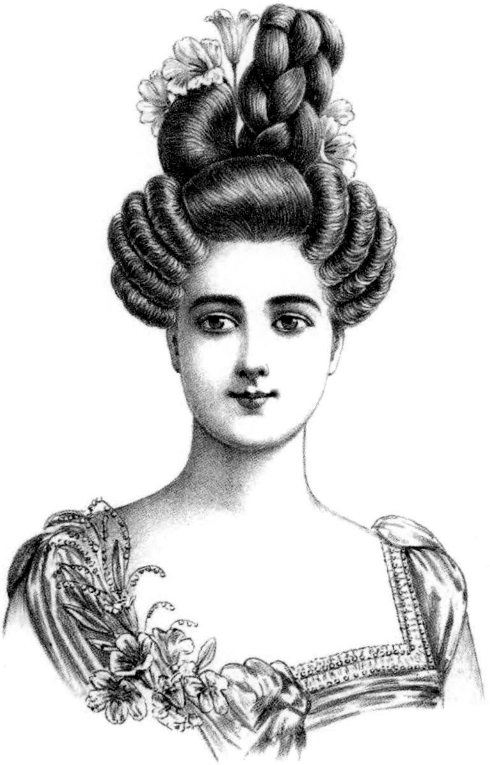

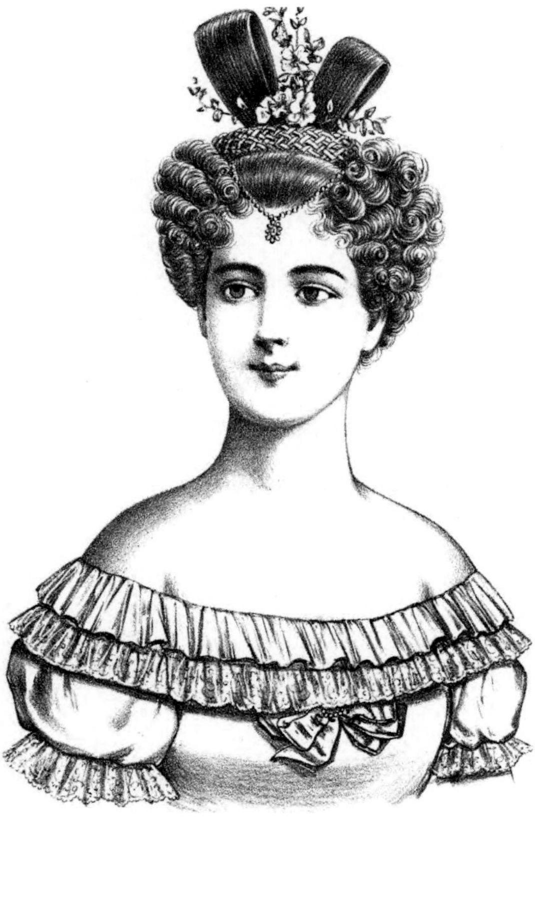

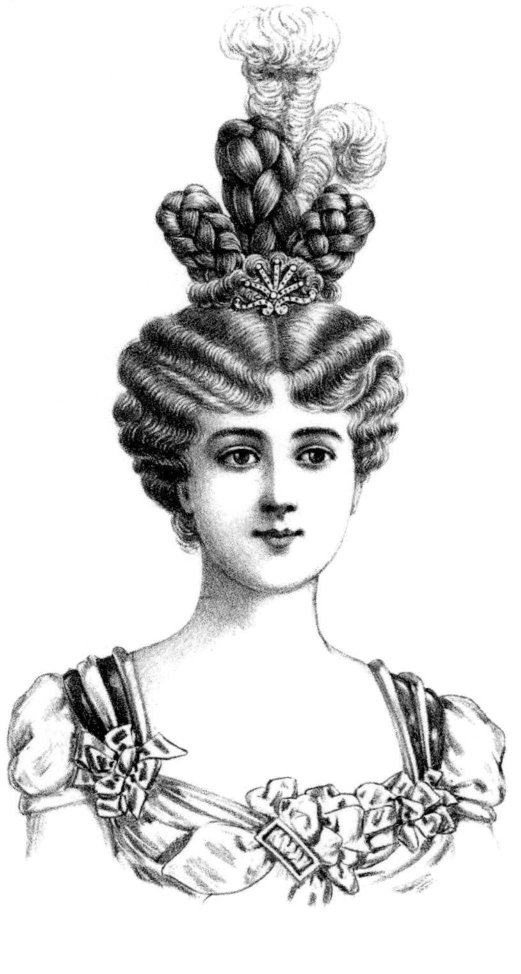

Hairstyles, 1830s, *Album Historischer und Phantasie-Frisuren*, Heinrich Moritz

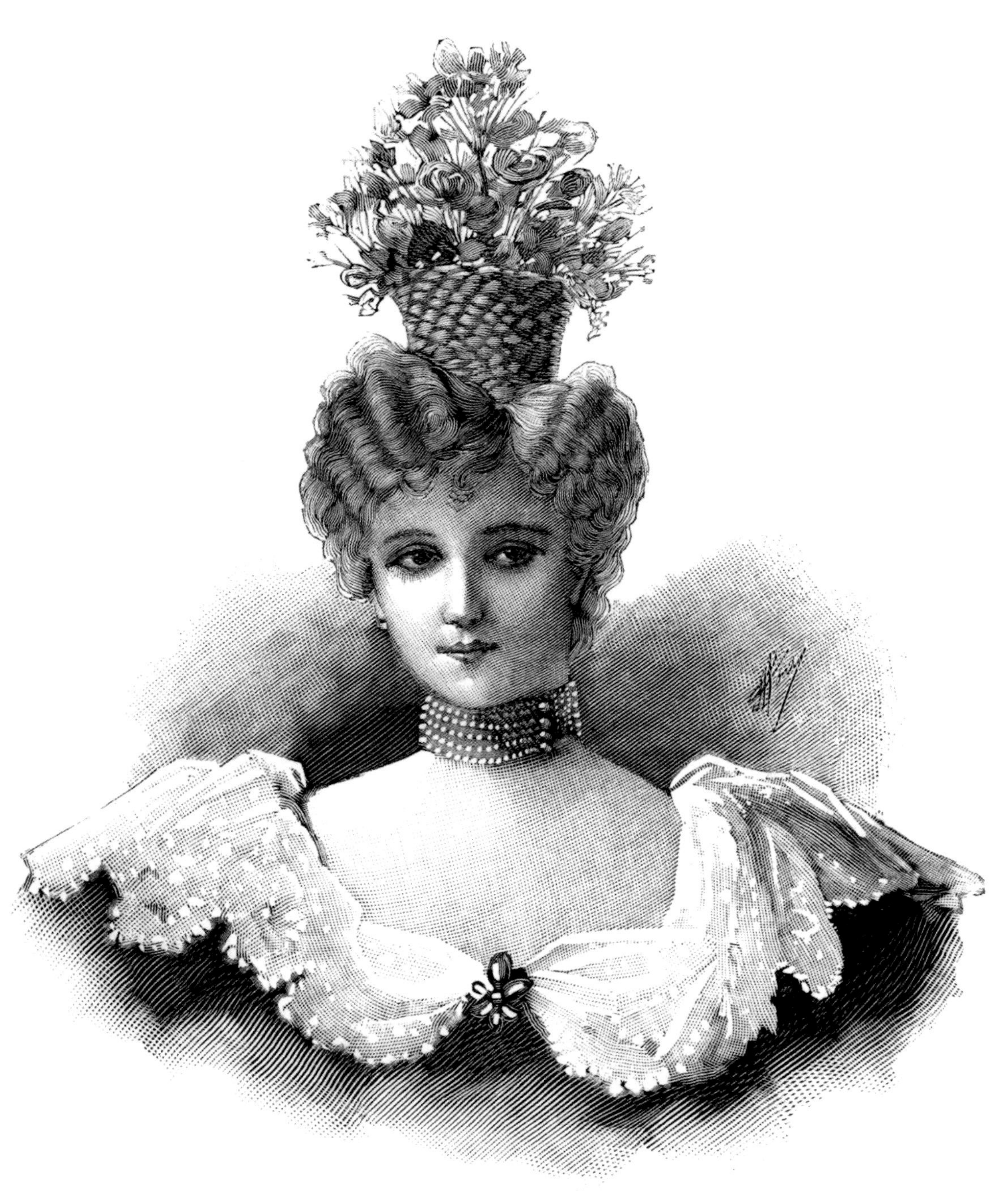

'Fantaisie' hairstyle, 1830,
L'Art de la Coiffure et de la Mode

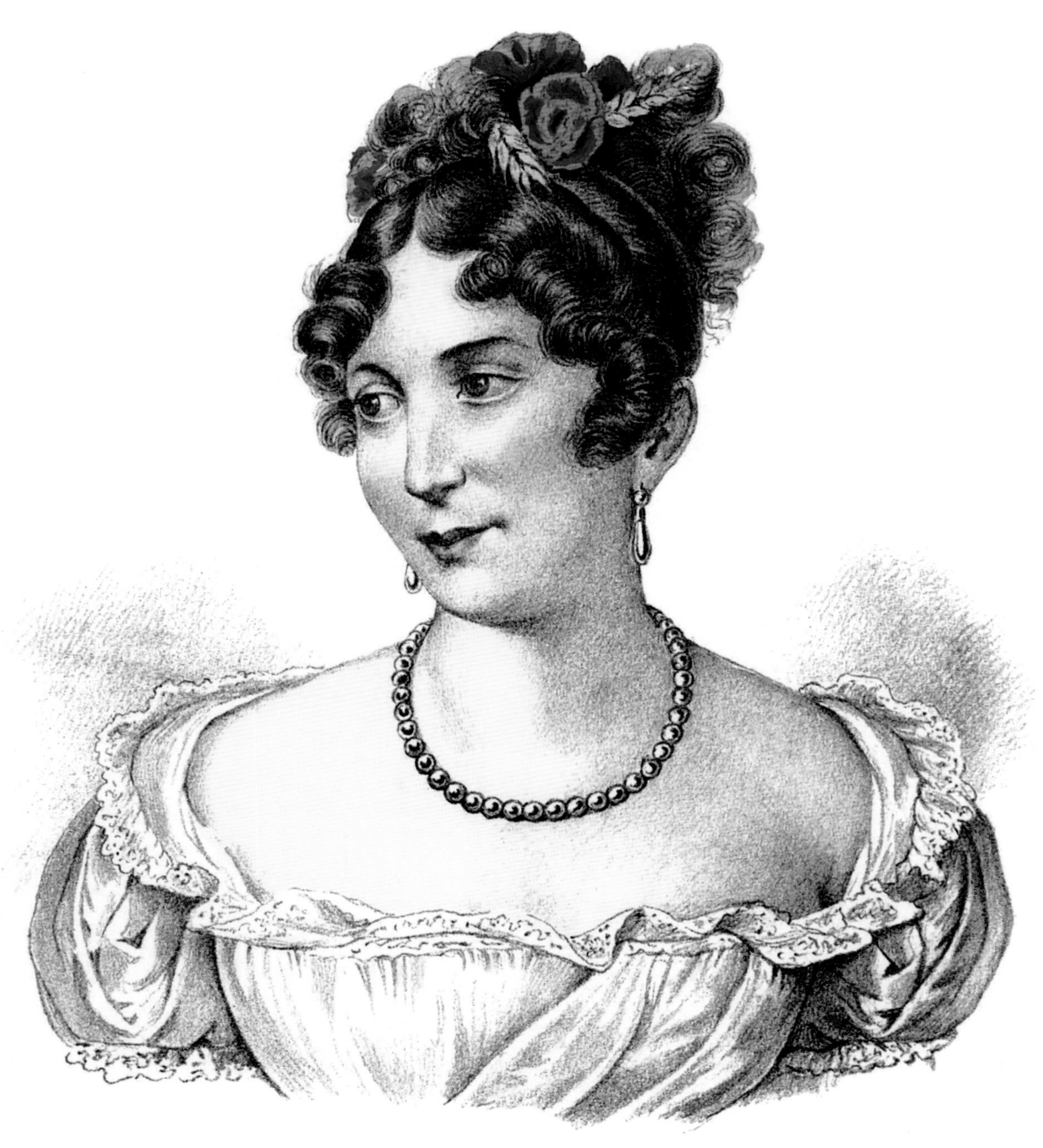

Coiffure First Empire, Mlle. Mars, 1840s,
Album de Coiffures Historiques, E. Nissy

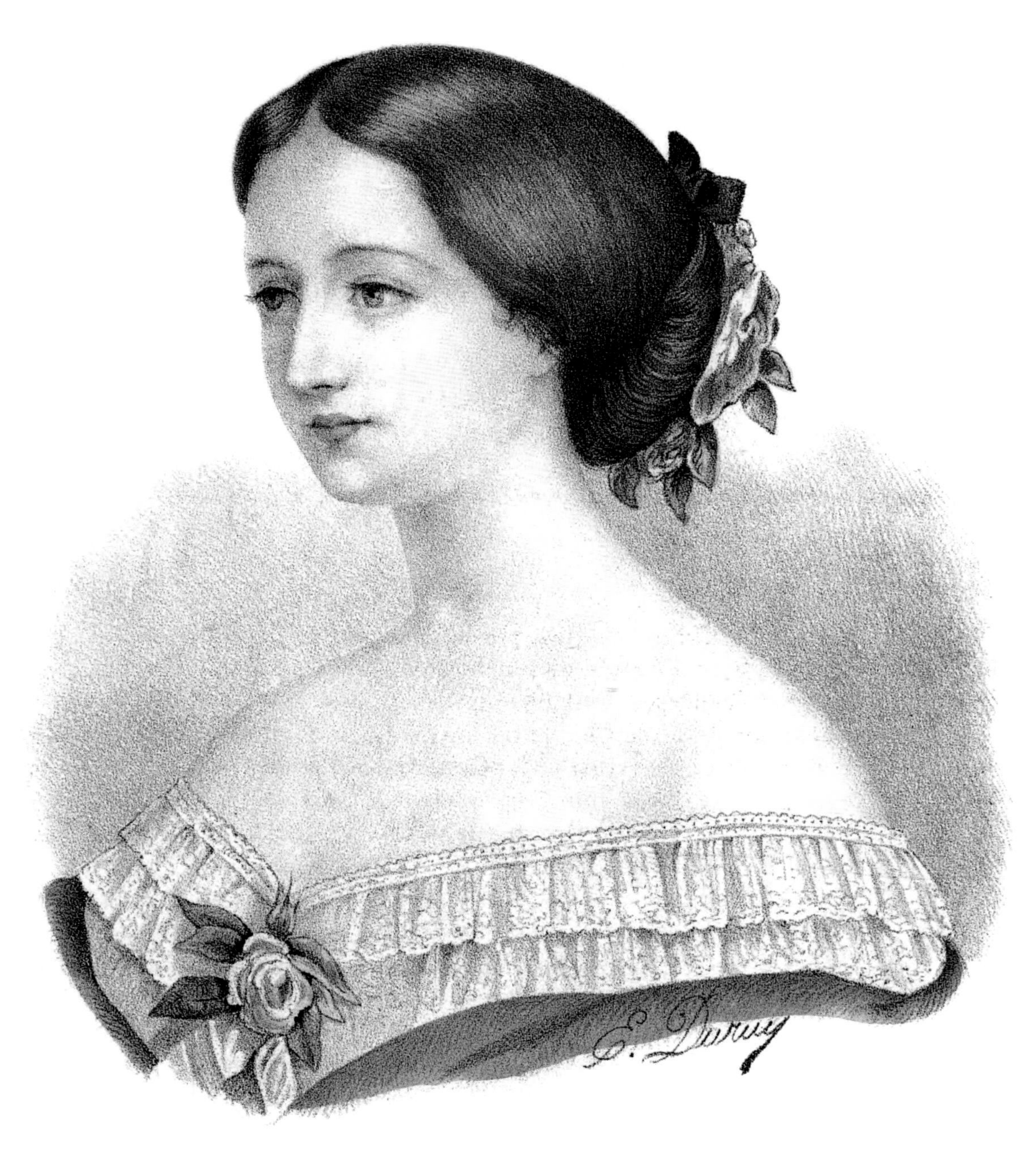

Coiffure Second Empire (Empress Eugénie, wife of Napoleon III), c.1850, *Album de Coiffures Historiques*, E. Nissy

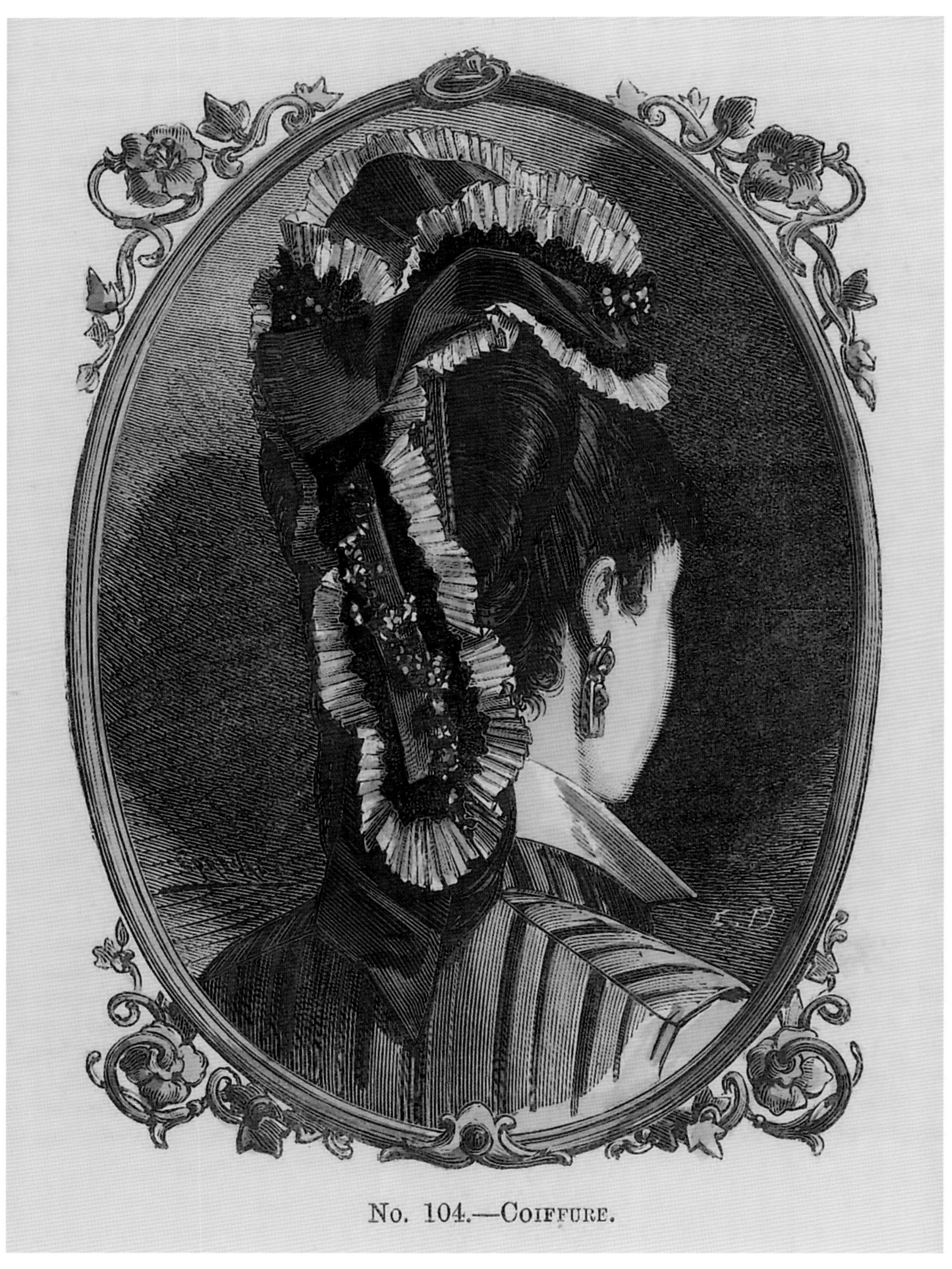

French hairstyle, 1865, *The Milliner and Dressmaker and Warehouseman's Gazette*

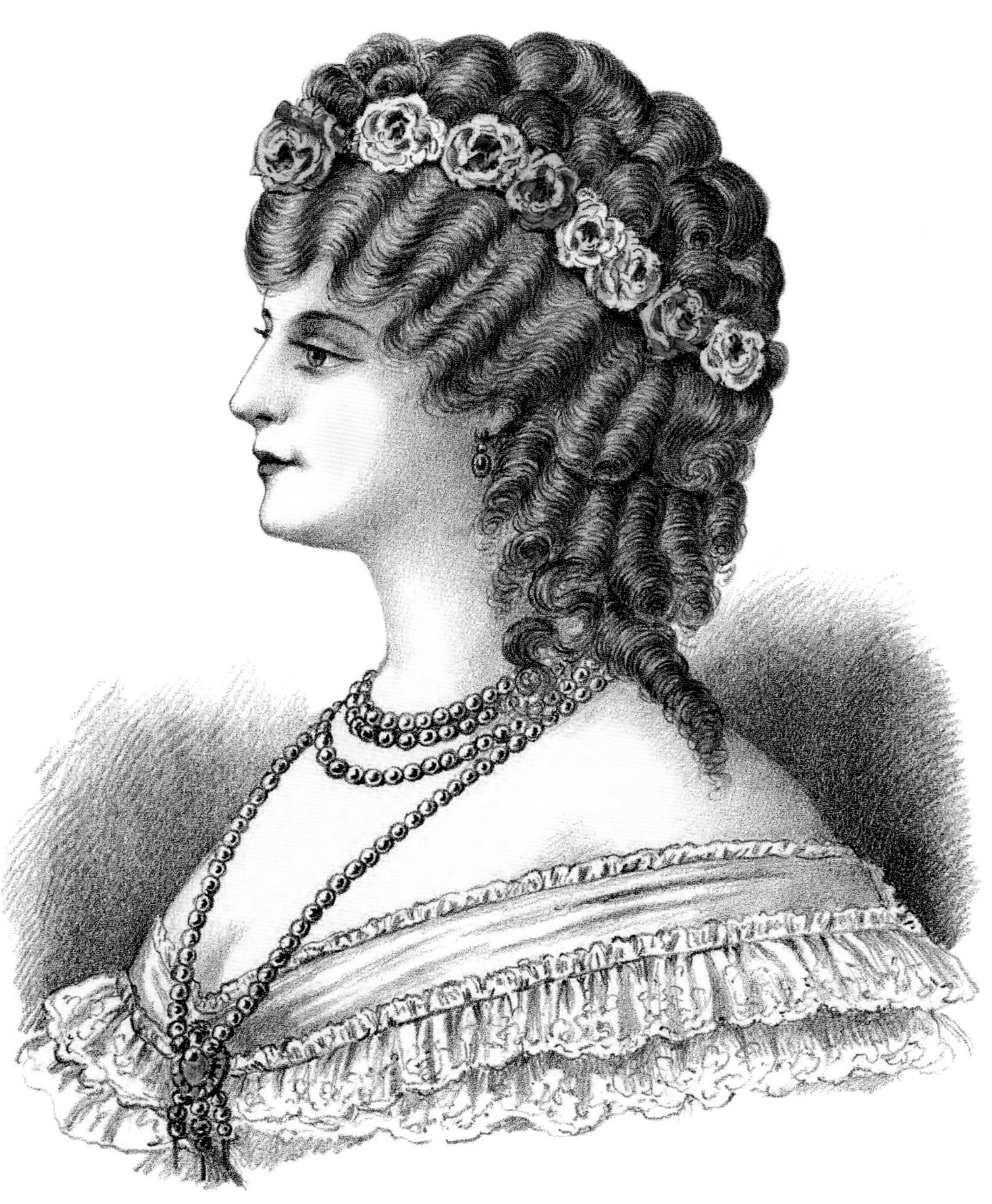

Second Empire hairstyle, La Baroutchi, 1867,
Album de Coiffures Historiques, E. Nissy

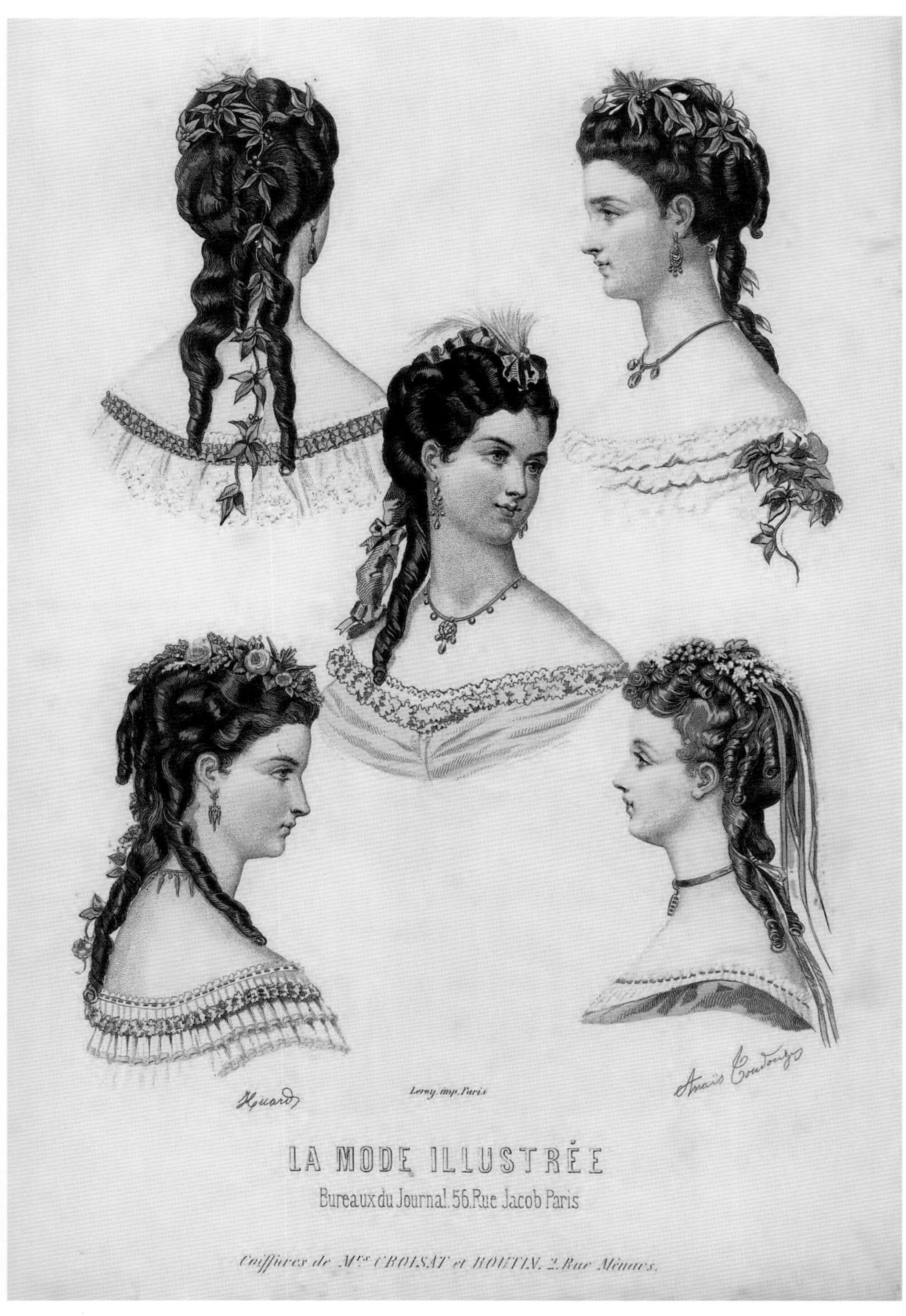

Hairstyles of Mr. Croizat and
Mr. Boutin, 1868, *La Mode Illustrée*

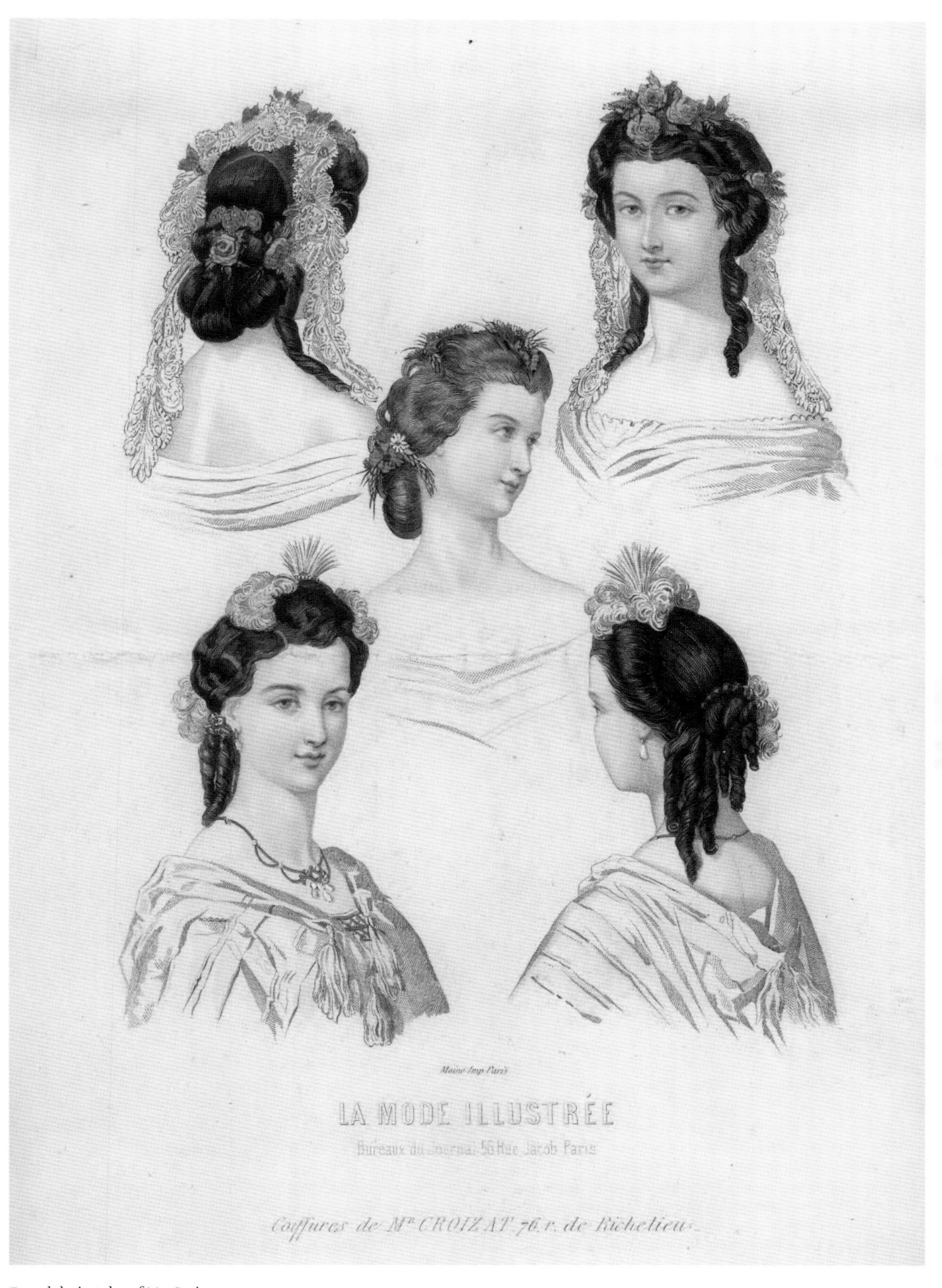

French hairstyles of Mr. Croizat,
1869, *La Mode Illustrée*

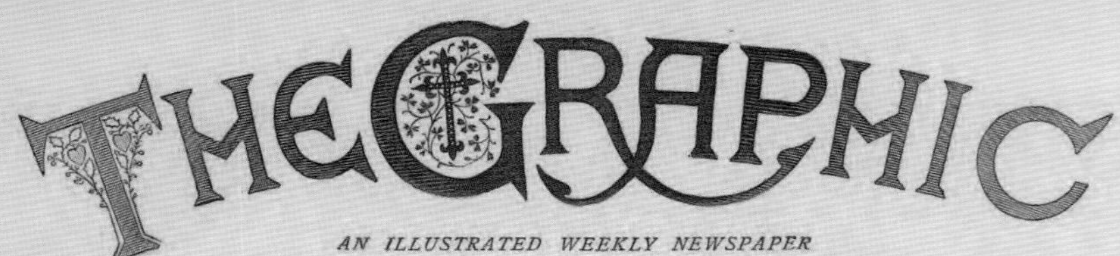

AN ILLUSTRATED WEEKLY NEWSPAPER

VOL. I—No. 26
Registered for Transmission Abroad

SATURDAY, MAY 28, 1870

PRICE SIXPENCE,
OR SEVENPENCE STAMPED

CHRONICLE

THE Government grant of one thousand pounds "on account of Dr. Livingstone's expedition" is a welcome sign of recognition from the State of that distinguished traveller's claim to public sympathy, but it can hardly be said to go further than this. The sum is paltry in itself, and is understood to be altogether inadequate to the purpose for which it is granted. Under these circumstances it is not surprising that Lord Clarendon's letter to Sir Roderick Murchison has given rise to some dissatisfaction. The ground on which the money is granted is that this illustrious explorer, who has already done so much to extend our knowledge of the great continent of Africa, has been struggling without aid or communication with England for the last three years; that from the last accounts he had reached a point from which he could neither advance nor retreat without supplies; and that, the money granted to him at his departure being exhausted, further sums are urgently required to provide a fresh equipment and the means of conveying it into the interior. After citing reasons so strong, it appears ridiculous to conclude

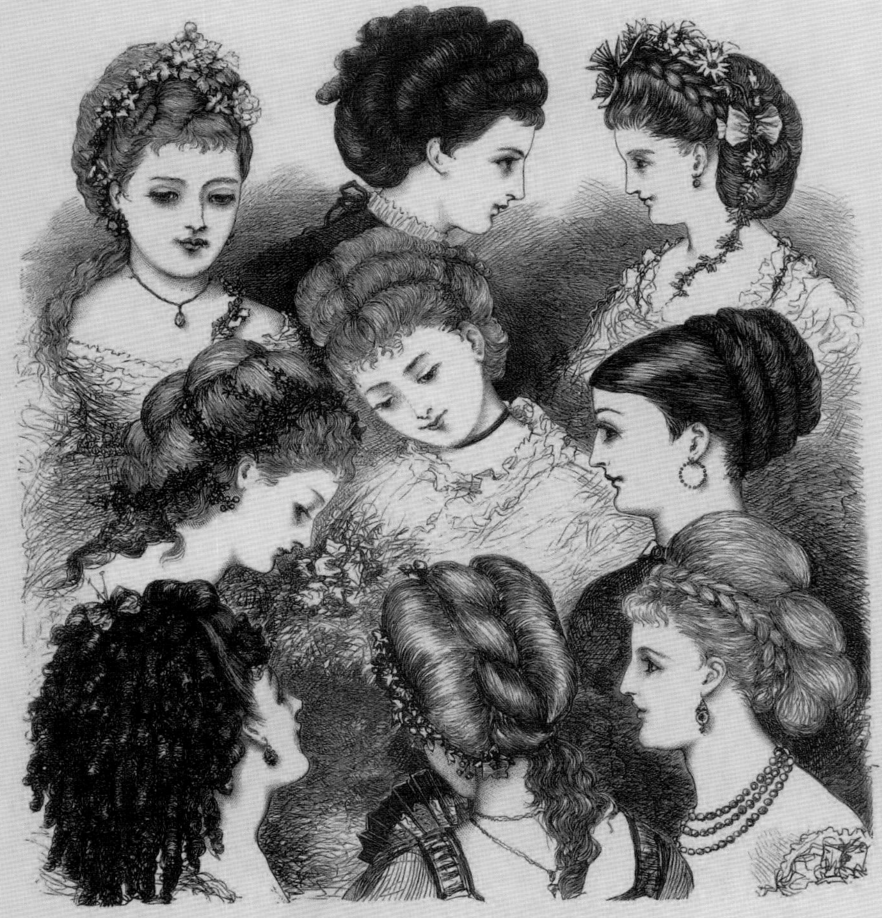

THE PRESENT FASHIONS IN HAIR

'The Present Fashions in Hair', 1870, *The Graphic*

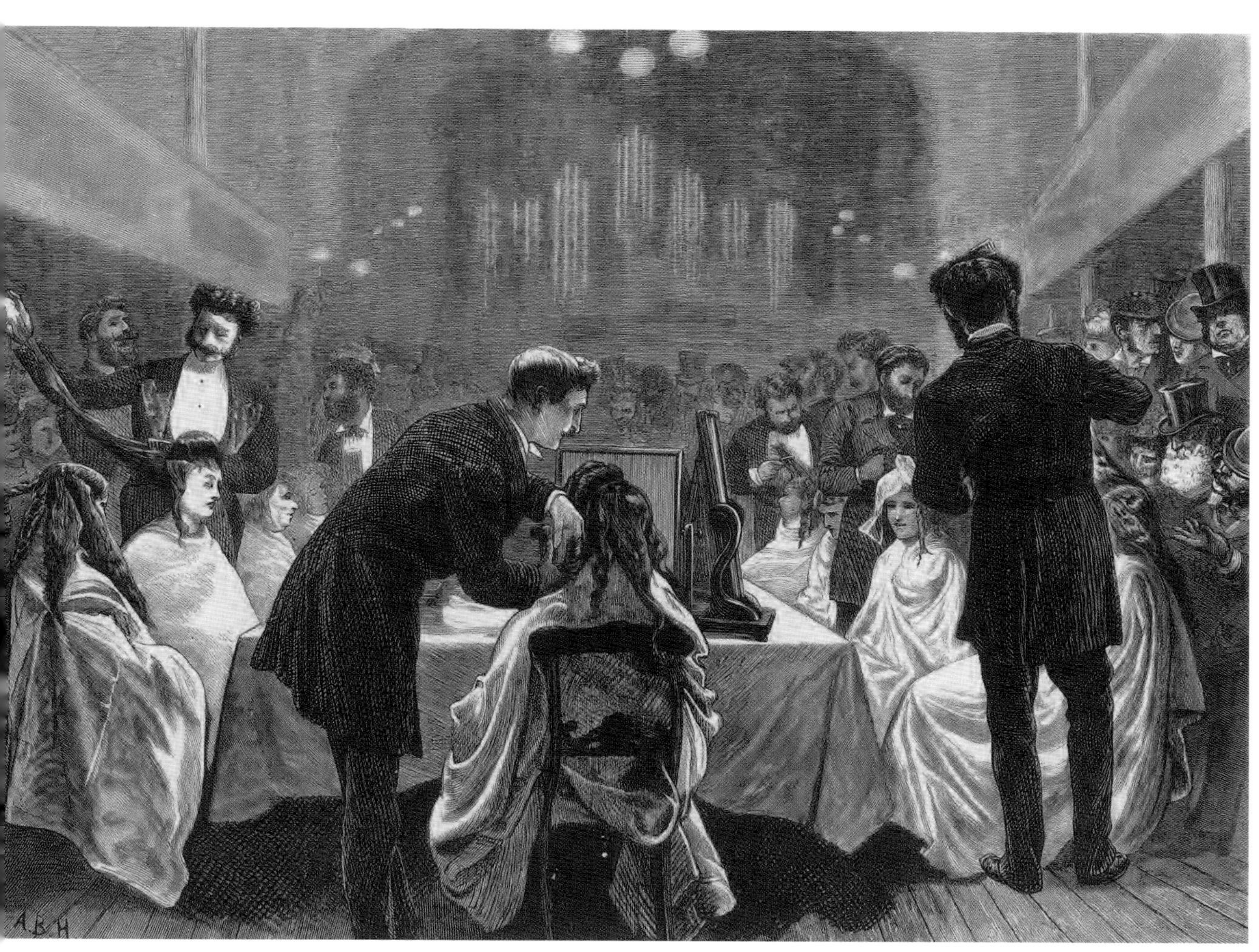

'A Hair-Dressing Exhibition',
1872, *The Graphic*

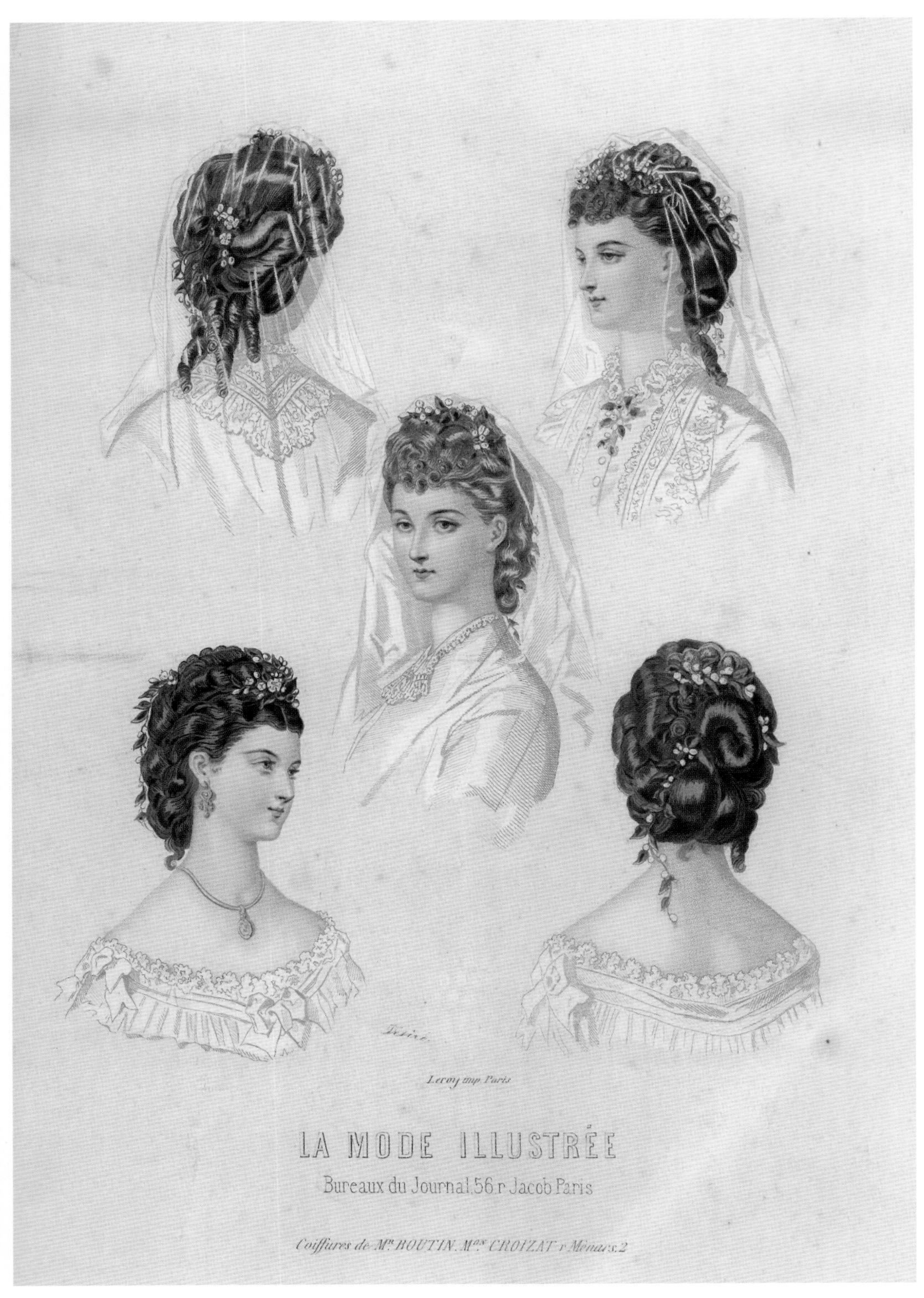

French wedding hairstyles by Mr. Croizat & Mr. Boutin, 1872, *La Mode Illustrée*

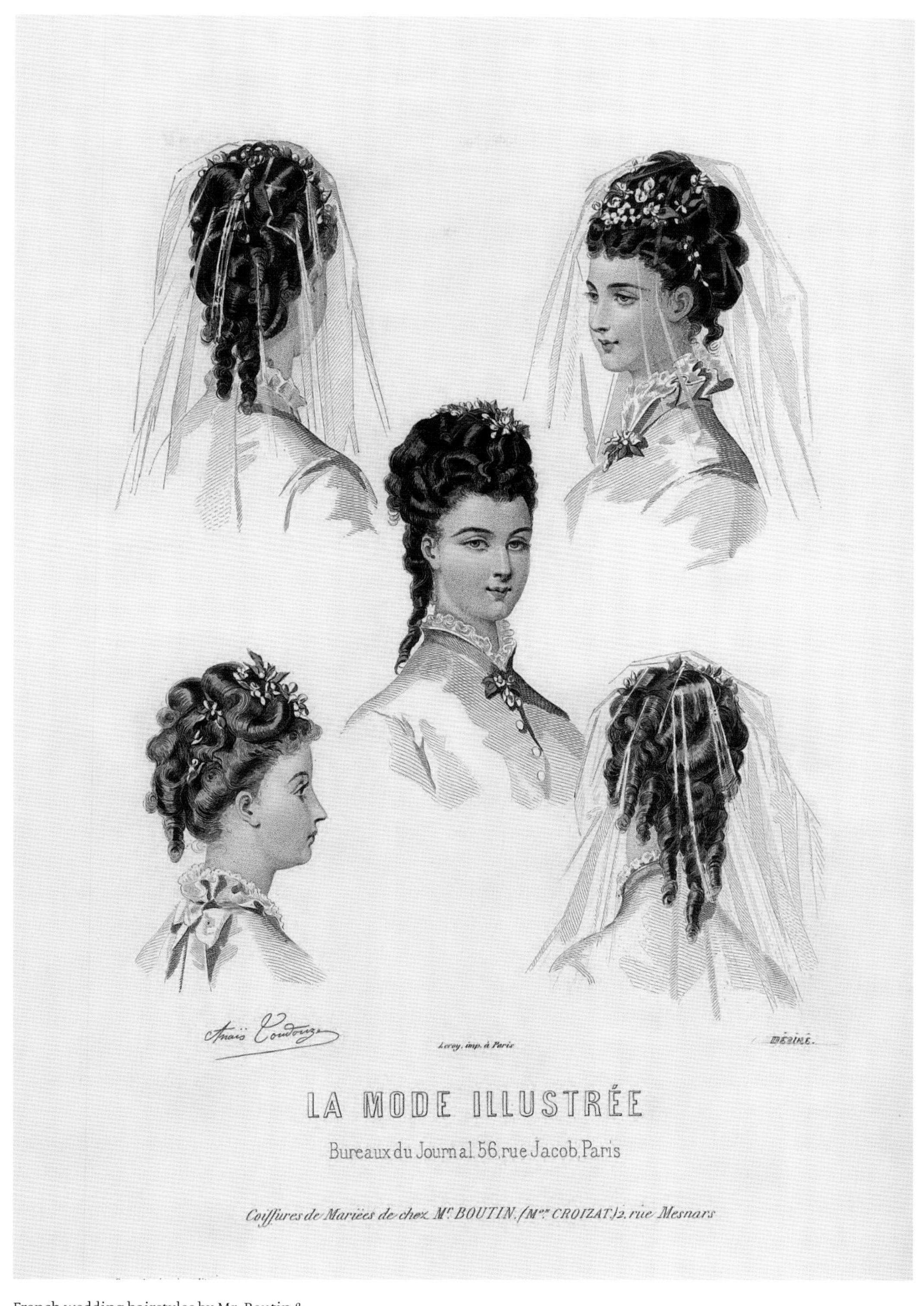

French wedding hairstyles by Mr. Boutin & Mr. Croizat, 1874, *La Mode Illustrée*

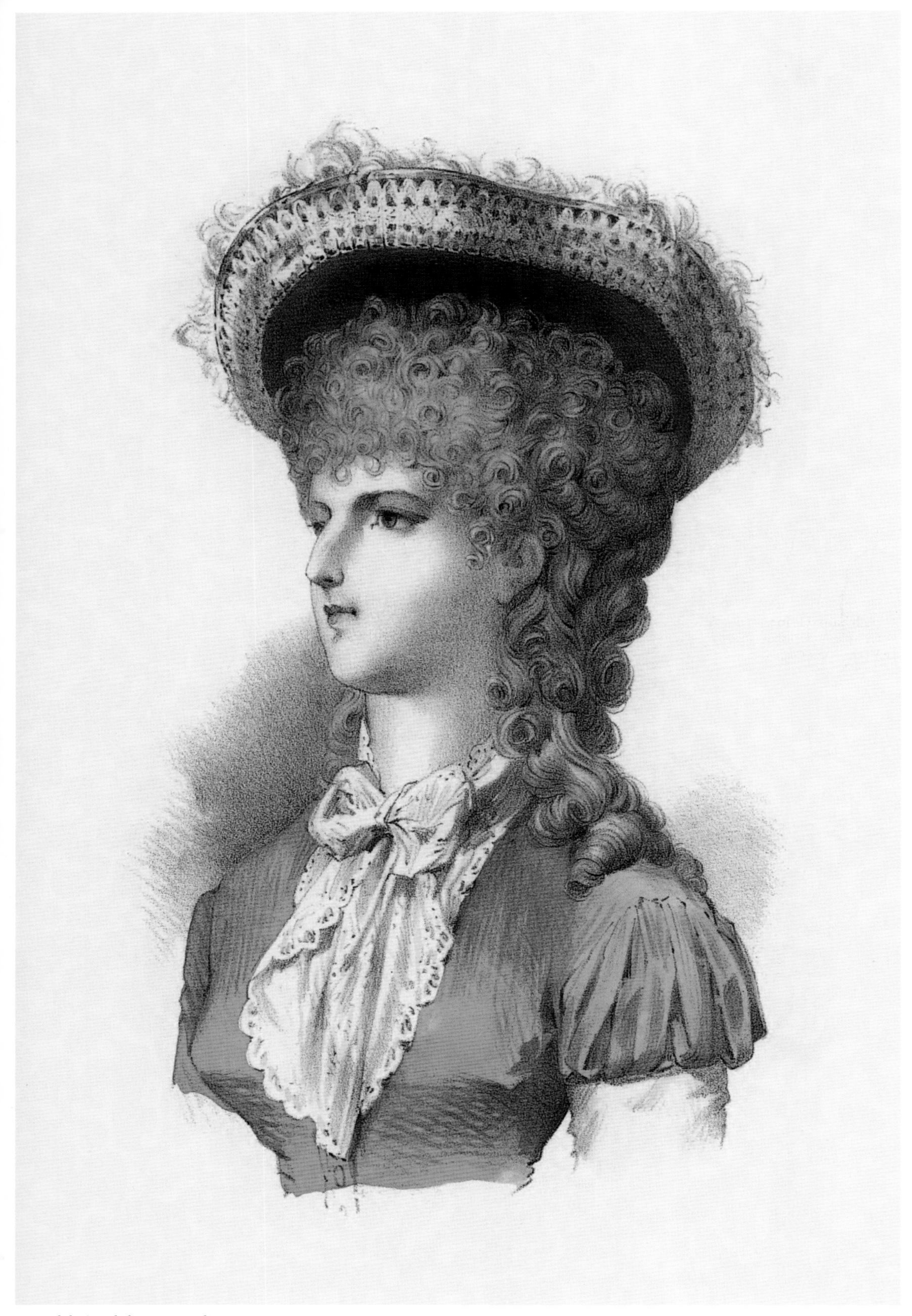

French hairstyle by Mr. Gourdeau, 1889, *Le Moniteur de la Coiffure*

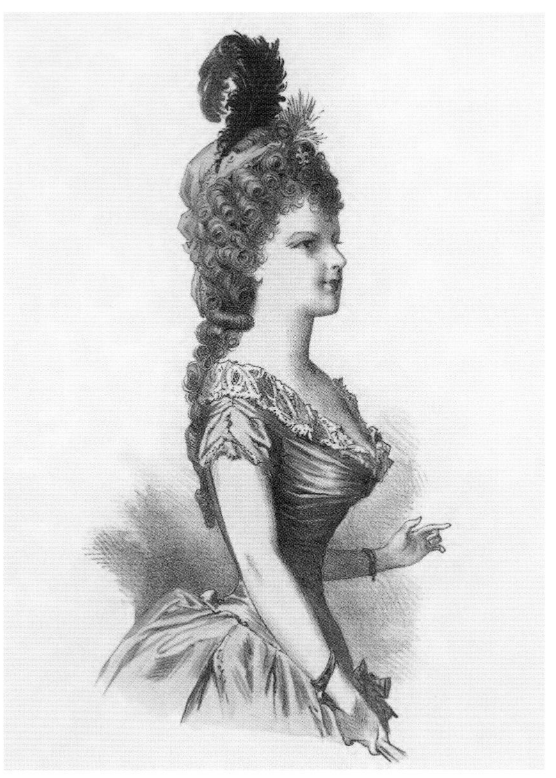

French hairstyle in the Directoire manner by Mr. Dubourg, 1890, *Le Moniteur de la Coiffure*

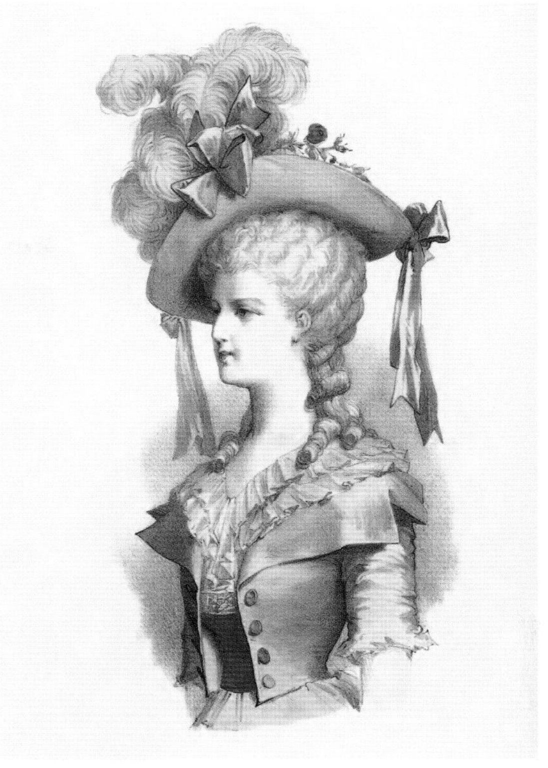

French hairstyle by Mr. Auguste Petit, 1889, *Le Moniteur de la Coiffure*

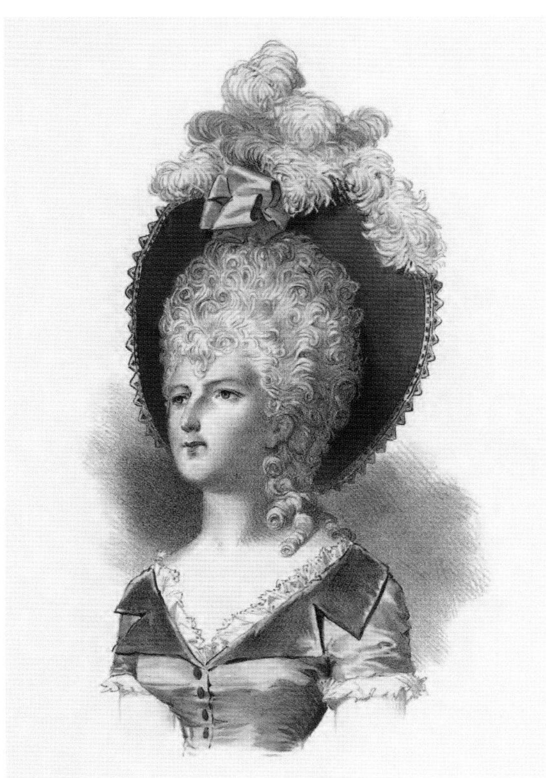

French hairstyle by Mr. Rey, 1889, *Le Moniteur de la Coiffure*

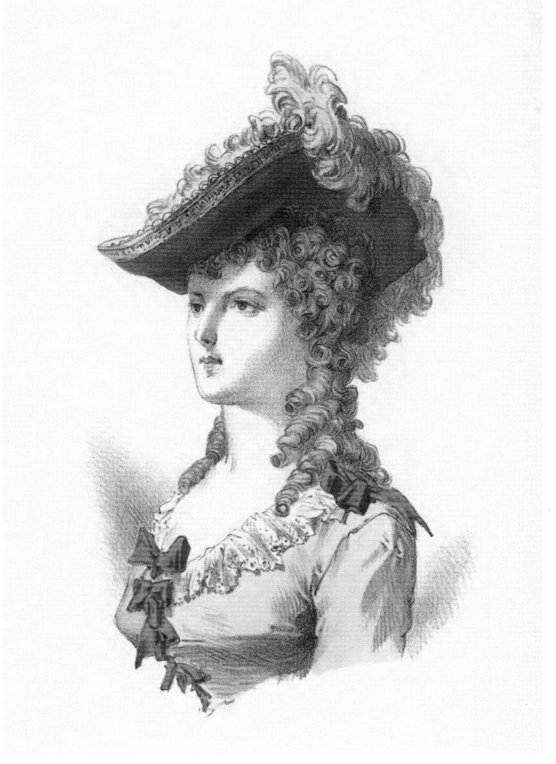

French hairstyle in the style of Louis XIV by Mr. Raoul, 1890, *Le Moniteur de la Coiffure*

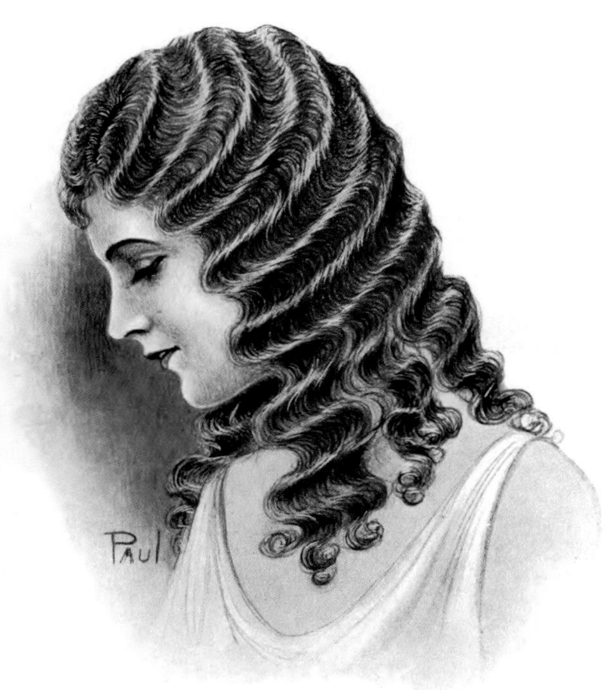

'Marcel Wave – A wave by Marcel at his best', 1880s, *The Art and Craft of Hairdressing*, Gilbert A. Foan

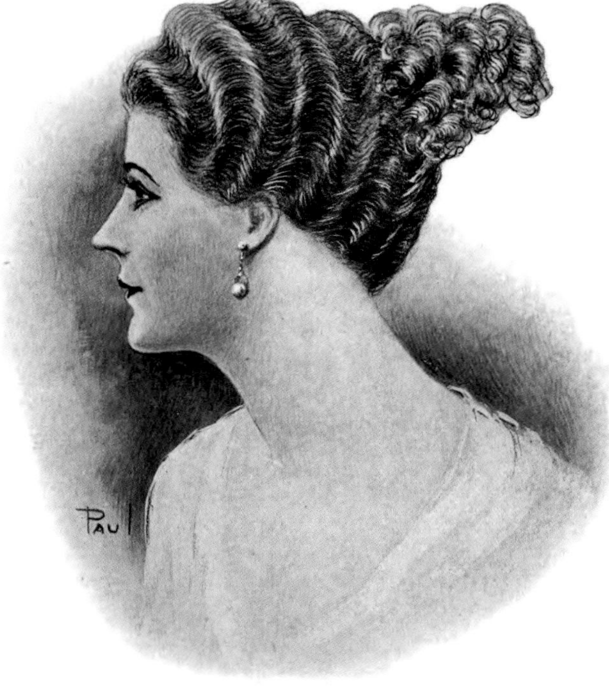

'Greek Dressing with Marcel Wave', 1890, *The Art and Craft of Hairdressing*, Gilbert A. Foan

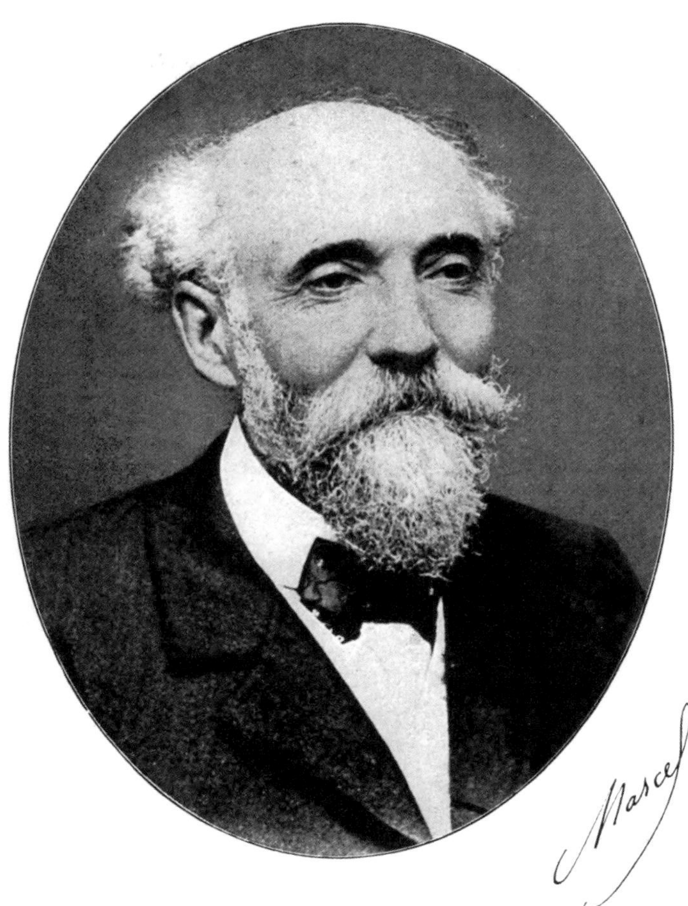

ortrait of Marcel (The celebrated
reator of the wave that bears his
name), 1890s

Marcel waving (original
method), 1880s, *The Art and Craft
f Hairdressing*, Gilbert A. Foan

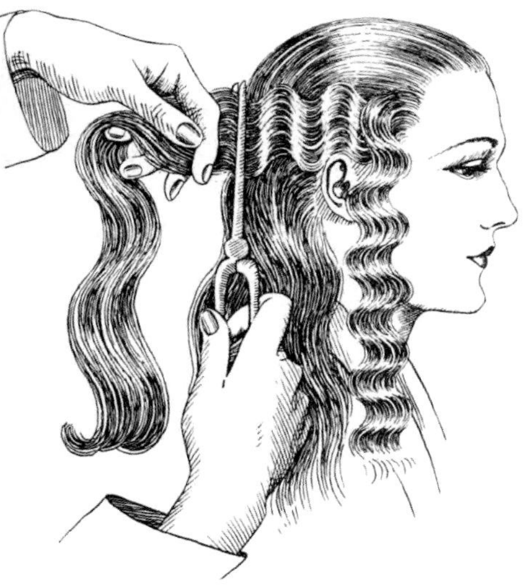

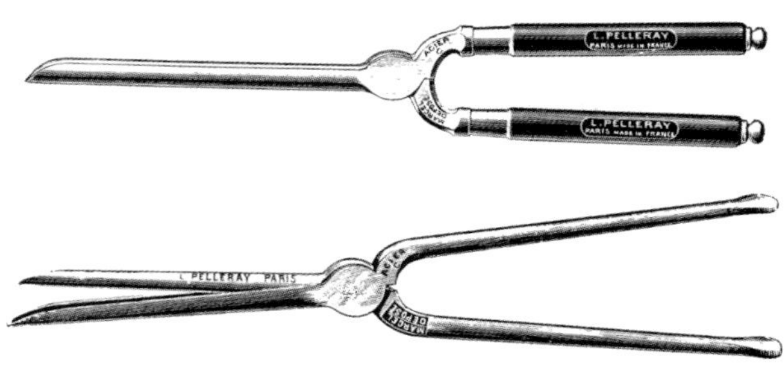

Types of irons used for
Marcel waving, 1880s

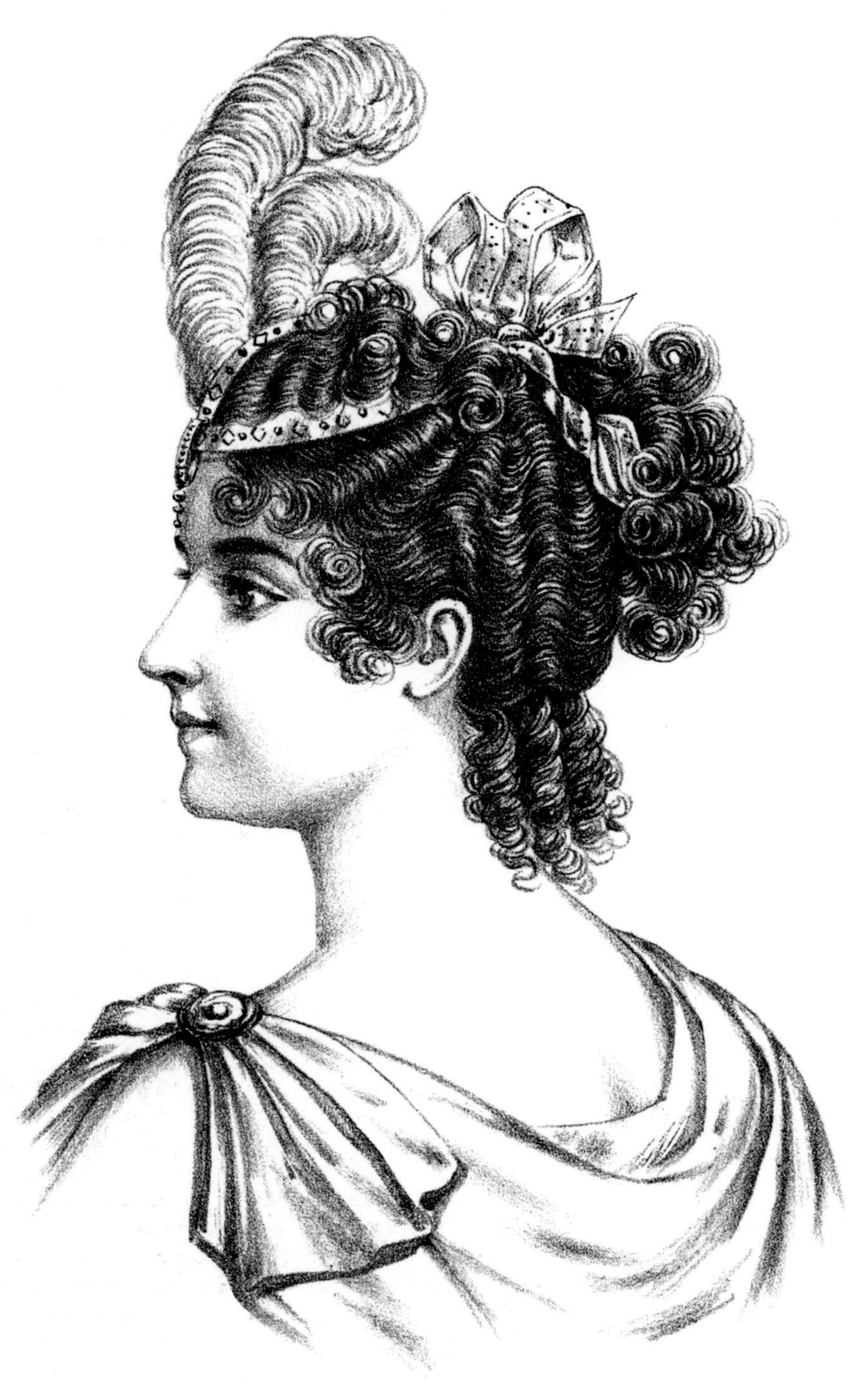

'Ancient Greek' fantasy hairstyle, c.1890, *Album Historischer und Phantasie-Frisuren*, Heinrich Moritz

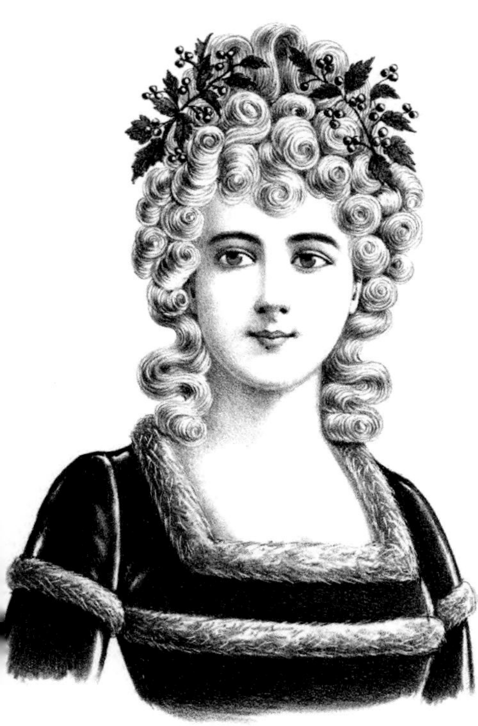

'inter' fantasy hairstyle, .890, *Album Historischer und ıntasie-Frisuren*, Heinrich Moritz

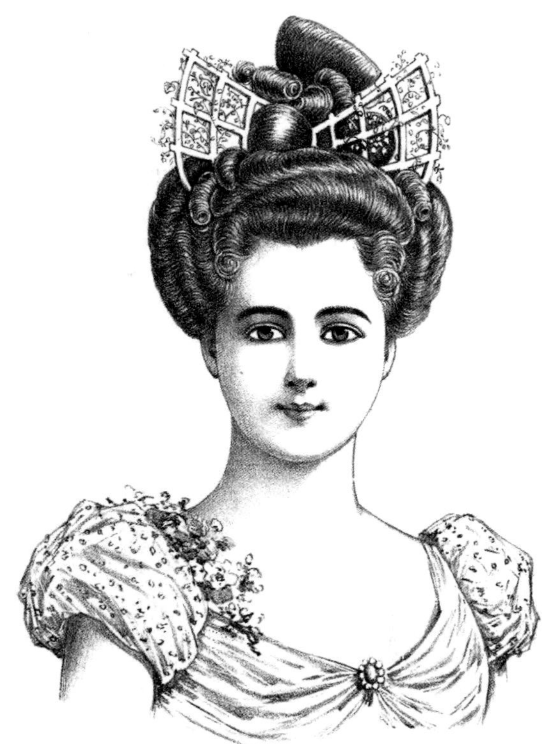

'Spring' fantasy hairstyle, c.1890, *Album Historischer und Phantasie-Frisuren*, Heinrich Moritz

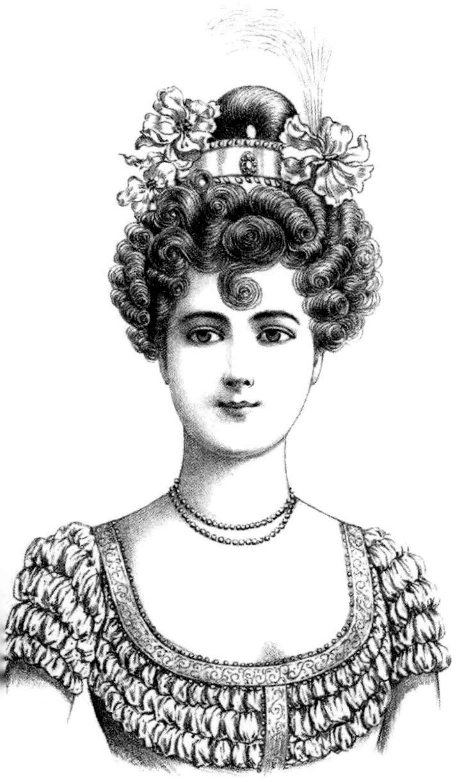

ımmer' fantasy hairstyle, ı890, *Album Historischer und ıntasie-Frisuren*, Heinrich Moritz

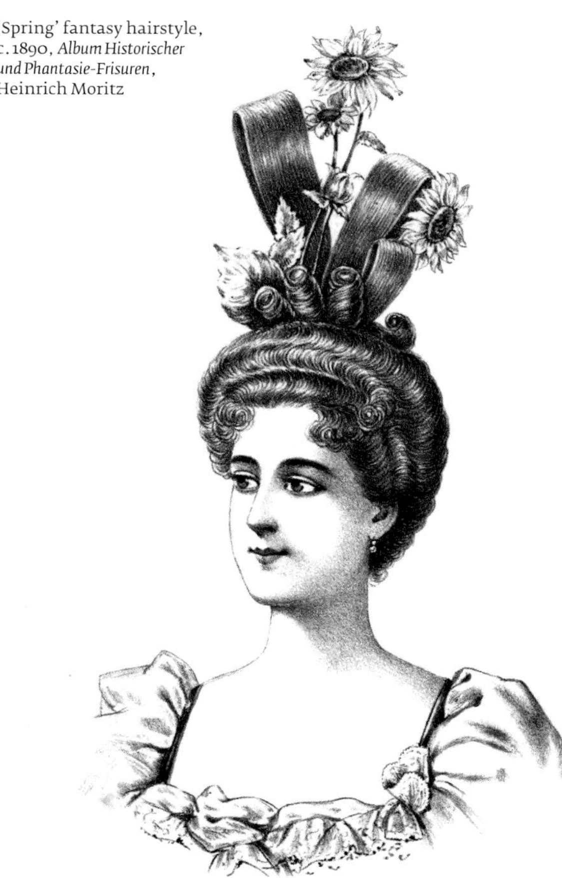

'Autumn' fantasy hairstyle, c.1890, *Album Historischer und Phantasie-Frisuren*, Heinrich Moritz

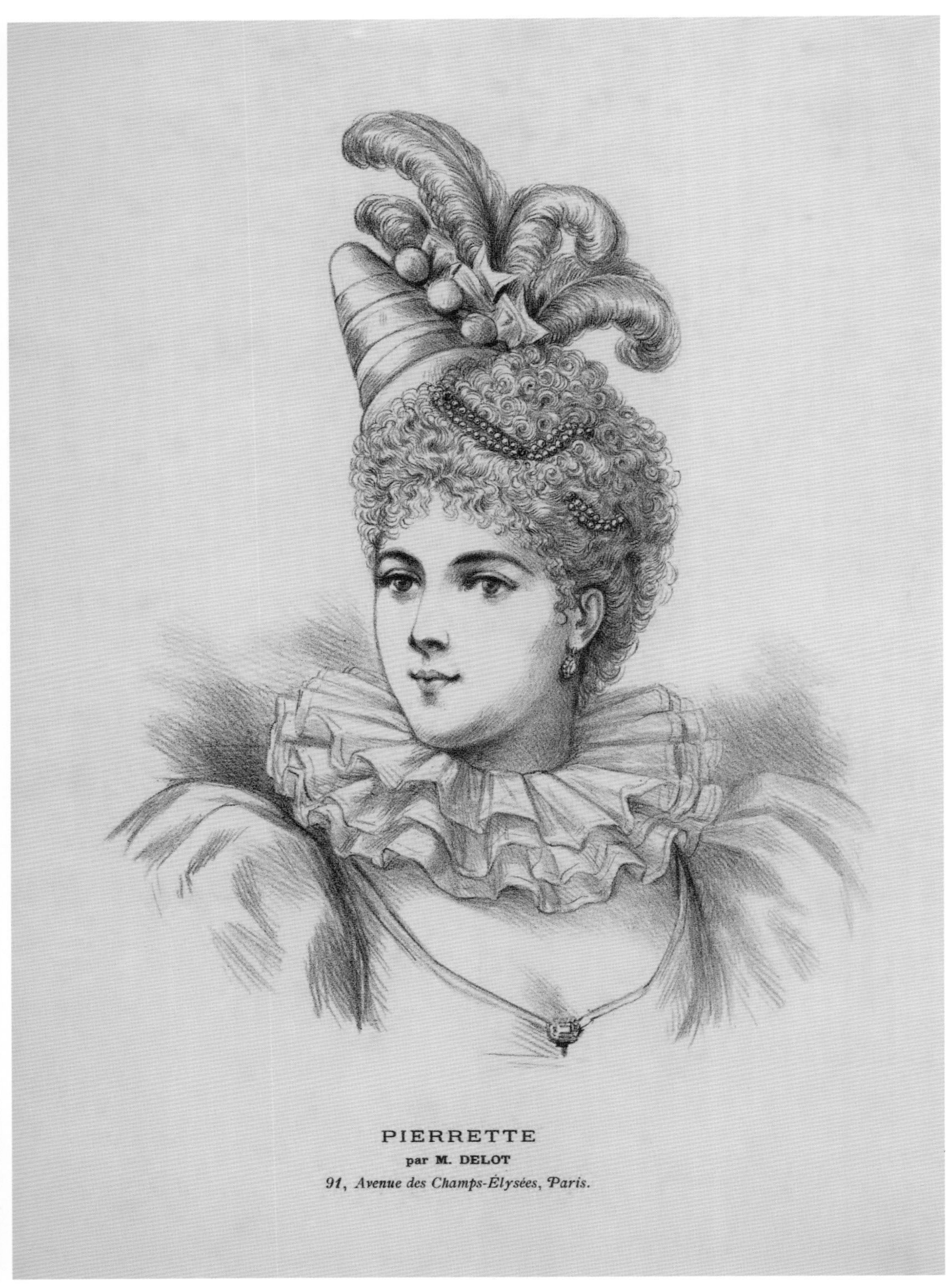

'Pierrette' hairstyle by Mr. Delot, Paris, c. 1894, *L'Art dans la Coiffure*, J. Caumont

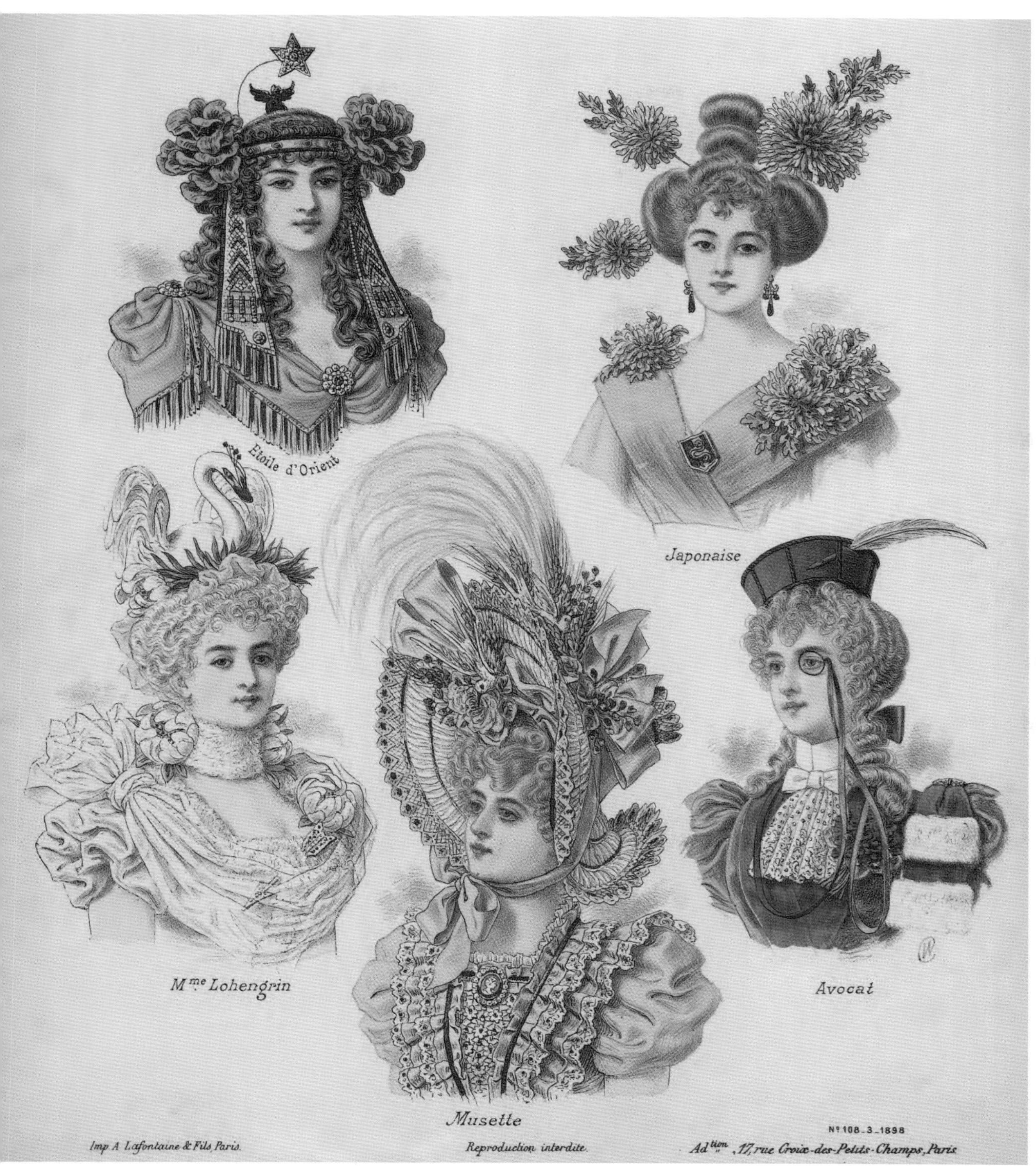

ench theatrical hairstyles, 'Etoile d'Orient', 'Japonaise',
vocat', 'Musette', 'Mme. Lohengrin', 1898, *La Coiffure Française*

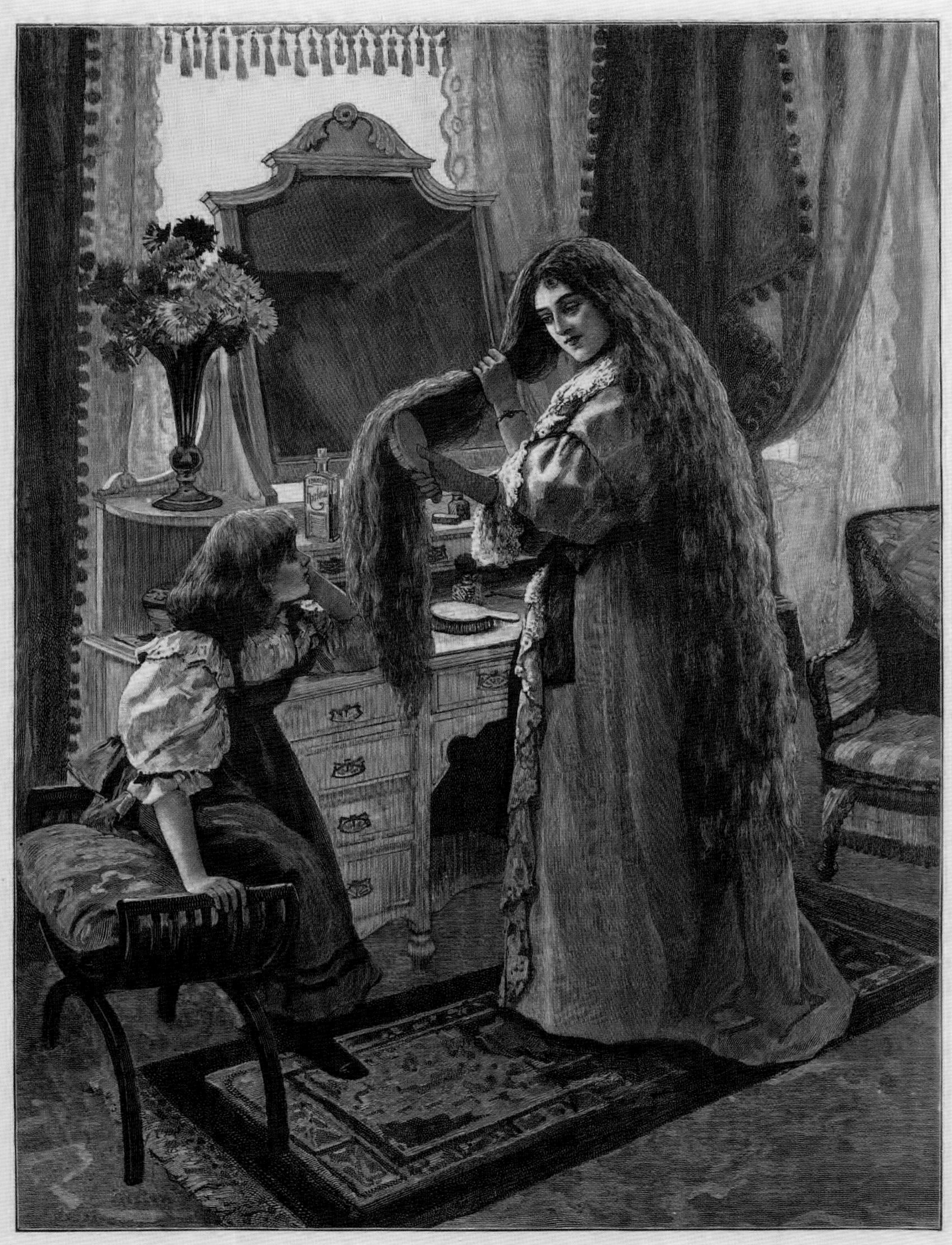

"Mamma, shall I have beautiful long hair like you when I grow up?"
"Certainly, my dear, if you use Edwards' 'Harlene.'"

Advertisement for Edwards' 'Harlene' hair product, 1895, *The Illustrated London News*

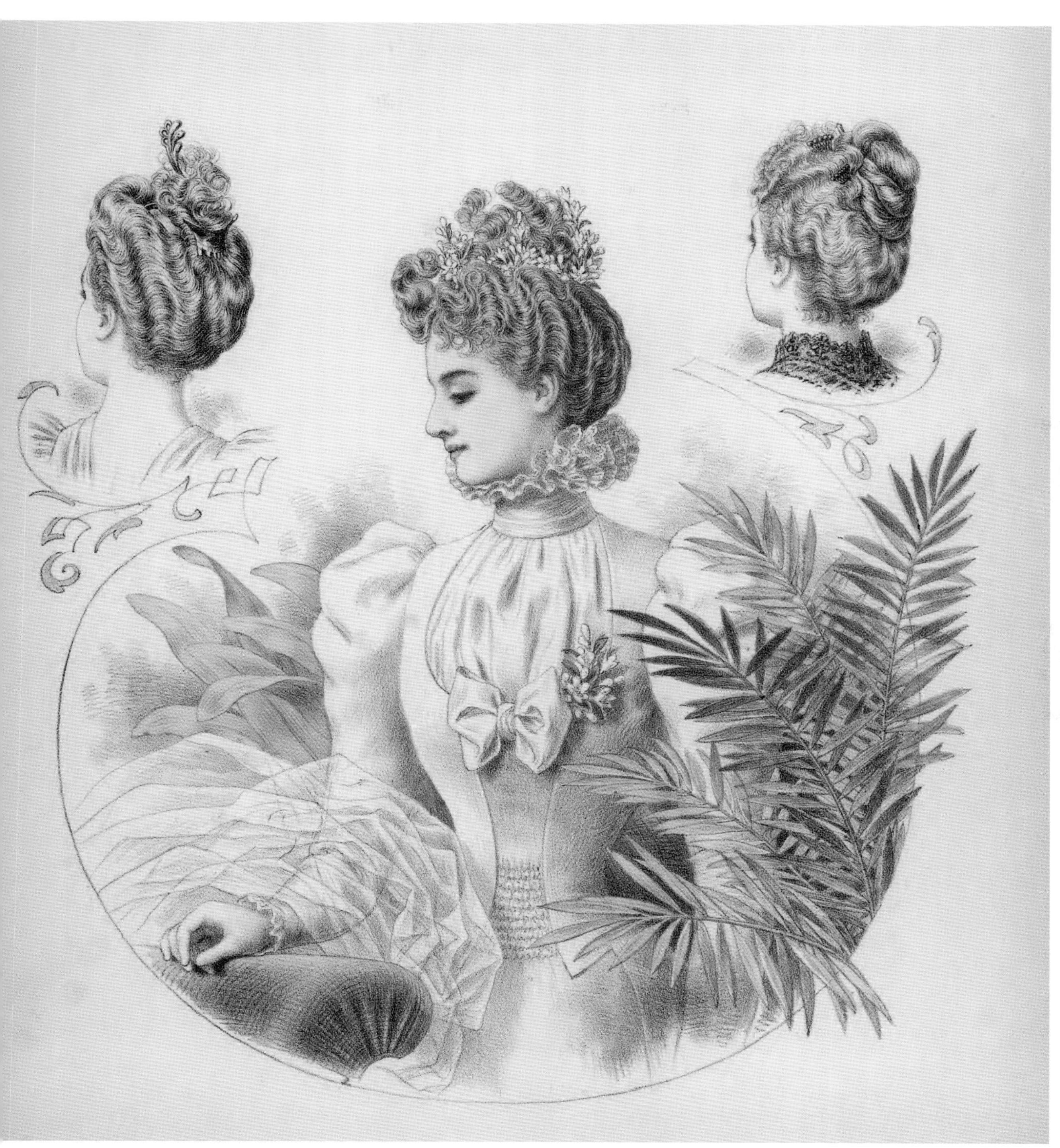

rench hairstyle, 1897,
e Coiffure Française

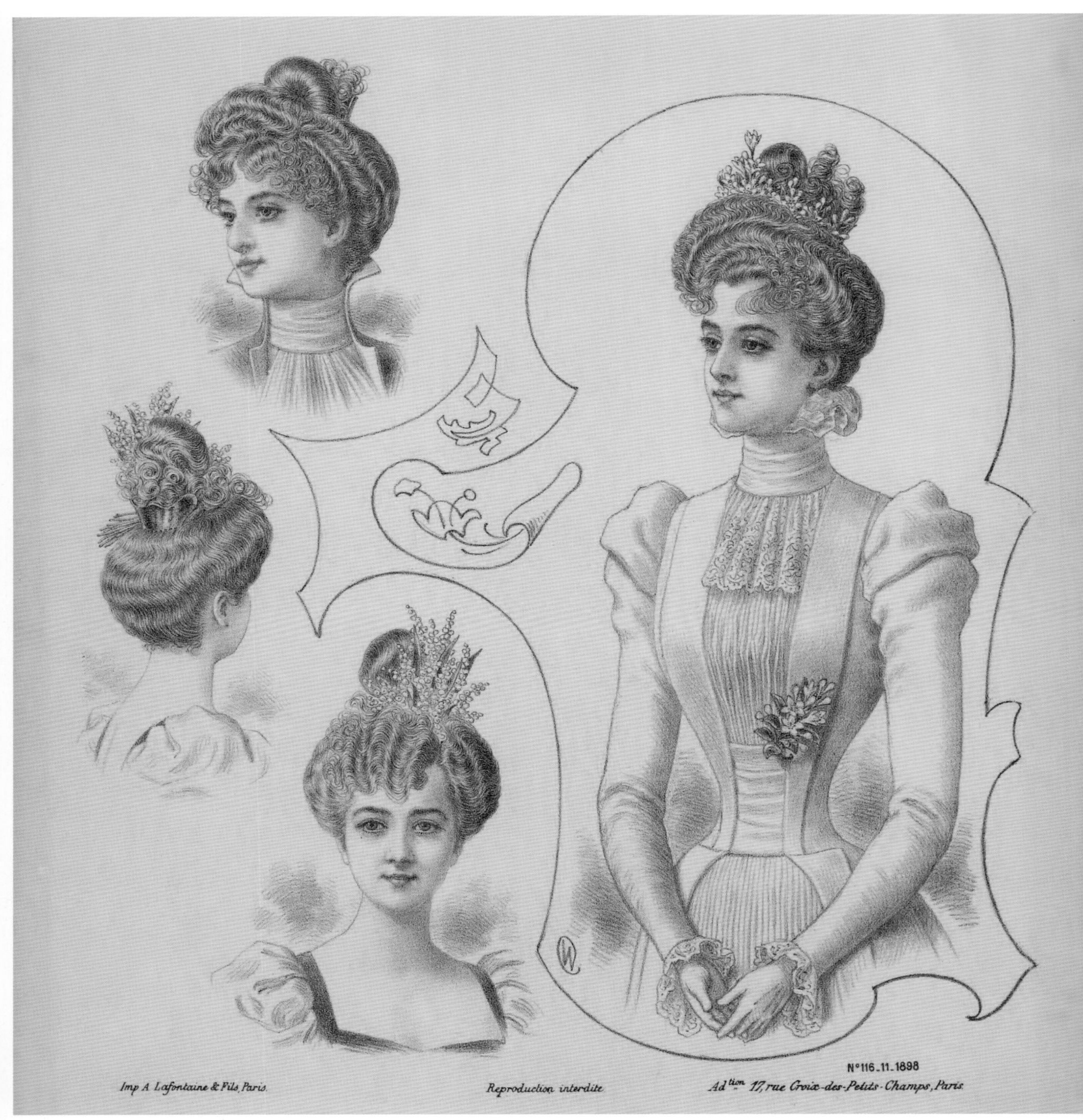

French hairstyles, 1898,
La Coiffure Française

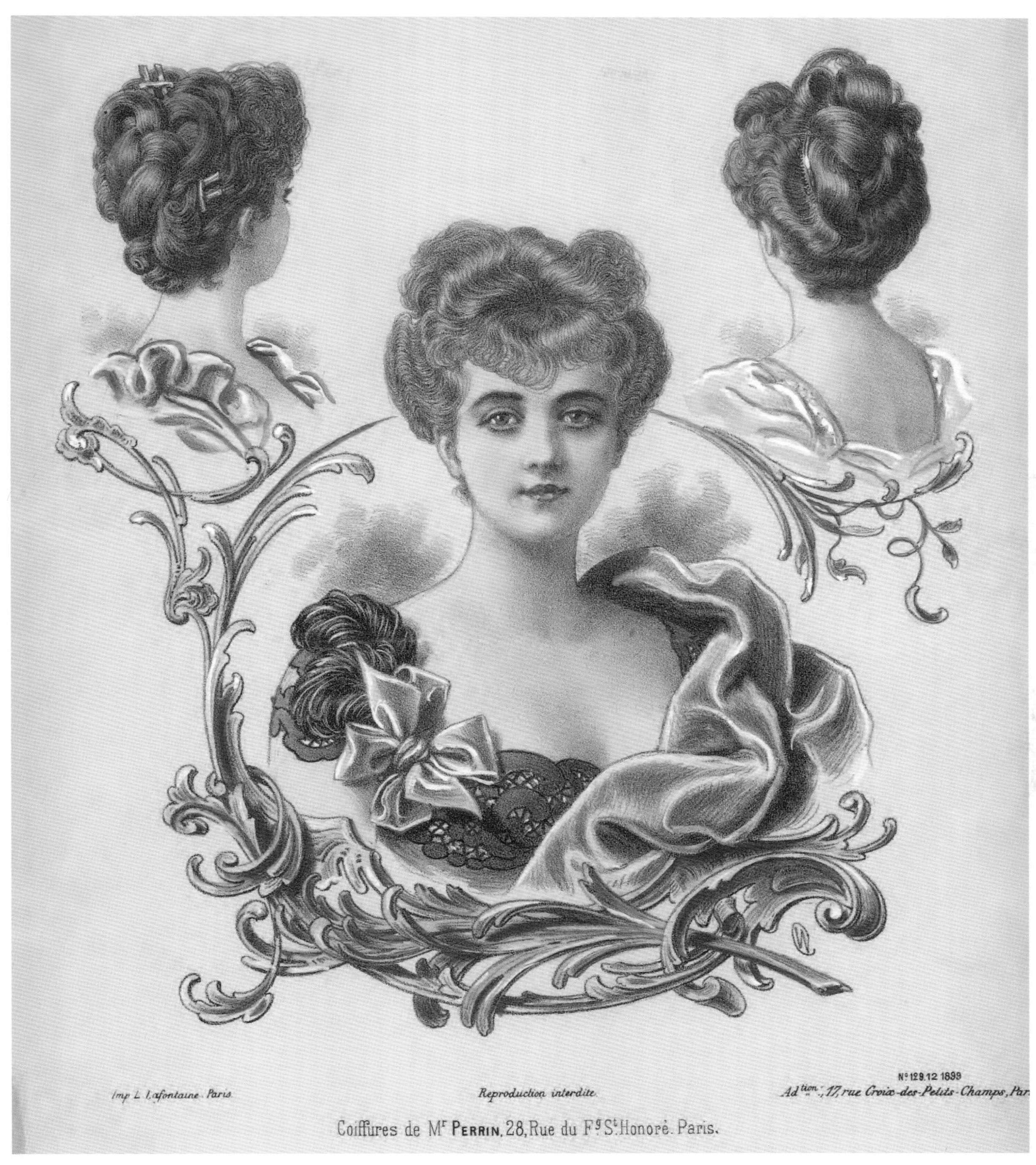

French hairstyles by Mr. Perrin, 1899, *Coiffure Française Illustrée*

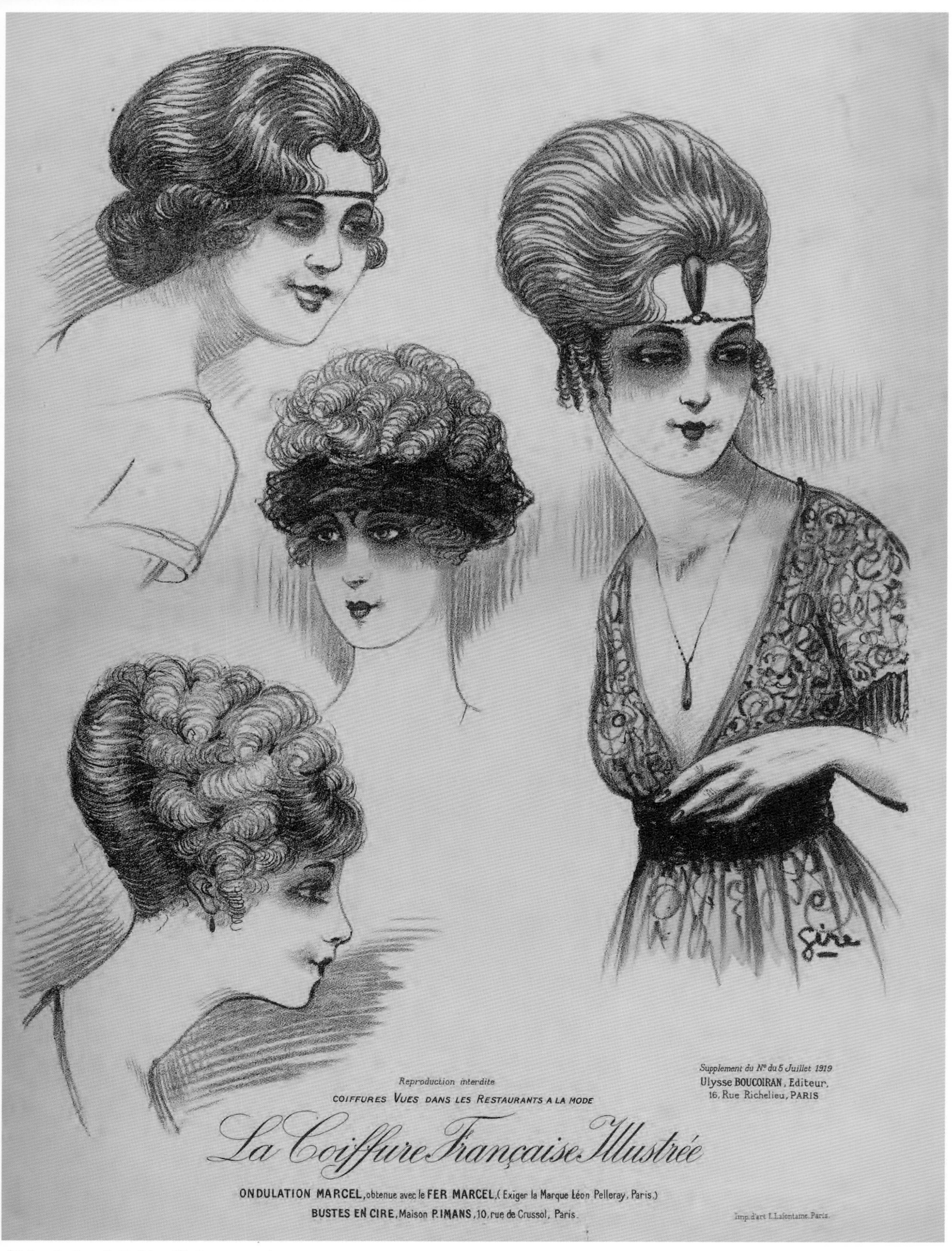

'Hairstyles Seen in Fashionable Restaurants', 1919, *La Coiffure Française Illustrée*

1900S, 1910S

In 1900 *The Strand Magazine* published an article titled "The Magic of Hairdressing" penned by Florence Burnley and Kathleen Schlesinger that noted, "If manners make the man, then surely hair makes the woman outwardly at least. The hairdresser is the wizard who with magic touch transforms woman." Certainly in the early years of the 20th century hairdressers continued to perform coiffured wizardry on their more than willing clients. Initially the fashion during the early Edwardian period was for seriously big hair, with naturally long hair being supplemented with postiches (small wiglets), false buns and pads to give a sense of quantity and mass. Unlike in Victorian times, the hair was made to look soft and full, an effect that was achieved through substantial backcombing. A product commonly known as a "Transformation" which was introduced in 1902 was also employed to create this new voluminous look – it was essentially a domed frame made from natural hair that acted as a base upon which the hair at the back of the head could be built up over. The front hair was normally dressed over pads to give a pompadour or loose puff look, while the hair on the back of the head was swept upwards and held in place over a "Transformation" with tortoiseshell combs and hairpins. Often highly decorated hair clasps and combs or feathers were worn, especially in the evenings, to further embellish a lady's coiffure.

In 1905, a new type of postiche began to be sold, which was a shaped band of hair that fitted over the forehead and which could be dressed in with the wearer's own natural hair. It was, however, a young French chemist, Eugène Schueller who would perhaps have the most lasting effect on hairdressing when, in 1907 he formulated a new hair-colour dye, which he christened Auréale. Two years later he registered his new company, the "Société Française de Teintures Inoffensives pour Cheveux", which would eventually become L'Oréal. A natural entrepreneur, the young Schueller was also on the editorial team of *La Coiffure de Paris* magazine (founded in 1909), and contributed to its science column, where he suggested for the first time that patch tests should be carried out before colouring hair. He also established in 1910 his own hair-colouring school in the Rue de Louvre, Paris, having recruited a hairdresser from the Russian court. Schueller used the school to give practical demonstrations of his new dyes in order to persuade other hairdressers to use his products. Importantly, L'Oréal dyes were longer-lasting and safer to use and, unlike earlier colourants, were not associated with hair loss.

By around 1910 there was a stylistic swing away from waved hair, and in its place new coiffures took hold that were characterised by a general flatness on the top of the head and the introduction of wide bandeau. In 1913 there was another distinctive shift in hair fashions with hair worn relatively full and then wrapped around the back of the head, terminating high on the crown. This style continued to enjoy popularity throughout the First World War although with many women carrying out essential war-work, big hair was something of an anachronism – it was not really practical for working in a factory environment. Another style that was to emerge during this period was the "Bob", first created in 1909 by Antoine de Paris when he chopped the French actress Eve Lavallière's hair short to make her look younger for a stage role. In 1913, the celebrated ballroom dancer and silent screen film star Irene Castle frustrated by hairpins falling out when she was vigorously dancing began wearing her hair in a similar blunt cut, which quickly become known as the "Castle Bob".

During this time the renowned couturier Paul Poiret also helped to make shingled bobs fashionable, as did Coco Chanel. In 1917, prior to going out Chanel singed her hair badly, but in her indomitable style instead of forgoing an evening of entertainment, she just chopped her remaining hair into her famous and highly influential straight bob. Although short bobs were occasionally worn by stylistically progressive women during the late 1910s, the vast majority of ladies opted for something much less daring and preferred their front of their hair set into tight waves or curls, while the hair on the back of their heads was worn relatively high with often Spanish-style fan-shaped mantilla combs used to complete the overall look.

The First World War wrought huge social, political, economic, and intellectual changes in Europe and the United States. Known as "the war to end all wars", it also produced a seismic shift in gender politics. During the war years, women had worked as nurses in the Armed Services, factory workers on the home front, or just held the proverbial family fort while their husbands and brothers were fighting overseas, and this had a dramatic empowering effect which they were not prepared to give up once the war had ended. Throughout this period the fight for women's suffrage was at its zenith and in 1918 women in Great Britain and Germany were finally given the vote; two years later women in the United States also won this hard-fought right. This new political freedom for women would in the coming decade find expression not just in the fashions they wore but also in the new hairstyles they adopted… new hairstyles for a new era…

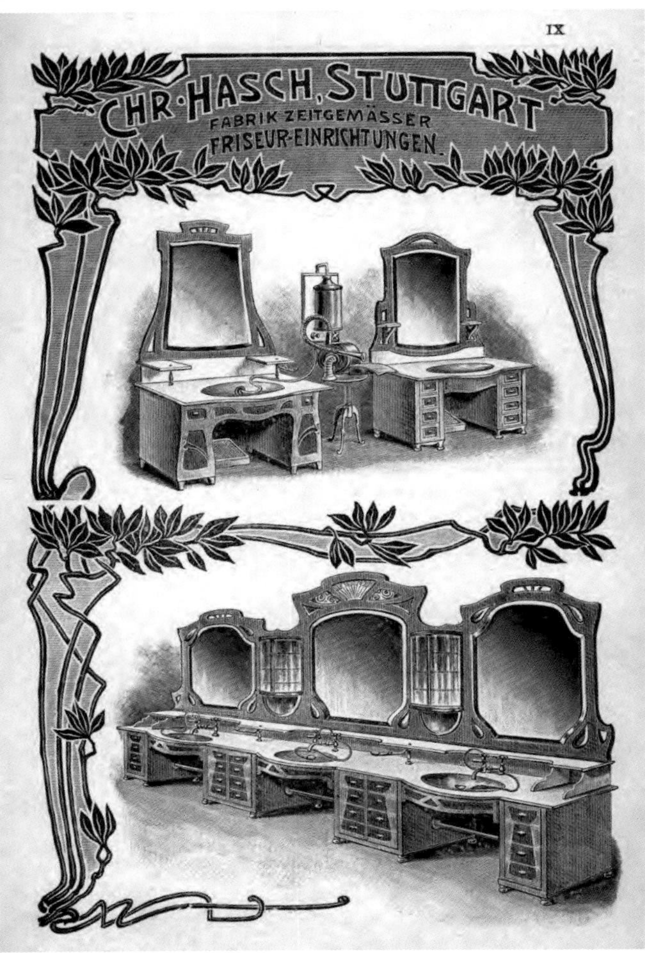

Advertisement for hair salon furnishings, Chr. Hasch of Stuttgart, c.1900

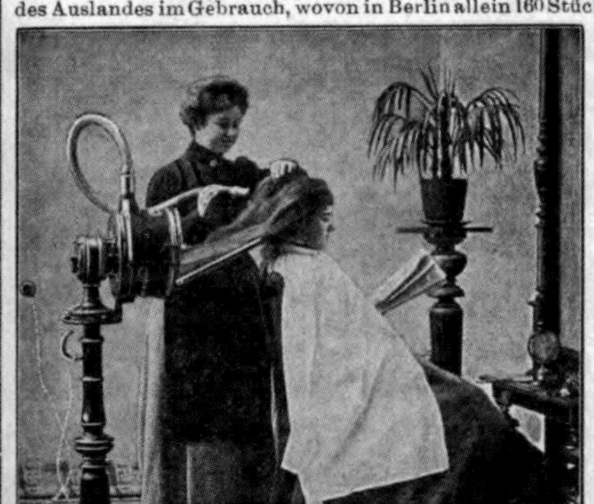

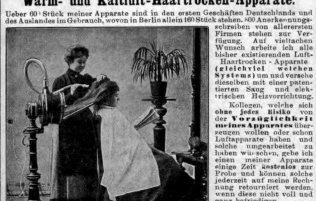

Advertisement for Jean Hornung's patented hairdryer, c.1900

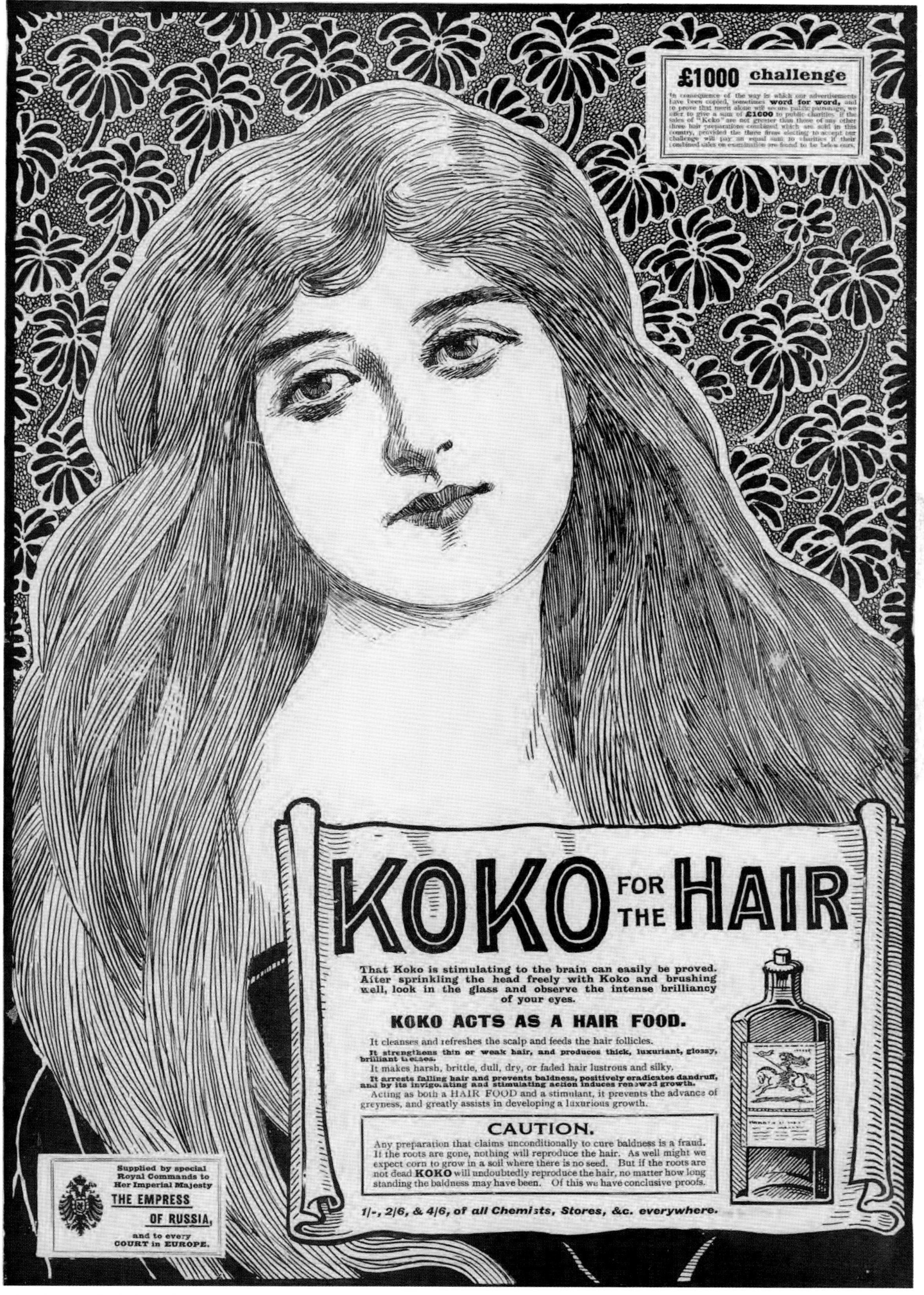

Advertisement for Koko Hair Product, 1901

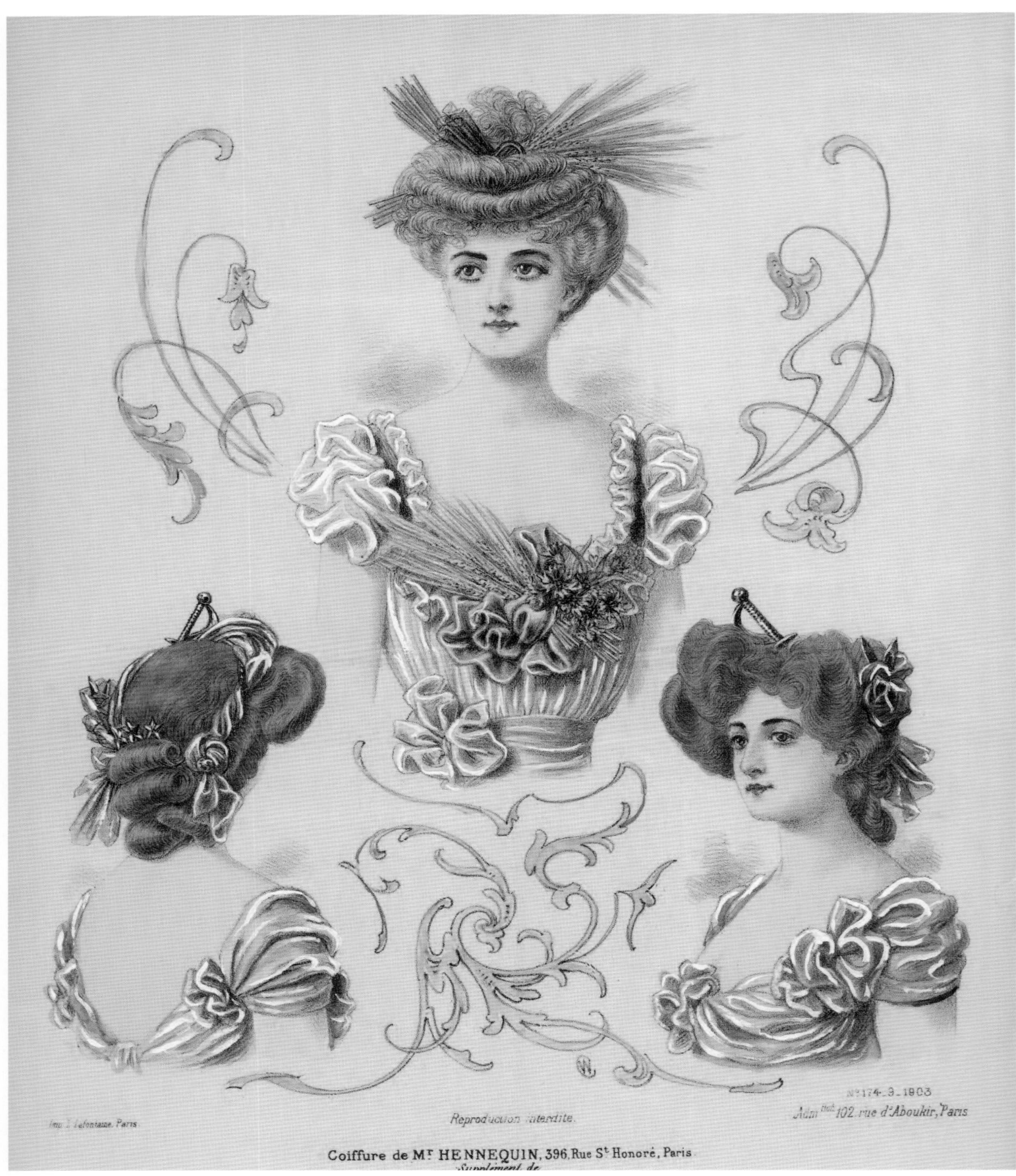

Hairstyles by Mr. Hennequin,
1903, *La Coiffure Française Illustrée*

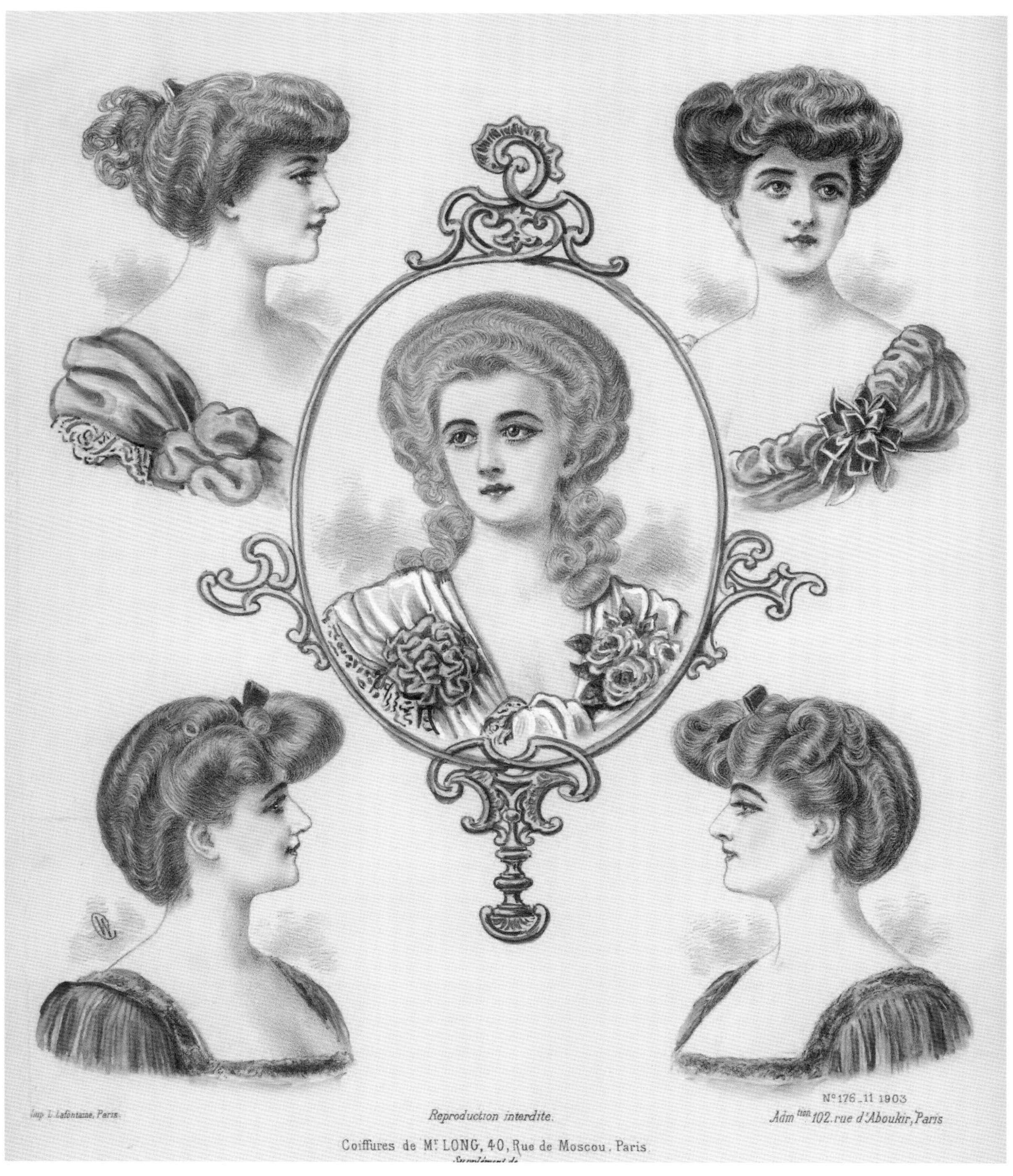

Hairstyles by Mr. Long, 1903,
La Coiffure Française Illustrée

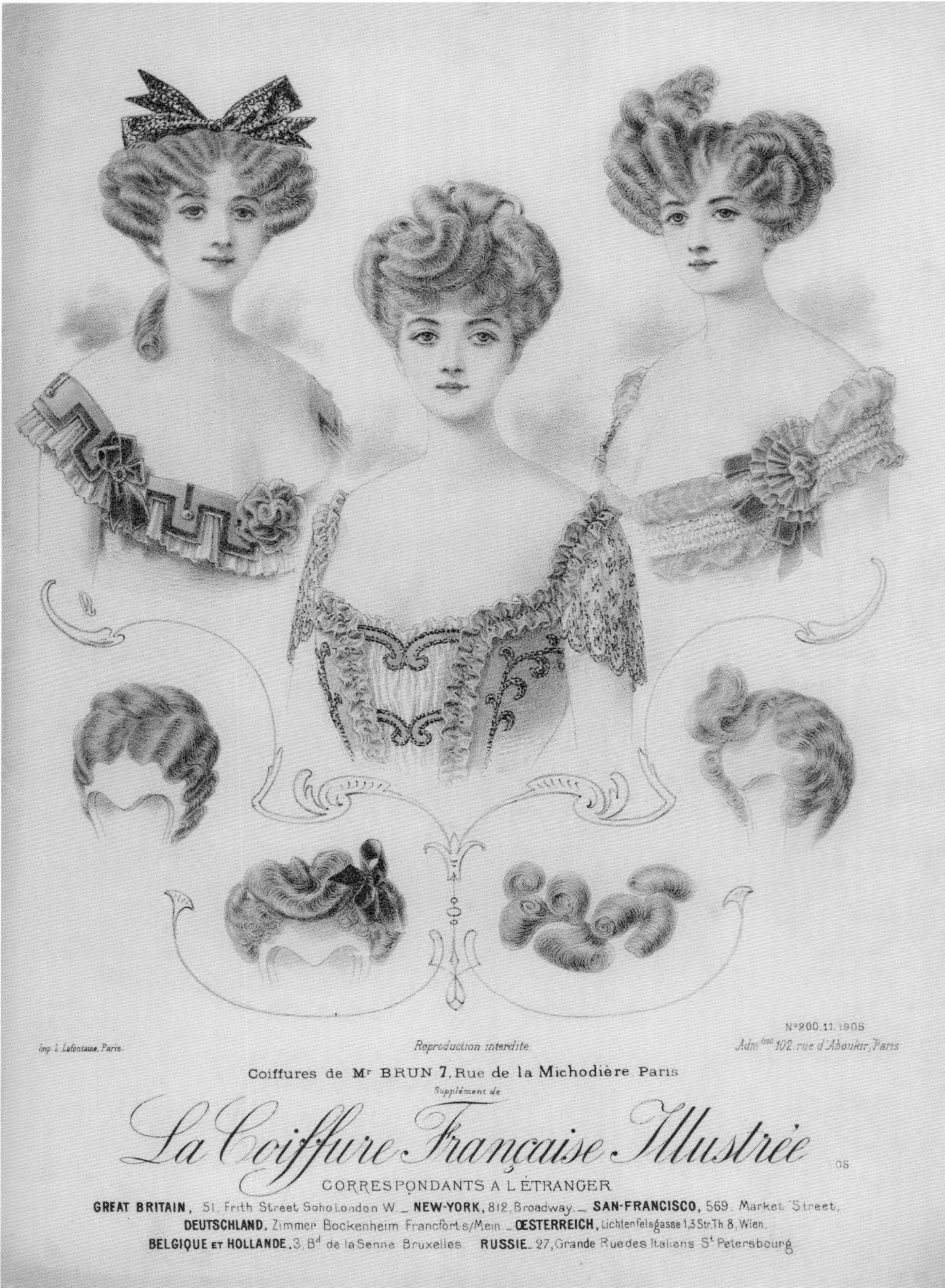

Hairstyles by Mr. Brun, 1905,
La Coiffure Française Illustrée

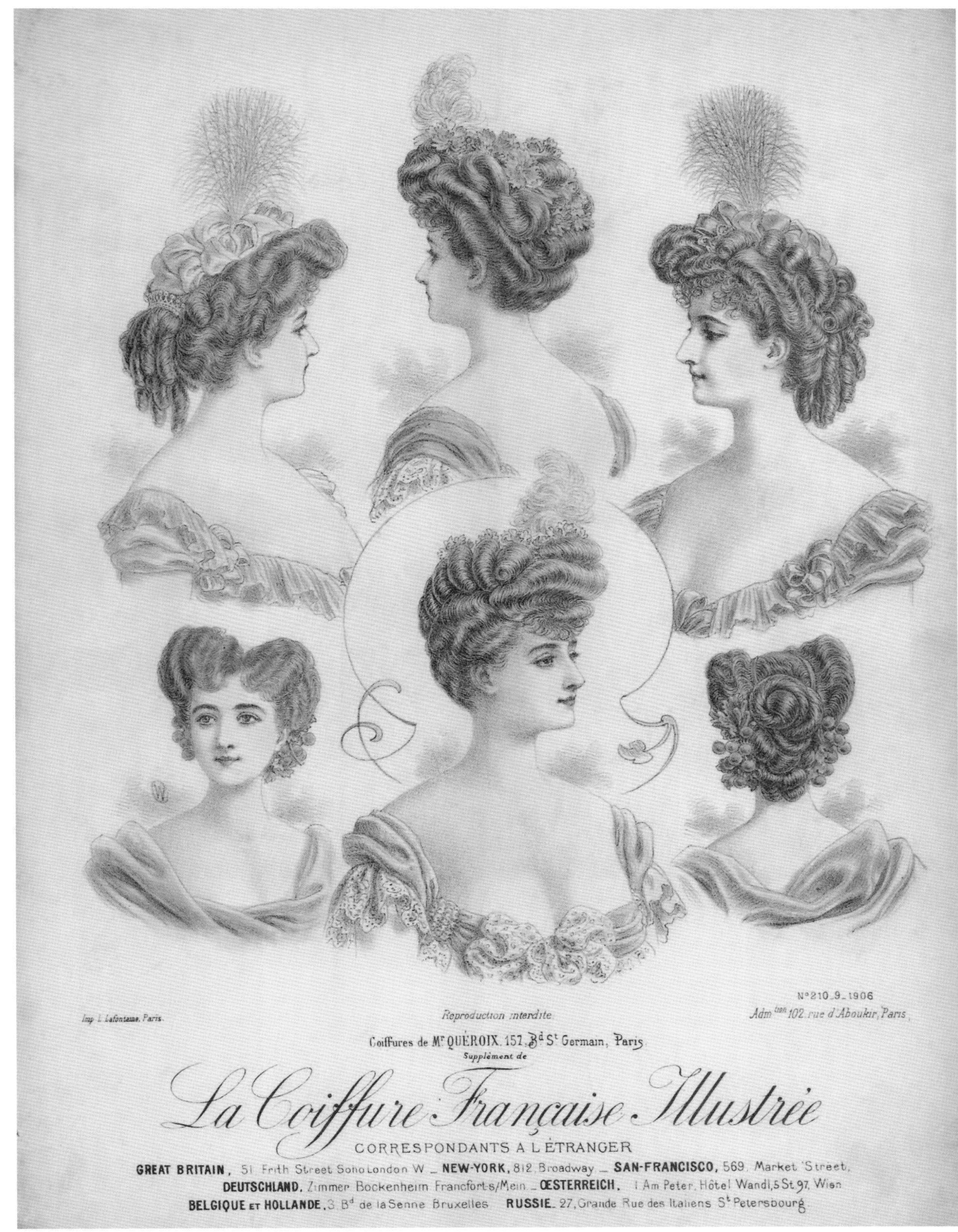

Hairstyles by Mr. Quéroix, 1906,
La Coiffure Française Illustrée

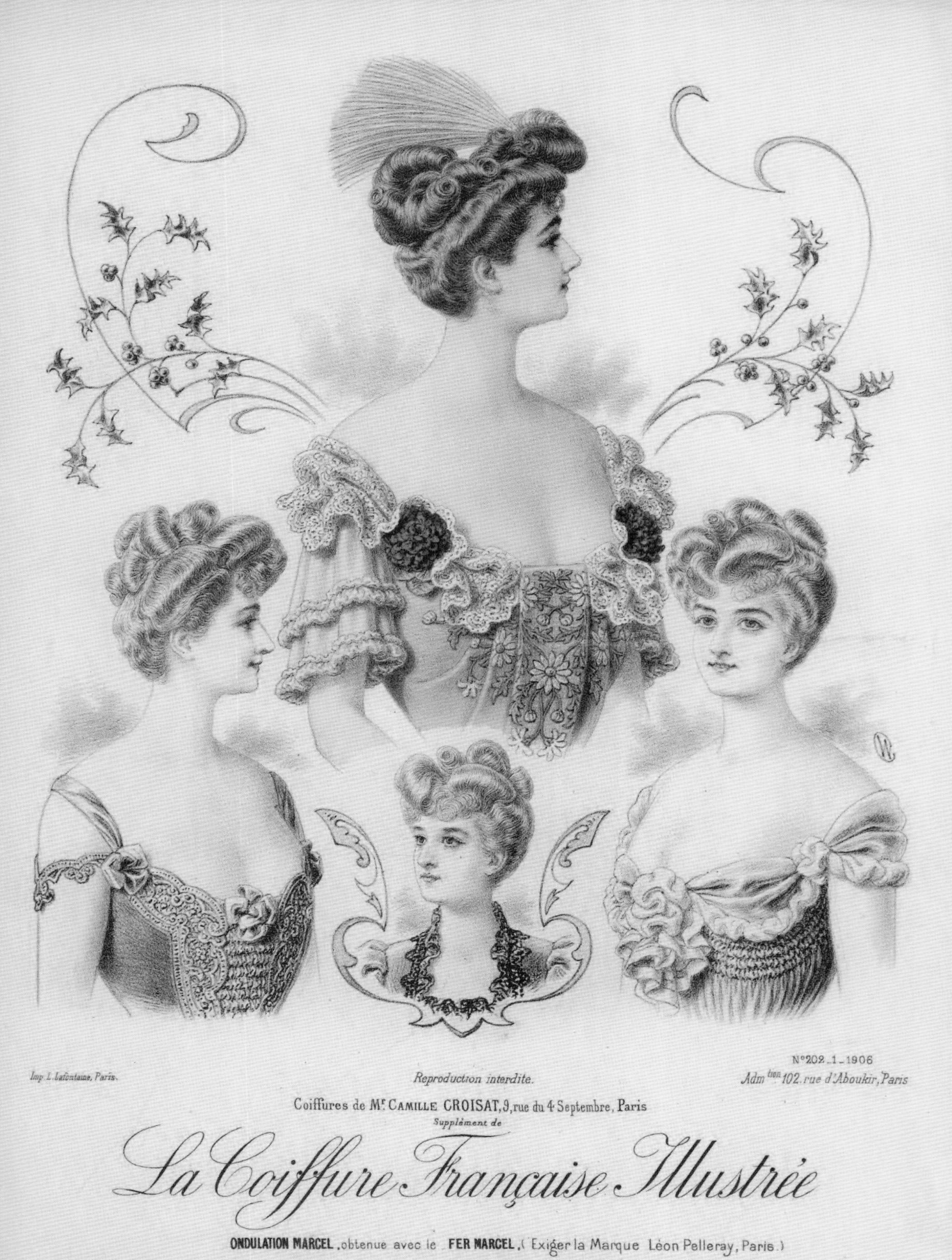

Hairstyles by Mr. Camille Croisat, 1906, *La Coiffure Française Illustrée*

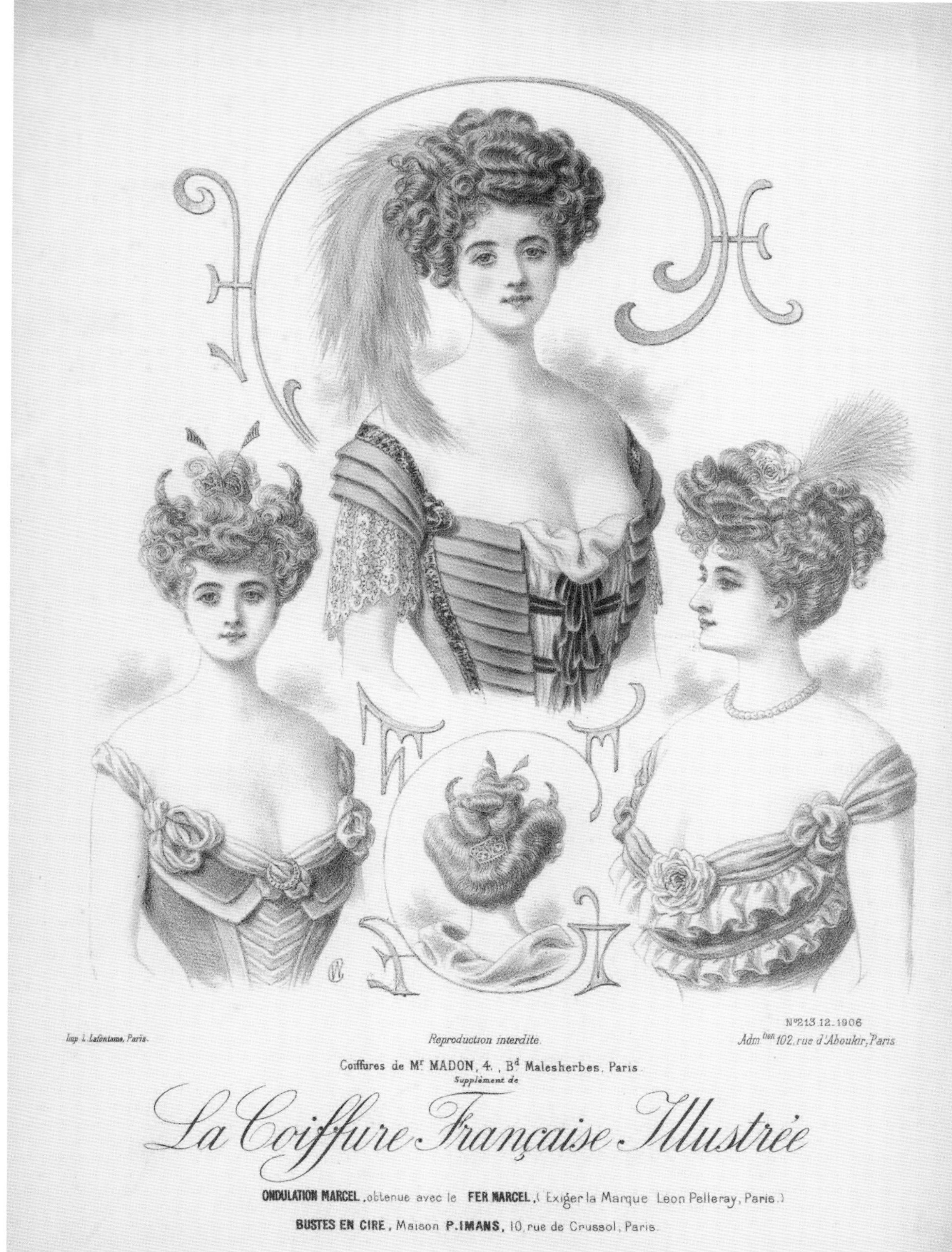

Hairstyles by Mr. Madon, 1906,
La Coiffure Française Illustrée

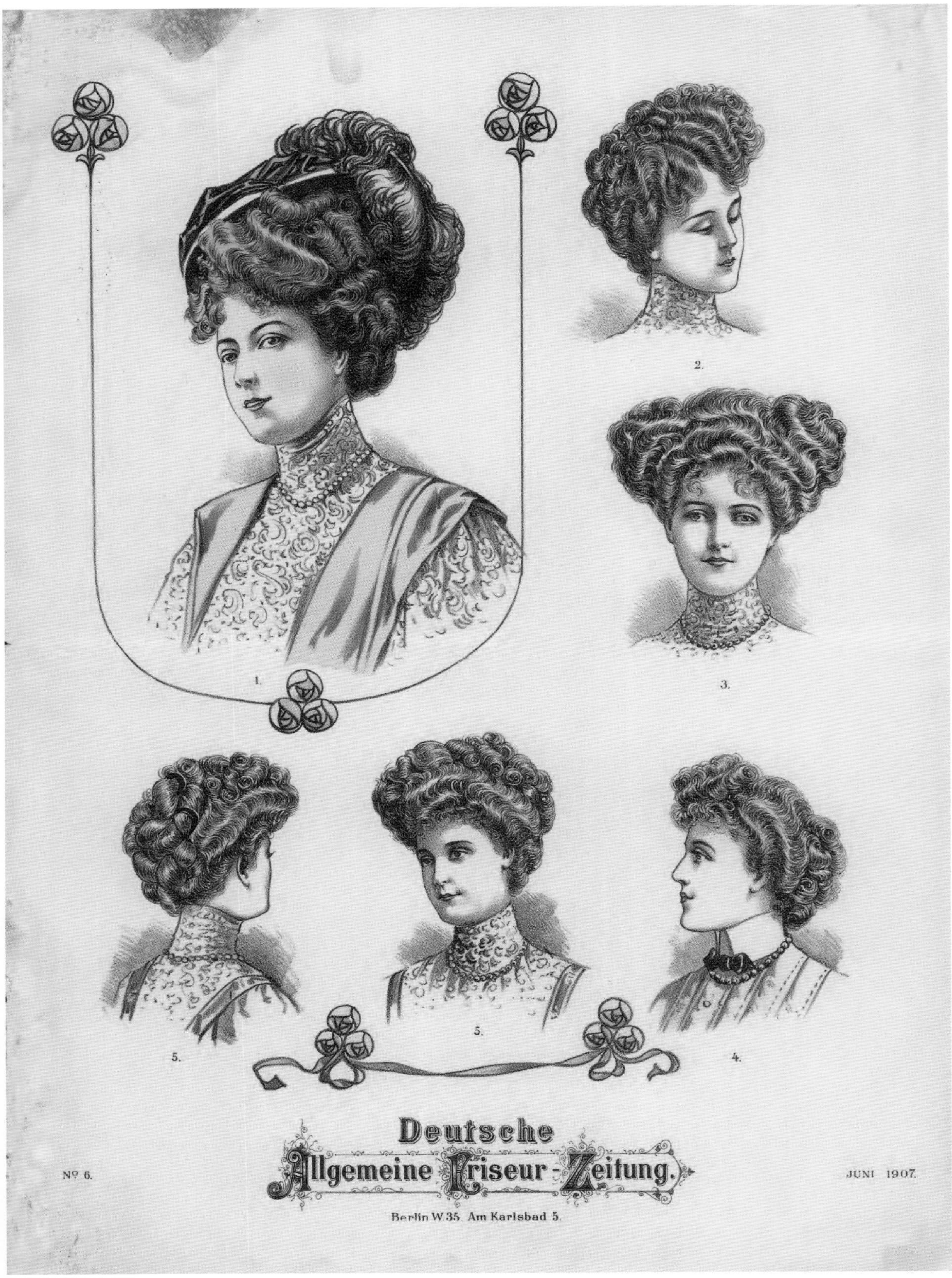

German hairstyles, June 1907,
Deutsche Allgemeine Friseur-Zeitung

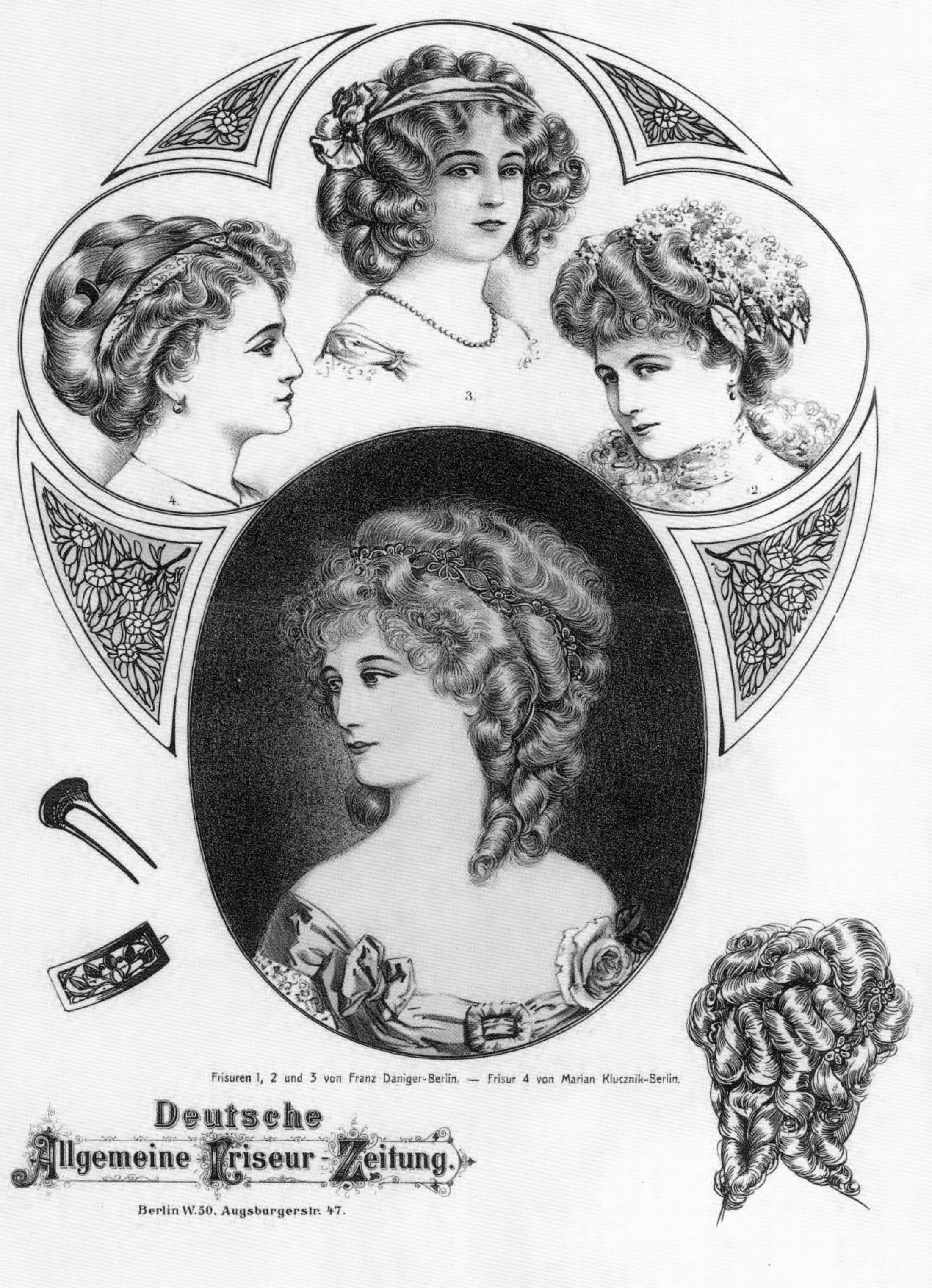
N° 4.
APRIL 1910.
3.
4.
2.
Frisuren 1, 2 und 3 von Franz Daniger-Berlin. — Frisur 4 von Marian Klucznik-Berlin.
Deutsche
Allgemeine Friseur-Zeitung.
Berlin W.50, Augsburgerstr. 47.

German hairstyles, April 1910,
Deutsche Allgemeine Friseur-Zeitung

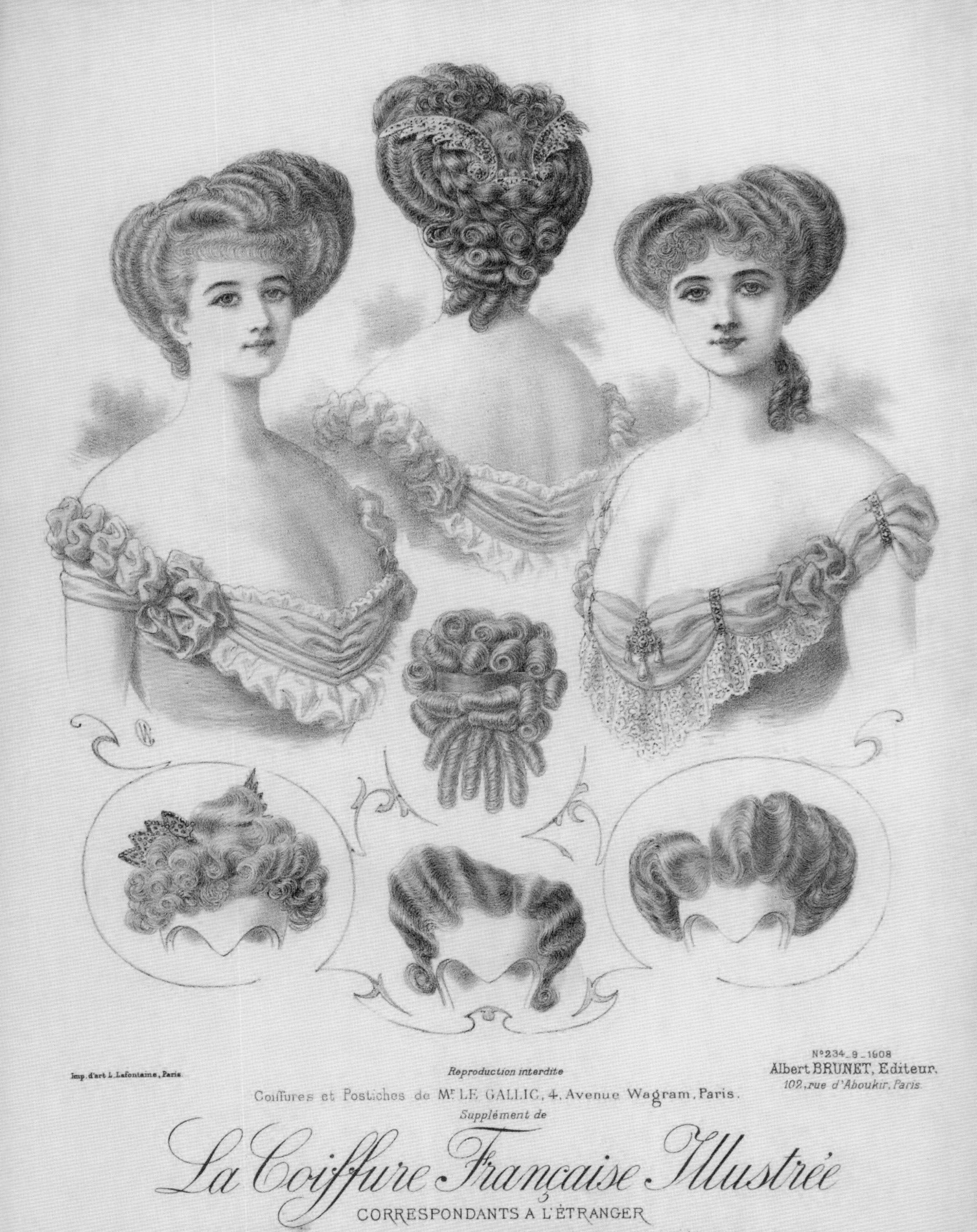

Hairstyles and hairpieces, by Mr. Le Gallic, 1908, *La Coiffure Française Illustrée*

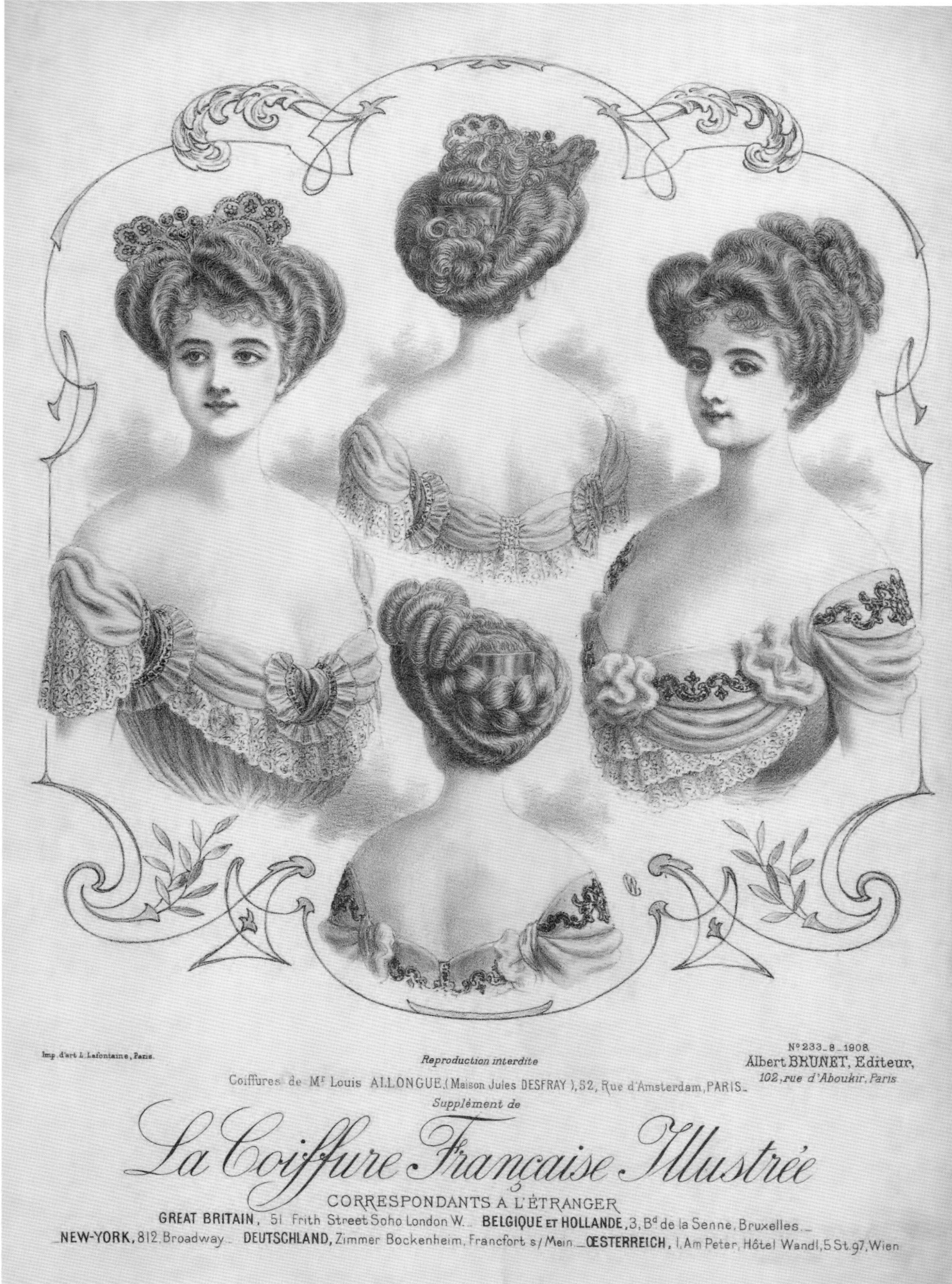

Hairstyles by Mr. Allongue,
1908, *La Coiffure Française Illustrée*

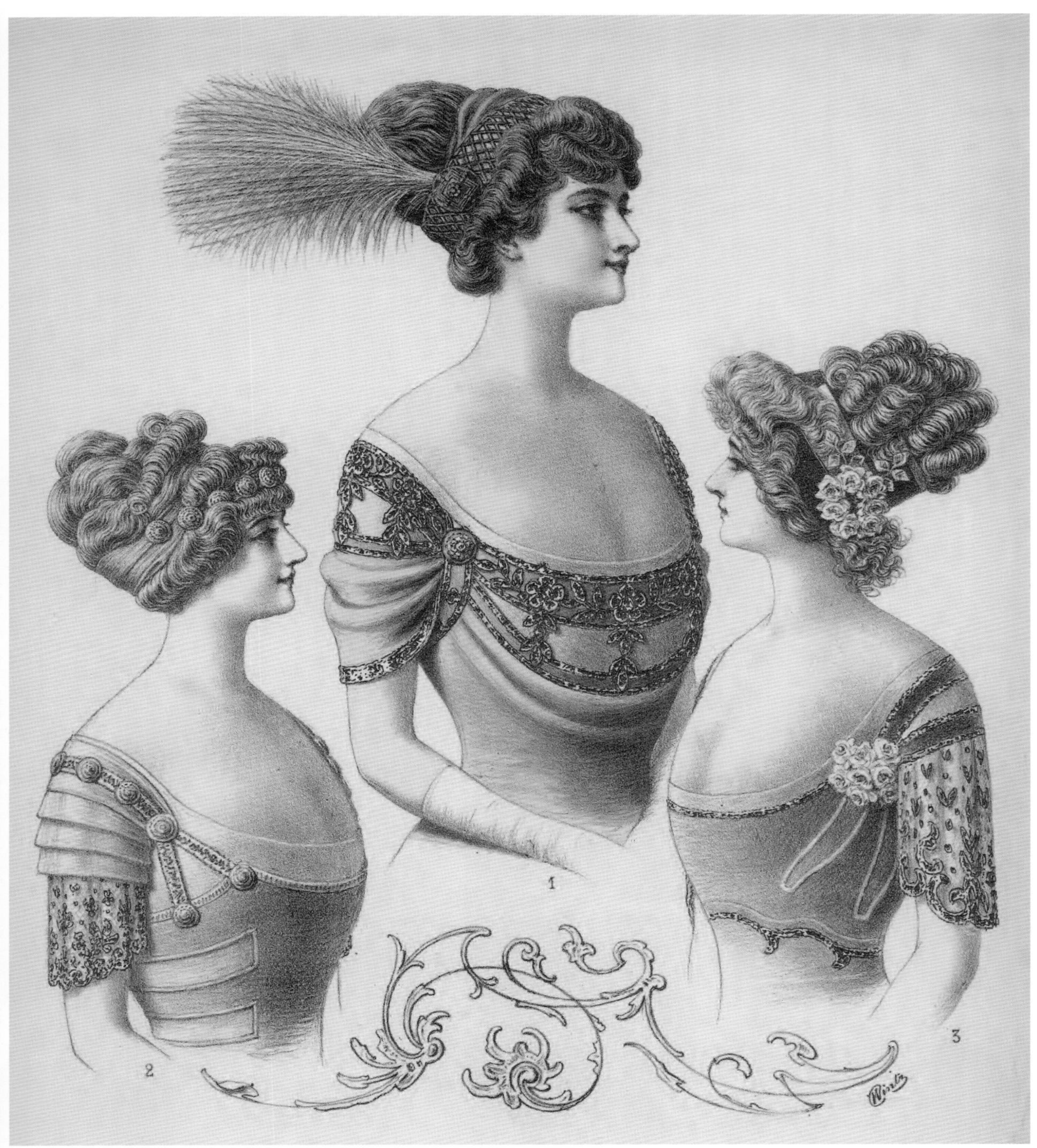

'Marcel Wave' hairstyles by Mr. Madon,
1911, *La Coiffure Française Illustrée*

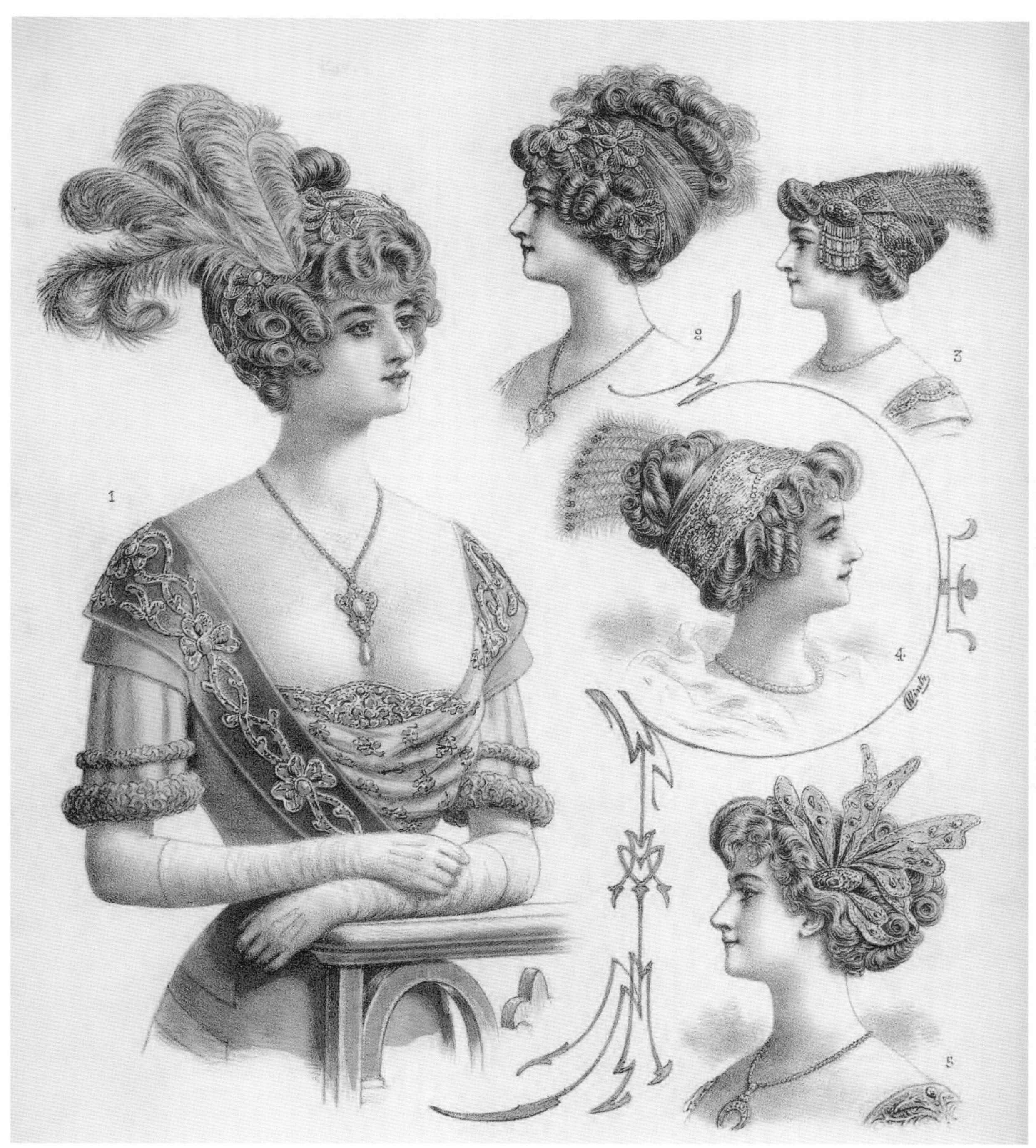

‘Marcel Wave’ hairstyles by Maison Raoul, 1911, *La Coiffure Française Illustrée*

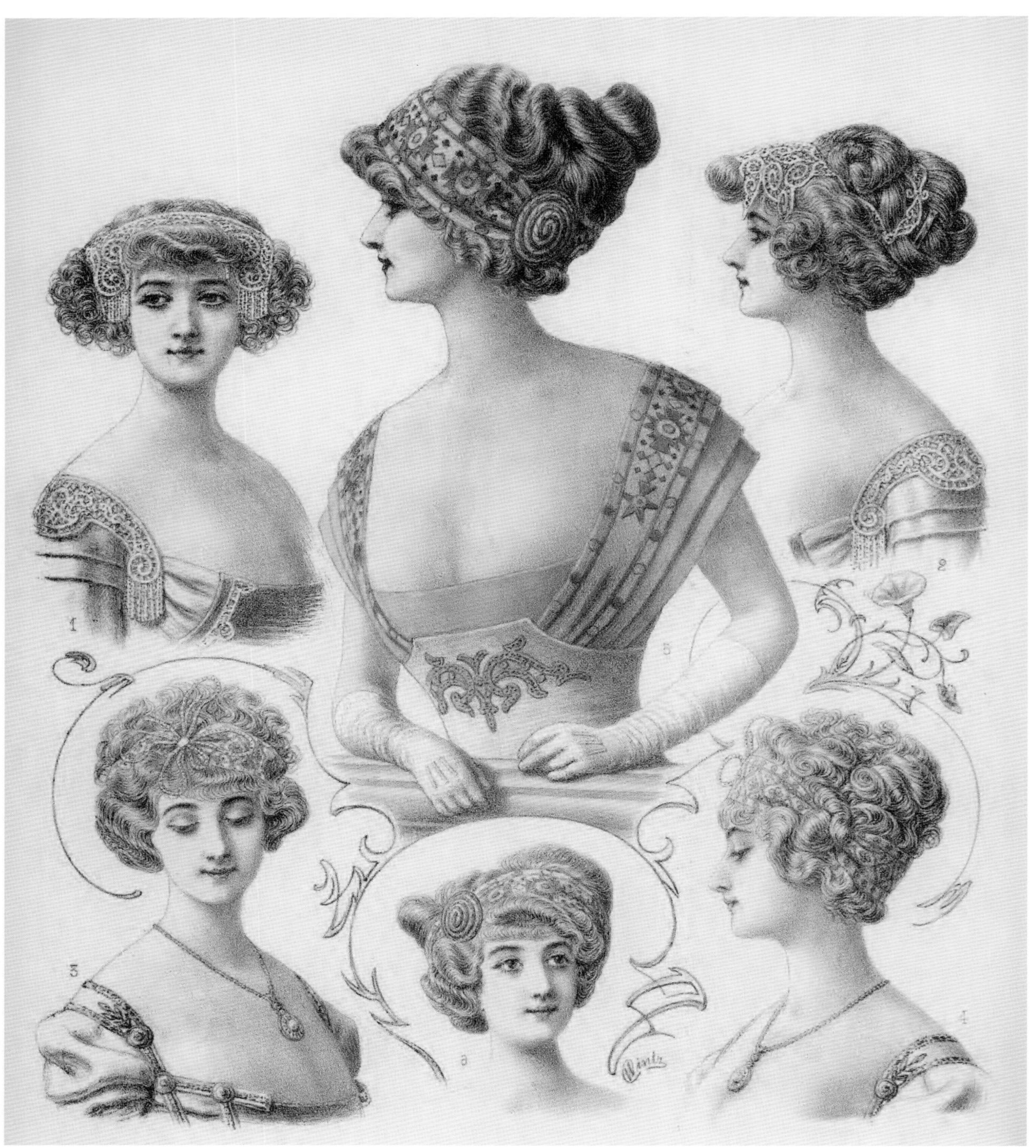

French hairstyles by Mr. Torac, 1911, *La Coiffure Française Illustrée*

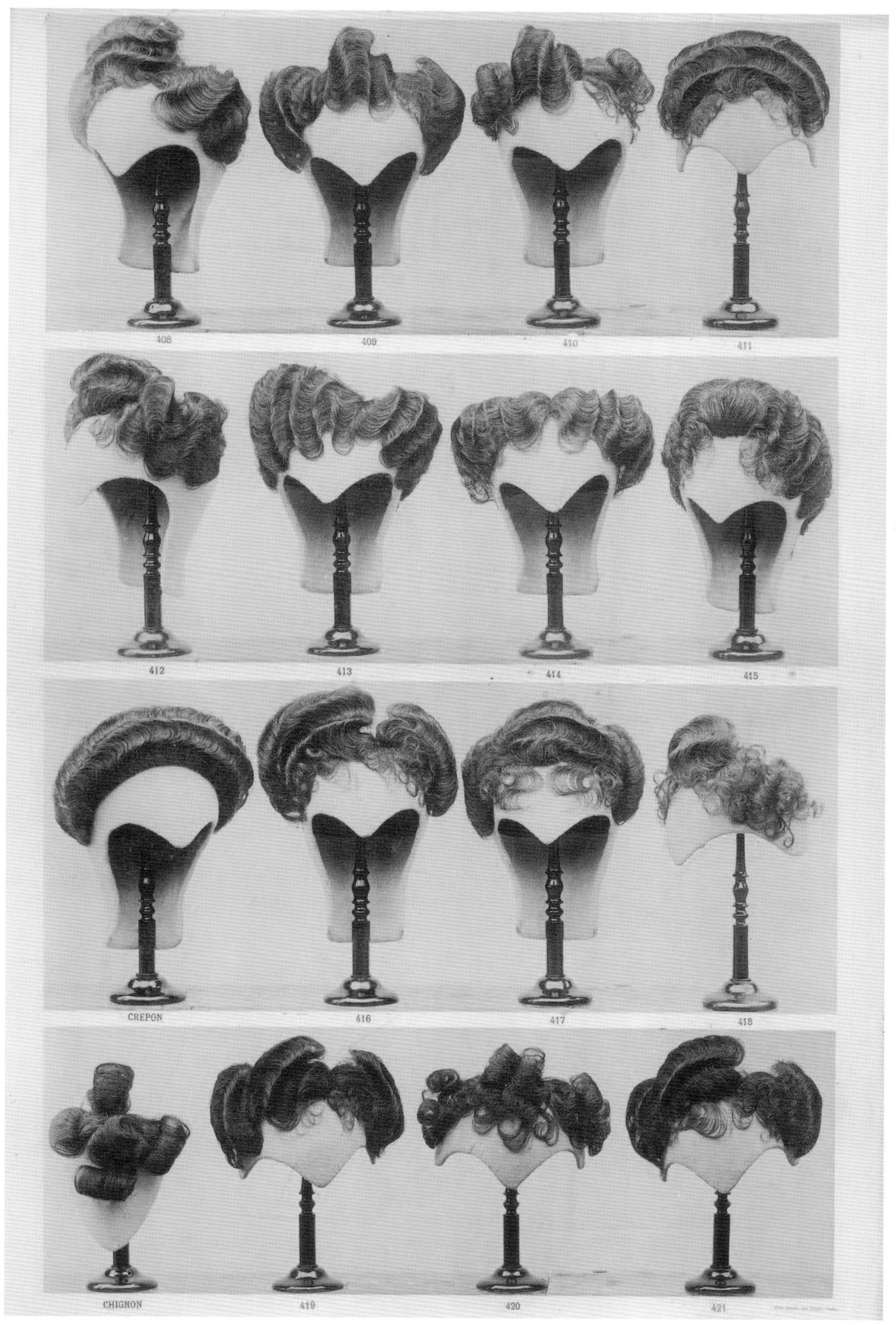

French wig styles, 1911, *La Toilette – Journal des Salons de Coiffure*

19 Février 1910 L'ILLUSTRATION Annonces — 11

GRAND MAGASIN DE CHEVEUX ⌀ POSTICHES D'ART

Nouvelle Création Sensationnelle de la Maison

Marius HENG

TÉLÉPHONE : 210-72 **33, rue Bergère, 33, PARIS** TÉLÉPHONE : 210-72

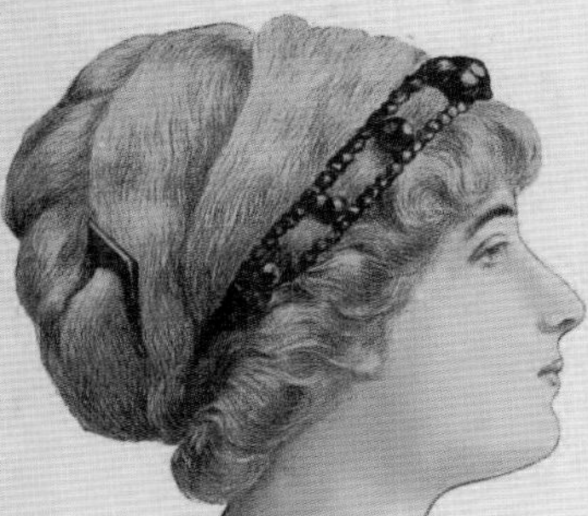

La coiffure nouvelle, faite avec le nouveau postiche *Le " Sans-Gêne "* (modèle déposé) — cette merveilleuse invention de la Maison HENG — est certainement le Postiche le plus pratique qu'on ait jamais fait ; car non seulement il coiffe élégamment et au goût du jour, non seulement il embellit, rajeunit et sied à tous les visages, mais encore il se place facilement et simplement.

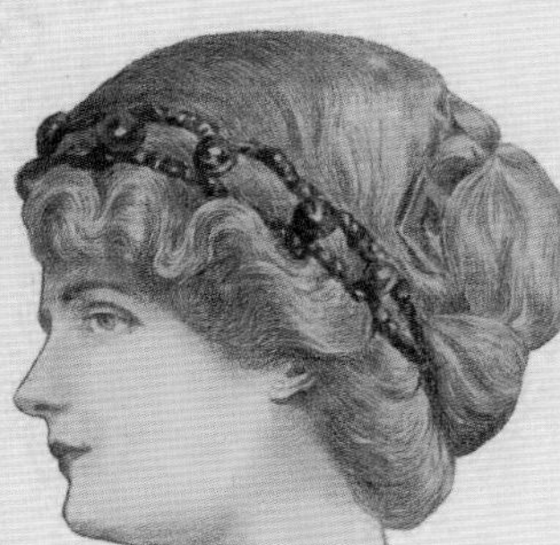

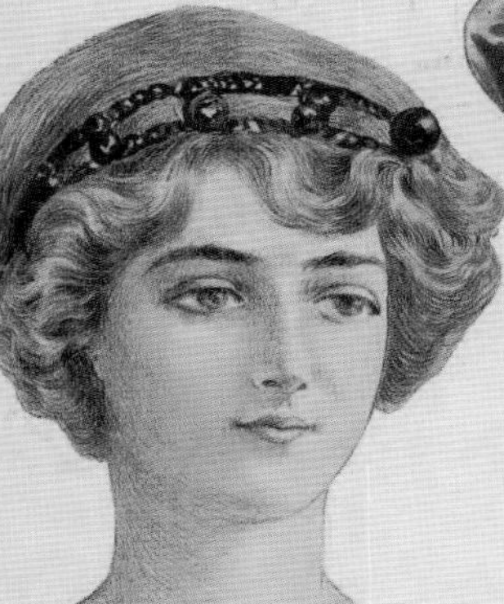

Manière de placer le "SANS-GÊNE" (Modèle déposé).

Il suffit, en effet, de le poser sur la tête, comme l'indique la gravure ci-dessus, et l'on est coiffée en un clin d'œil.

En outre de tous ces avantages, il en est un autre qui n'est pas à dédaigner et que vous saurez apprécier, Madame, c'est son extrême légèreté, sa monture complètement à jour dont une partie seulement — de la grosseur d'un fil — touche la tête. Madame, vous ne serez vraiment coiffée à la mode que lorsque vous aurez un *" Sans-Gêne "* (modèle déposé) de la MAISON

Marius HENG, 33, rue Bergère, PARIS

(Reproduction interdite) ENVOI FRANCO DU CATALOGUE SUR DEMANDE (Reproduction interdite)

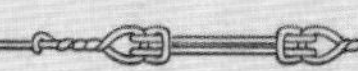

Advertisement for 'Sans-Gêne' wig from Maison Marius Heng, 1910, *L'Illustration*

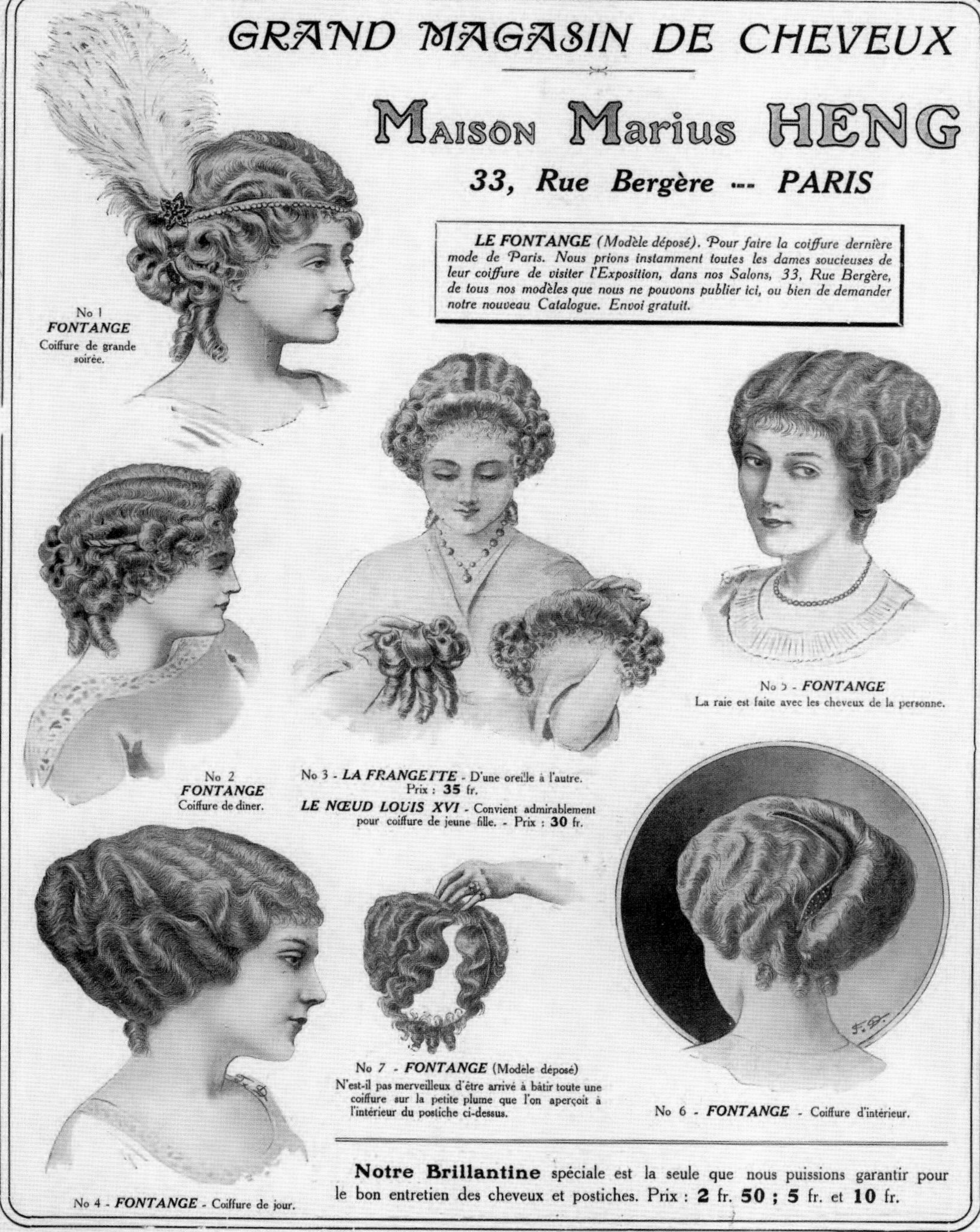

Advertisement for Wigs from Maison Marius Heng, 1. Fontange Formal Evening, 2. Fontange Dinner Party, 3. La Frangette and the Louis XVI knot, 4. Fontange Day time, 5. Fontange with the hair of the person, 6. Indoor Hairstyle, 1911, *L'Illustration*

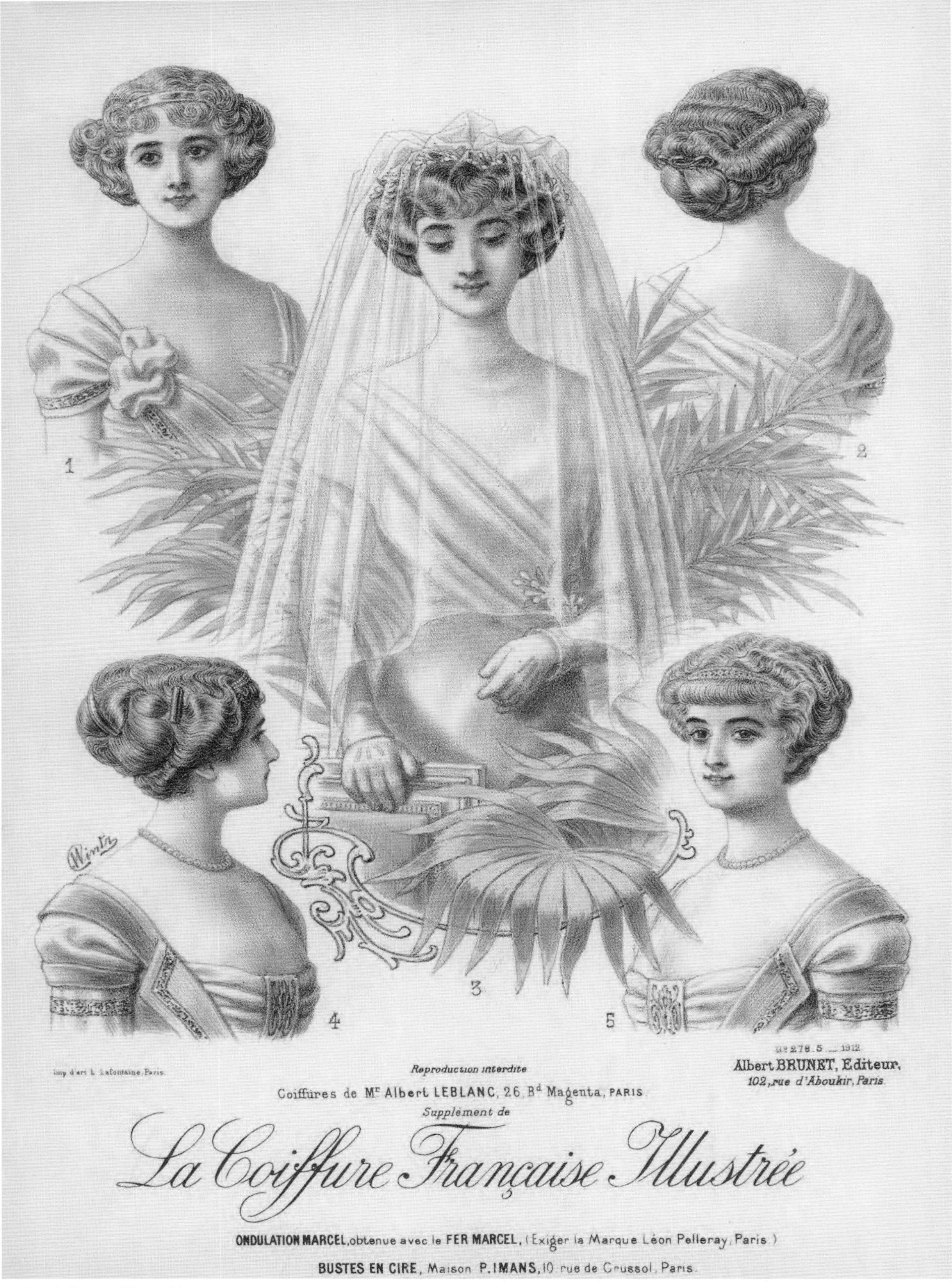

Hairstyles by Mr. Albert Leblanc,
1912, *La Coiffure Française Illustrée*

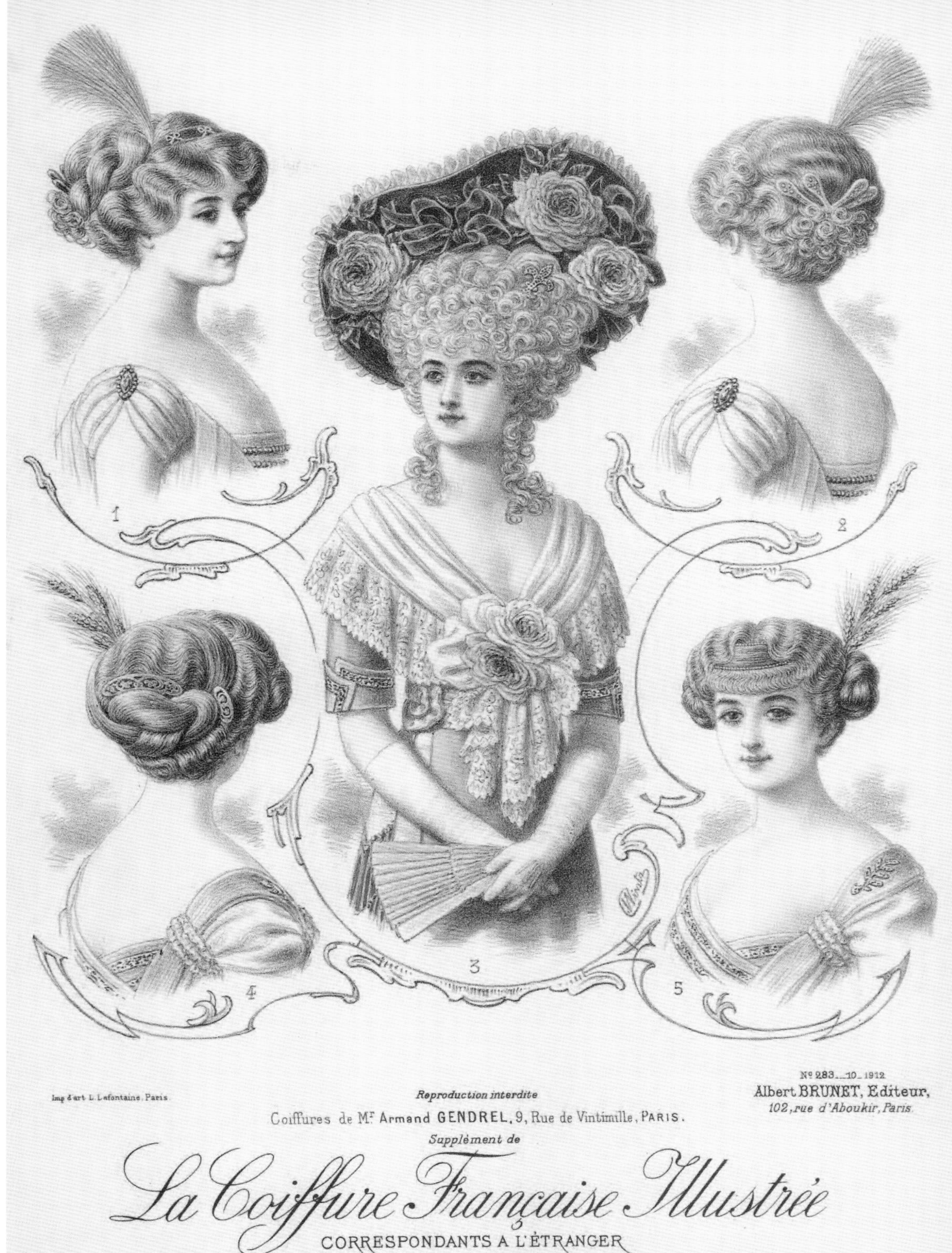

Hairstyles by Mr. Armand Gendrel,
1912, *La Coiffure Française Illustrée*

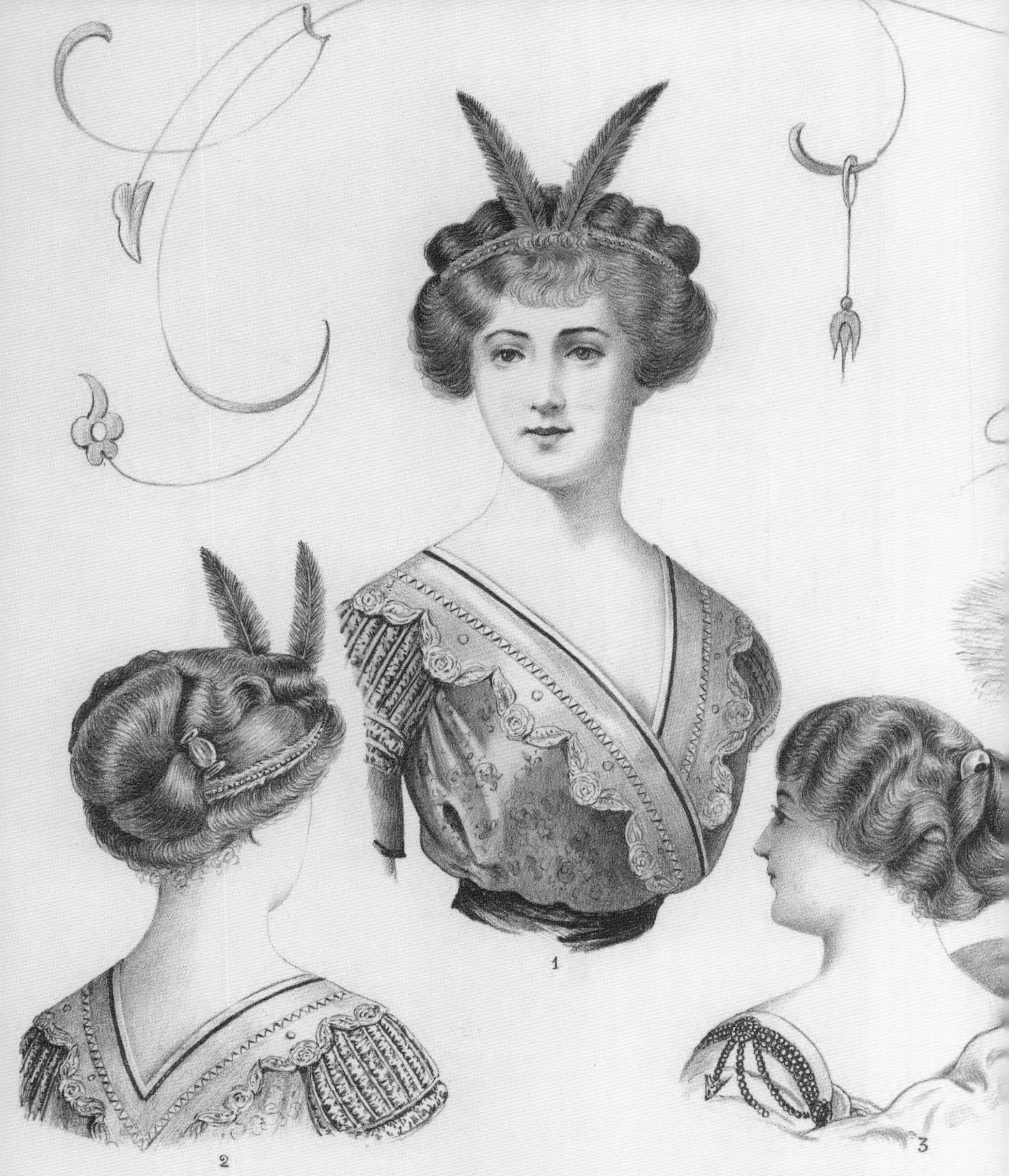

Imp. d'art L. Lafontaine, Paris.

Coiffures vues à la Grande Fête don

au profit de « L'ŒUVRE H

La Coiffure

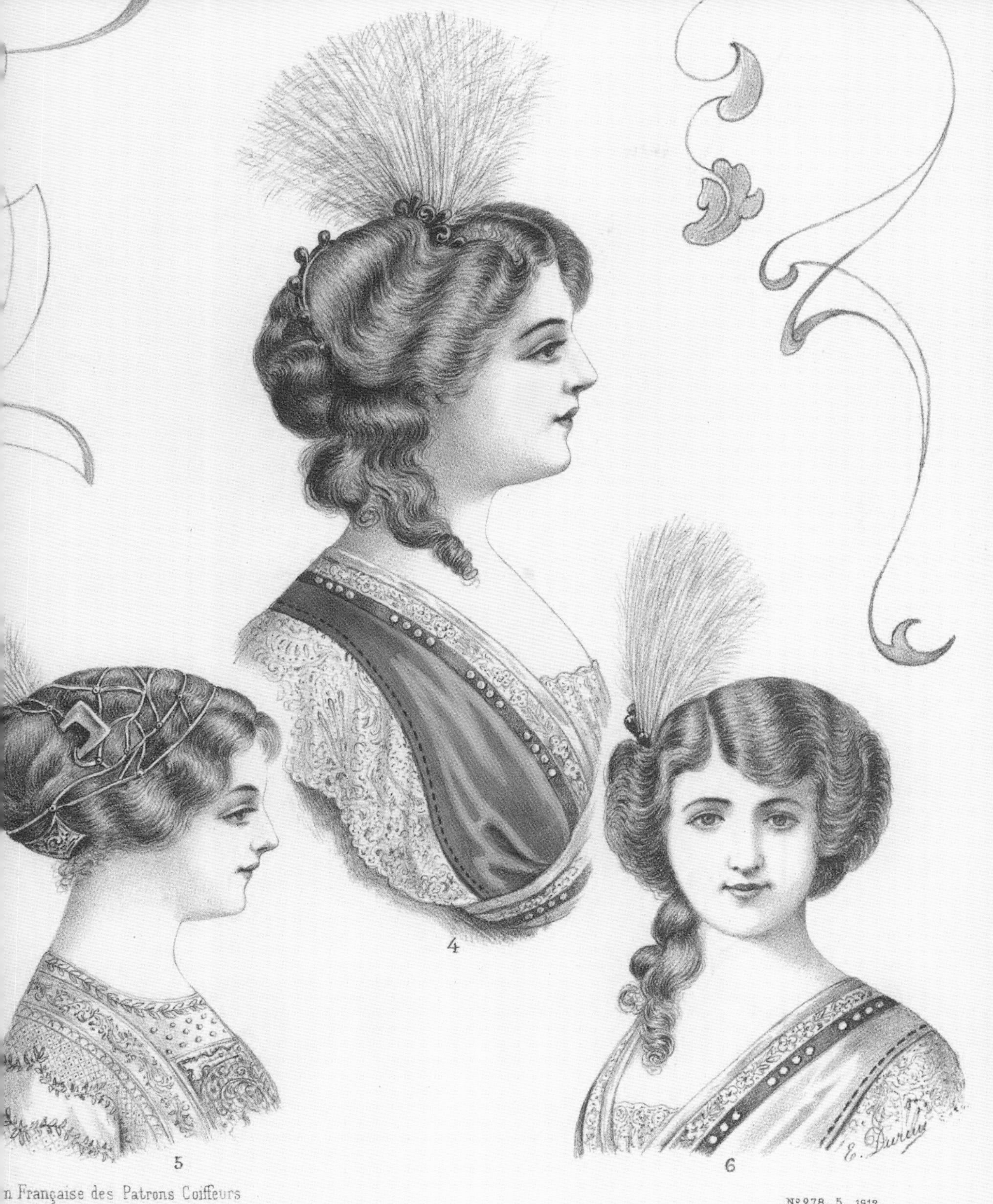
4
5
6
E. Durin
n Française des Patrons Coiffeurs
de Secours pour les Coiffeurs)
Nº 278._5._1912.
Albert BRUNET, Editeur,
102, rue d'Aboukir, Paris.
aise Illustrée

Previous spread: Hairstyles seen at the ball given by the Fédération Française des Patrons Coiffeurs, 1912

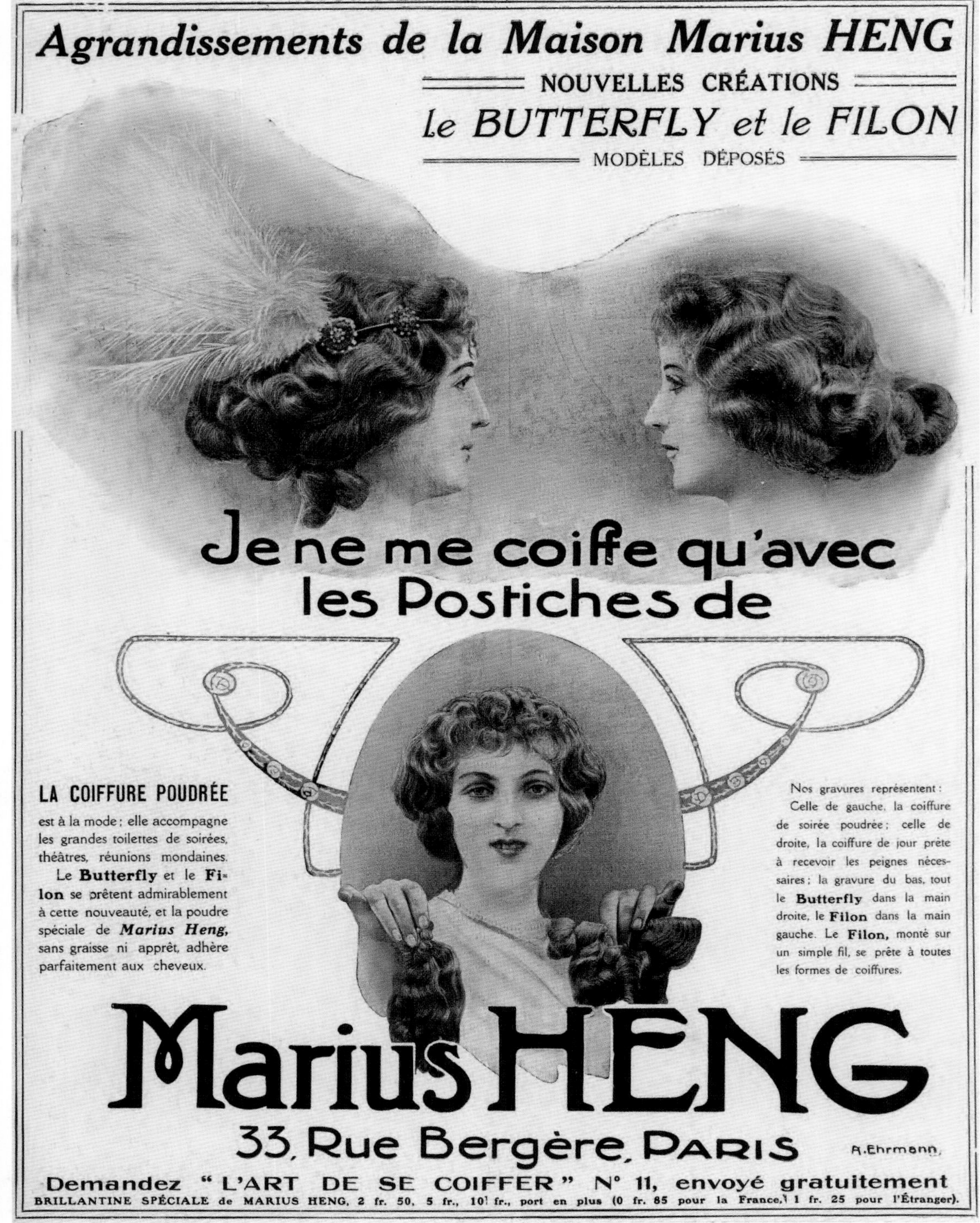

Advertisement for wigs by Maison Marius Heng, 1912, *L'Illustration*

Mon LÉON PELLERAY

Maison fondée en 1830
TÉLÉPHONE 123-71

EM. BOISSEAU, Succr

Adresse télégraphique :
RAYPELLE-PARIS

PARIS, 17, rue Croix-Petits-Champs. — BRUXELLES, 11, rue du Canal (Demander prix spéciaux)

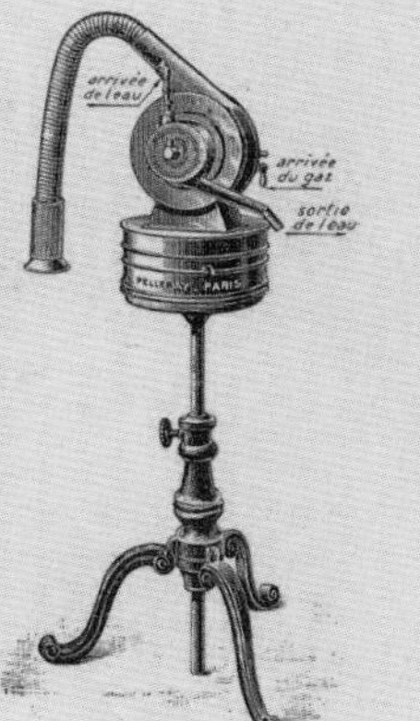

SÉCHOIR HYDRAULIQUE

Le plus économique

La ventilation se fait au moyen de l'eau et la chaleur est produite par le gaz

N° 5799. **Séchoir hydraulique** sur consoles en fonte et devant être fixées au mur. . **68.** »

N° 4675. **Séchoir hydraulique** monté sur tige et pied fonte vernie noire. . . . . **80.** »

N° 5800. **Séchoir hydraulique** monté sur sellette façon noyer . . . . . . **80.** »

Sur sellette laquée blanc.

Supplément . . . . **3.** »

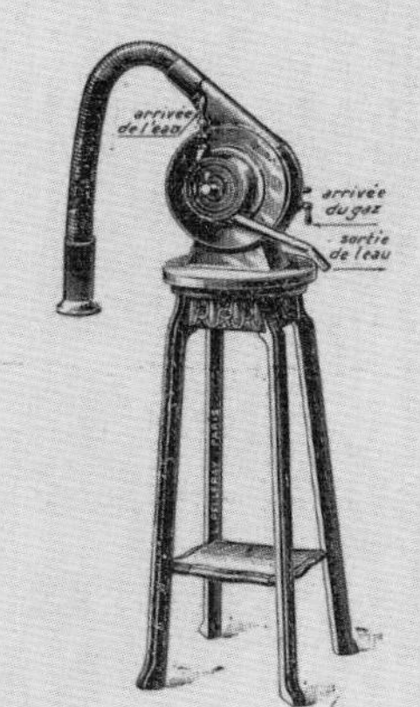

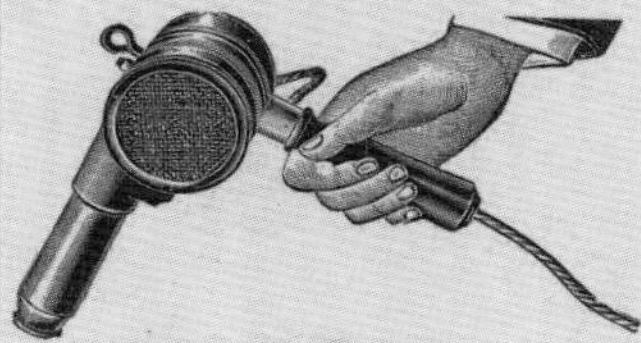

SÉCHOIR ÉLECTRIQUE PORTATIF PLIANT

N° 4668. **Séchoir électrique portatif** donnant air chaud ou froid à volonté . . . **60** »

N° 4647. **Gaine cuir** pour appareil 4668 pièce **9.75**

SÉCHOIR ÉLECTRIQUE "ÉCLAIR,,

AVEC RÉGULATEUR DONNANT TROIS VITESSES

Chauffage au gaz ou à l'électricité

Tube métallique flexible avec poignée cuir

L'INSCRIPTION en lettres émaillées : **Séchoir Electrique,** est offerte gratuitement à tout acheteur.

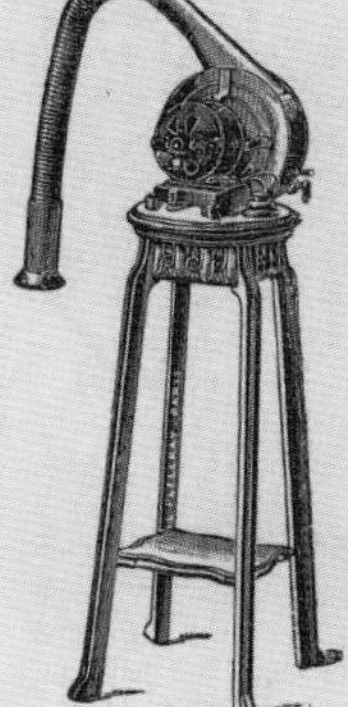

SUR CONSOLE

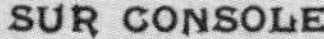

Chauffage au gaz

N° 5820. Courant **continu** 110 ou 220 volts . . . . . . **125.** »

N° 5821. Courant **alternatif** 110 ou 220 volts (50 périodes). **132.** »

Chauffage à l'électricité

N° 5822. Courant **Continu** 110 ou 210 volts . . . . . . **148.** »

N° 5823. Courant **alternatif** 110 ou 220 volts (50 périodes) . **155.** »

SUR PIED (fonte vernie)

Chauffage au gaz

N° 4735. Courant **continu** 110 ou 220 volts. **138.** »

N° 4736. Courant **alternatif** 110 ou 220 volts (50 périodes) . . . . **145.** »

Chauffage à l'électricité

N° 4757. Courant **continu** 110 ou 220 volts. **162.** »

N° 4758. Courant **alternatif** 110 ou 220 volts (50 périodes). . . . . . . **169.** »

SUR SELLETTE (façon noyer)

Chauffage au gaz

N° 5805. Courant **Continu** 110 ou 220 volts **135.** »

N° 5806. Courant **internatif** 110 ou 220 volts (50 périodes) . . . . **142.** »

Chauffage à l'électricité

N° 5807. Courant **Courant** 110 ou 220 volts. **159.** »

N° 5808. Courant **internatif** 110 ou 220 volts (50 périodes) . . . . **166.** »

Avec Selette **LAQUÉE BLANC.** Supplément : **3 fr.**

NOTA. — Prière de bien indiquer la nature du courant et le voltage.

Monsieur Léon Pelleray advertisement for electric and hydraulic hairdryers, 1913, *La Coiffure de Paris*

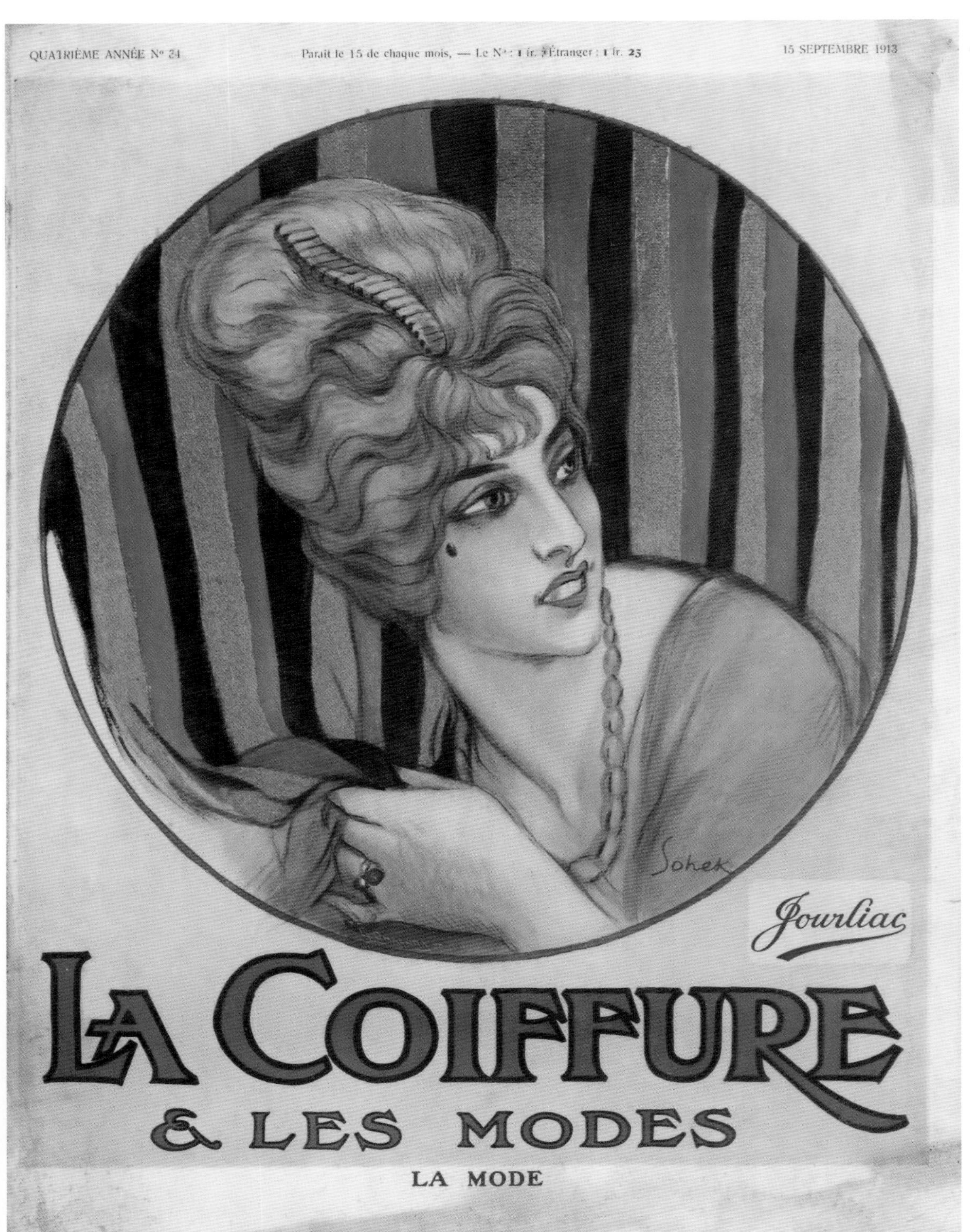

La Coiffure et les Modes magazine cover, 1913

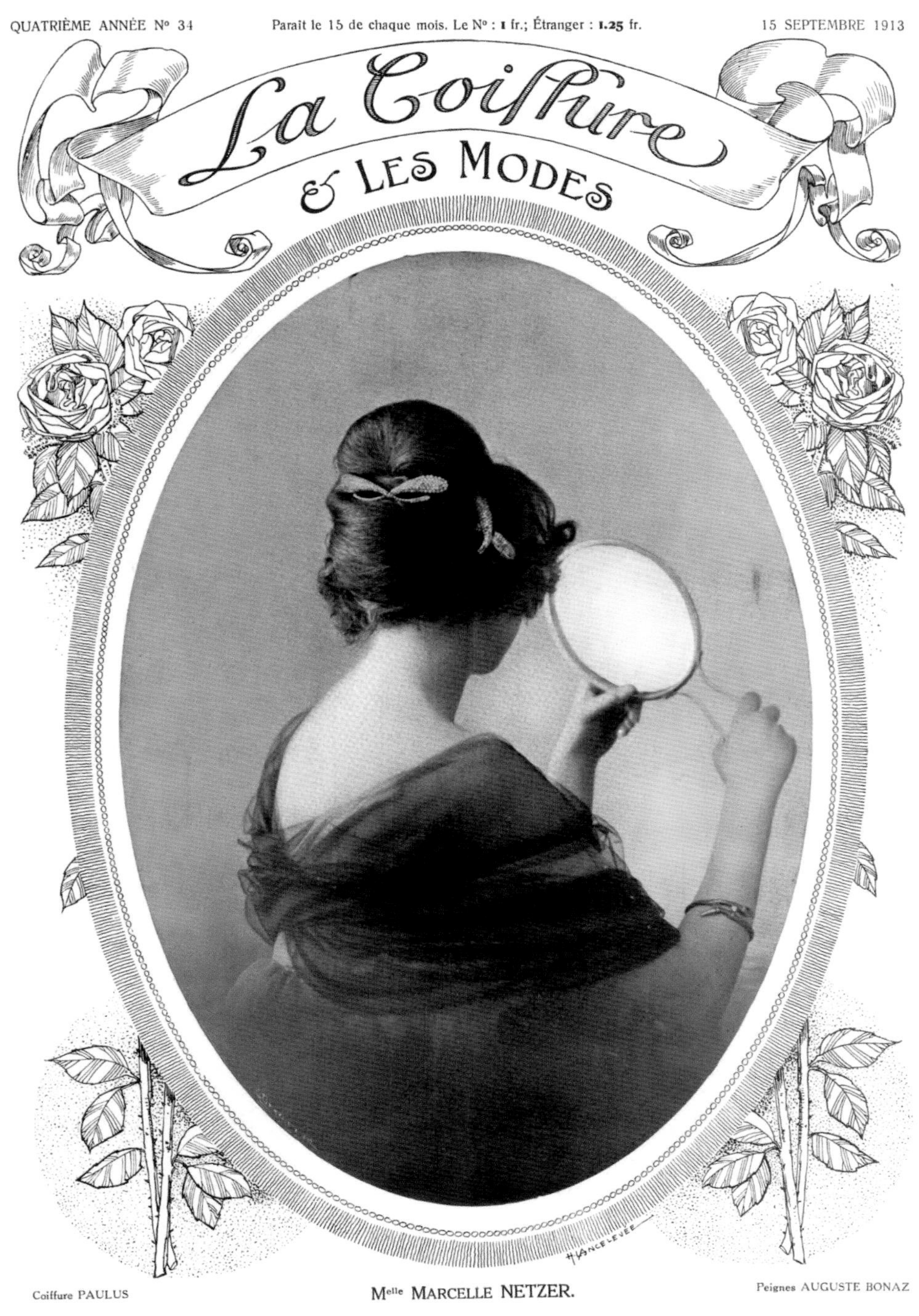

Miss Marcelle Netzer, 1913, *La Coiffure et les Modes*

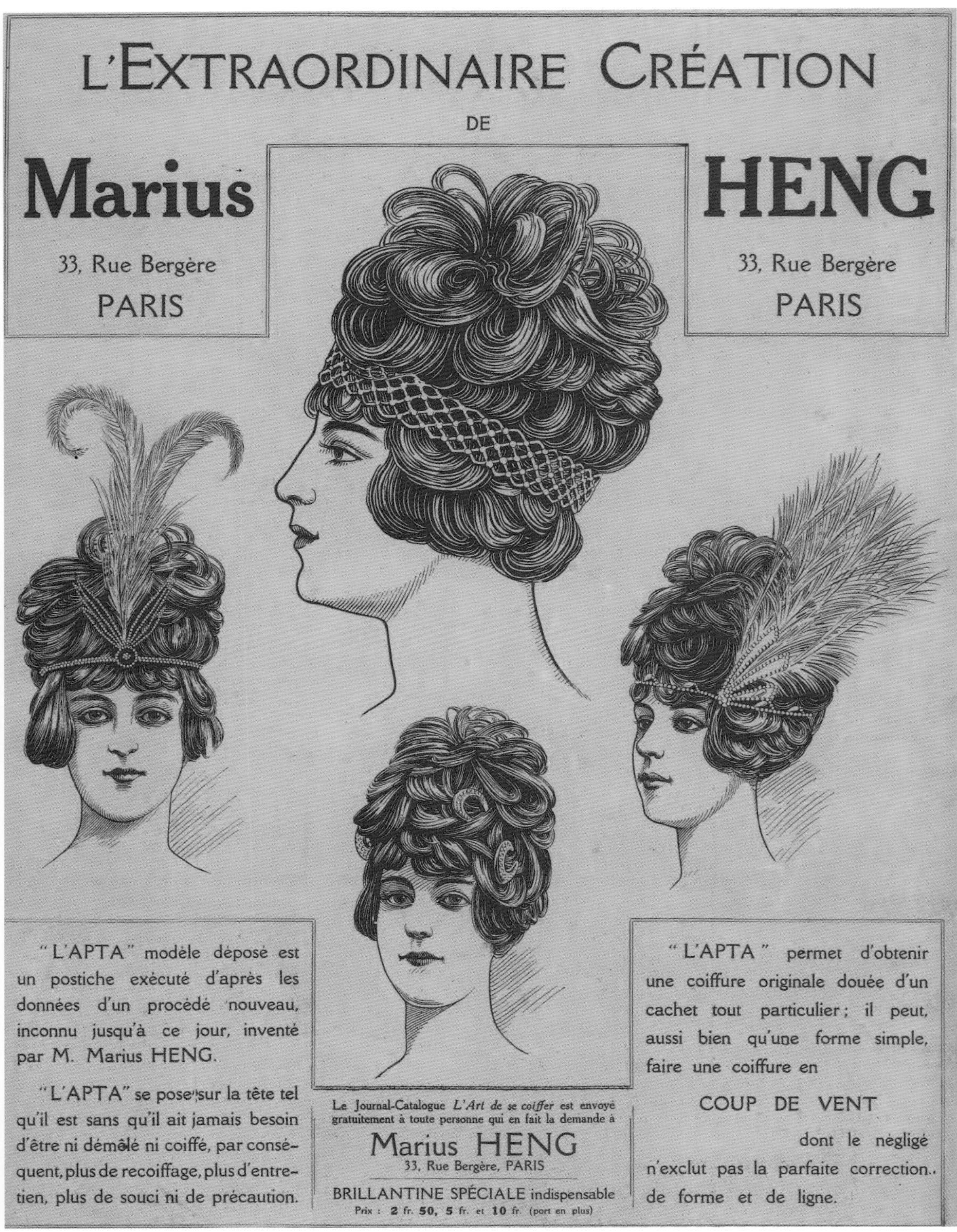
L'EXTRAORDINAIRE CRÉATION
DE
Marius
HENG
33, Rue Bergère
PARIS
33, Rue Bergère
PARIS
"L'APTA" modèle déposé est un postiche exécuté d'après les données d'un procédé nouveau, inconnu jusqu'à ce jour, inventé par M. Marius HENG.
"L'APTA" se pose sur la tête tel qu'il est sans qu'il ait jamais besoin d'être ni démêlé ni coiffé, par conséquent, plus de recoiffage, plus d'entretien, plus de souci ni de précaution.
Le Journal-Catalogue L'Art de se coiffer est envoyé gratuitement à toute personne qui en fait la demande à
Marius HENG
33, Rue Bergère, PARIS
BRILLANTINE SPÉCIALE indispensable
Prix : 2 fr. 50, 5 fr. et 10 fr. (port en plus)
"L'APTA" permet d'obtenir une coiffure originale douée d'un cachet tout particulier ; il peut, aussi bien qu'une forme simple, faire une coiffure en
COUP DE VENT
dont le négligé n'exclut pas la parfaite correction.. de forme et de ligne.

Advertisement for the 'L'Apta' wig by Marius Heng, 1912, *L'Illustration*

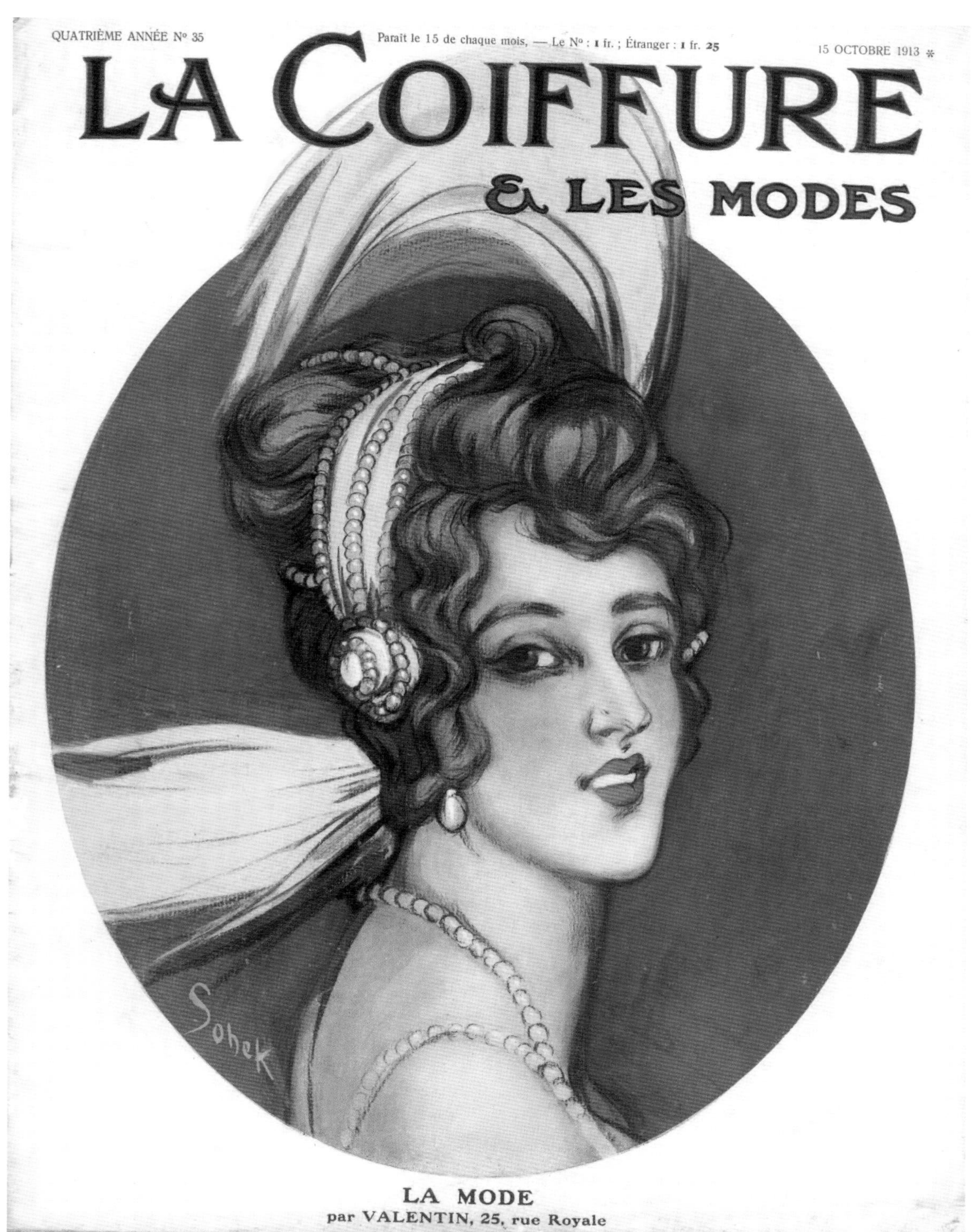
QUATRIÈME ANNÉE N° 35
Paraît le 15 de chaque mois, — Le N° : 1 fr. ; Étranger : 1 fr. 25
15 OCTOBRE 1913

LA COIFFURE
& LES MODES

LA MODE
par VALENTIN, 25, rue Royale

La Coiffure & les Modes magazine cover, Paris, 1913

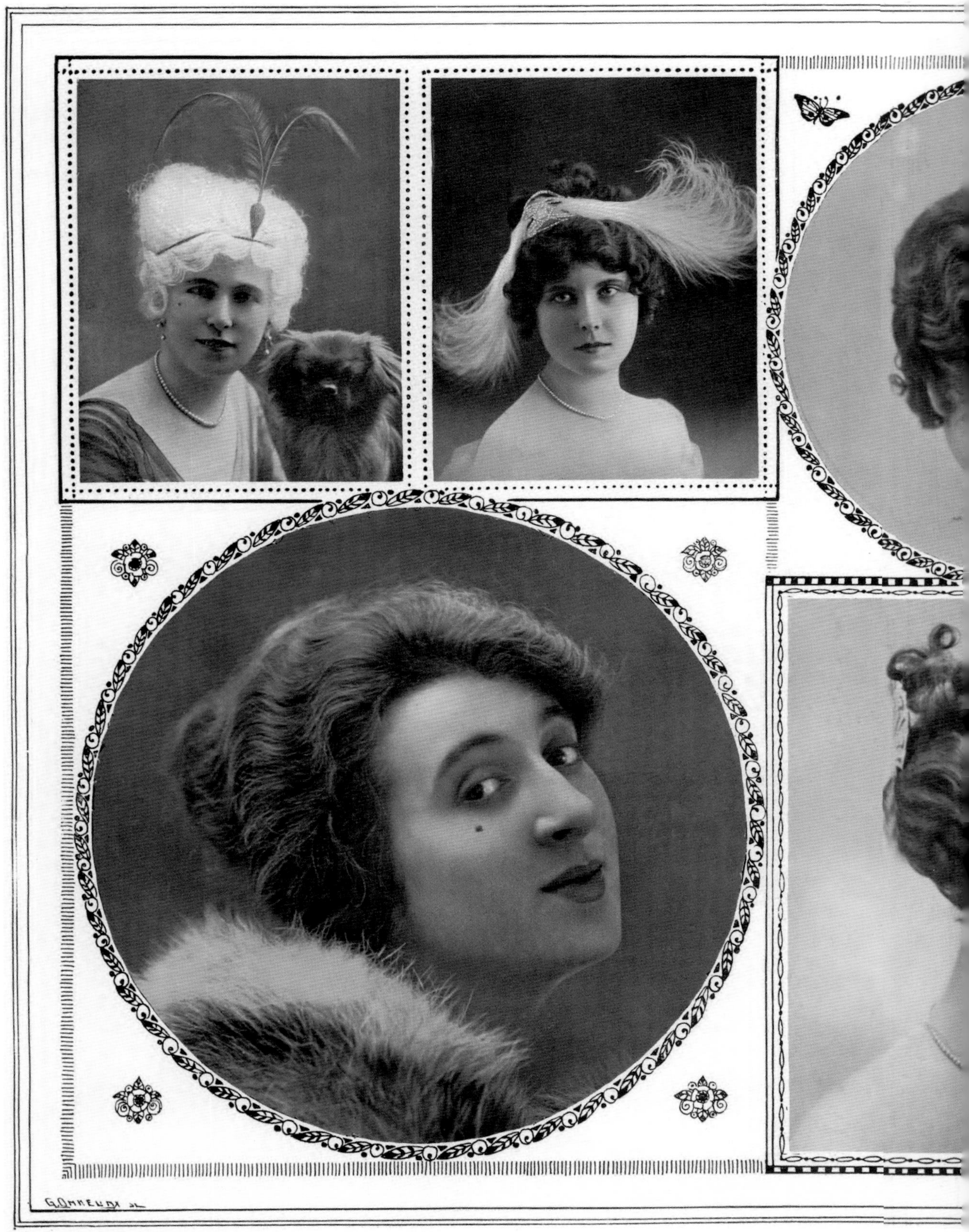

Jeanne Provost and Sylvia, hairstyles by Valentin, Paris, 1914, *La Coiffure et les Modes*

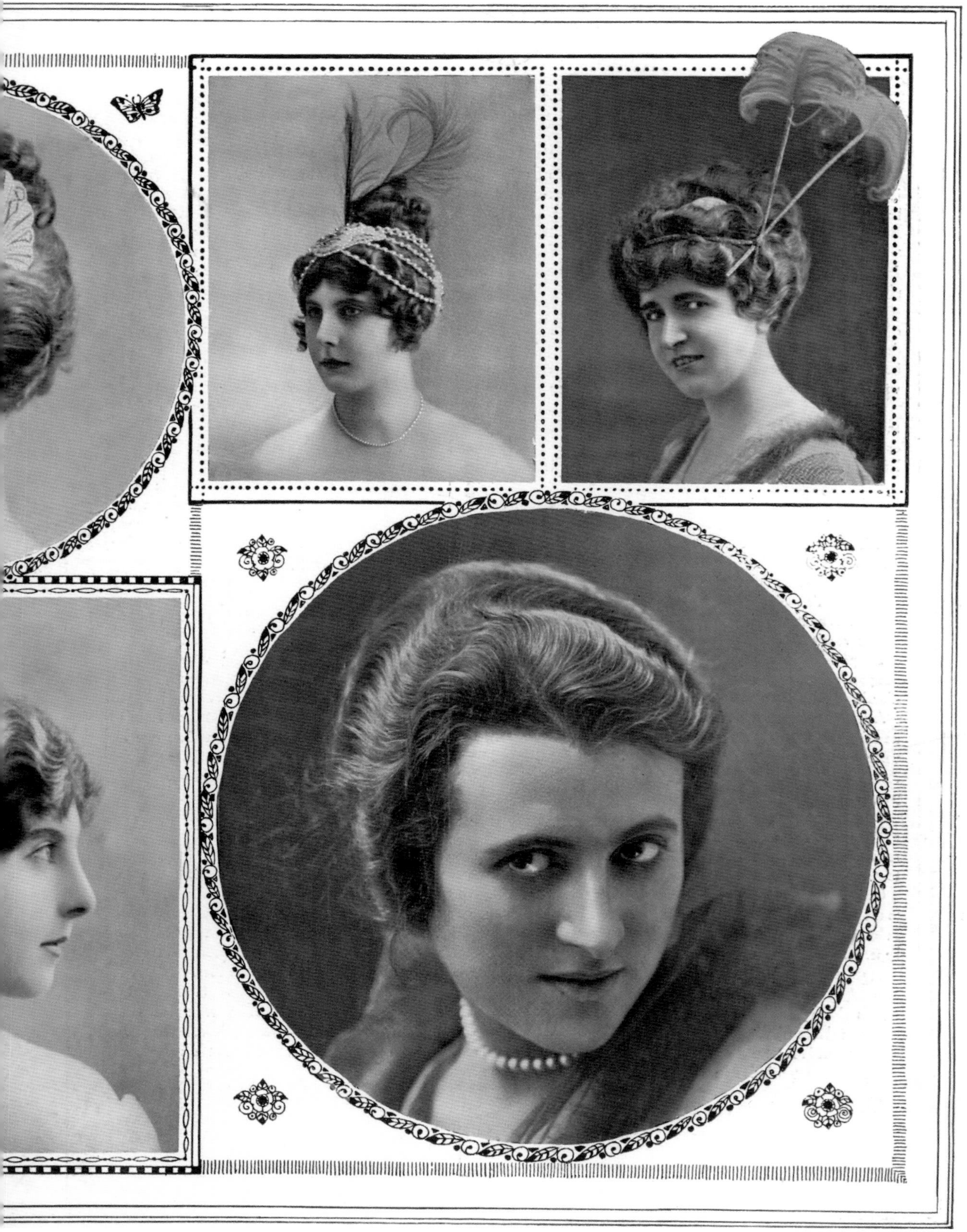

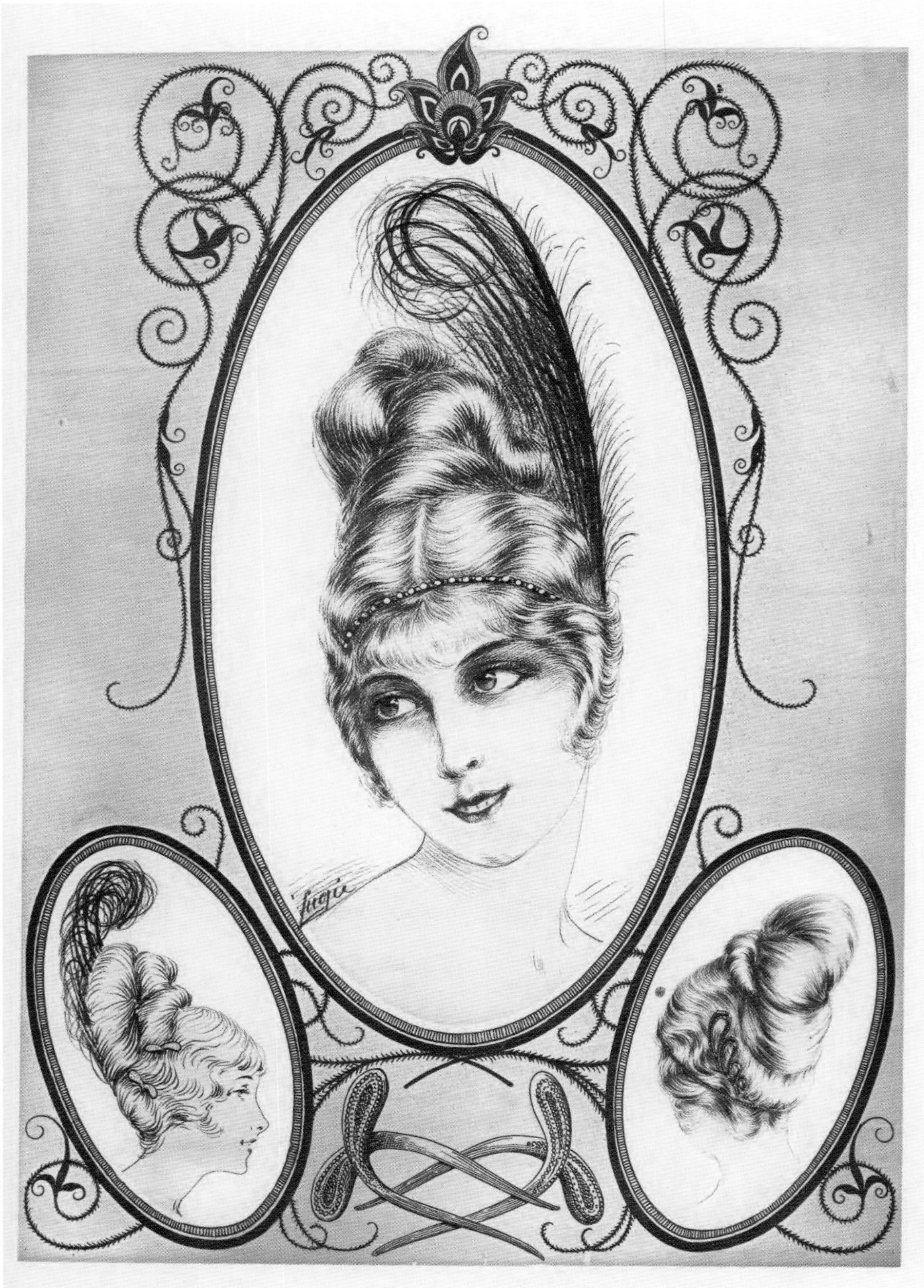

Hairstyles with feathers, Paris, 1914, *La Coiffure et les Modes*

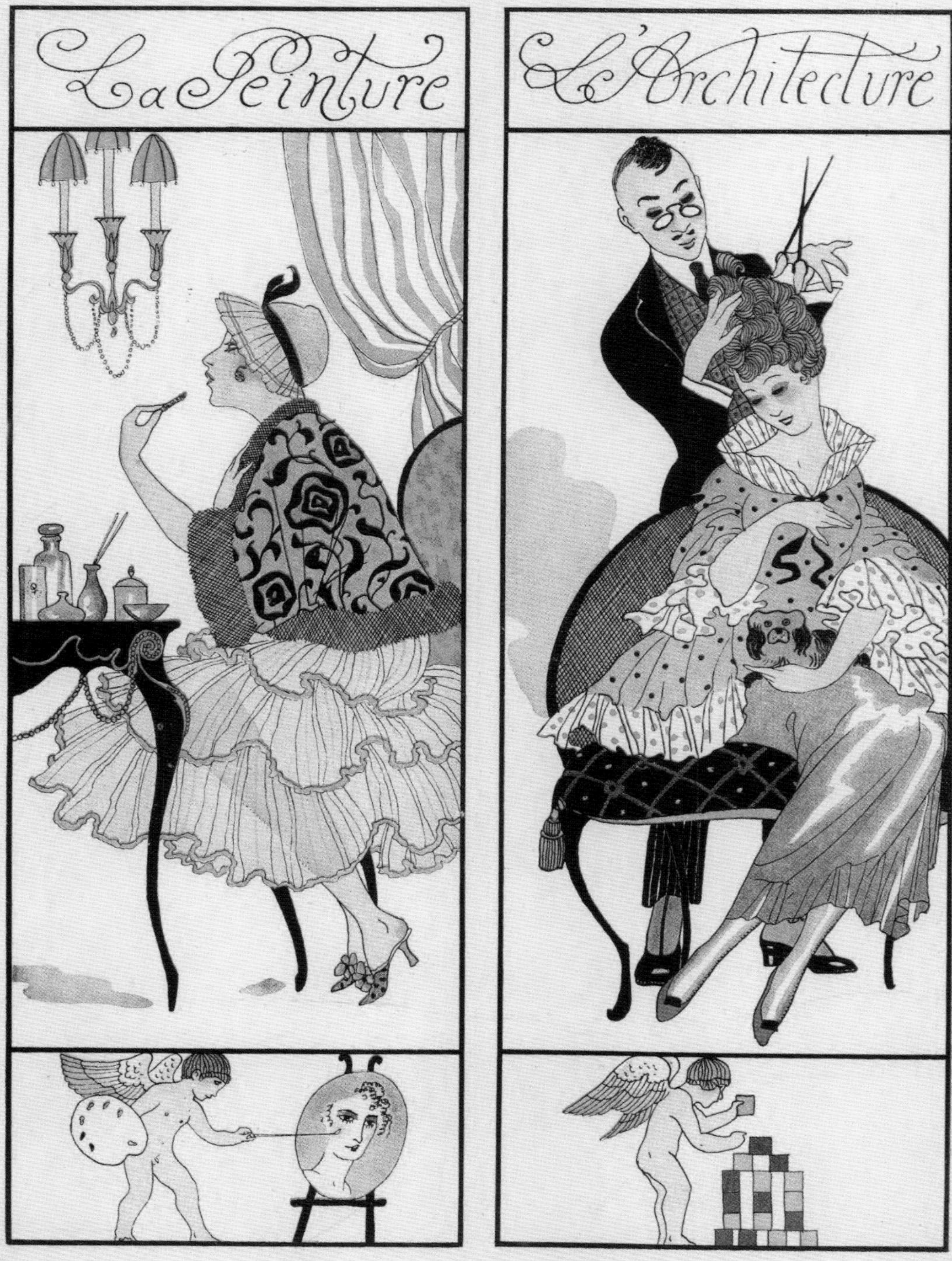

'La Peinture, L'Architecture', drawing by Georges Barbier, 1910s, *La Vie Parisienne*

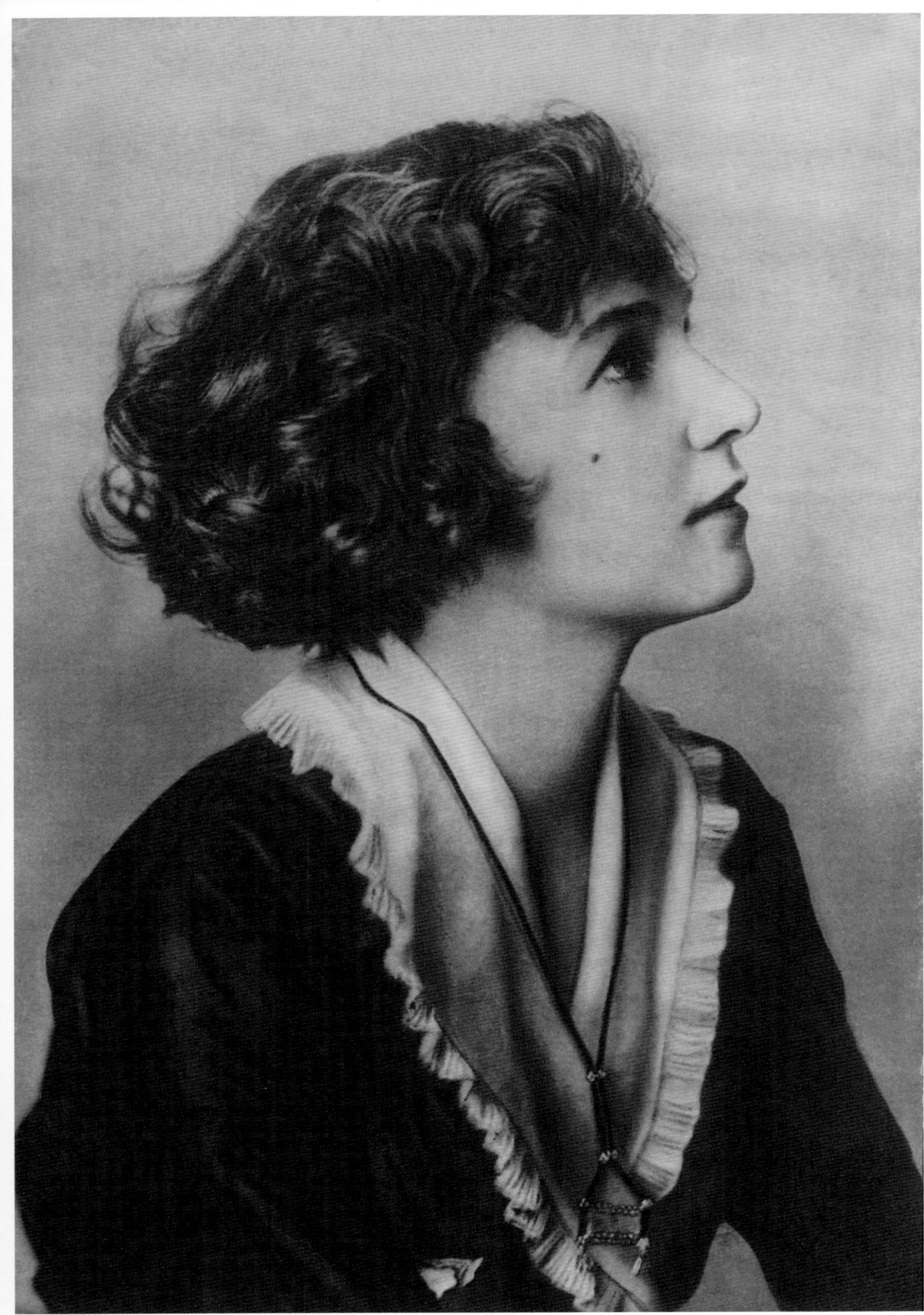

Irene Castle with her hair cut
into a 'Castle Bob', c. 1913–15

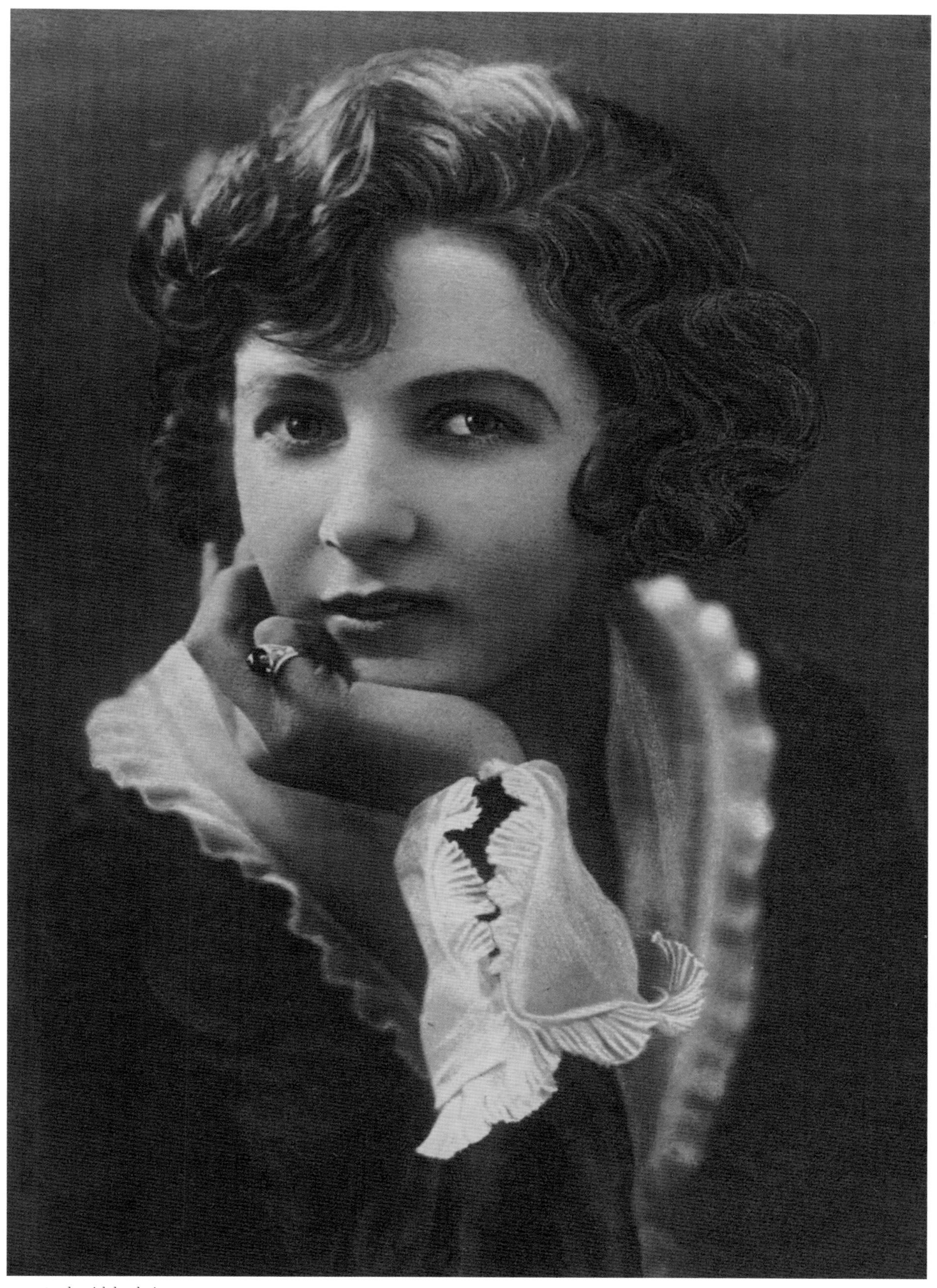

Irene Castle with her hair cut into a 'Castle Bob', c. 1913–15

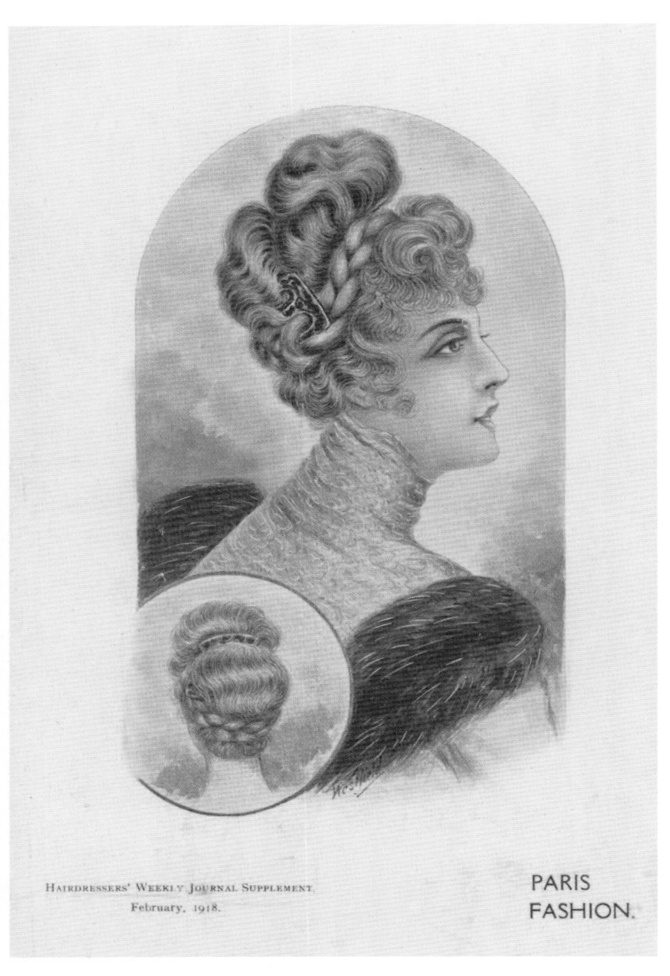

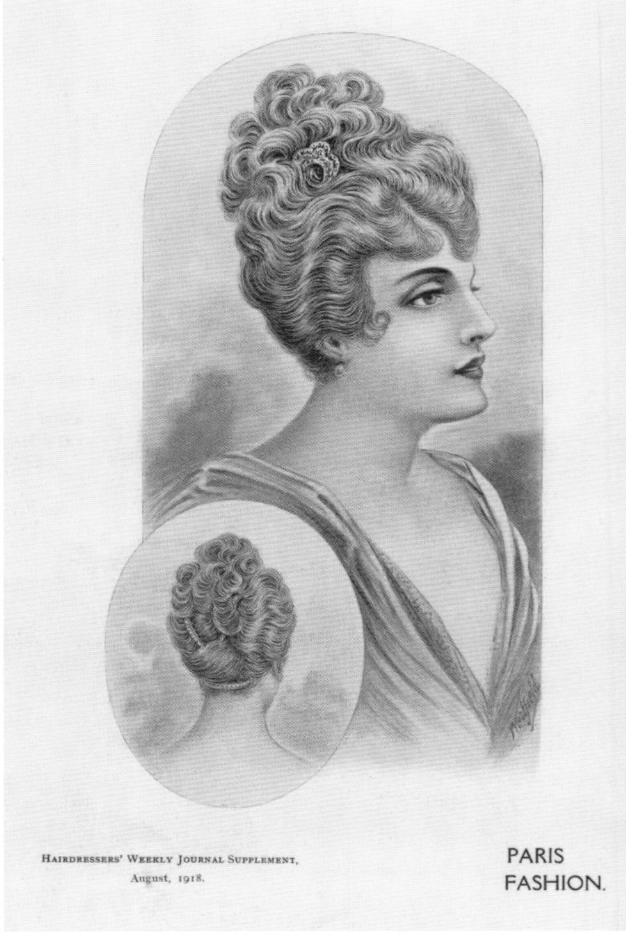

French hairstyles, 1918, 'Paris Fashion', *Hairdressers' Weekly Journal* supplement

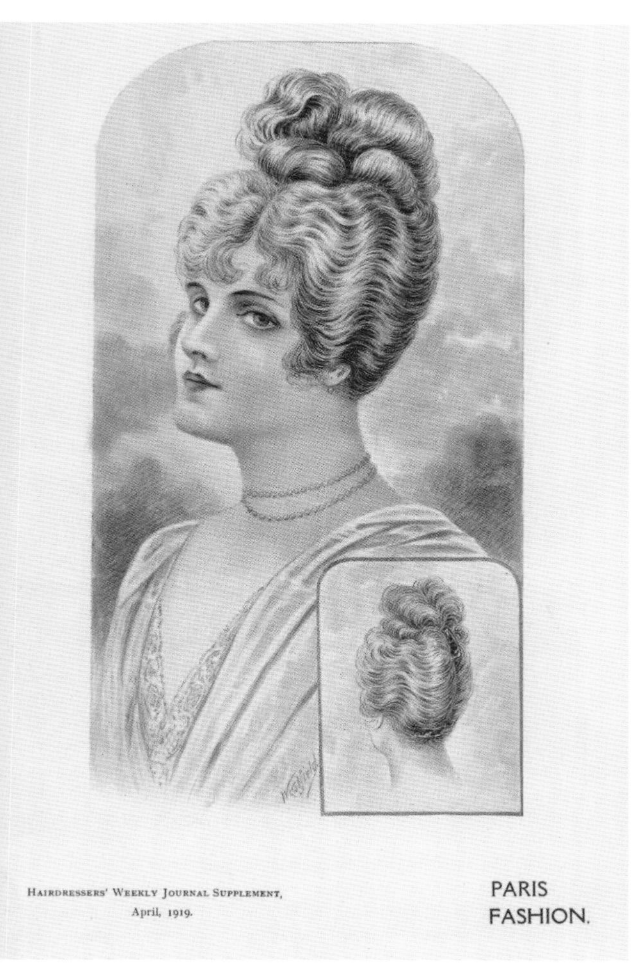

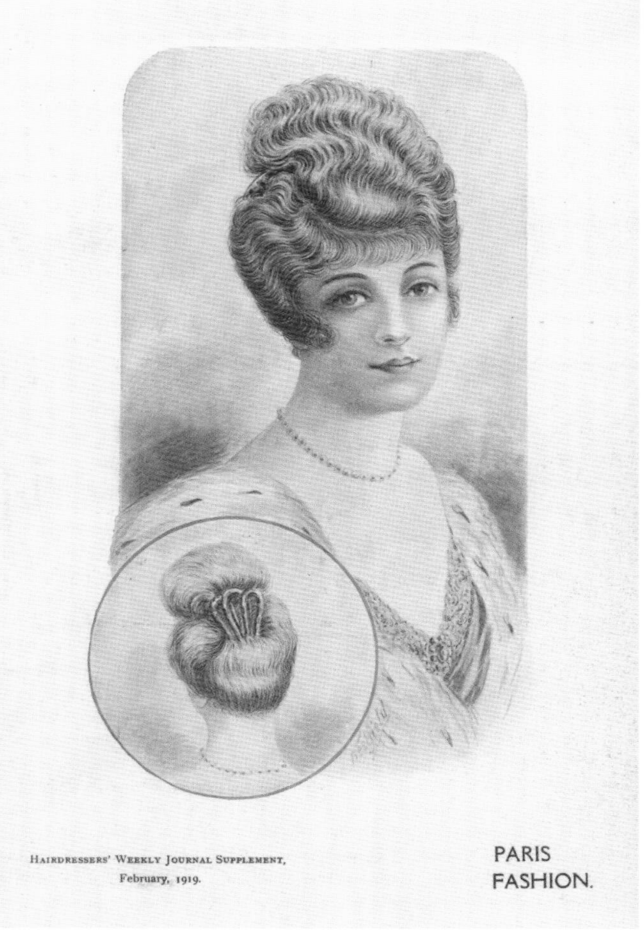

rench hairstyles, 1919, 'Paris Fashion',
airdressers' *Weekly Journal* supplement

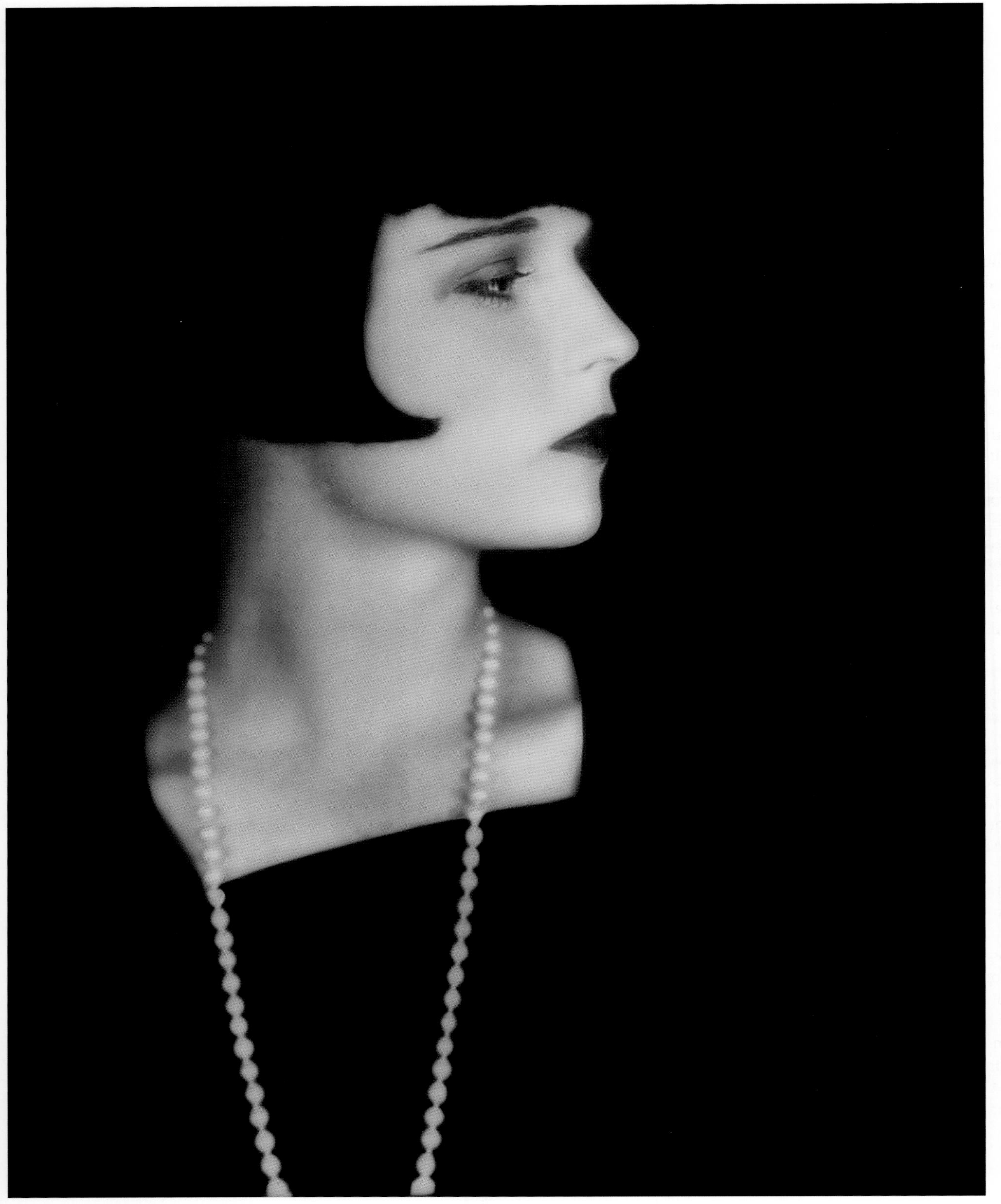

Louise Brooks with 'Japanese Bonnet Style Bob', c. 1929

1920S

The Roaring Twenties was a time of unbridled optimism and economic confidence, with young women enjoying their newfound social and political freedoms. While only the fashionable elite had worn the short bob in the previous decade, in the 1920s it became a widespread phenomenon that transcended class and geography. Young women also found themselves in the enviable position of being able to work and therefore earn money – the number of women working during this period rose an astonishing 51% in the United States, with one in four women over the age of 16 in some form of employment. With larger amounts of disposable income, women naturally used their money to keep fashionably up-to-date; indeed it was an era where fashion finally became democratised. The 1920s vogue for the short bob connects directly with the idea of female emancipation – even the word "Bob" signifies an edgy cultural gender play. Although most hairdressers initially resisted the introduction of the bob, this eye-catching style actually helped to further establish the profession of women's hairdressing, because it necessitated some skill and was not just a quick dry cut.

During the 1920s the use of shampoo became more widespread and the era also saw the introduction of numerous new permanent waving machines. The "perm" had actually been previously invented in the 1880s by Marcel Grateau, and the technique had been further refined by Karl Ludwig Nessler in 1909 with his introduction of the first permanent wave machine – this involved soaking the hair in an alkaline solution of sodium hydroxide and then winding it round electrically heated brass rollers. It was not until the 1920s, however, that perms became more prevalent. Importantly the perm made short hair eminently stylish, and this new fashion for short, easy-to-wear wavy hair proved to be a nice little earner for hairdressers – every six months a woman would need to get her hair repermed at often quite a considerable cost. The perm also "added value" to the vocation of hairdressing because it was too technically complex to undertake at home and therefore necessitated a visit to a "professional" salon.

Hairdressers enjoyed great prosperity thanks to the vogue for bobs, which were principally worn by young women who were proud of their financial autonomy. Certainly the bob caused quite a stir and was even seen by some detractors as the paganisation of Christian women, while others fussed that by wearing their hair in a bob, women might start going bald or begin growing a beard. Certainly the bob echoed the fashion in clothes for an androgynous curveless profile, while its provocative girlish look celebrated a sporty youth culture that countered the matronly style of the pre-war era. Simpler and less confining, the bob had a coquettish charm especially when worn by the young demimonde of flappers and boyish "garçonnes".

Although throughout the Twenties, short hair with Marcel waves was ubiquitous, by the end of the decade a more severe straight-cut bob in the "Japanese Bonnet Style" began replacing this type of rippled bob. This new type of helmet-like bob was popularised by the silent movie star Louise Brooks, who starred in two sexually progressive films in 1929 – *Pandora's Box* and *Diary of a Lost Girl* – both made by the German director, Georg Wilhelm Pabst. It was the inherent seductiveness, rebelliousness and uninhibited sexuality of the characters she played that appealed to young female movie-goers and underscored the underlying symbolism of the bob: the freer hairstyle, the freer woman.

During this era of unprecedented liberation and economic boom, women started entering the hairdressing profession and one saw the feminisation of what had once been a predominantly male trade. Many of their clients were women who could spend their own money as they liked, and as such spent a lot of their incomes on having their hair shampooed, permanently waved and cut into the fashionable styles of the day. The Twenties was also the time when a new professionalism entered the teaching of cosmetology as young women were taught the craft and science of the hairdressing trade. Significantly, as perhaps the most seminal era in the history of hair, the 1920s saw an utter paradigm shift towards shorter and less fussy hairstyles, which were utterly in accord with the wider society's desire for a new and liberal Modernity that would once and for all sweep away the poignant memories of war in its pursuit of Machine-Age progress.

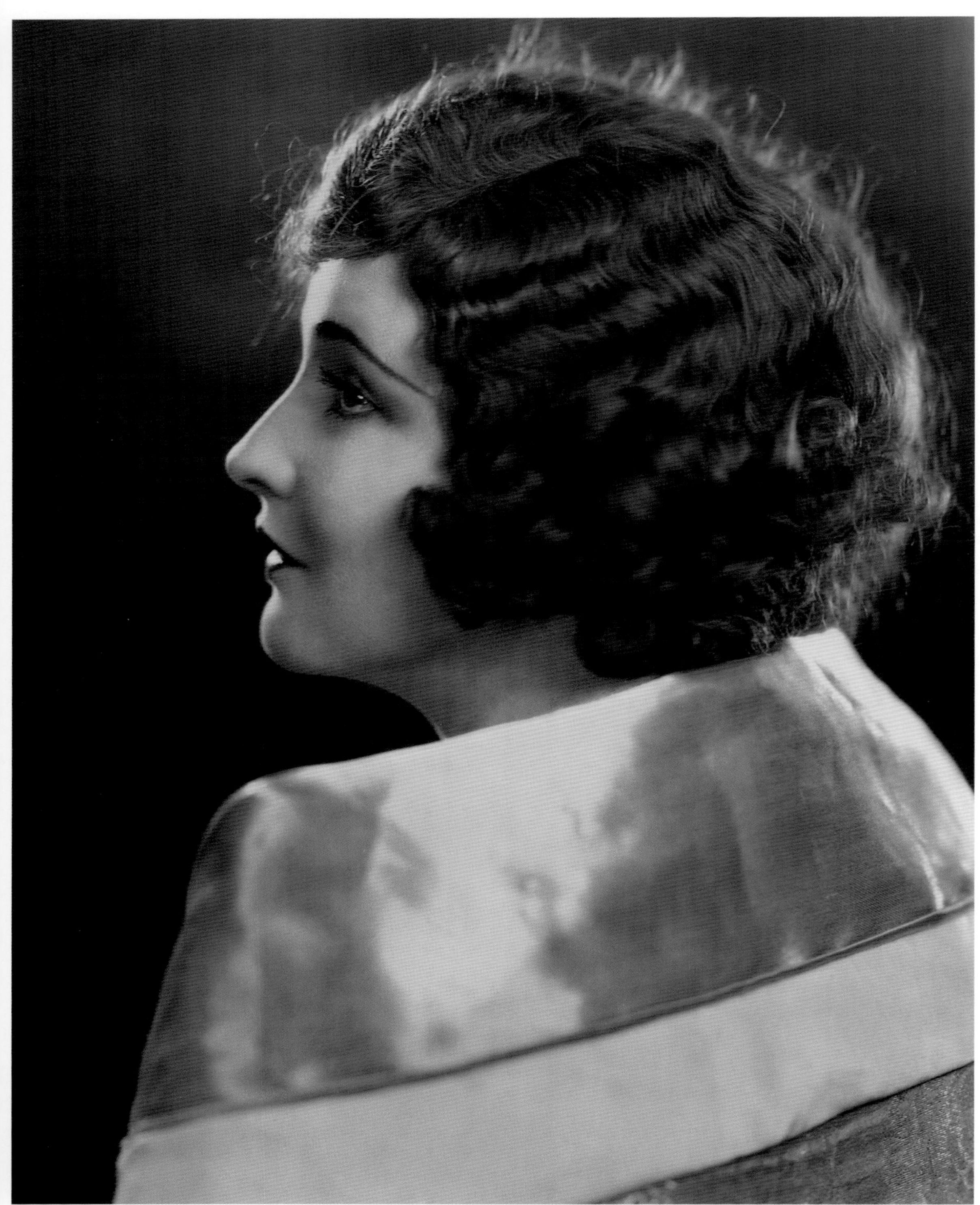

Portrait of Agnes Ayres, Paramount Pictures actress, 1920s, photographed by Eugene Robert Richee

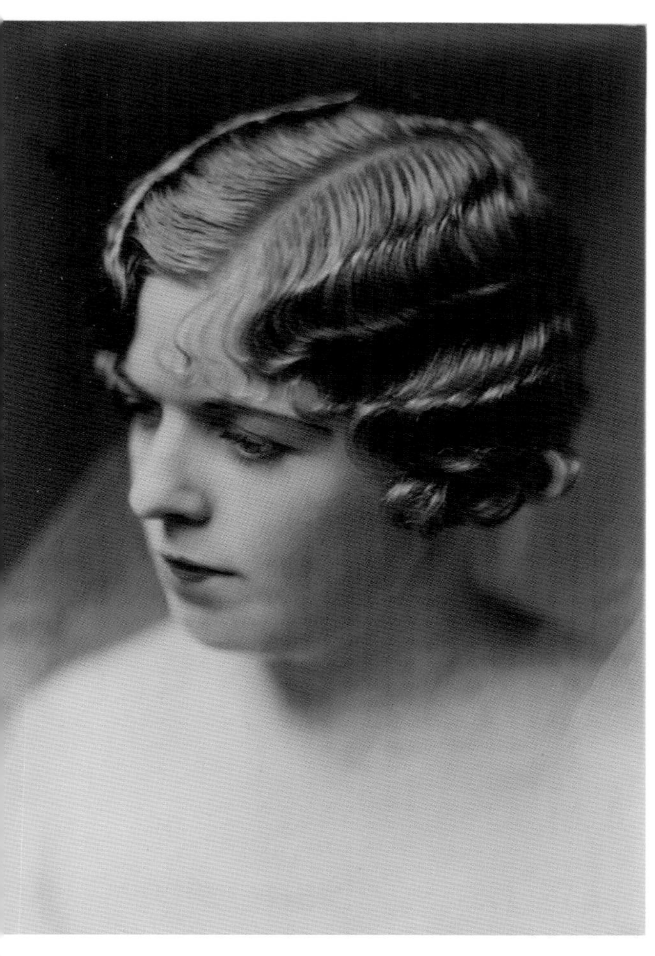
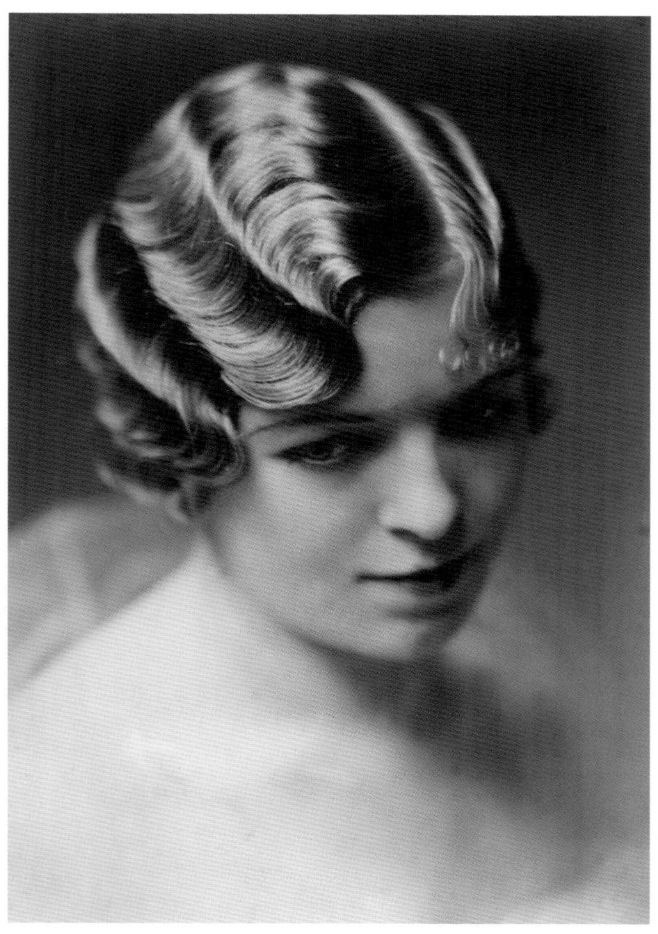

American "Marcel Wave" hairstyle, 1920s, C. Myland

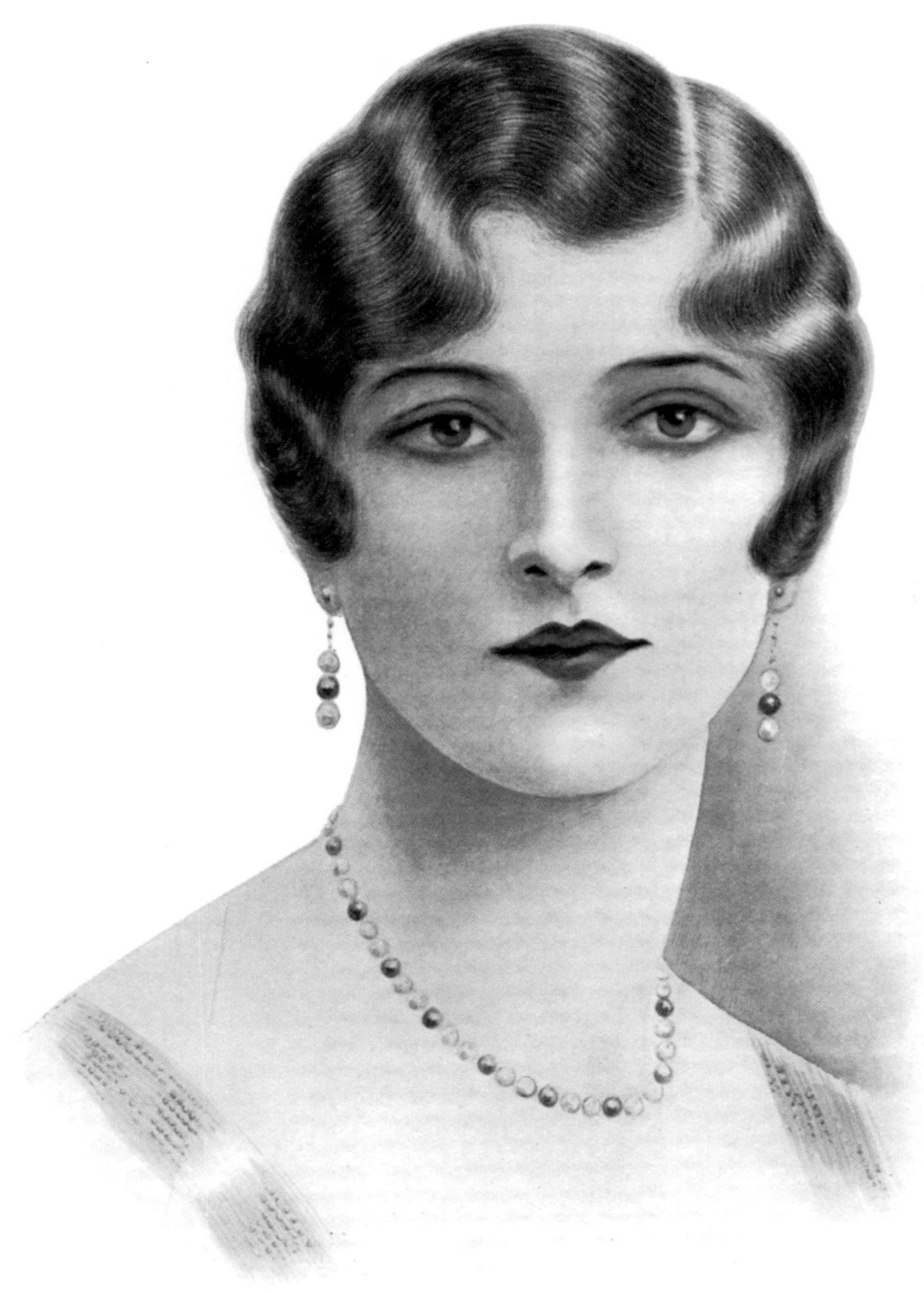

Marcel Waved bob, 1920s, *Album of Period Coiffures: Historical and Modern*, H. Serventi

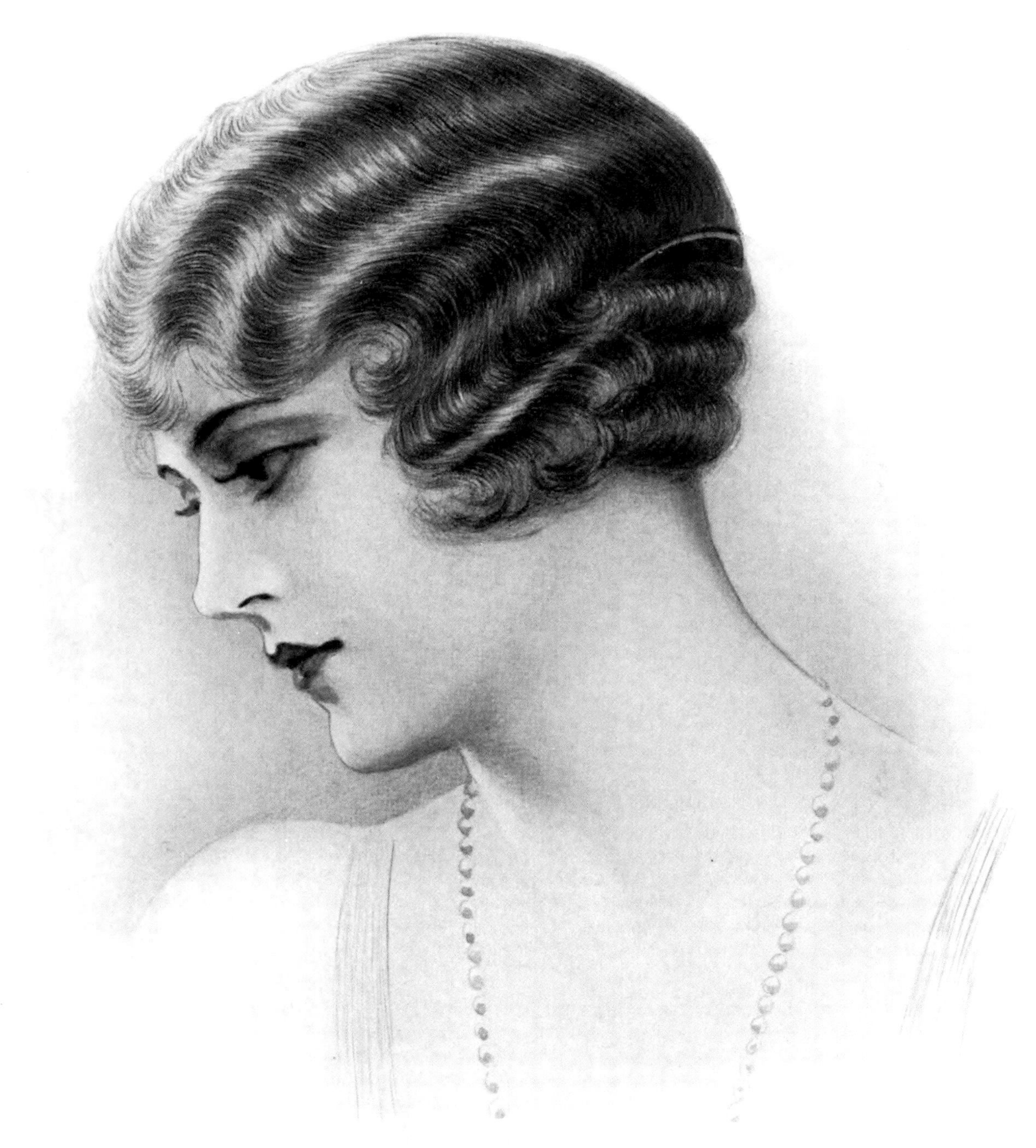

A Semi-Bobbed hairstyle, 1920s, *Album of Period Coiffures: Historical and Modern*, H. Serventi

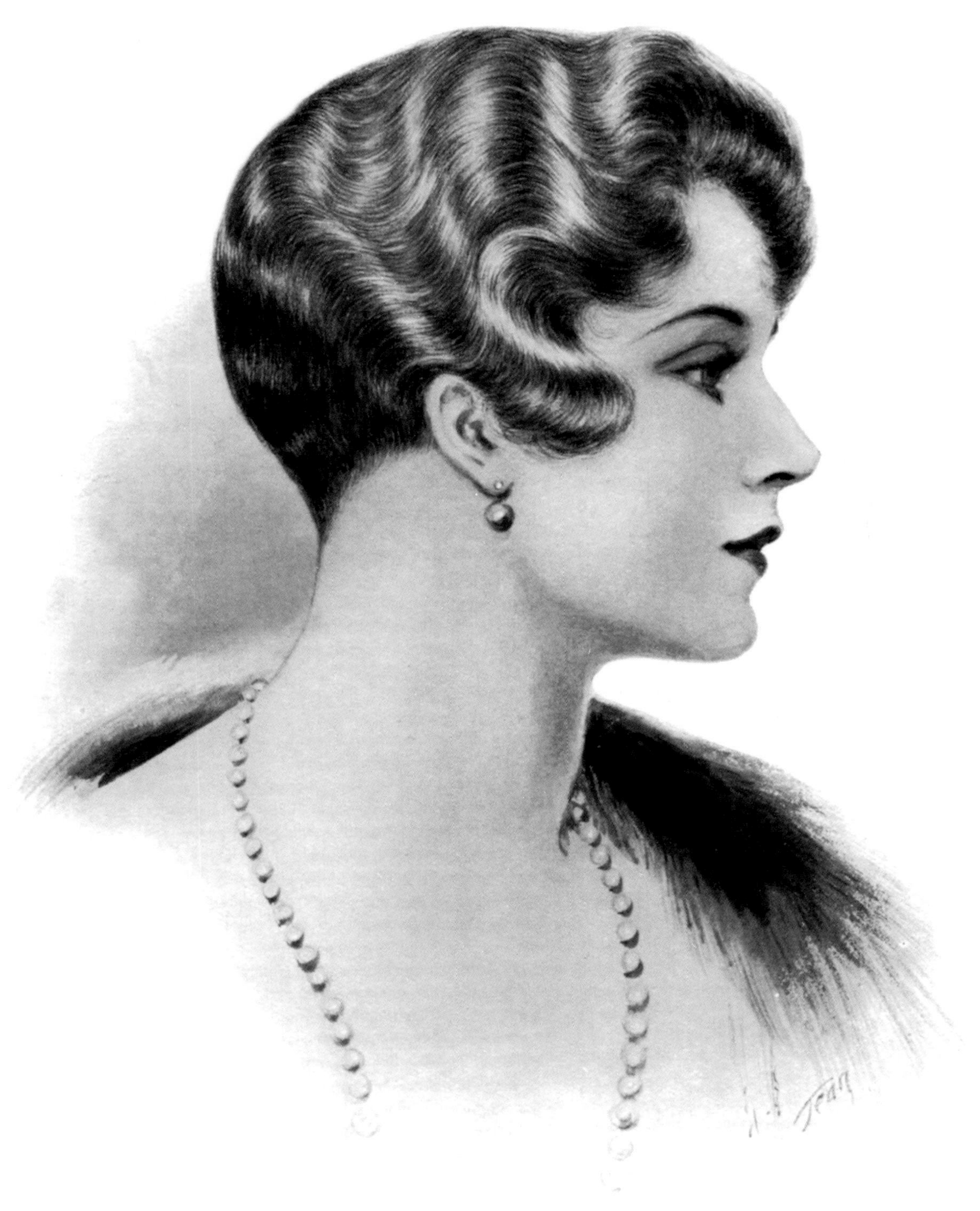

Permanently waved shingled bob, 1920s, *Album of Period Coiffures: Historical and Modern*, H. Serventi

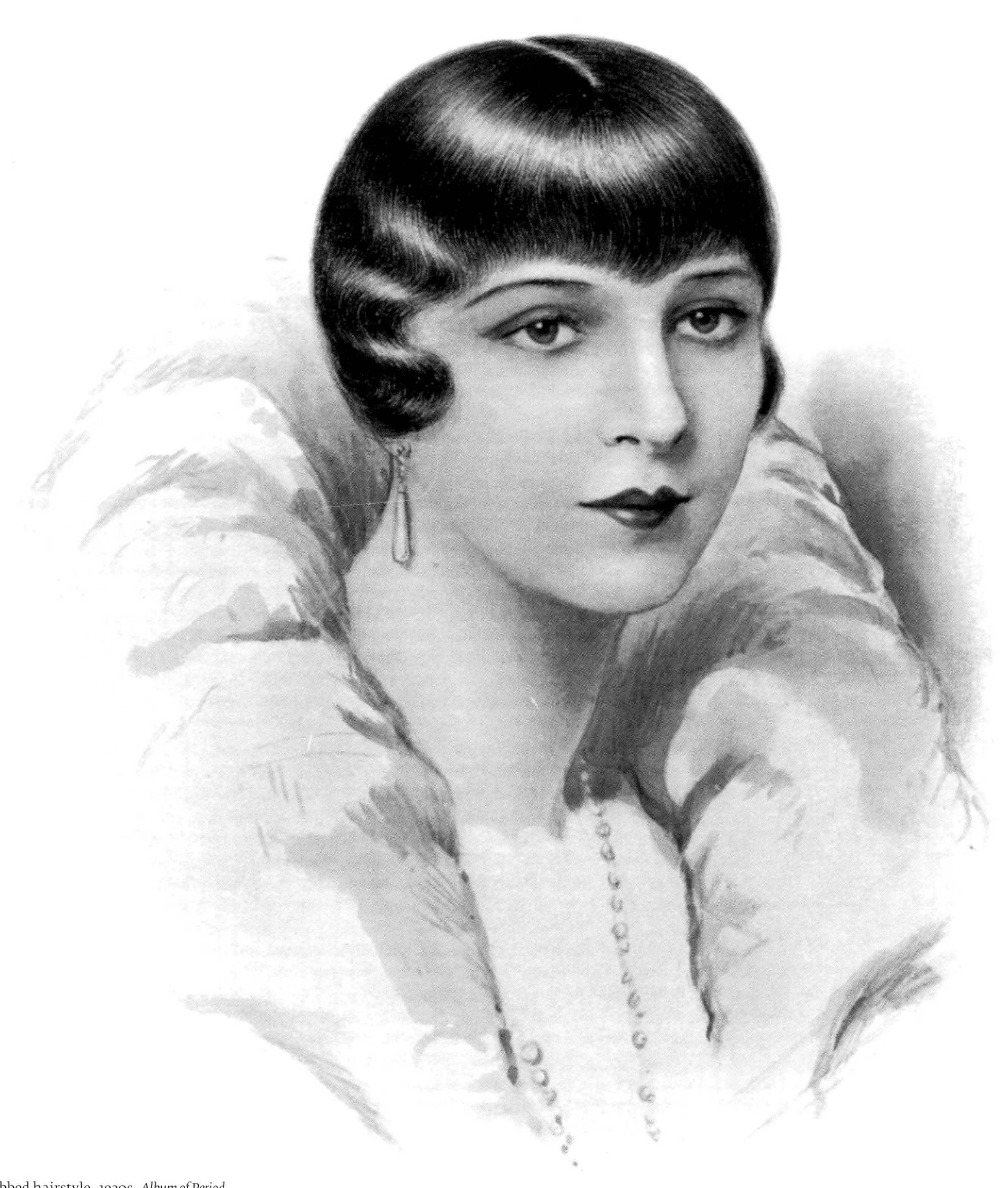

Bobbed hairstyle, 1920s, *Album of Period Coiffures: Historical and Modern*, H. Serventi

THE DELINEATOR, August, 1922 — Page 39

THE HAIR-FREE COIFFURE AND ITS AFTERMATH

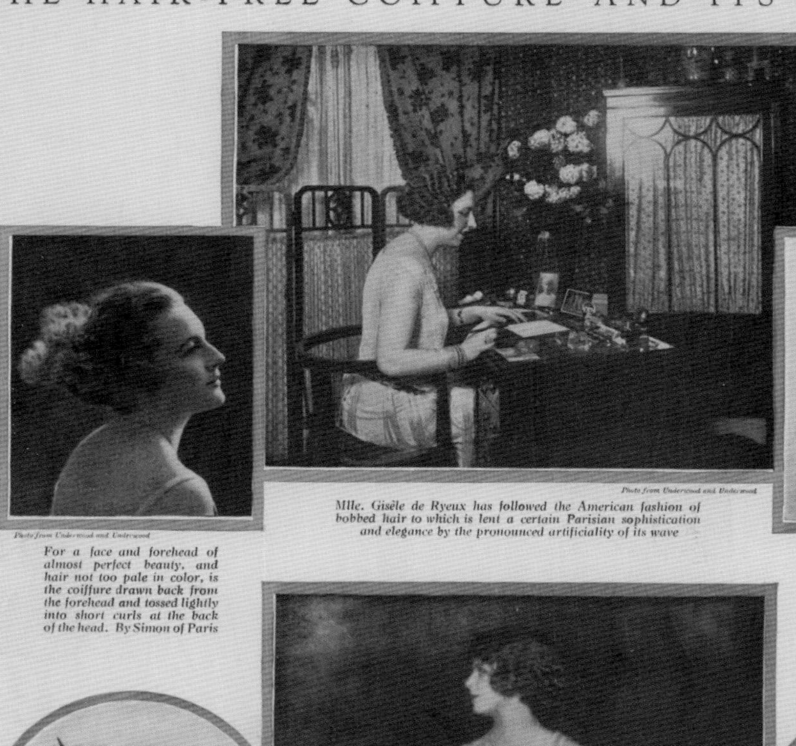

Photo from Underwood and Underwood

Mlle. Gisèle de Ryeux has followed the American fashion of bobbed hair to which is lent a certain Parisian sophistication and elegance by the pronounced artificiality of its wave

Photo from Underwood and Underwood

For a face and forehead of almost perfect beauty, and hair not too pale in color, is the coiffure drawn back from the forehead and tossed lightly into short curls at the back of the head. By Simon of Paris

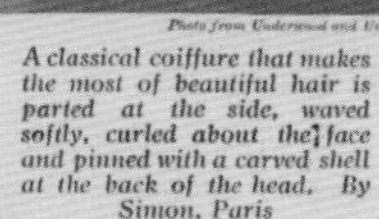

Photo from Underwood and Underwood

A classical coiffure that makes the most of beautiful hair is parted at the side, waved softly, curled about the face and pinned with a carved shell at the back of the head. By Simon, Paris

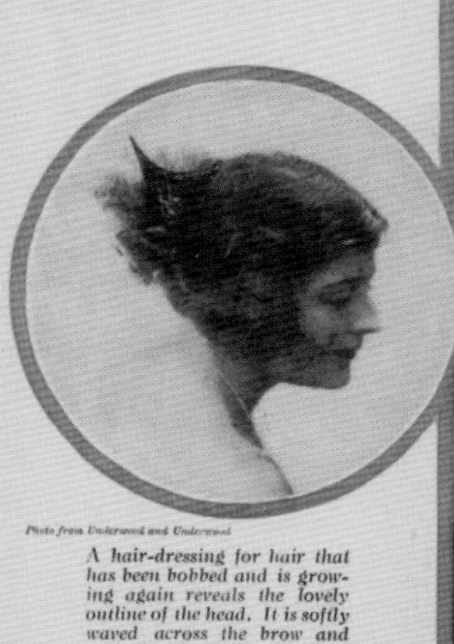

Photo from Underwood and Underwood

A hair-dressing for hair that has been bobbed and is growing again reveals the lovely outline of the head. It is softly waved across the brow and curled at the sides and back. The coiffure is by Simon of Paris

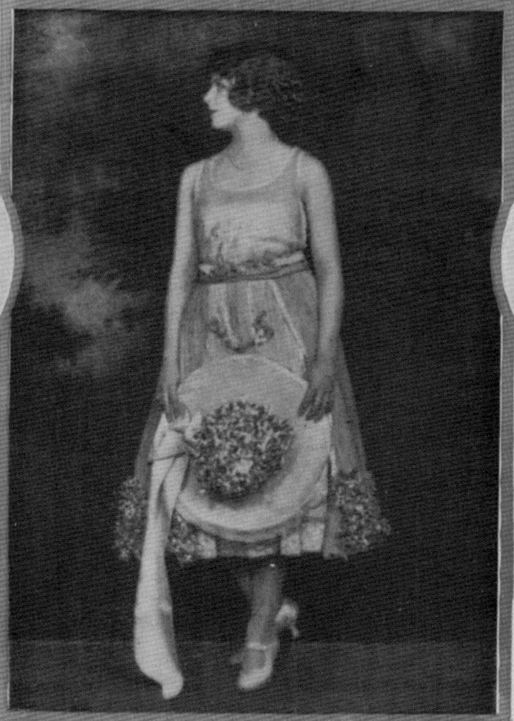

Photo by The White Studio

The short cut is usually an experimental matter. The length and arrangement must suit the face and straight hair in most cases must be curled. For Grace La Rue in "The Blue Kitten" the hair is curled in short baby-like curls

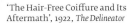

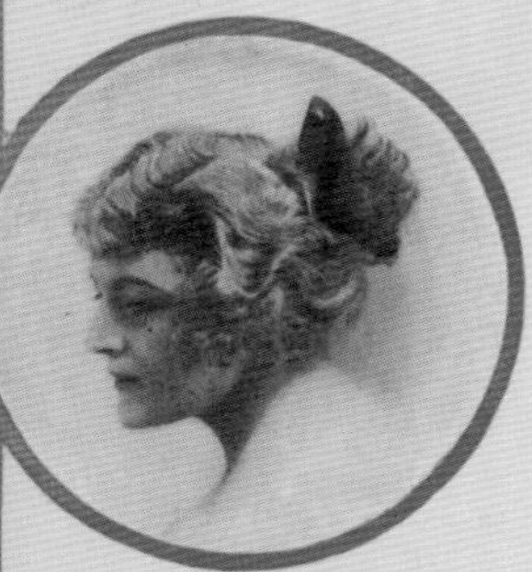

Photo from Underwood and Underwood

Hair that is "going up" after being cut off in its youth takes naturally to a psyche-like knot of curls at the back of the head. For most women the hair has more light and beauty if it is slightly waved. Coiffure by Simon, Paris

'The Hair-Free Coiffure and Its Aftermath', 1922, *The Delineator*

SUPPLÉMENT DE
LA COIFFURE DE PARIS

DIRECTION :
37, rue J.-J. Rousseau
Paris

PRIX DU NUMÉRO :
France..... 3 fr.
Étranger ... 4.25

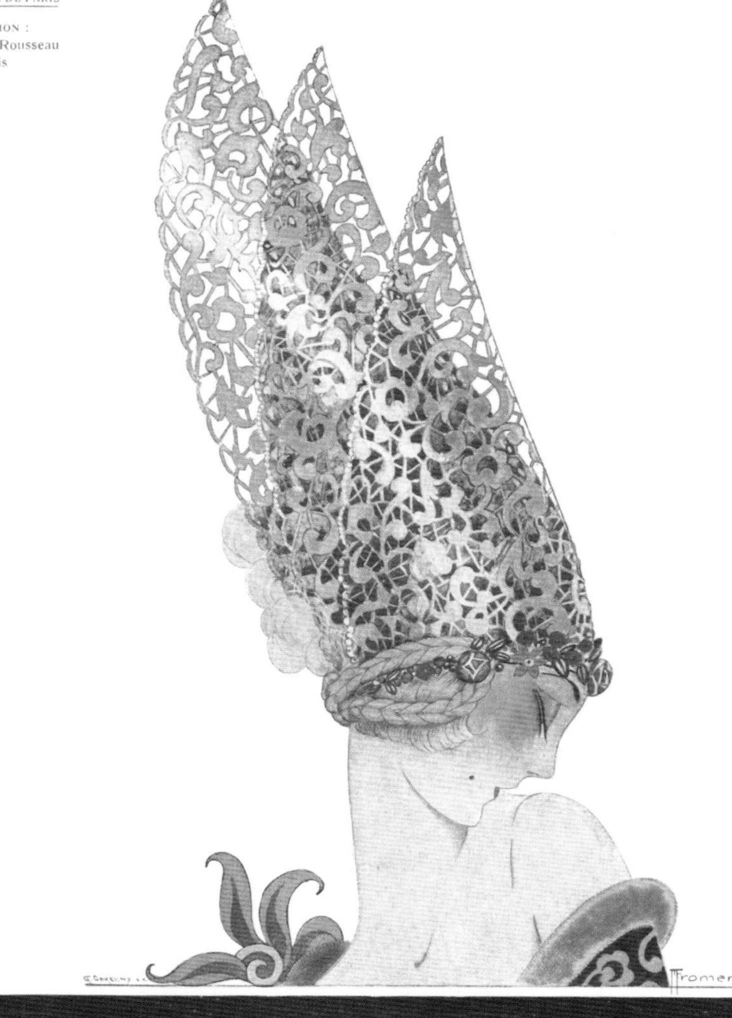

LA COIFFURE
et les Modes

11e ANNÉE - No 153
NOVEMBRE 1922

COIFFURE DESFOSSÉ
DESSIN DE FROMENTI

ABONNEMENT :
France ... 25 fr.
Étranger .. 35 fr.

La Coiffure et les Modes magazine cover, hairstyle by Desfossé, illustration by Fromenti, Paris, 1922

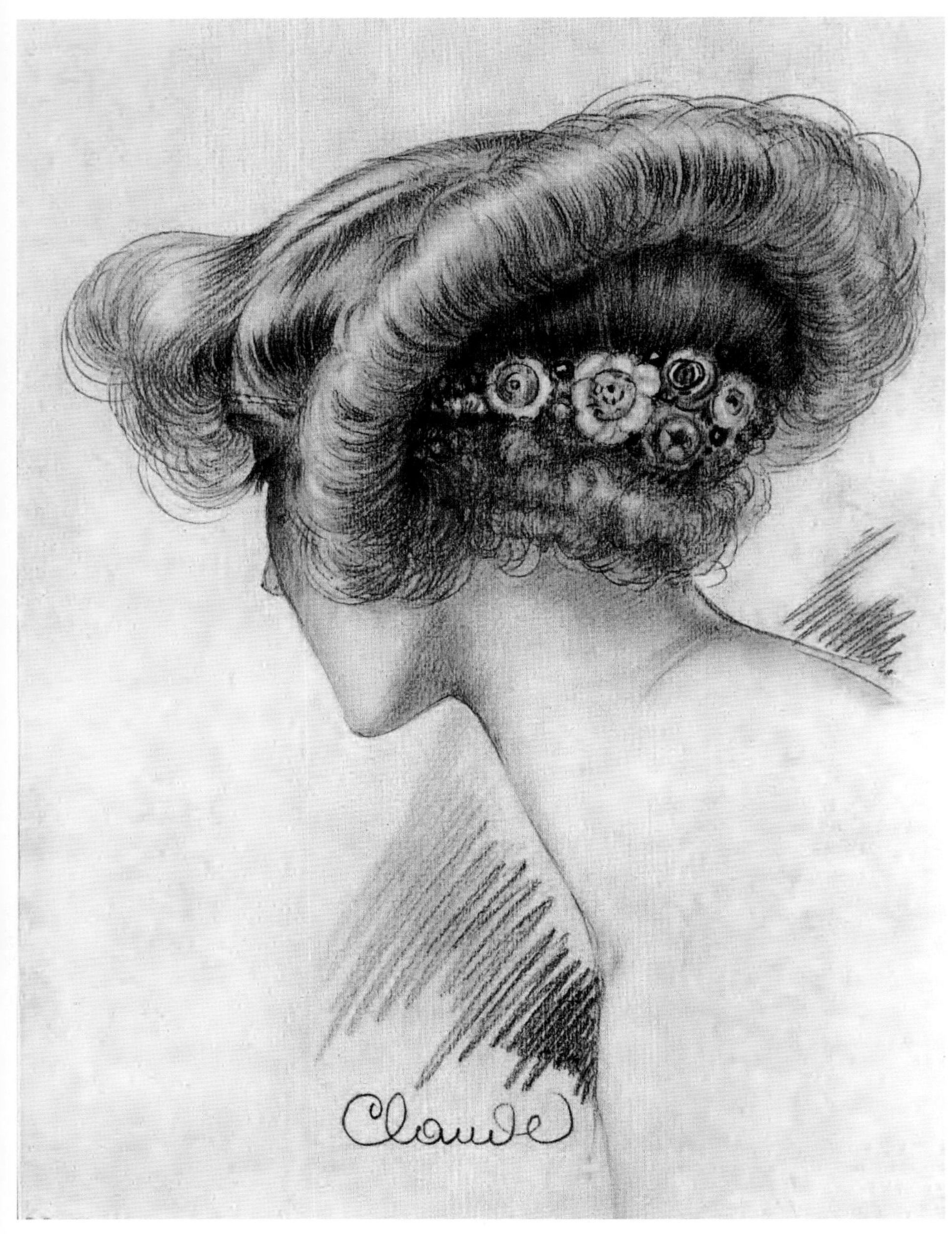

'An entirely new look', hairstyle
by Léon Agostini, Paris, 1922,
La Coiffure et les Modes

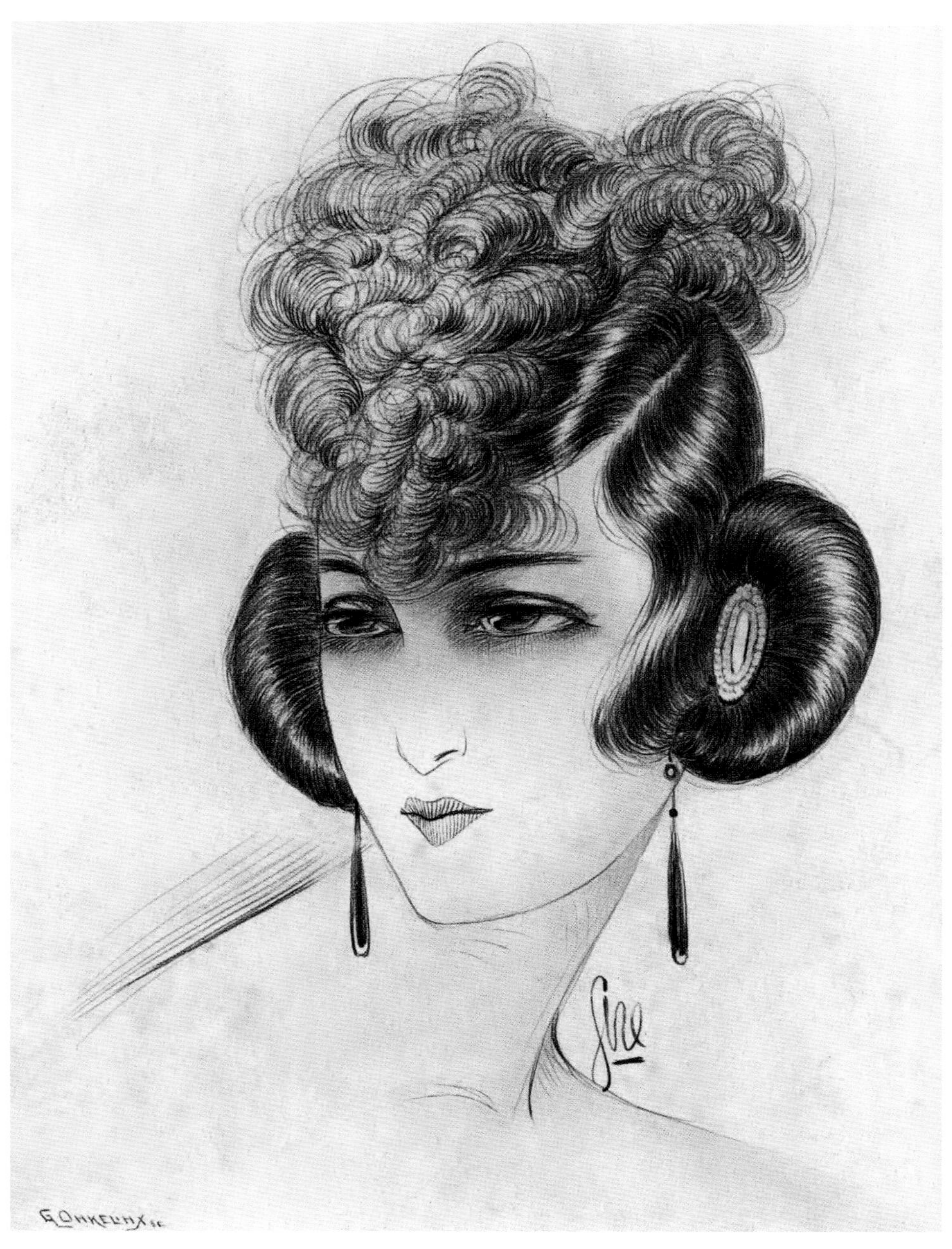

'Hairstyle seen at a competition',
Paris, 1922, *La Coiffure et les Modes*

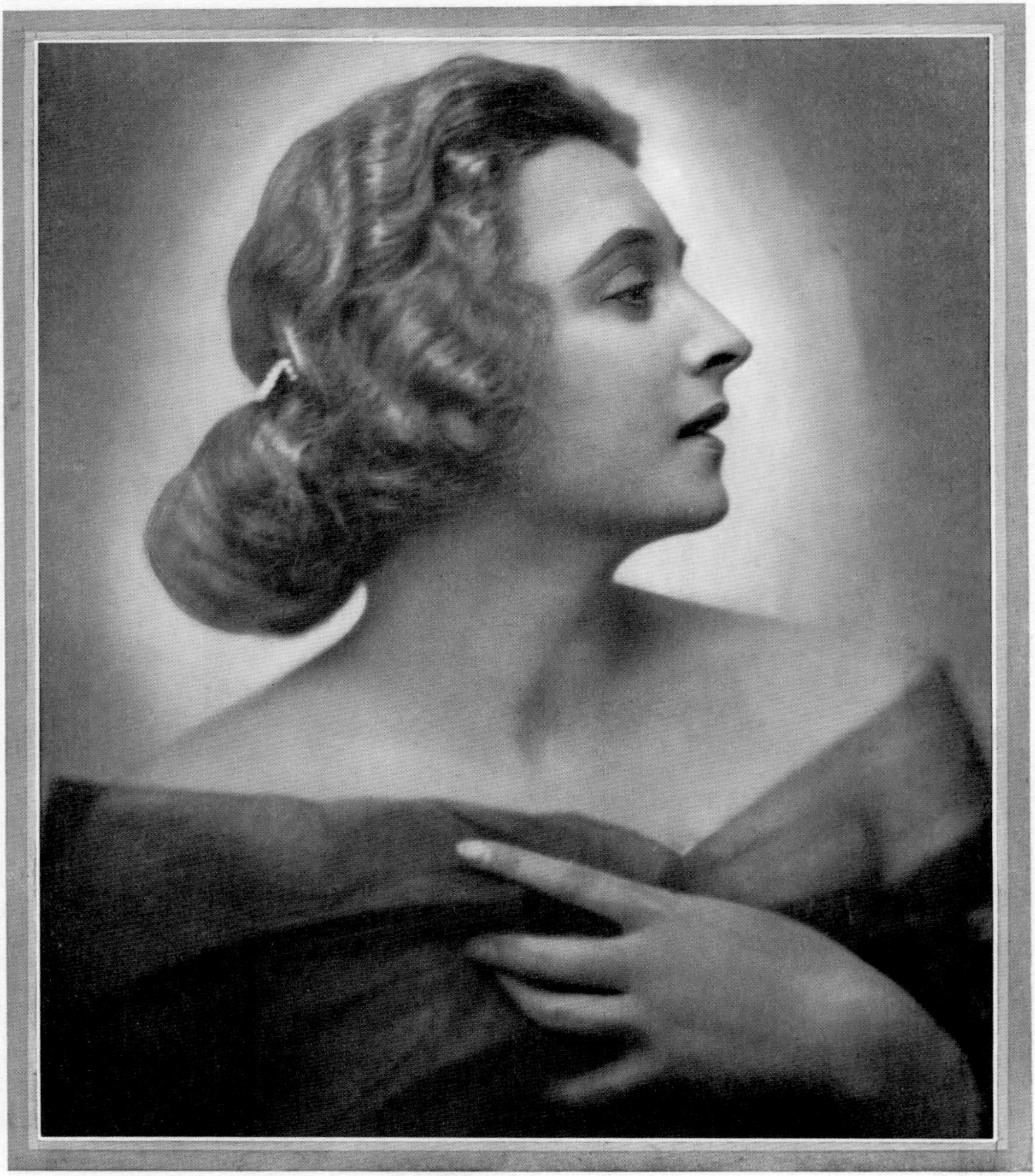

Photo Talbot.

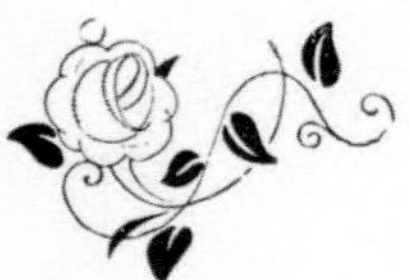

LA COIFFURE PRÉFÉRÉE

PORTÉE PAR Mlle CLAUDE FRANCE

Oui, cette coiffure, simple, naturelle, presque sans apprêt, avec son chignon bas, épais, ses ondulations floues qui élargissent à peine le volume de la tête, c'est celle que préfère encore la Parisienne.

'La Coiffure Préférée', worn by Miss Claude France, 1922, *La Coiffure et les Modes*

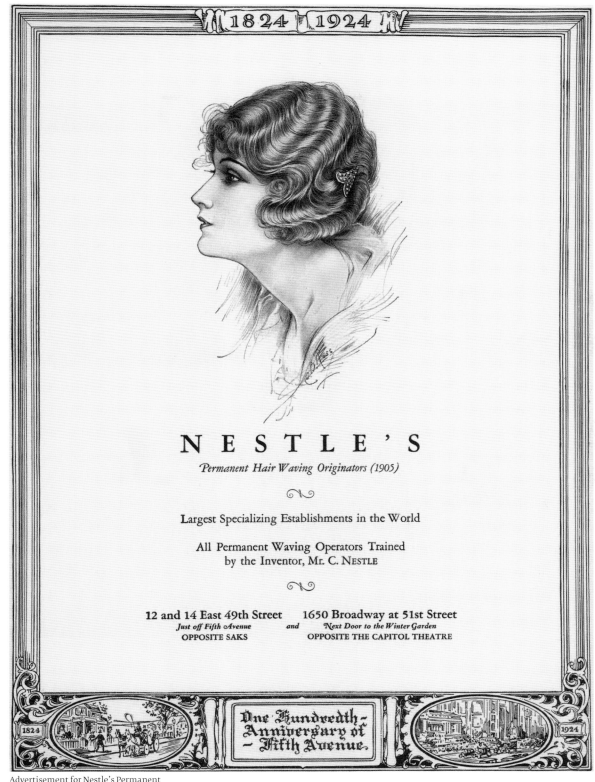

Advertisement for Nestle's Permanent Hair Waving Originators (1905), 1924

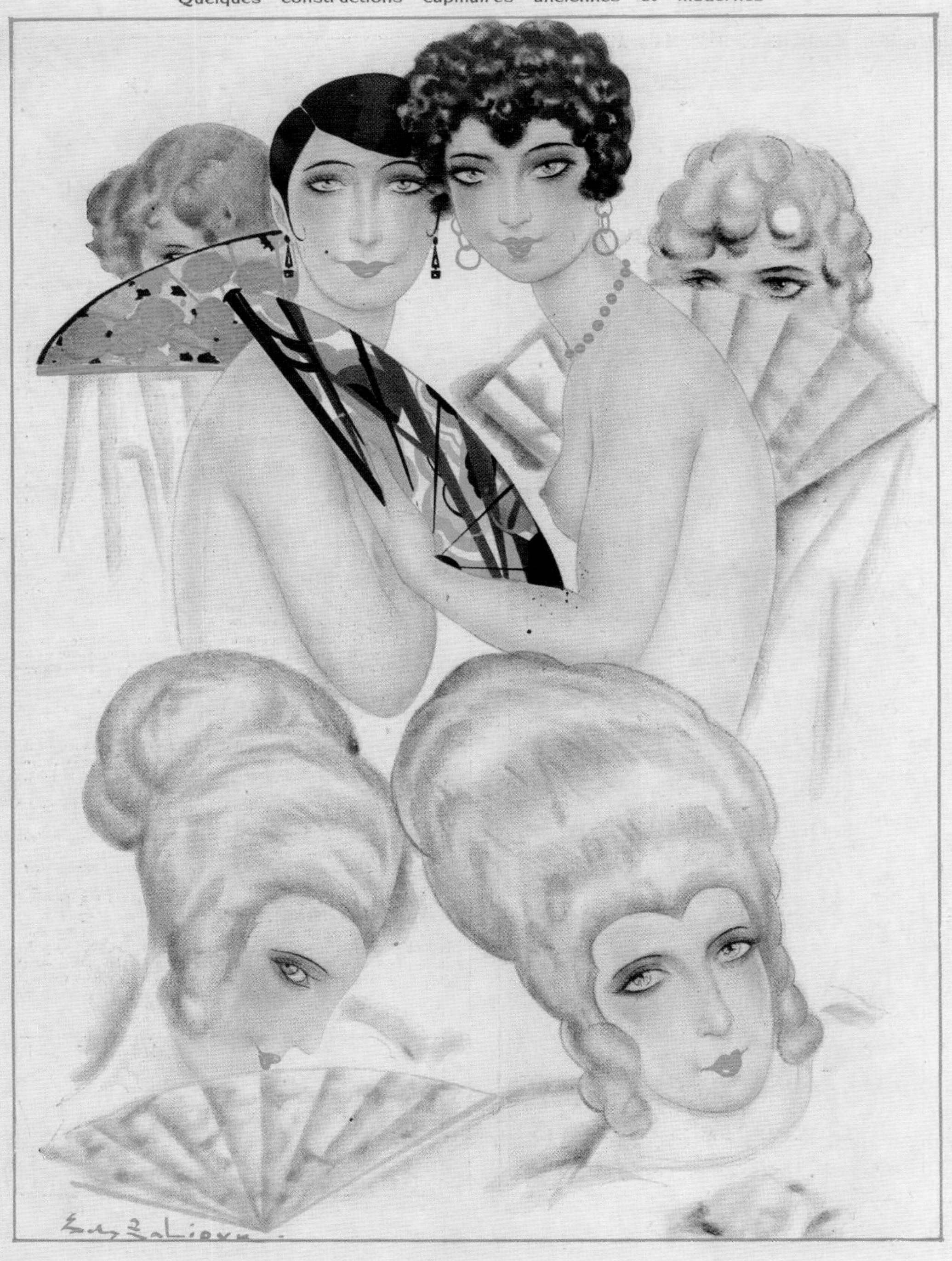

'La Mode Saisie Par les Cheveux', a few examples of ancient and modern hairstyles, drawing by Zaliouk, 1925, *La Vie Parisienne*

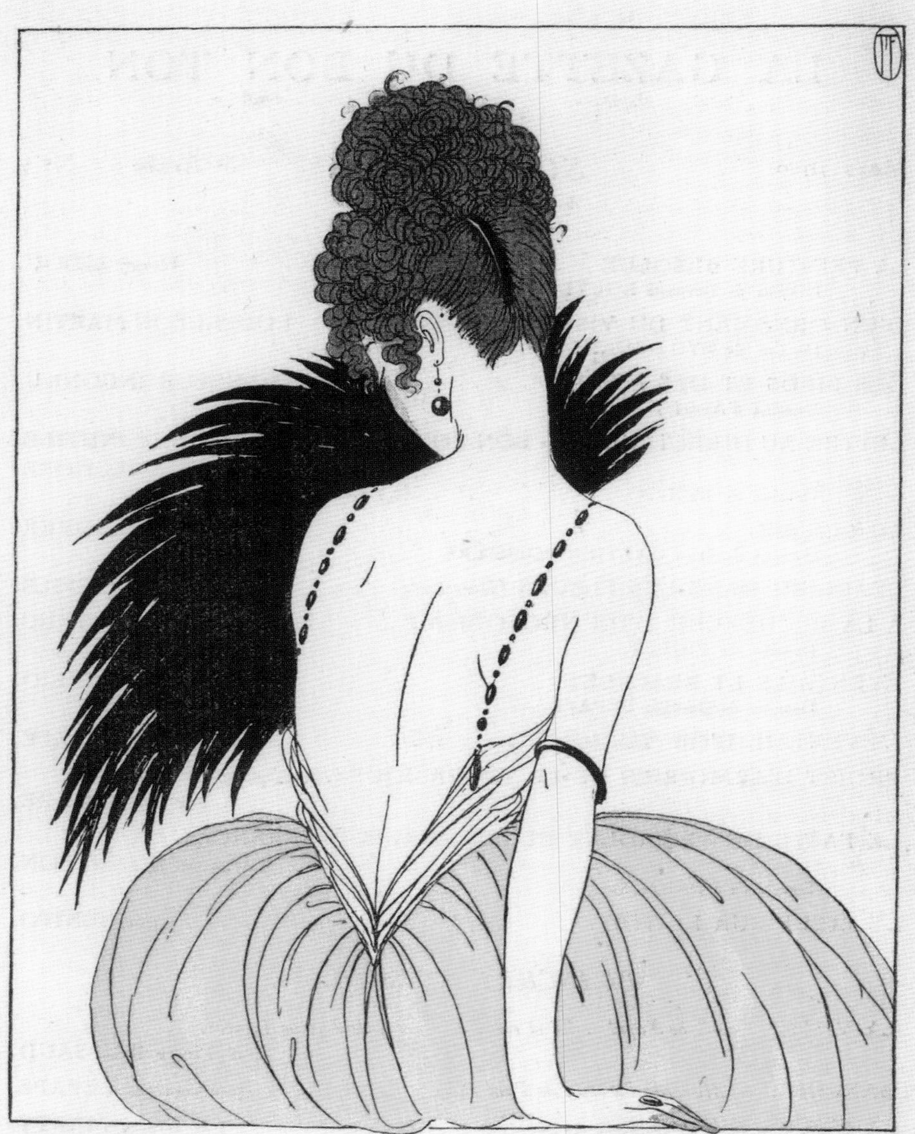

vertisement for hairstyles by
nile Ltd., London & Paris, 1920s

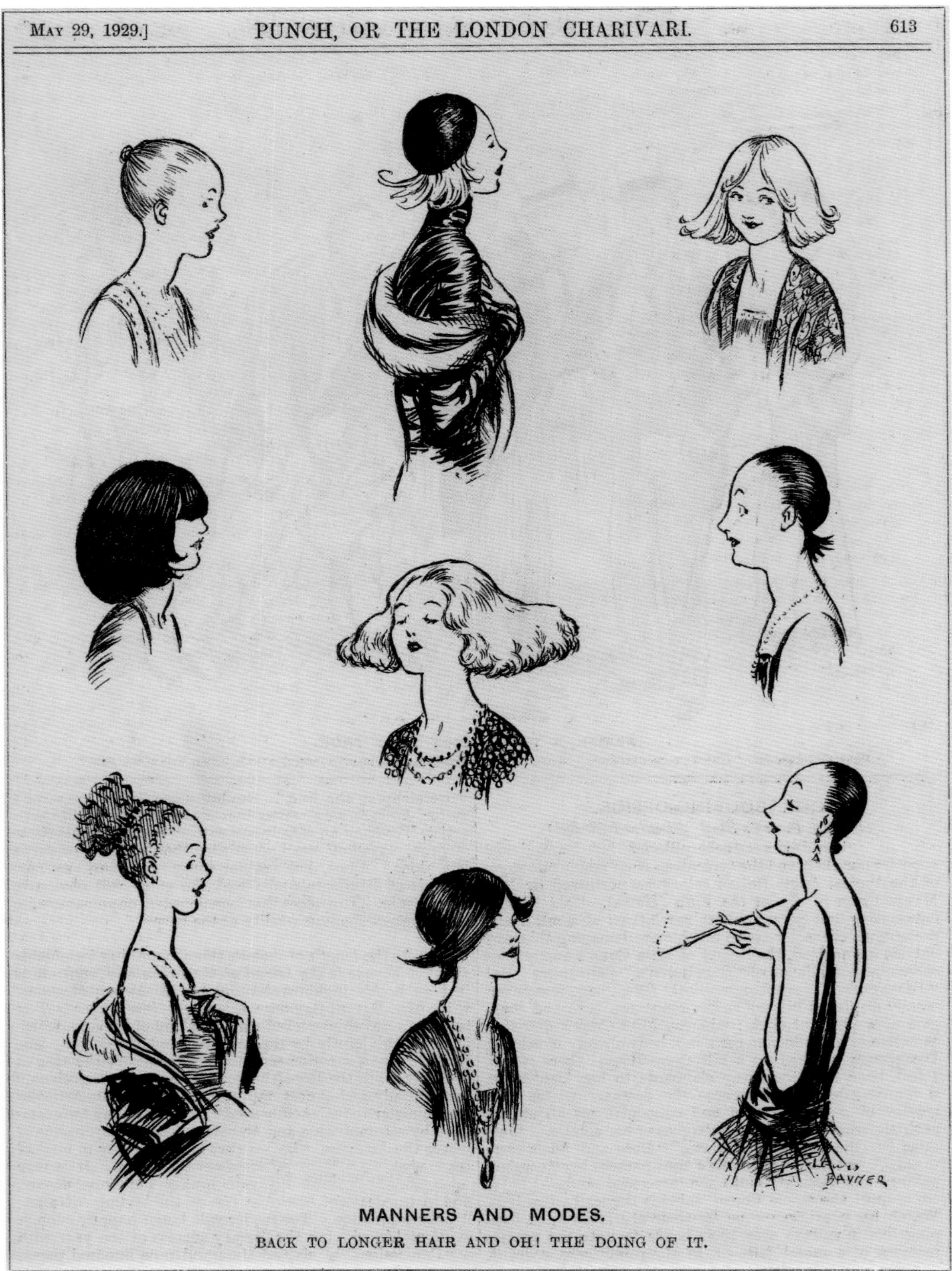

MAY 29, 1929.] PUNCH, OR THE LONDON CHARIVARI. 613

MANNERS AND MODES.

BACK TO LONGER HAIR AND OH! THE DOING OF IT.

Hairstyles, London, 1929, *Punch*

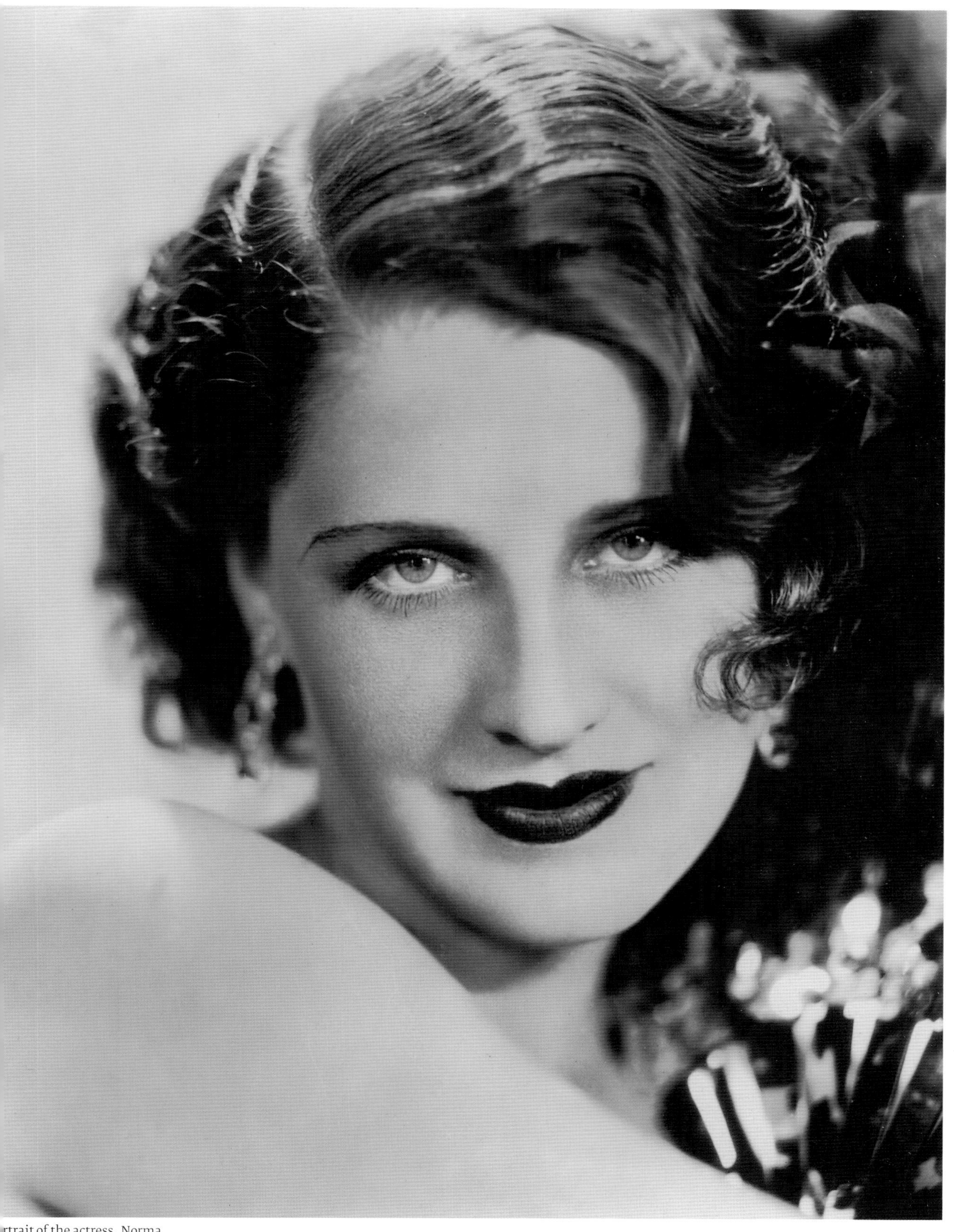

rtrait of the actress, Norma
earer with waved hair, c.1929

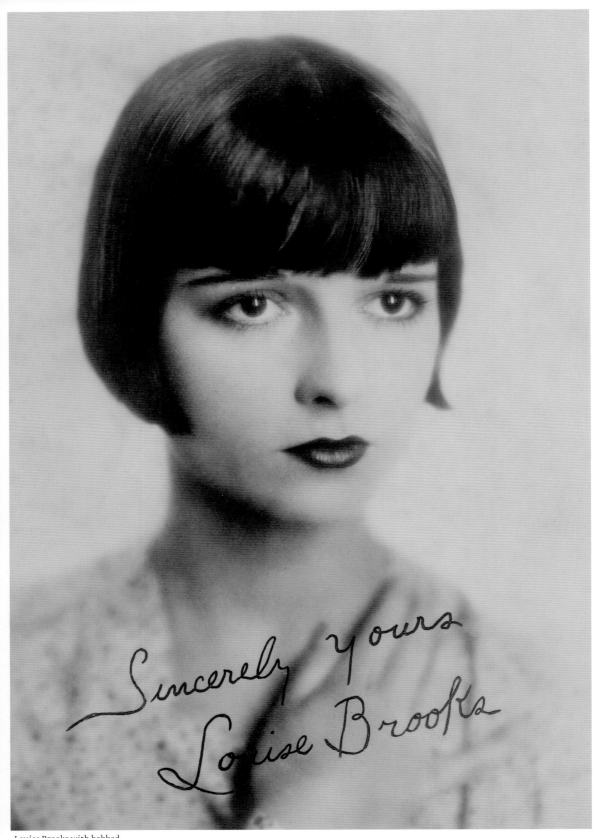

Louise Brooks with bobbed hairstyle, c.1929

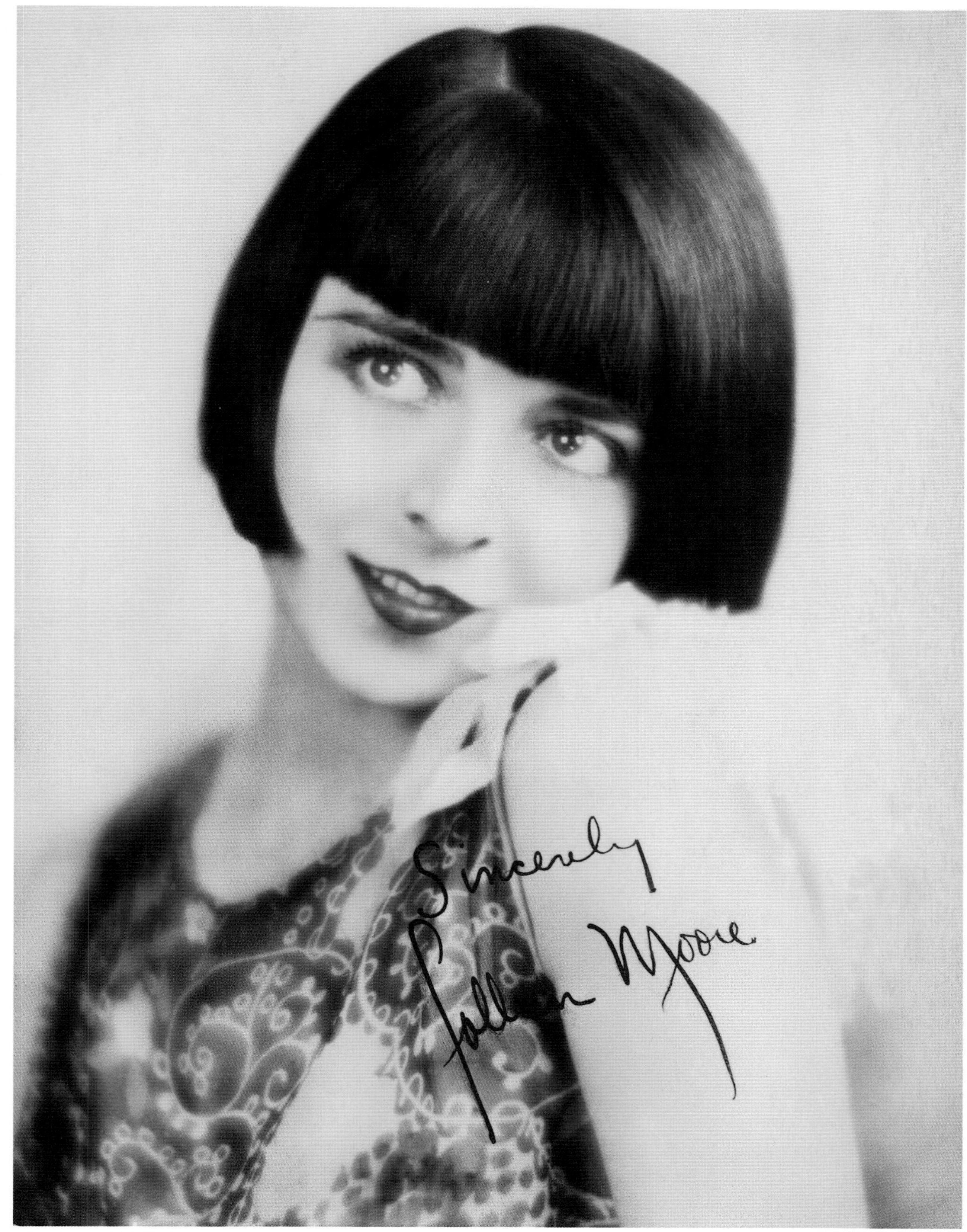

Colleen Moore with bobbed hairstyle, c. 1929

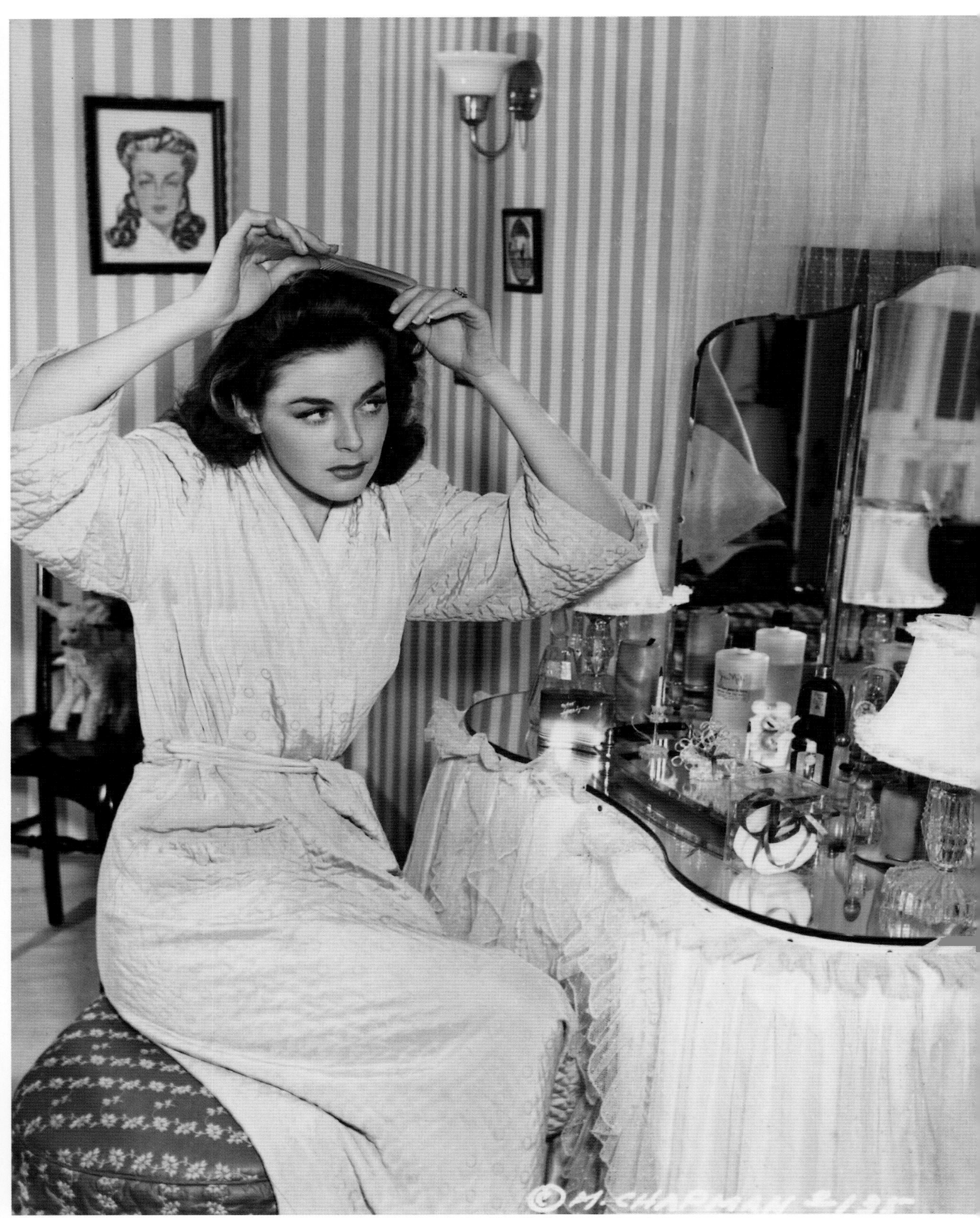

Actress Marguerite Chapman attending to her coiffure, 1935, photographed by Don English

1930S, 1940S

orn in Poland, in 1925 "Monsieur Antoine" (Antek ierplikowski) opened his famous Antoine de Paris salon in Saks ifth Avenue department store. By the 1930s he had become ne of the most influential and important hairdressers in the orld, with his famous "shingle" being worn by women across ne globe. A complete showman, "Monsieur Antoine" dyed is own hair, as well as that of his poodle, a fetching shade of lac, and was the world's first celebrity hairdresser of any note. o create his distinctive shingle haircut, the hair was cut into taper running from the nape of the neck to the level of the ar, and then was waved or curled. During the 1930s, Monsieur ntoine also introduced the use of blonde streaks to accent ne hair.

In 1931, *The Art and Craft of Hairdressing* (edited by Gilbert A. Foan) as published as a practical guide to the techniques of odern hairdressing and "a book written by hairdressers for airdressers". In this weighty tome numerous bobbed, semi-obbed and shingled hairstyles are illustrated, progressing om the severely masculine "Eton Crop" to the femininely ousled "Claudine" shingle. Another popular coiffure of the eriod was the "Cringle", which had the hair tapered short n the top of the head and sides but left longer at the neck. uring this period it became fashionable to use plastic and cquer dressings in order to fix the rippled curls in place. or plastic dressings, coloured powders were dabbed onto ne hair and then allowed to set under a hood-drier; it was nen popular for a fine metallic dust, either gold or silver in ppearance, to be sprinkled over the hairstyle to add an extra ouch of sparkle. Sometimes differently coloured powders and encils were used to create astonishing effects. Lacquered ressings were also used extensively to created sophisticated yles that incorporated a great number of curls or waves. As ilbert A. Foan noted, "The hardness of plastic and lacquer nables the hairdresser to place his waves and curls in position ith the certainty that they will stay there. Hence, the most nconventional and fantastic results can be fearlessly aimed at." lthough such hairstyles had a crisp-looking sophistication, they must have felt like hard, impenetrable helmets.

During the 1930s there was an increasing demand for extremely blonde hair that was worn slightly longer. This trend was generated by the silver-screen goddesses of the period, including Jean Harlow who became known as the "Platinum Blonde" and the "Blonde Bombshell", and whose bleached locks were responsible for skyrocketing sales of peroxide during this period. However, Harlow's mysterious death from renal failure at the tender age of 26 led to speculation of hair dye poisoning and the fashion for platinium blonde hair subsequently waned. Veronica Lake was another Hollywood actress whose distinctive blonde "peek-a-boo" shoulder-length hairstyle was widely imitated during the early 1940s. Her "One-Eyed Hairdo" or "Witch-Lock" was, however, deemed to be unsuitable during the war years and, in a *US News Review* titled "Safety Styles", she was shown having her luscious tresses shorn and then rolled and pinned into a "simple but becoming fashion" more appropriate for a war production plant.

Needless to say, the Second World War saw the demise of highly dressed coiffures and instead women began to wear their hair in practical styles that were rolled and pinned out of harm's way, captured in net-like snoods or tied up into a scarf in the land girl style. In 1945 a long pageboy roll became fashionable and, over the next three years, haircuts just got shorter and shorter. In 1948 and 1949, a new and very short urchin style was introduced that was almost shingled at the back and left with shaggy curls at the front, while some younger women adopted a simple fringe and ponytail combo. Another fashion was for short cuts that were side-parted, semi-quiffed over the forehead with small kiss-curls gently emerging from the sides and the back. Just like the early interwar years, the hairstyles during the immediate post-war years reflected a changing shift in how women saw themselves, and it is unsurprising that many who had experienced the make-do-and-mend ethos of the war years subsequently opted for shorter or more youthful hairstyles that symbolised, perhaps subconsciously, the beginning of a brave new world.

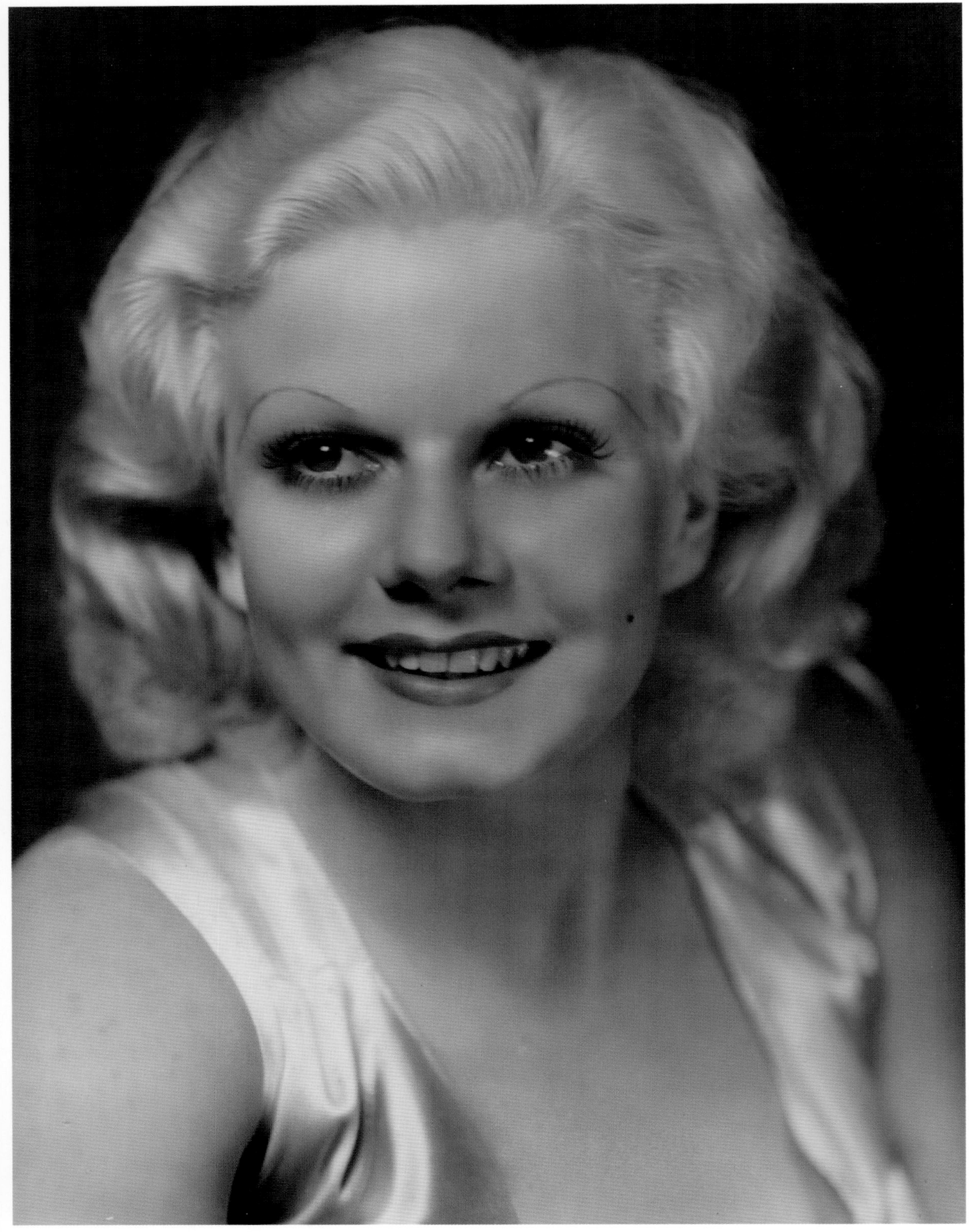

Jean Harlow with platinum-
blonde locks, early 1930s

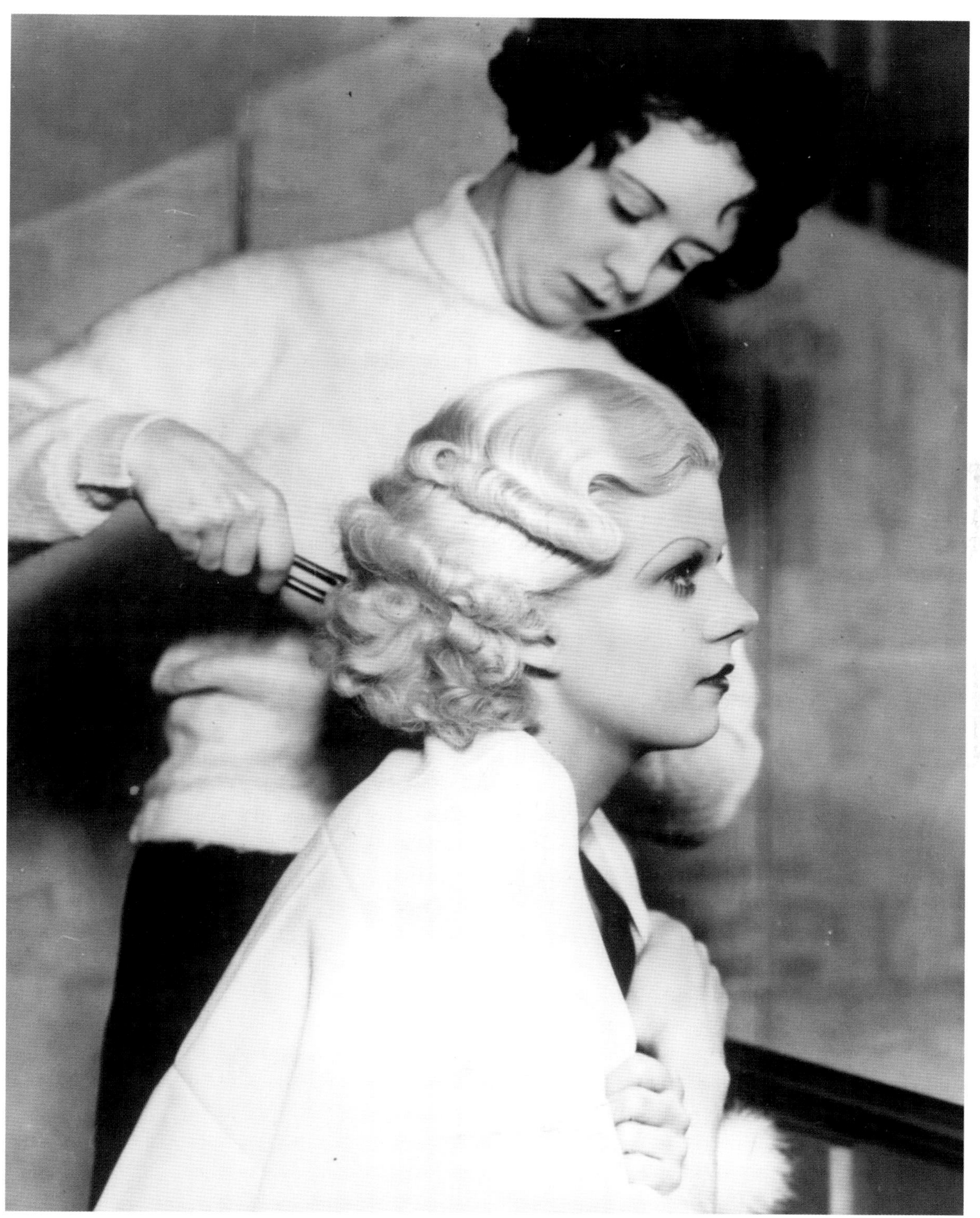

Jean Harlow having her famous platinum blonde hair set, 1933

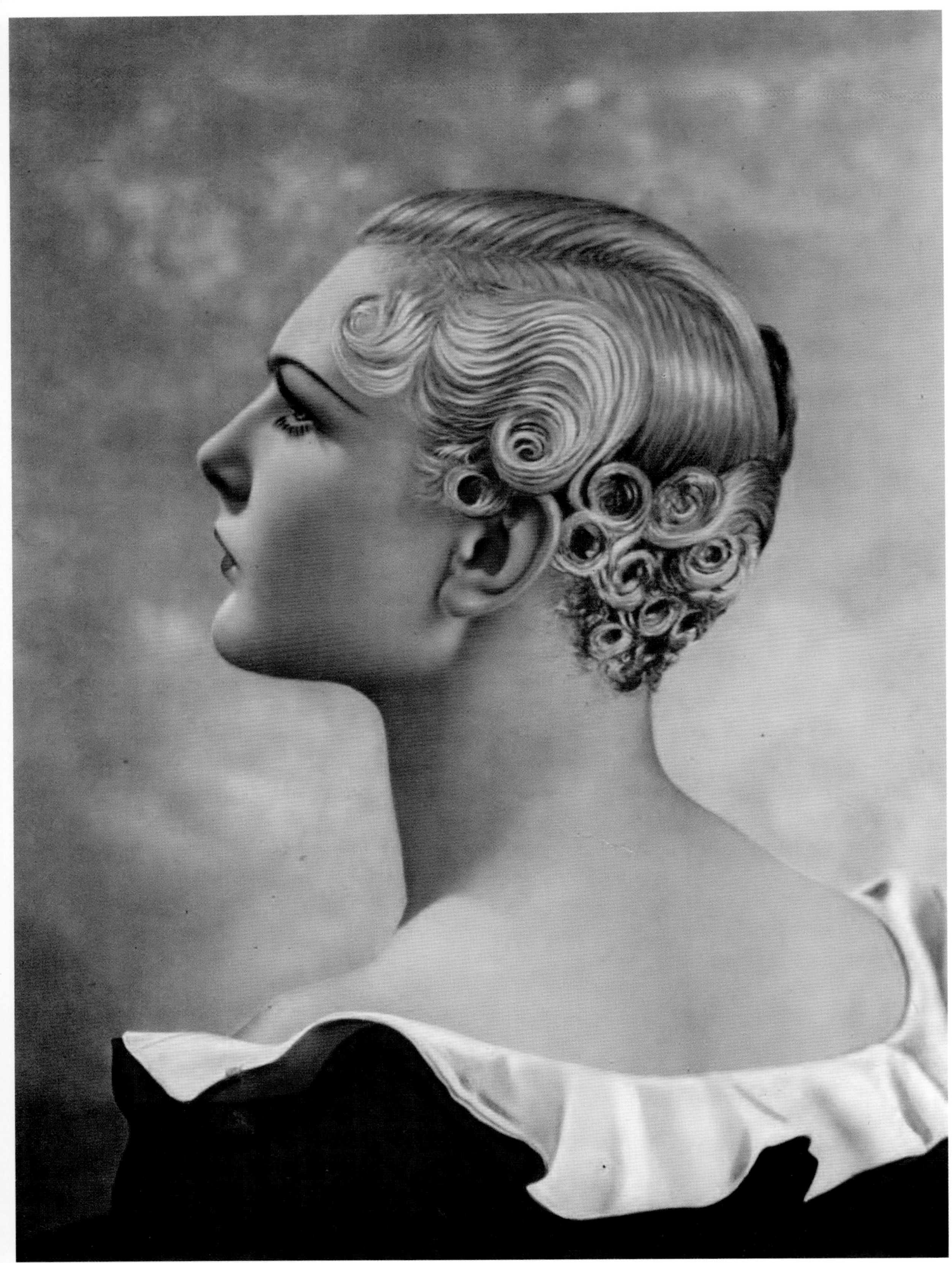

An Icall Plastic Dressing by Messrs I. Calvete Ltd., 1936, *The Art and Craft of Hairdressing*, Gilbert A. Foan

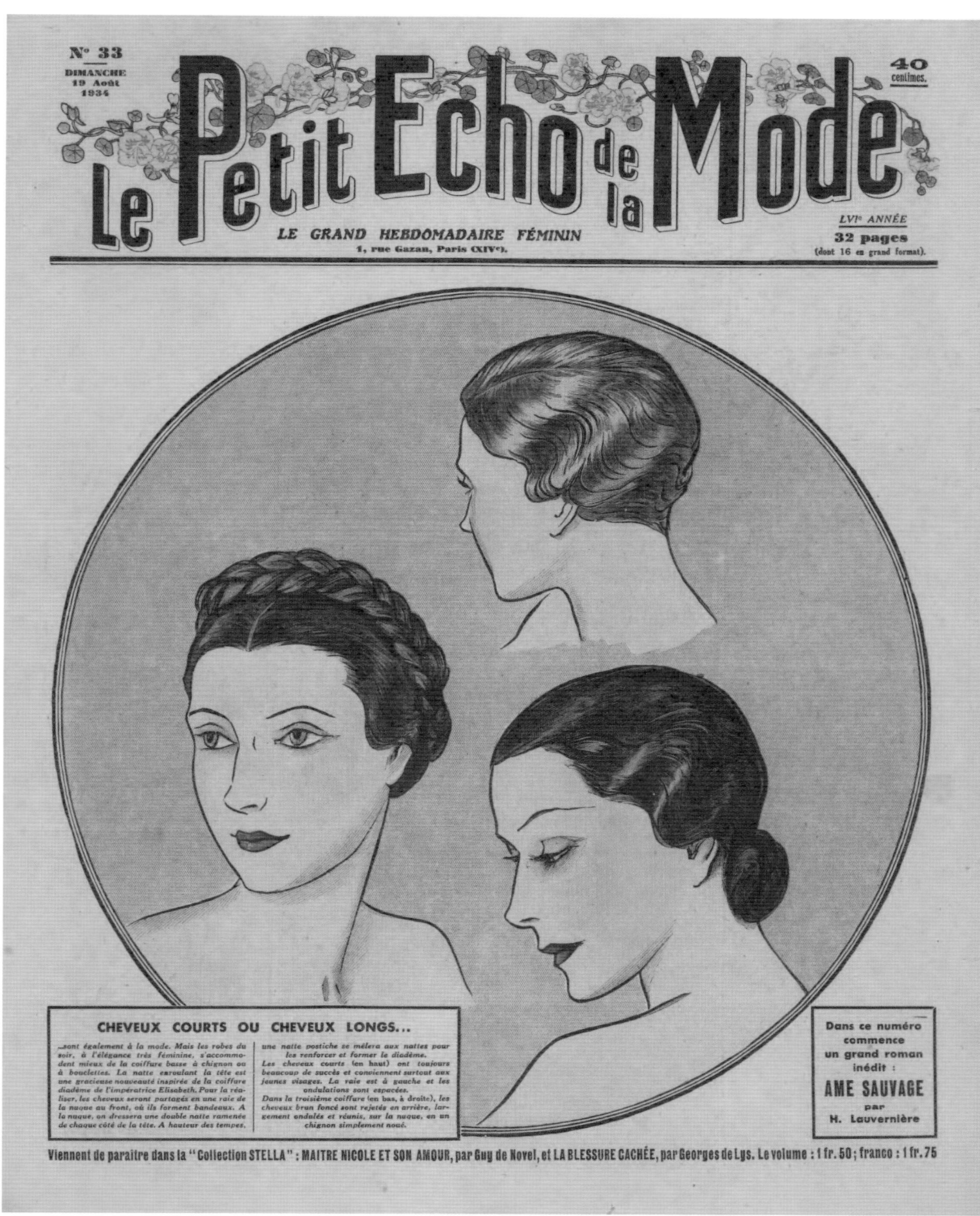

N° 33

DIMANCHE 19 Août 1934

Le Petit Echo de la Mode

40 centimes.

LE GRAND HEBDOMADAIRE FÉMININ

1, rue Gazan, Paris (XIVe).

LVIe ANNÉE

32 pages (dont 16 en grand format).

CHEVEUX COURTS OU CHEVEUX LONGS...

...sont également à la mode. Mais les robes du soir, à l'élégance très féminine, s'accommodent mieux de la coiffure basse à chignon ou à bouclettes. La natte enroulant la tête est une gracieuse nouveauté inspirée de la coiffure diadème de l'impératrice Elisabeth. Pour la réaliser, les cheveux seront partagés en une raie de la nuque au front, où ils forment bandeaux. A la nuque, on dressera une double natte ramenée de chaque côté de la tête. A hauteur des tempes, une natte postiche se mêlera aux nattes pour les renforcer et former le diadème.

Les cheveux courts (en haut) ont toujours beaucoup de succès et conviennent surtout aux jeunes visages. La raie est à gauche et les ondulations sont espacées.

Dans la troisième coiffure (en bas, à droite), les cheveux brun foncé sont rejetés en arrière, largement ondulés et réunis, sur la nuque, en un chignon simplement noué.

Dans ce numéro commence un grand roman inédit :

AME SAUVAGE

par

H. Lauvernière

Viennent de paraître dans la "Collection STELLA" : MAITRE NICOLE ET SON AMOUR, par Guy de Novel, et LA BLESSURE CACHÉE, par Georges de Lys. Le volume : 1 fr. 50 ; franco : 1 fr. 75

'Short or Long Hair...', Paris, 1934,
Le Petit Echo de la Mode

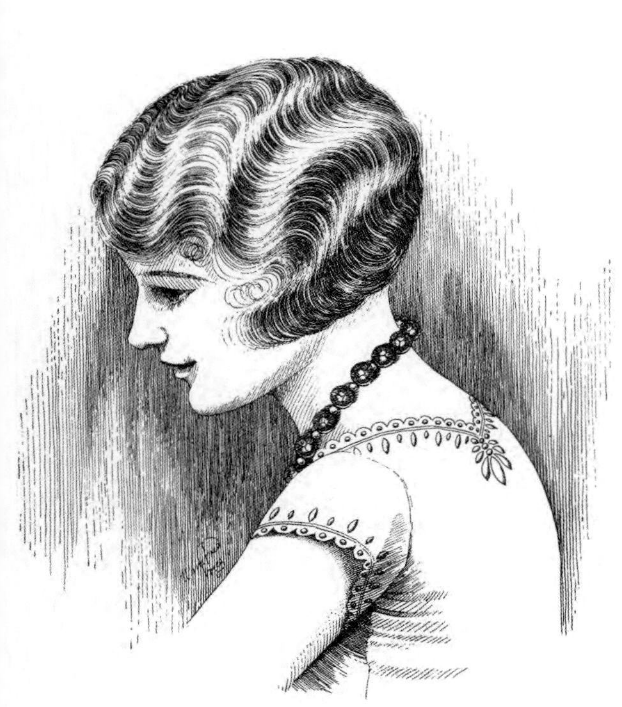

'Modern Shingle, Simple Mode, Waved', 1936, *The Art and Craft of Hairdressing*, Gilbert A. Foan

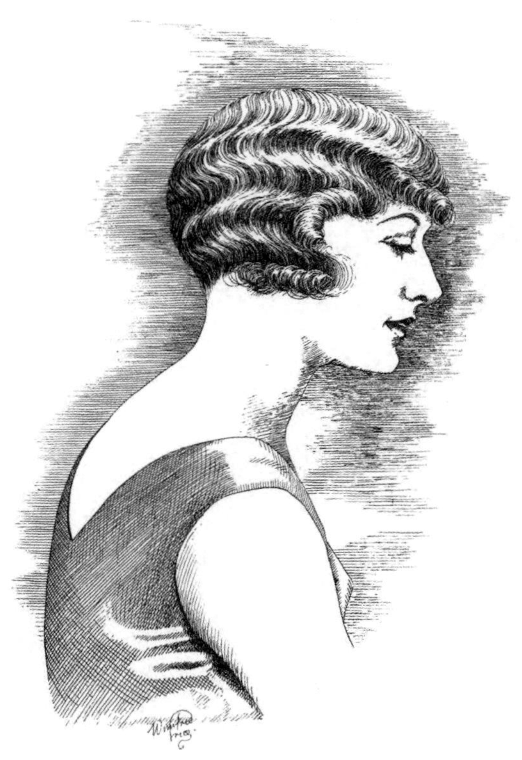

'Modern Shingle, Simple Mode, Waved and Curled', 1936, *The Art and Craft of Hairdressing*, Gilbert A. Foan

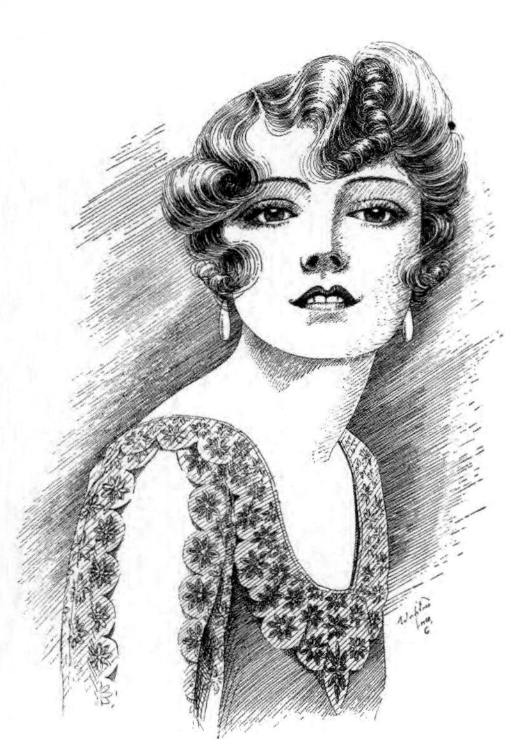

'Extra Waved Shingled Coiffure with Deep Curls', 1936, *The Art and Craft of Hairdressing*, Gilbert A. Foan

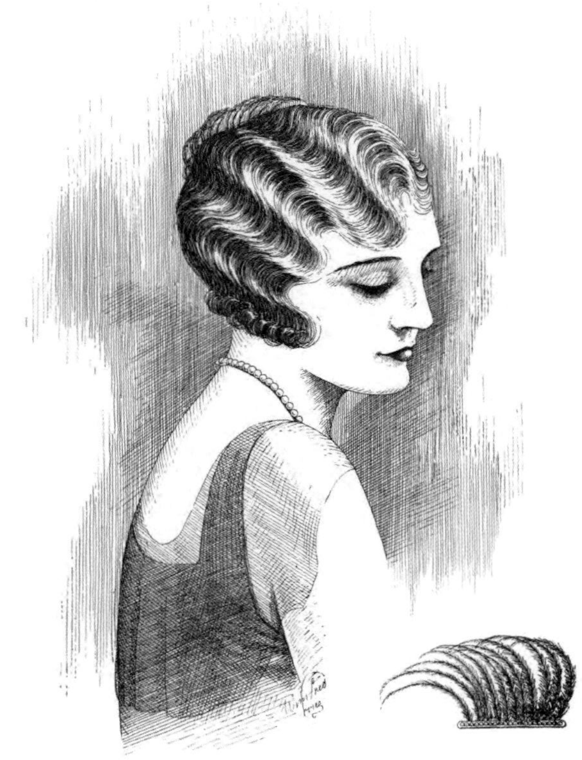

'Deeply-Waved Shingled Coiffure with Roll Curls and Back Ornament', 1936, *The Art and Craft of Hairdressing*, Gilbert A. Foan

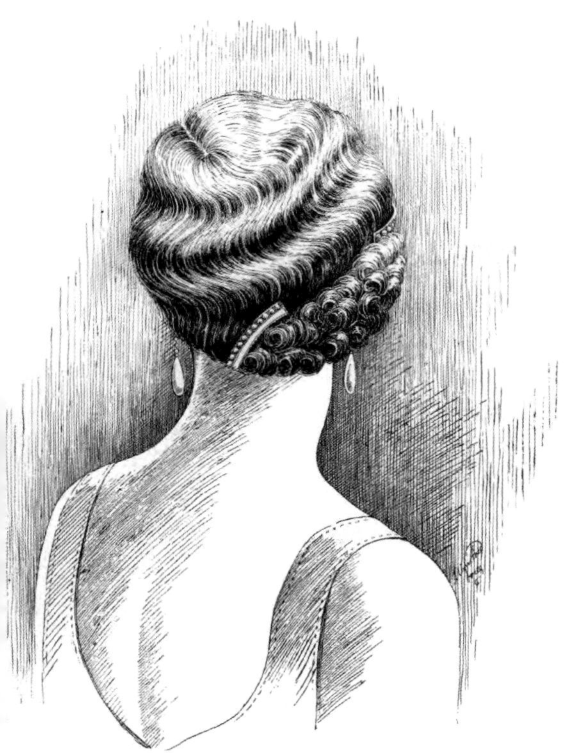

'Low Shingled Coiffure', 1936, *The Art and Craft of Hairdressing*, Gilbert A. Foan

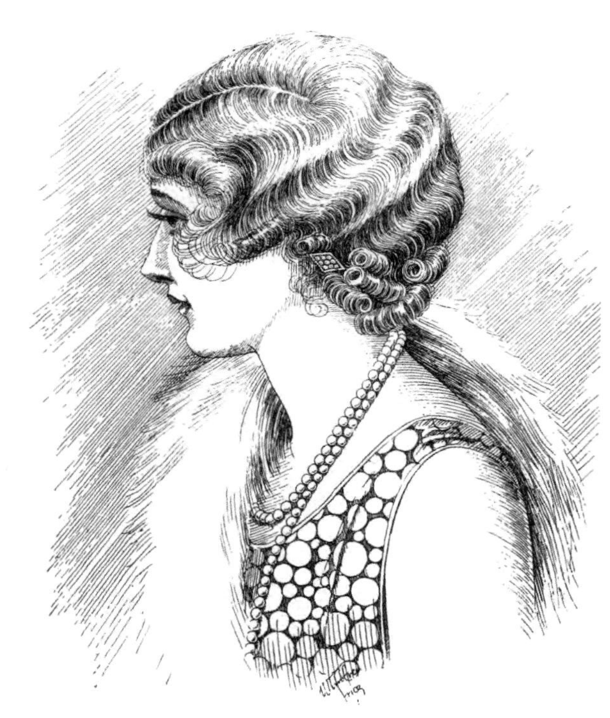

'Shingled Coiffure with Circular Wave', 1936, *The Art and Craft of Hairdressing*, Gilbert A. Foan

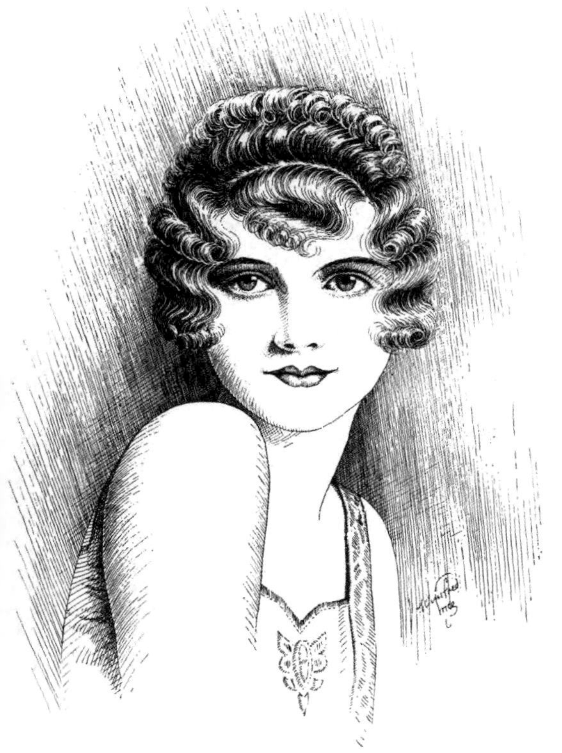

'Shingled Coiffure, Divisional Mode, with Pompadour Effect', 1936, *The Art and Craft of Hairdressing*, Gilbert A. Foan

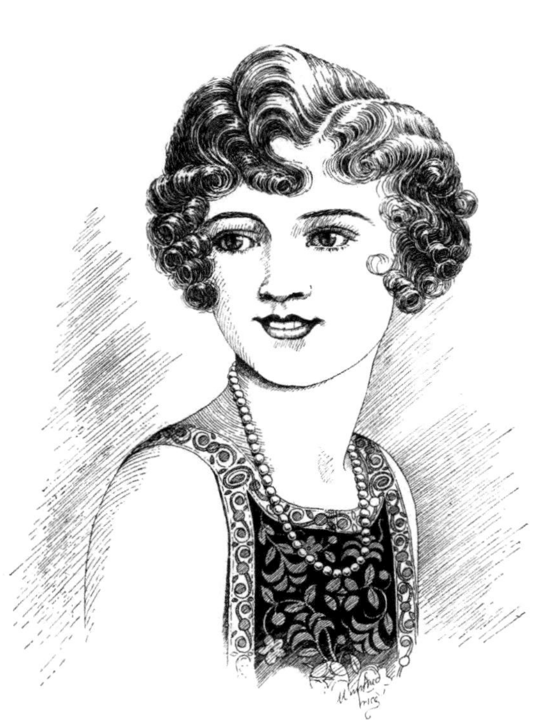

'Shingled Coiffure, Divisional Mode, with Marteaux', 1936, *The Art and Craft of Hairdressing*, Gilbert A. Foan

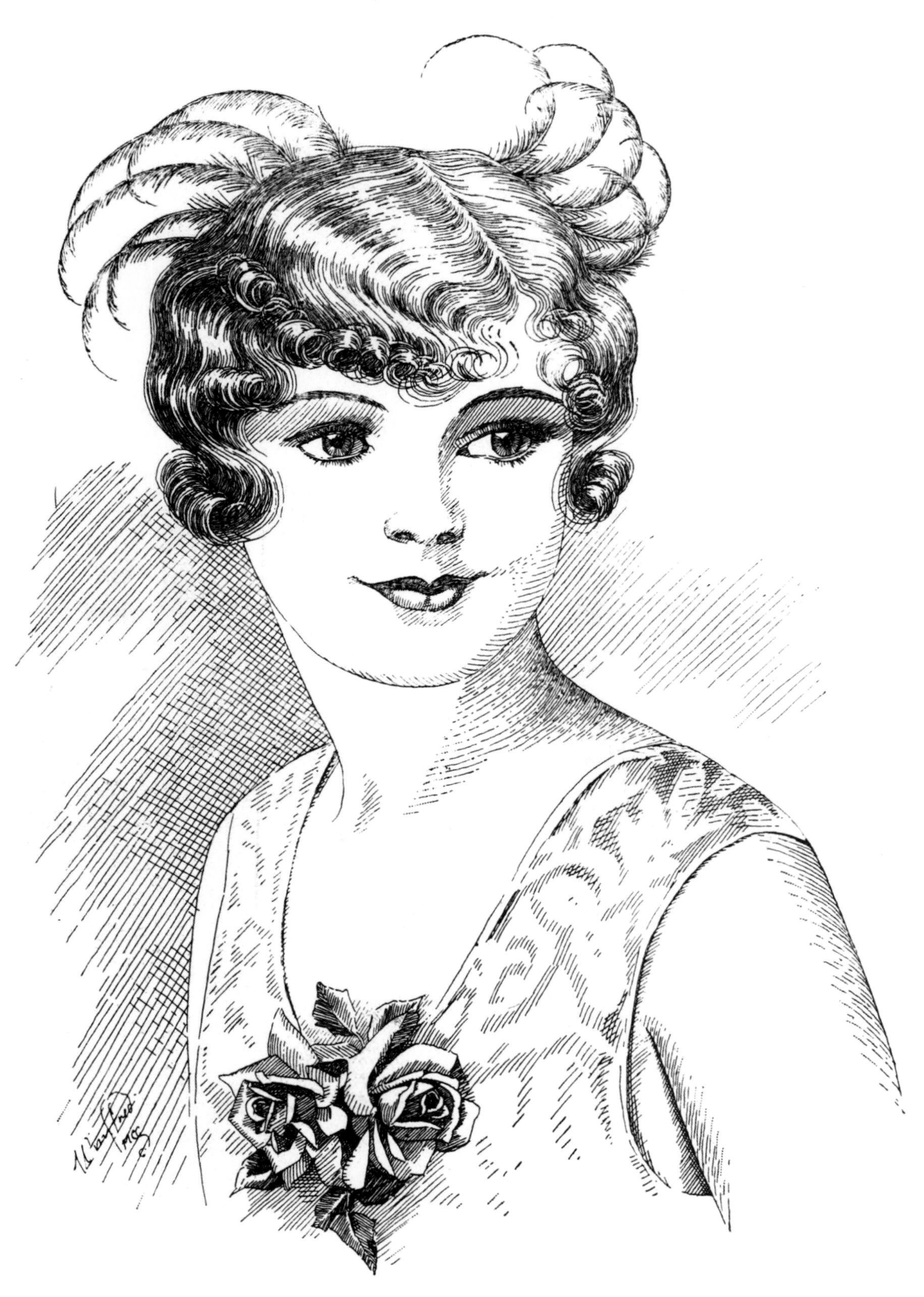

'Softly Waved Coiffure with Torsade', 1936,
The Art and Craft of Hairdressing, Gilbert A. Foan

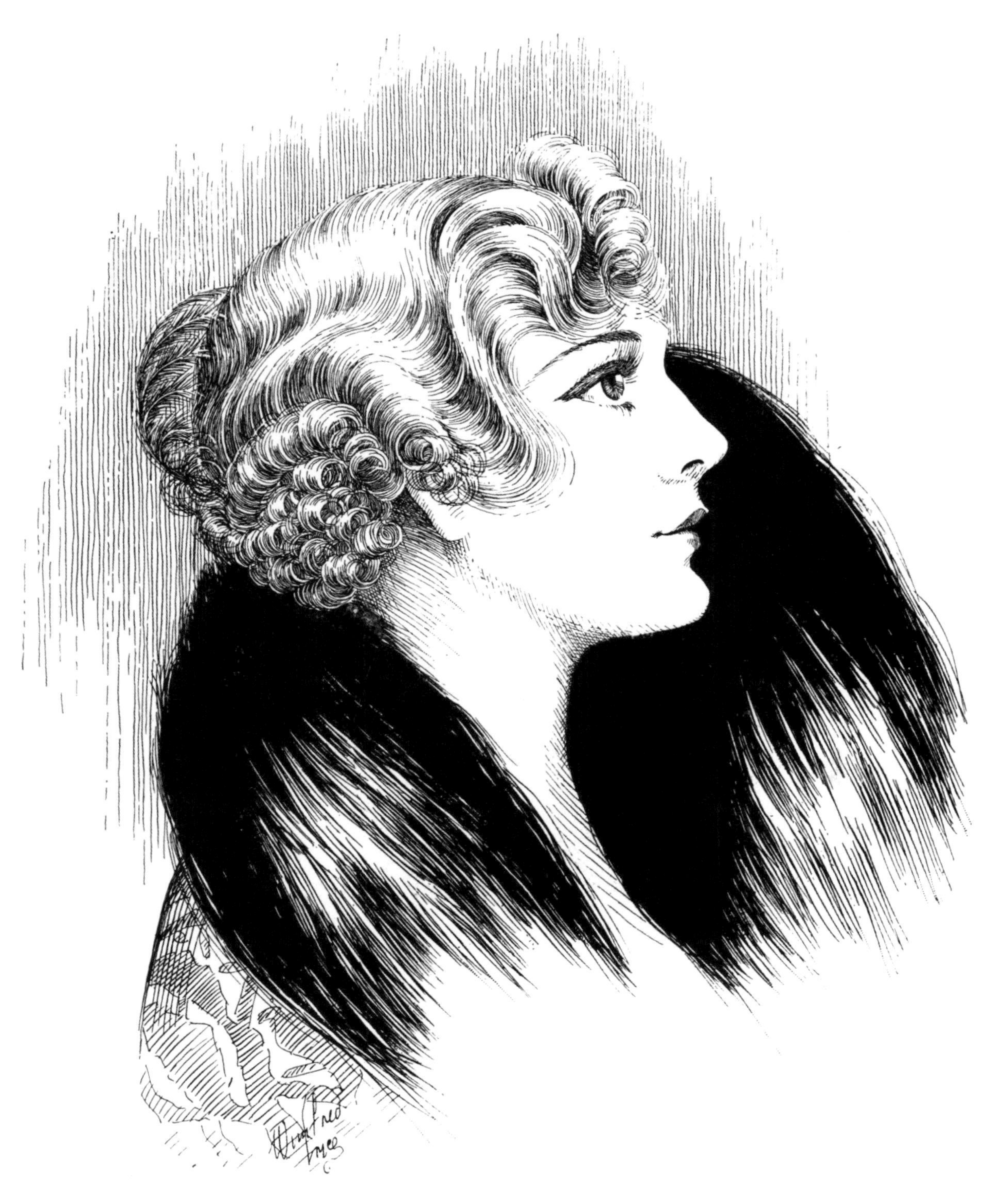

hingled Coiffure with Pronounced Waves and Curls',
36, *The Art and Craft of Hairdressing*, Gilbert A. Foan

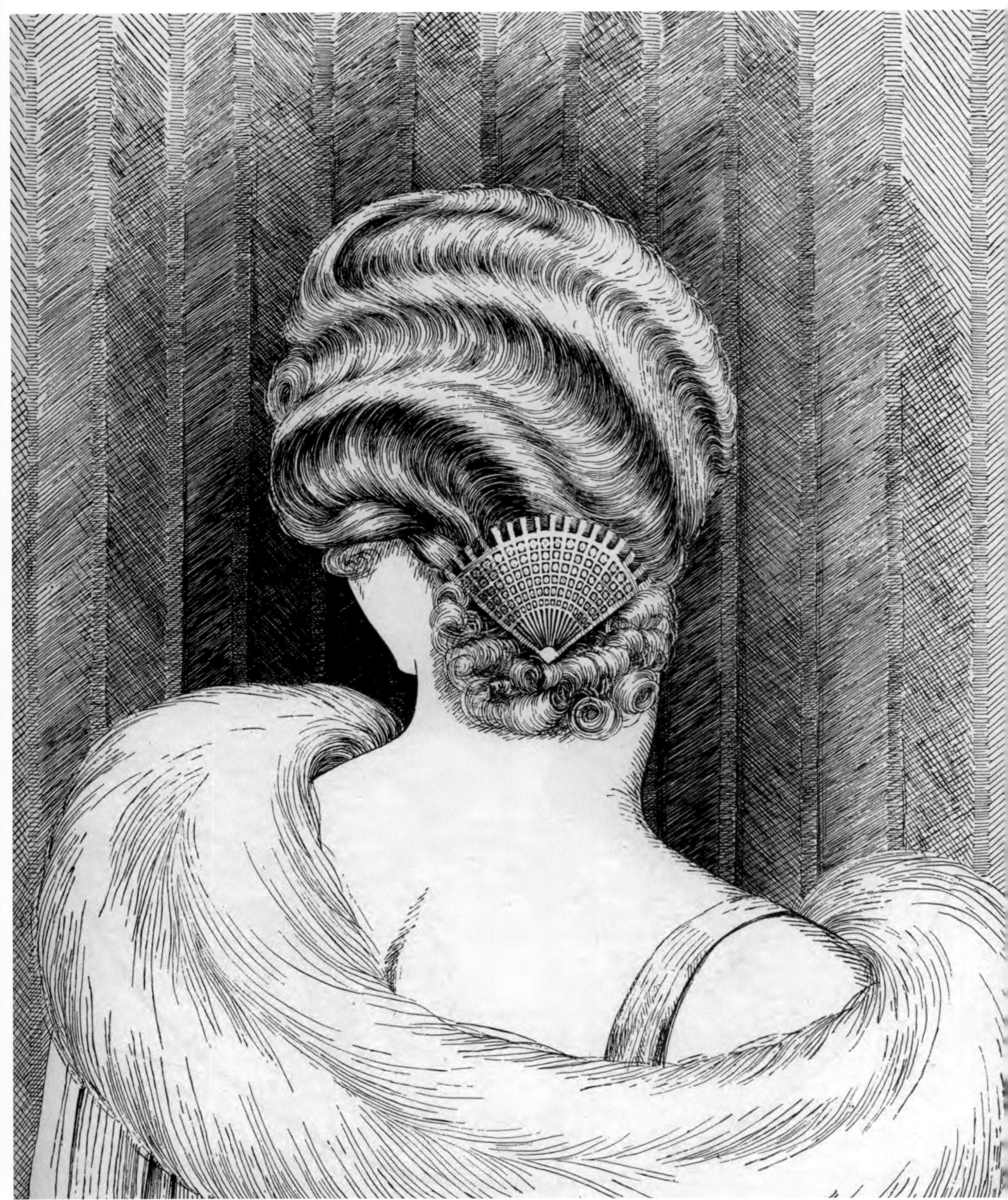

'Coiffure with Slanting Waves and Low-Neck Dressing', 1936, *The Art and Craft of Hairdressing*, Gilbert A. Foan

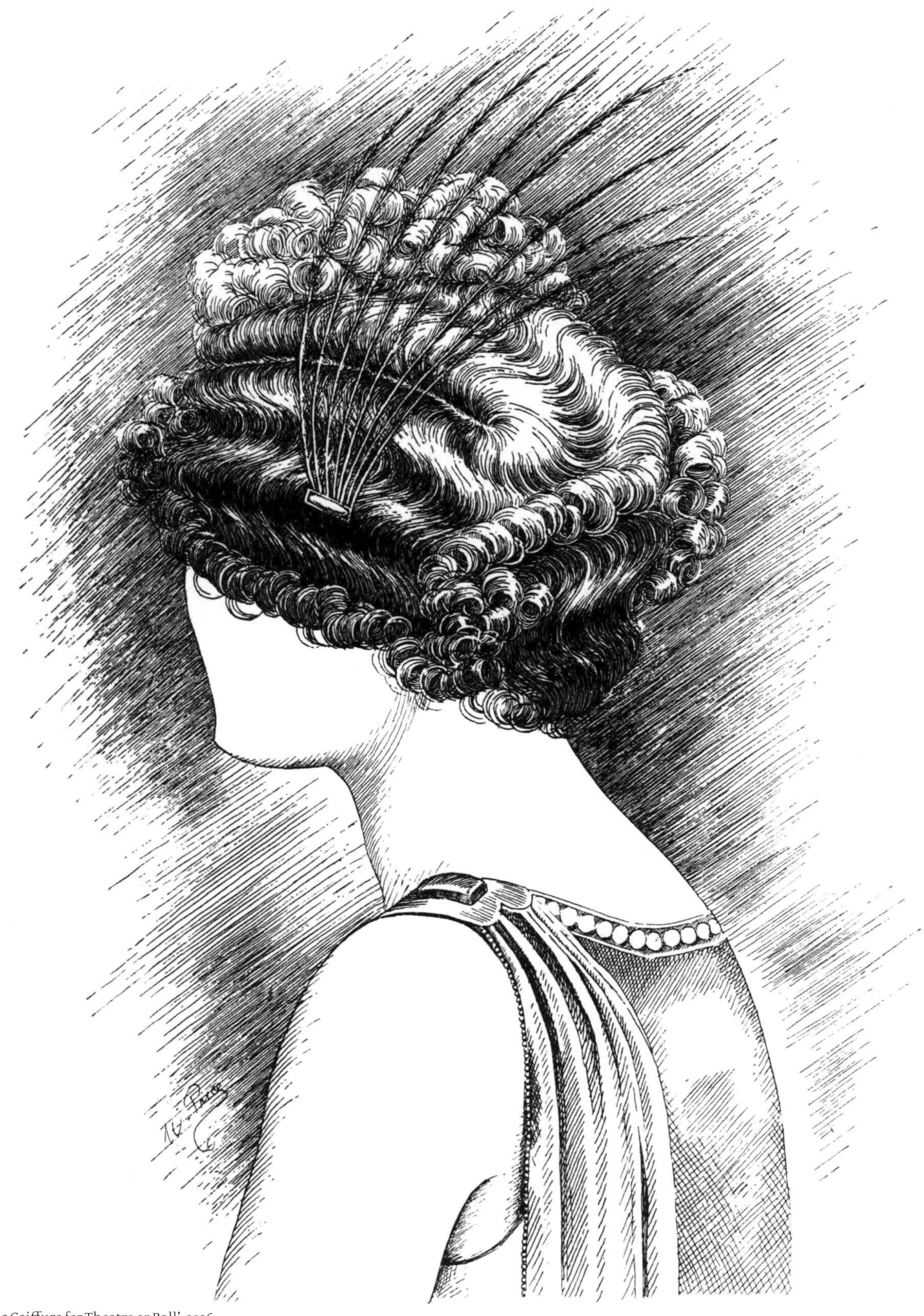

emi-Fantastic Coiffure for Theatre or Ball', 1936,
1e Art and Craft of Hairdressing, Gilbert A. Foan

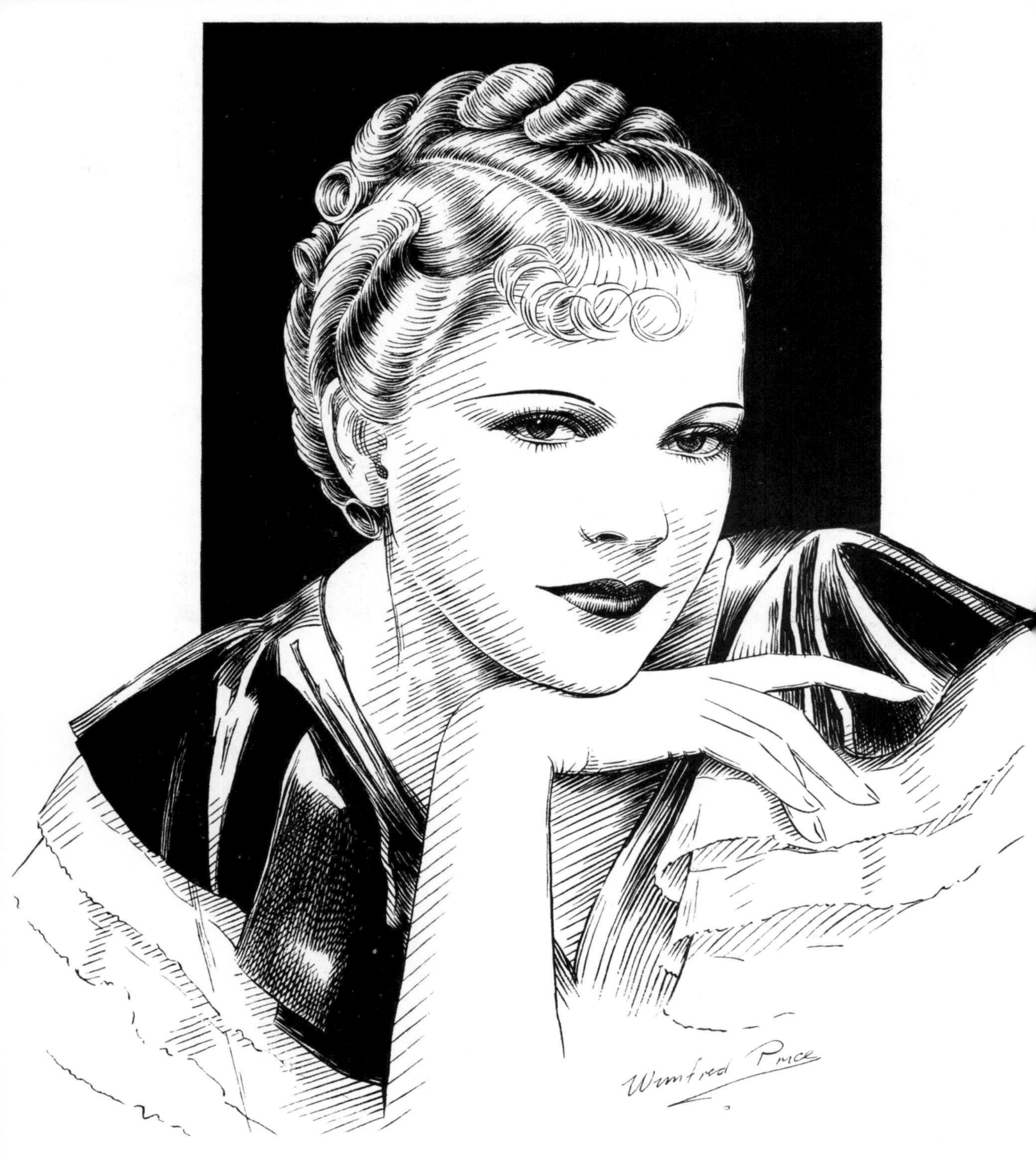

'An Angled Parting with Turn-Over at the Temple', 1936, *The Art and Craft of Hairdressing*, Gilbert A. Foan

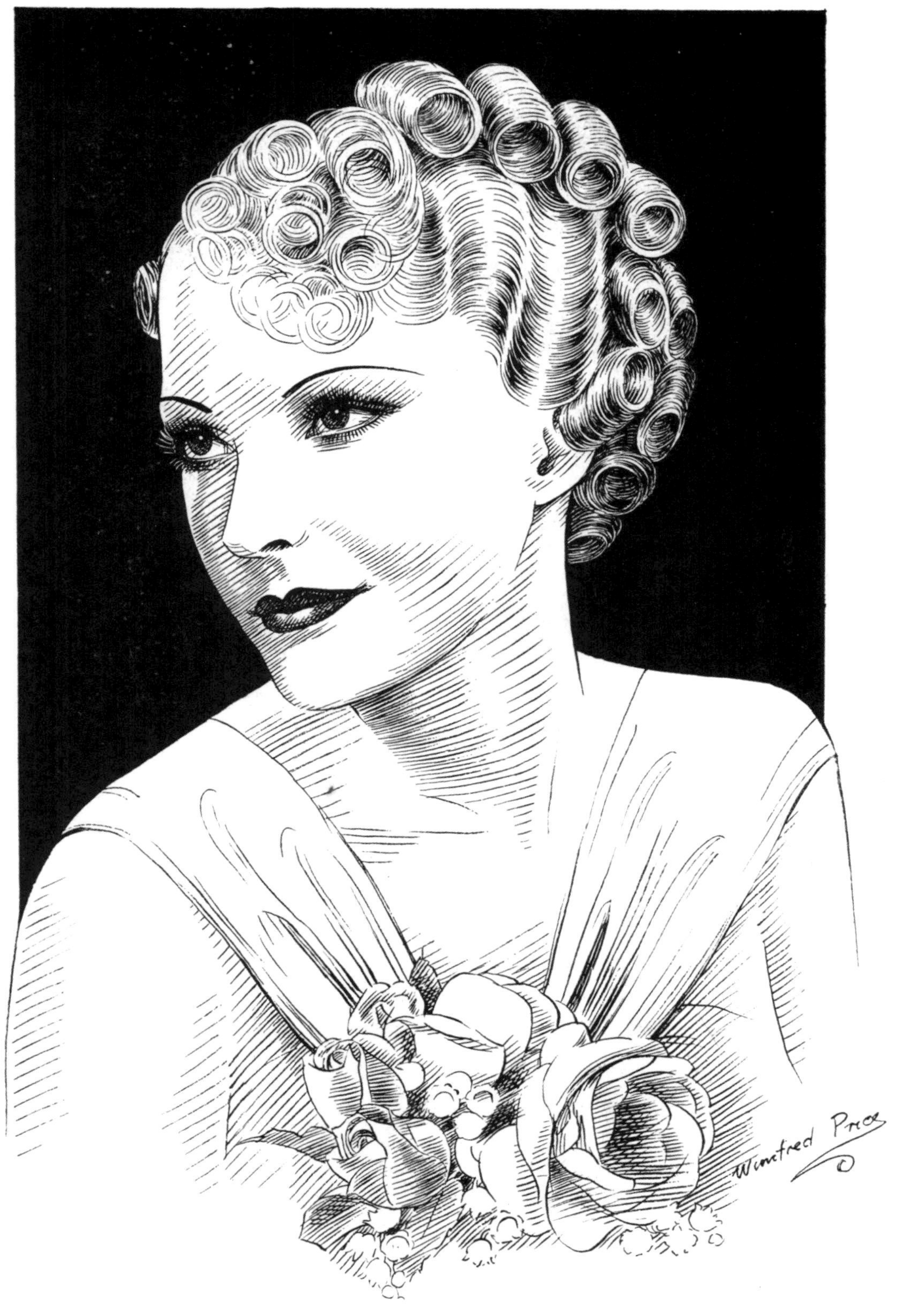

'An Evening Coiffure, Blonde and Delicate', 1936,
The Art and Craft of Hairdressing, Gilbert A. Foan

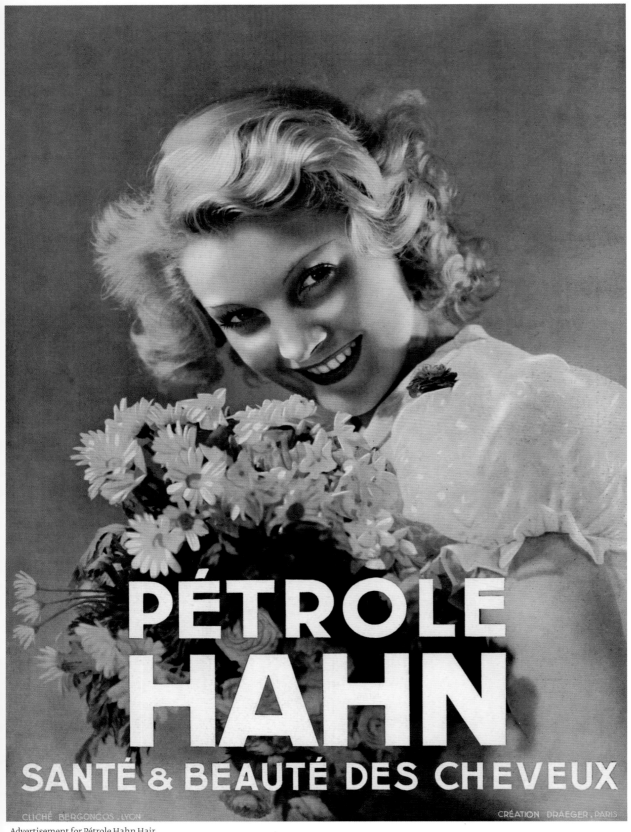

Advertisement for Pétrole Hahn Hair Care & Beauty, France, 1937, *L'Illustration*

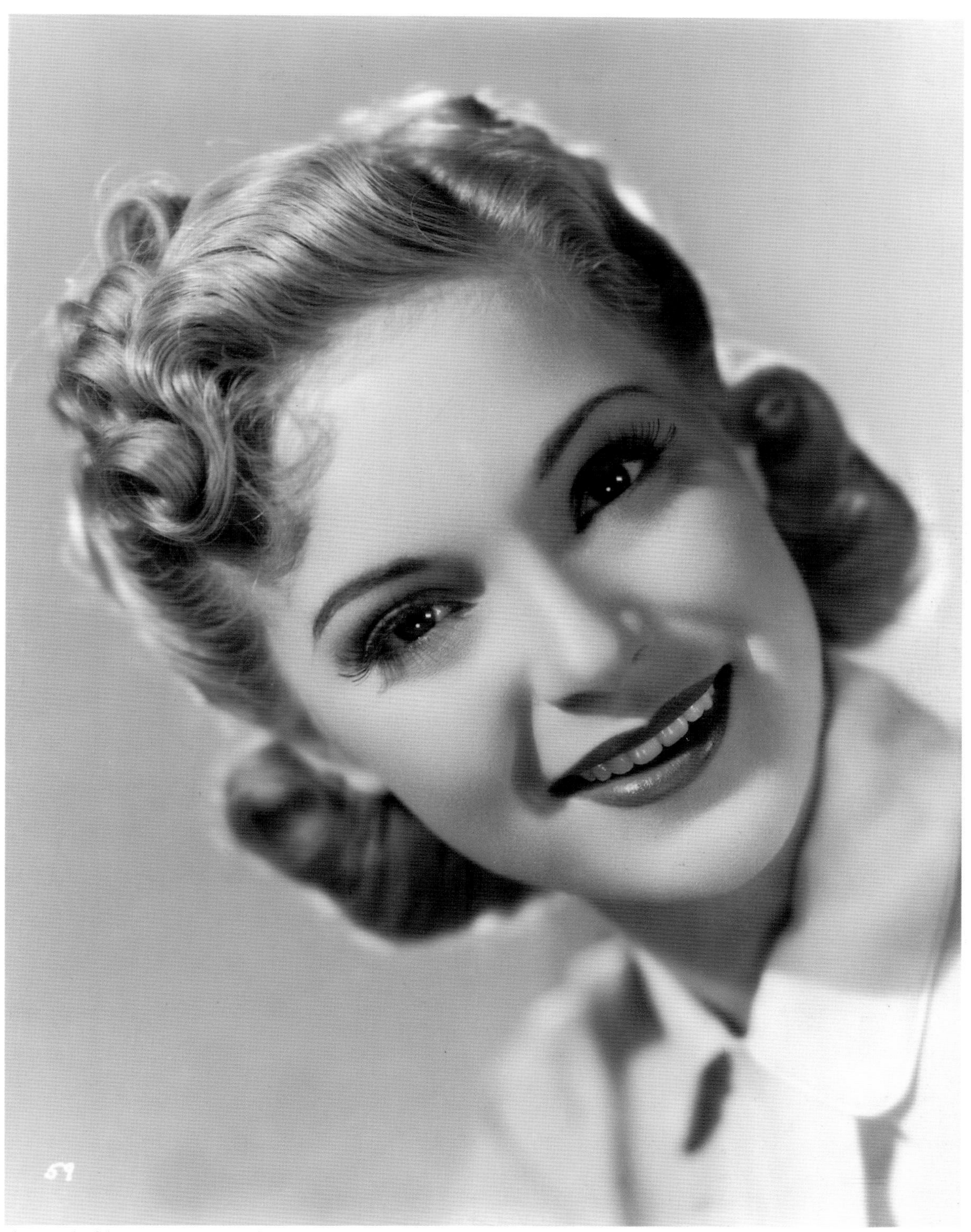

Photograph of the actress, Nan Grey, showing high hair- do with long back roll, 1938

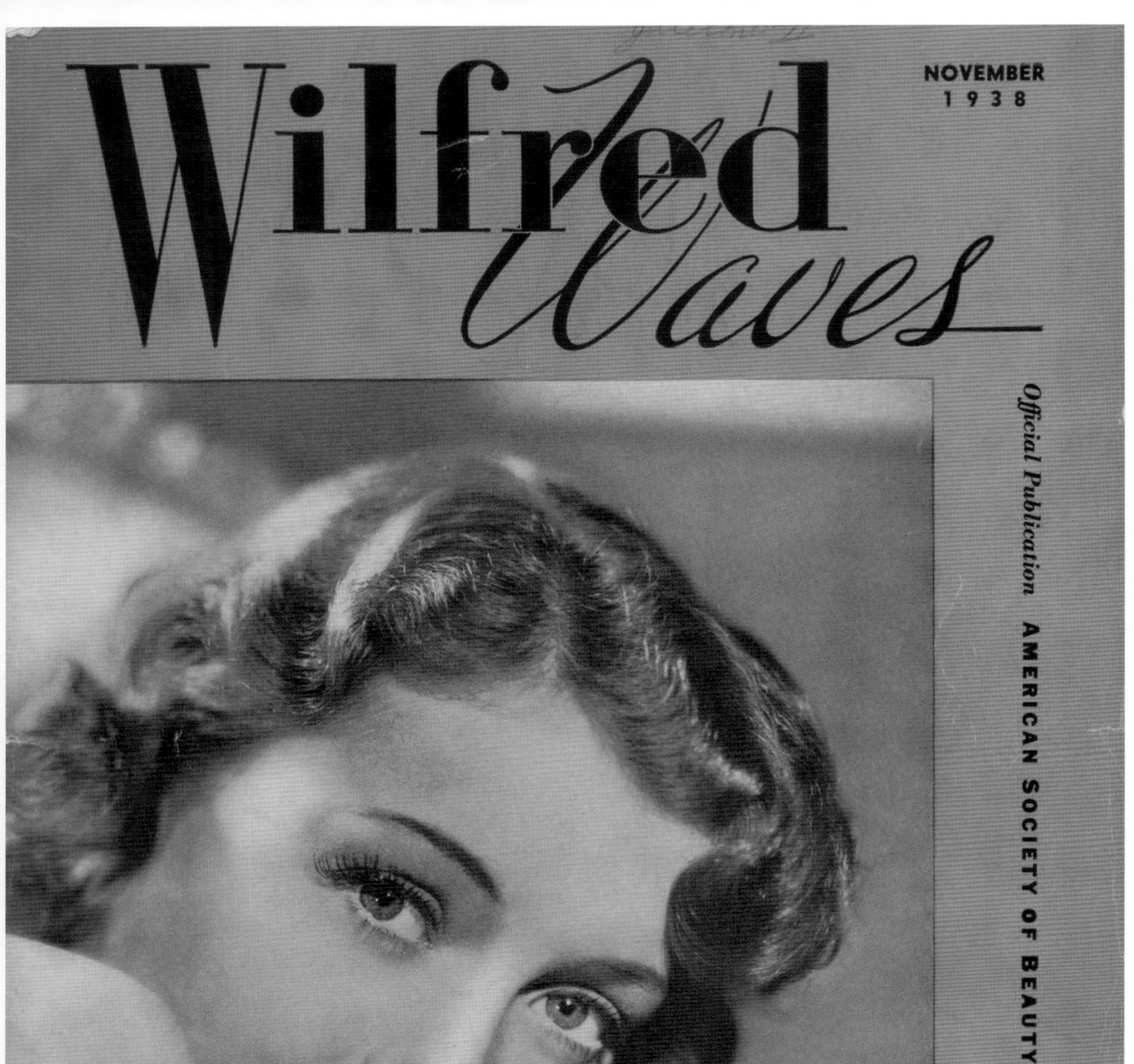

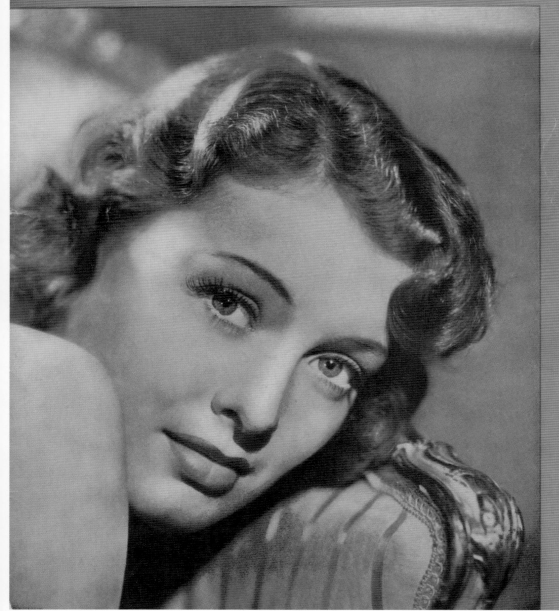

Wilfred Waves magazine cover, American Society of Beauty Culturalists, 1938

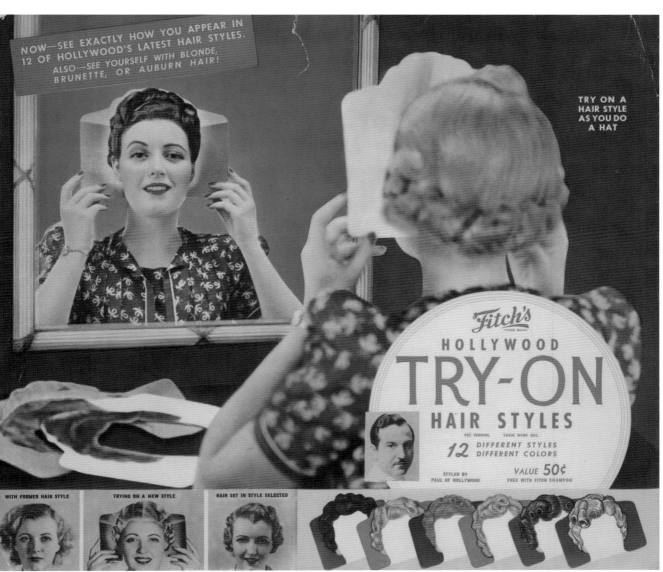

Fitch's Hollywood Try-On Hairstyles, styled by Paul of Hollywood, American Advertising and Research Corp. 1939

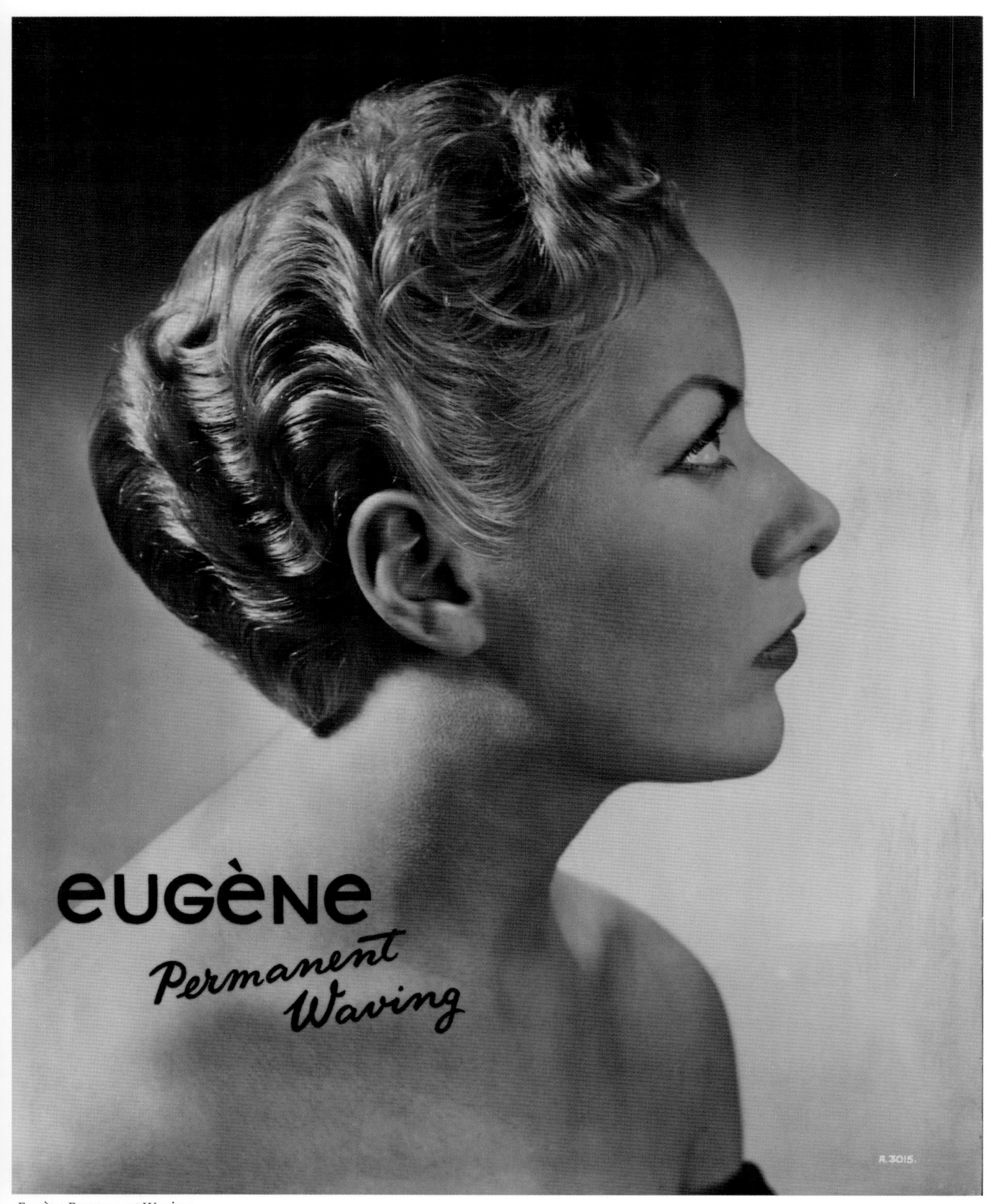

Eugène Permanent Waving
advertisement, 1930s

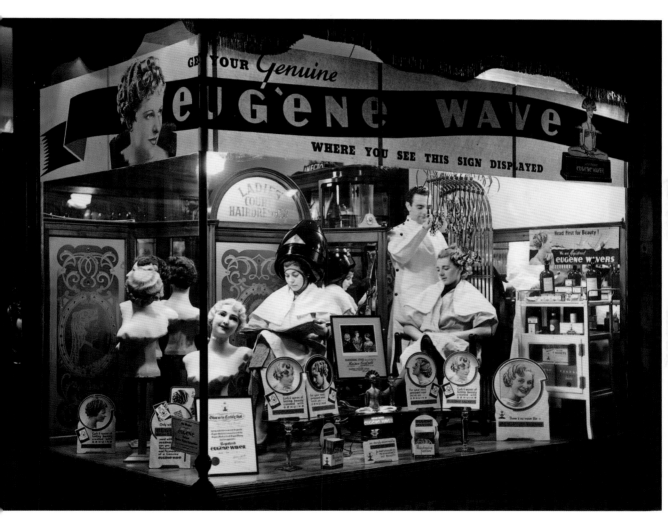

Hairdressing salon with Eugène Wave display in window and stylist demonstrating the use of the Eugène Wave machine, Blackpool, 1941, photographed by M. & R. Saidman

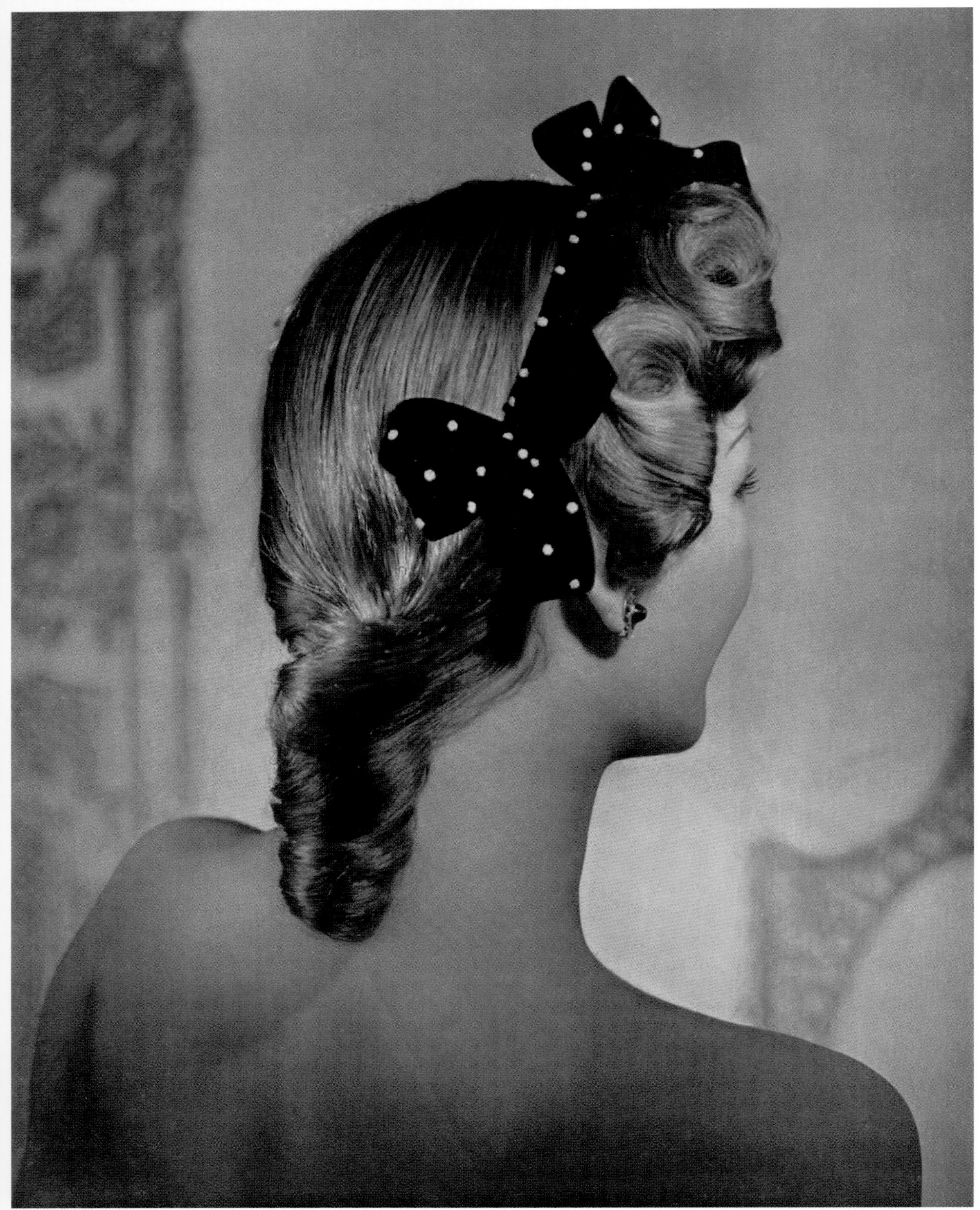

Coiffure by Guillaume of Paris, 1940, *The Home* (Australia)

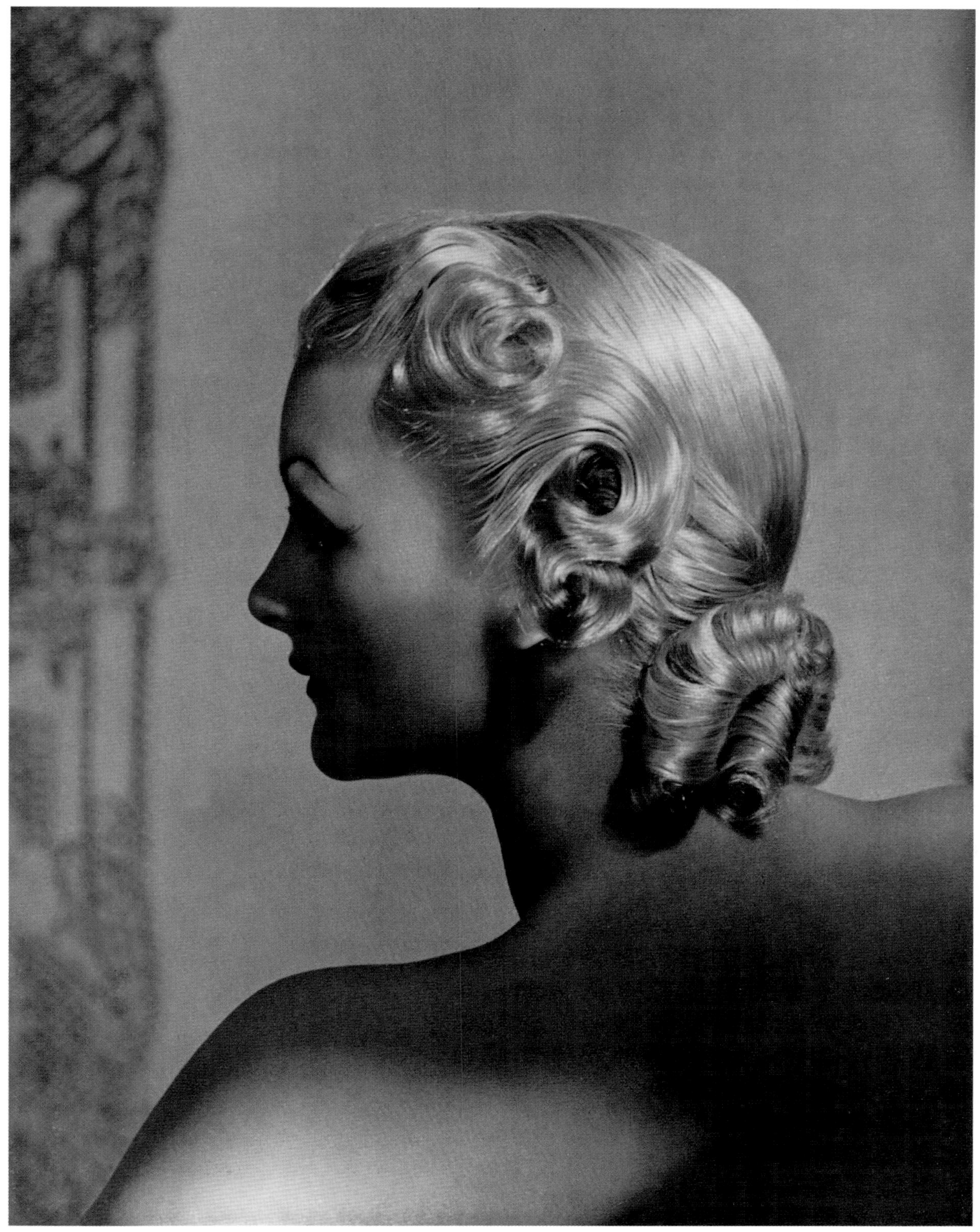

Coiffure by Guillaume of Paris, 1940, *The Home* (Australia)

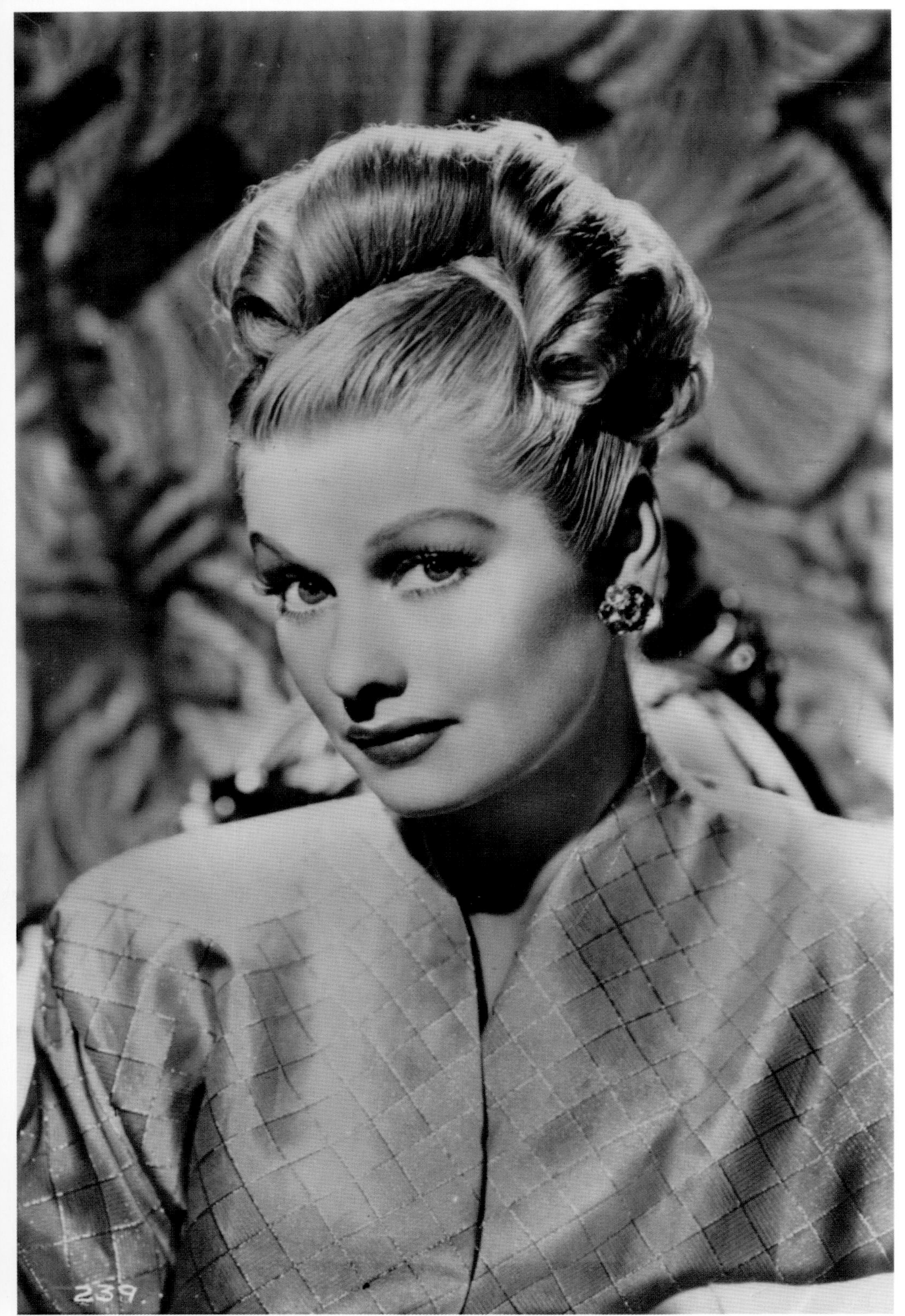

Actress Lucille Ball with hairstyle by Irma Kusely, MGM hairstylist, c.1940s

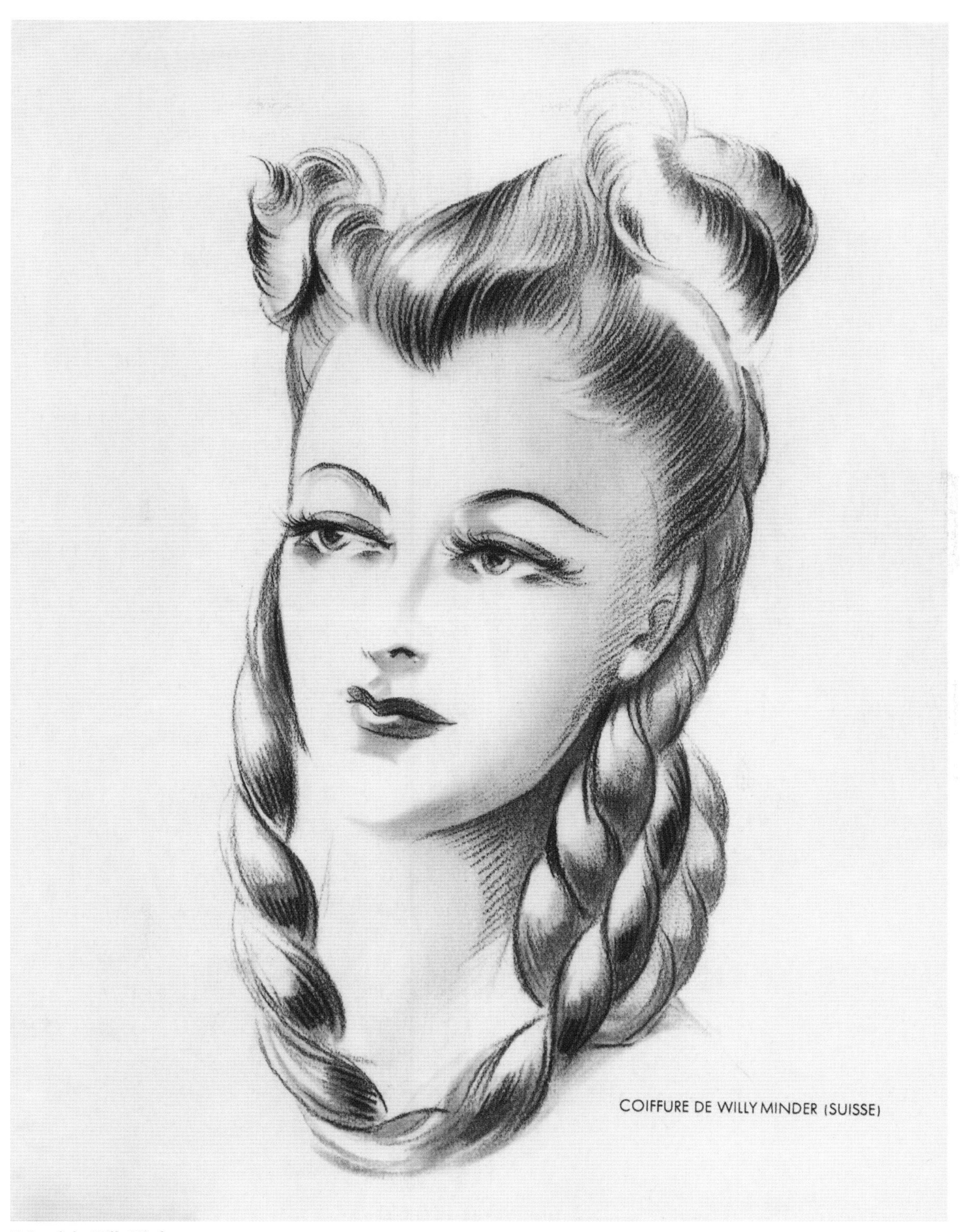

Hairstyle by Willy Minder,
Switzerland, 1940s

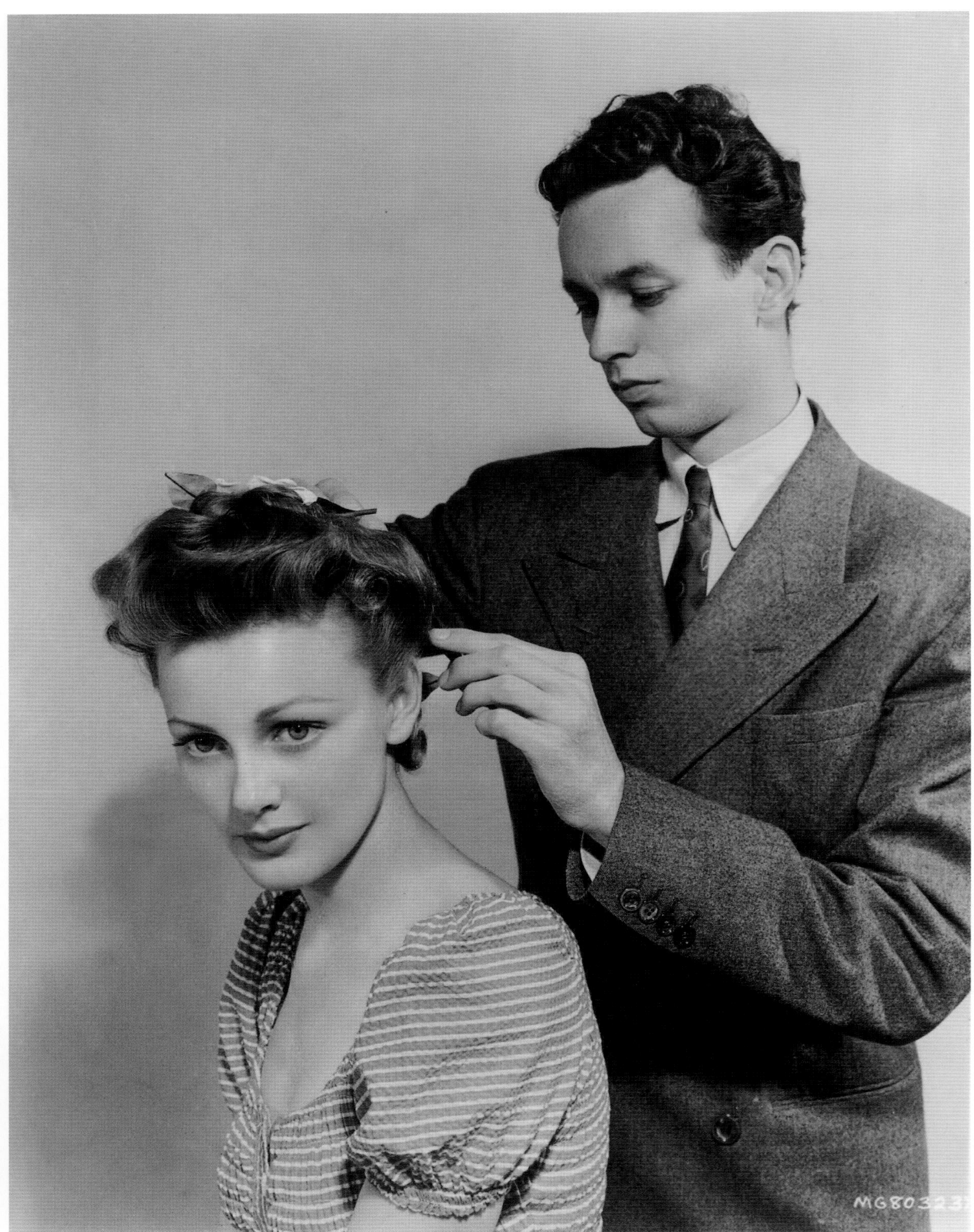

Short hairstyle created for the actress Virginia Grey by MGM stylist Larry Germaine, 1940

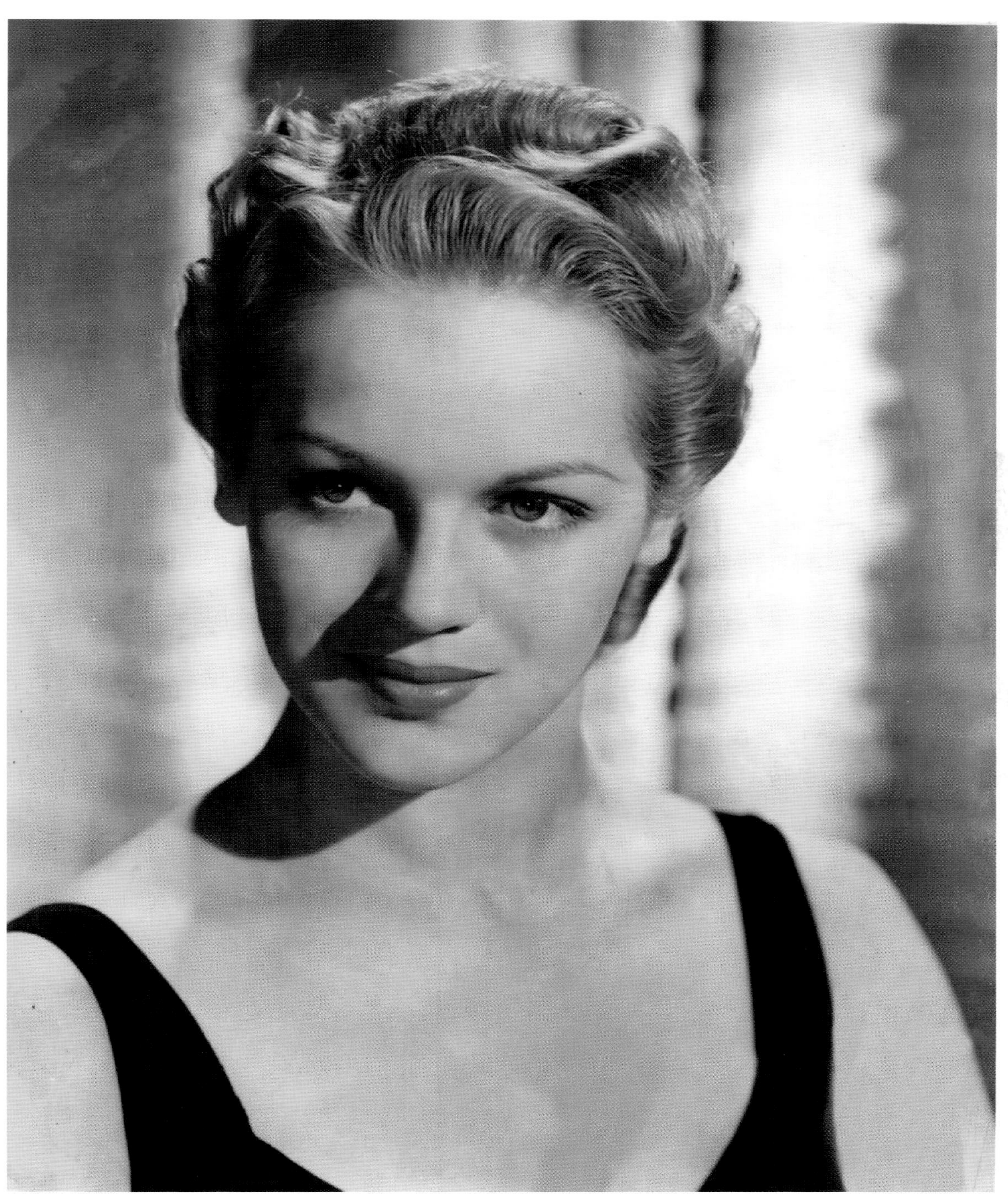
Virginia Grey with short waved hairstyle, 1941

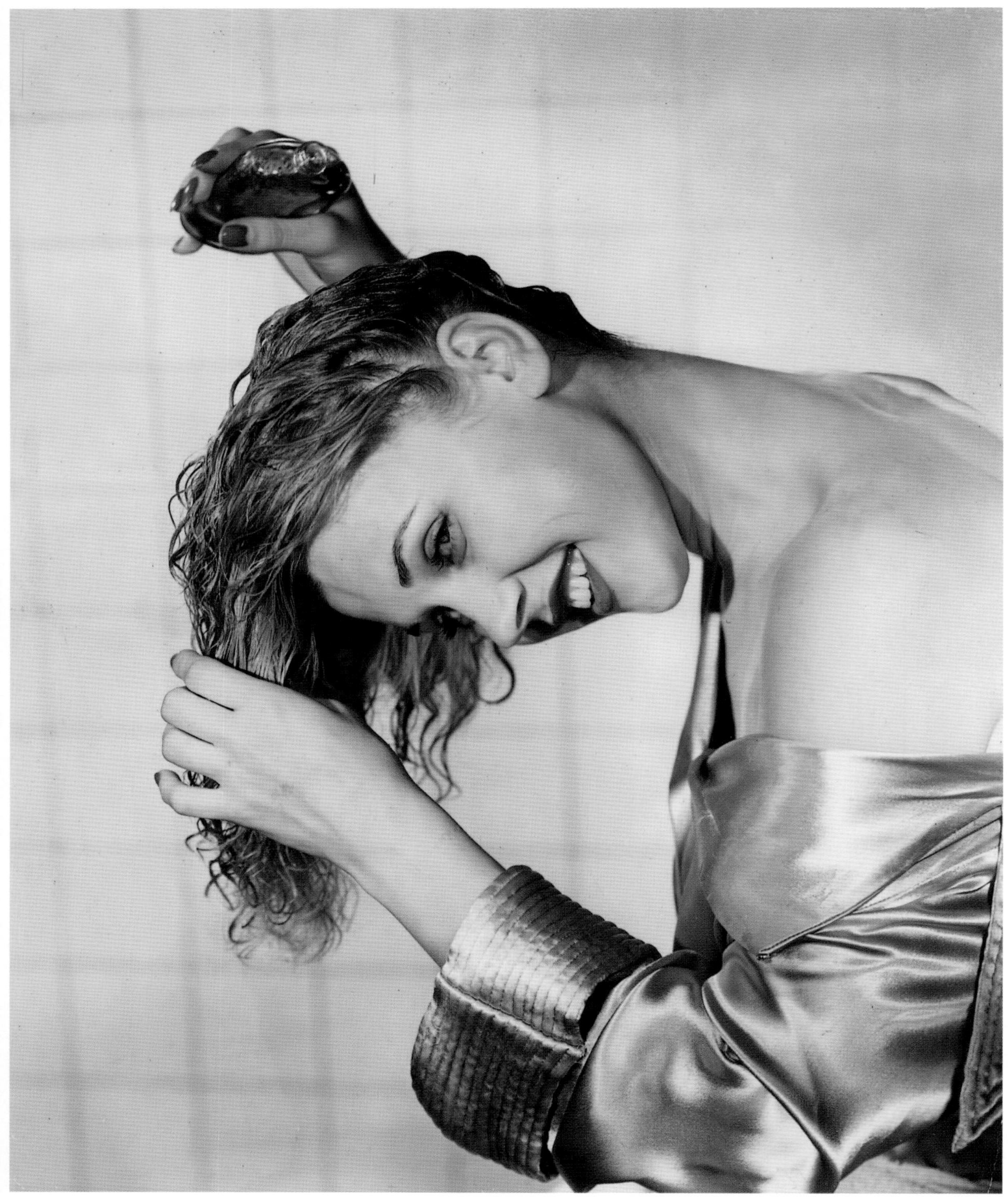

Advertising photograph for Liquid Soapless Shampoo with Hair Conditioner added, 1930s

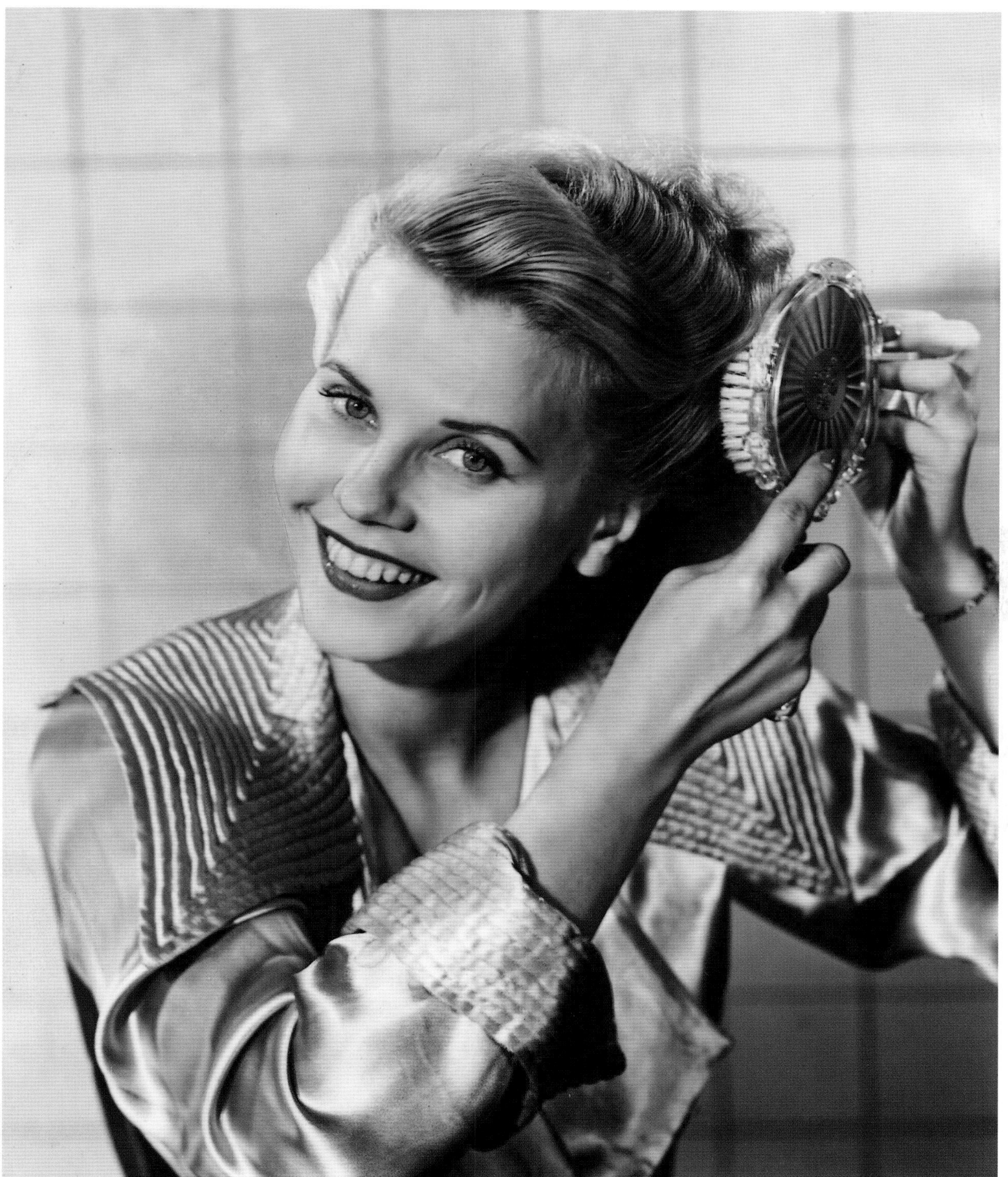

Advertising photograph for Liquid Soapless Shampoo with Hair Conditioner added, 1930s

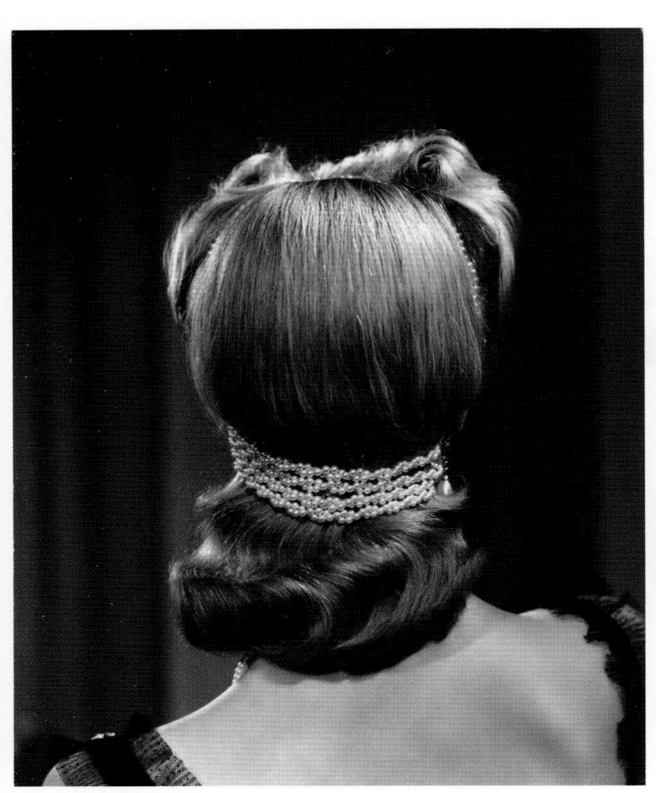

Anita Louise's hairdo with pearls twined about it, 1941, photographed by Schuyler Crail for Warner Bros.

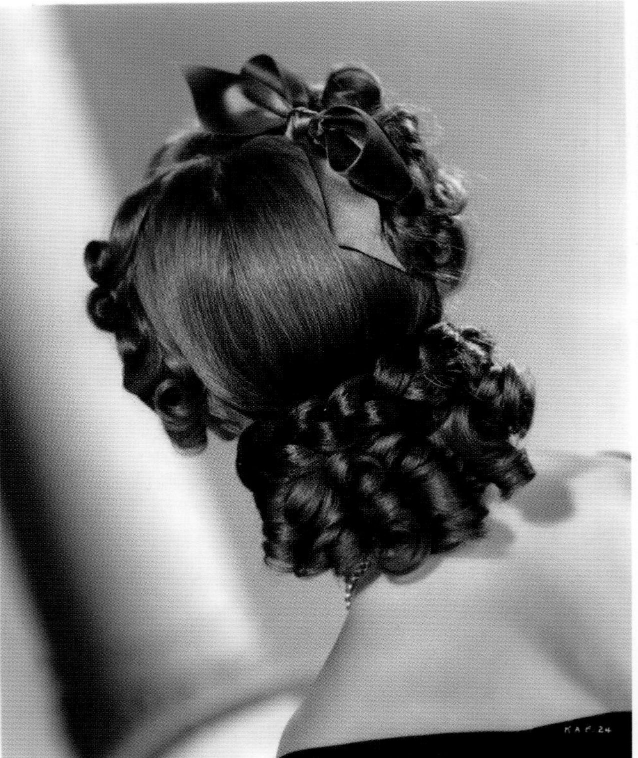

'A hair mode of modern quaintness is adopted by Kathryn Adams who enacts one the the leading roles in Universal's Argentine Nights', 1941, photographed by Ray Jones

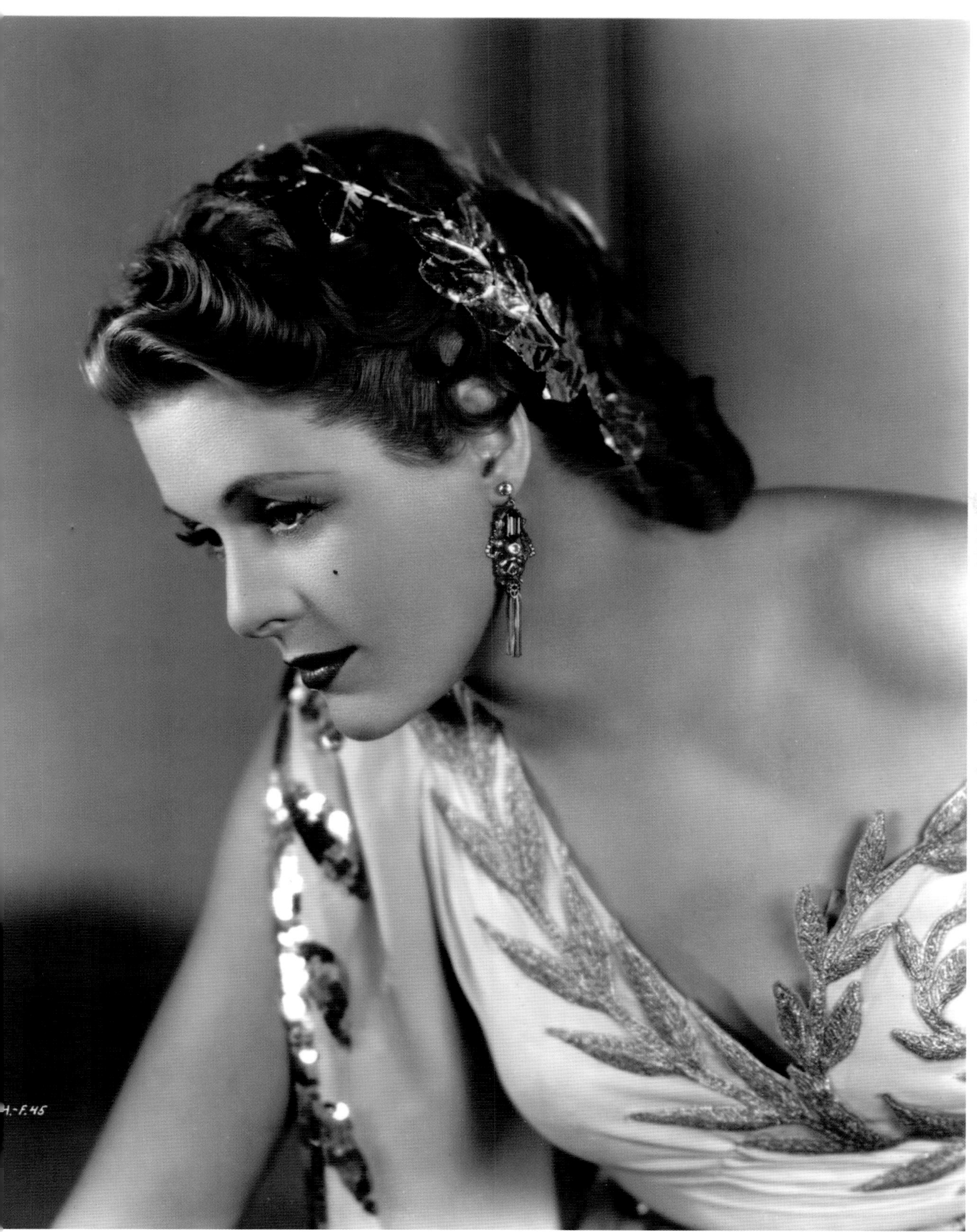

ne Hervey, Hairstyle by Emily Moore,
iversal Studios hairstylist, 1941

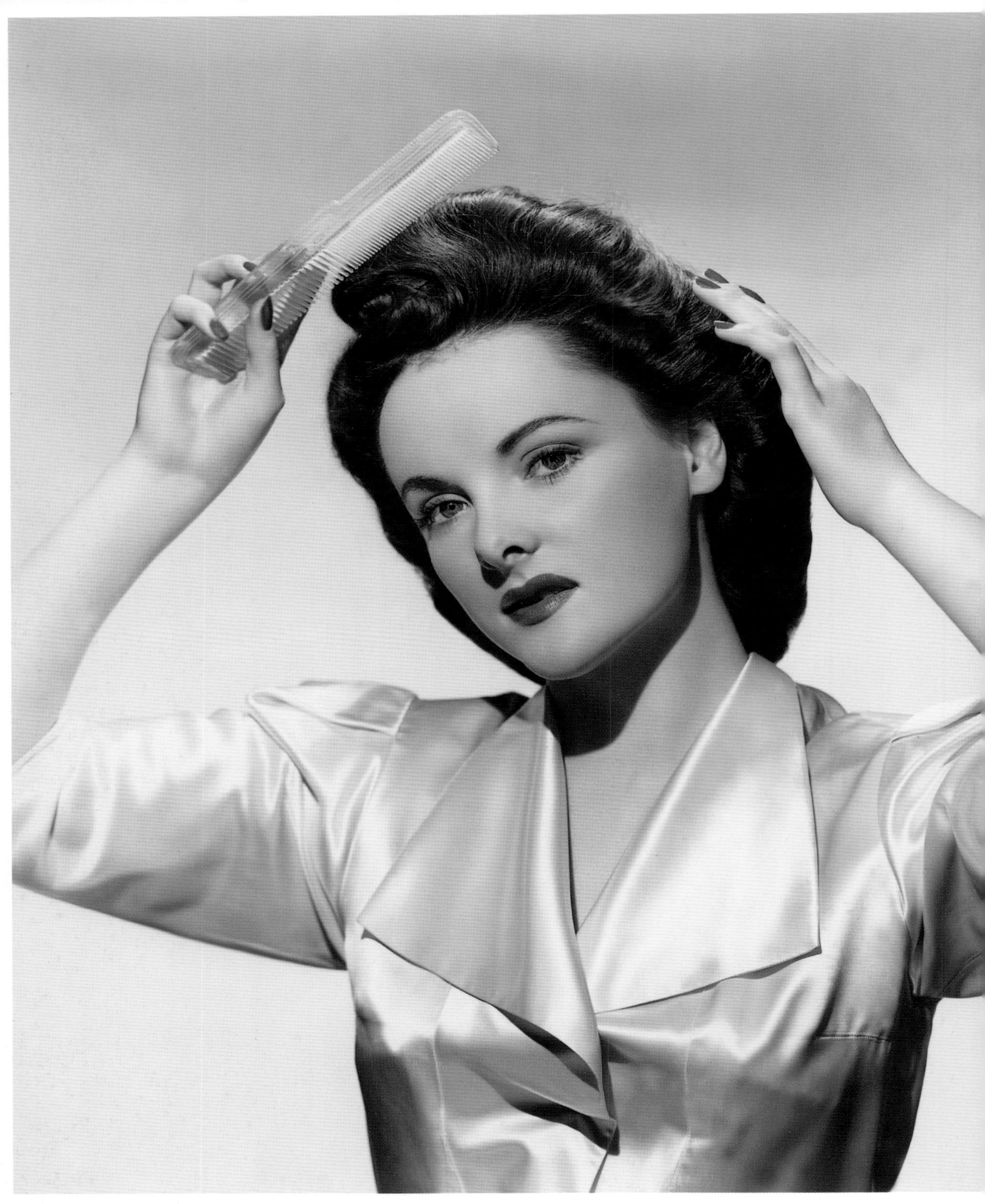

Actress Peggy Diggins combing her hair into a pinned roll, 1942

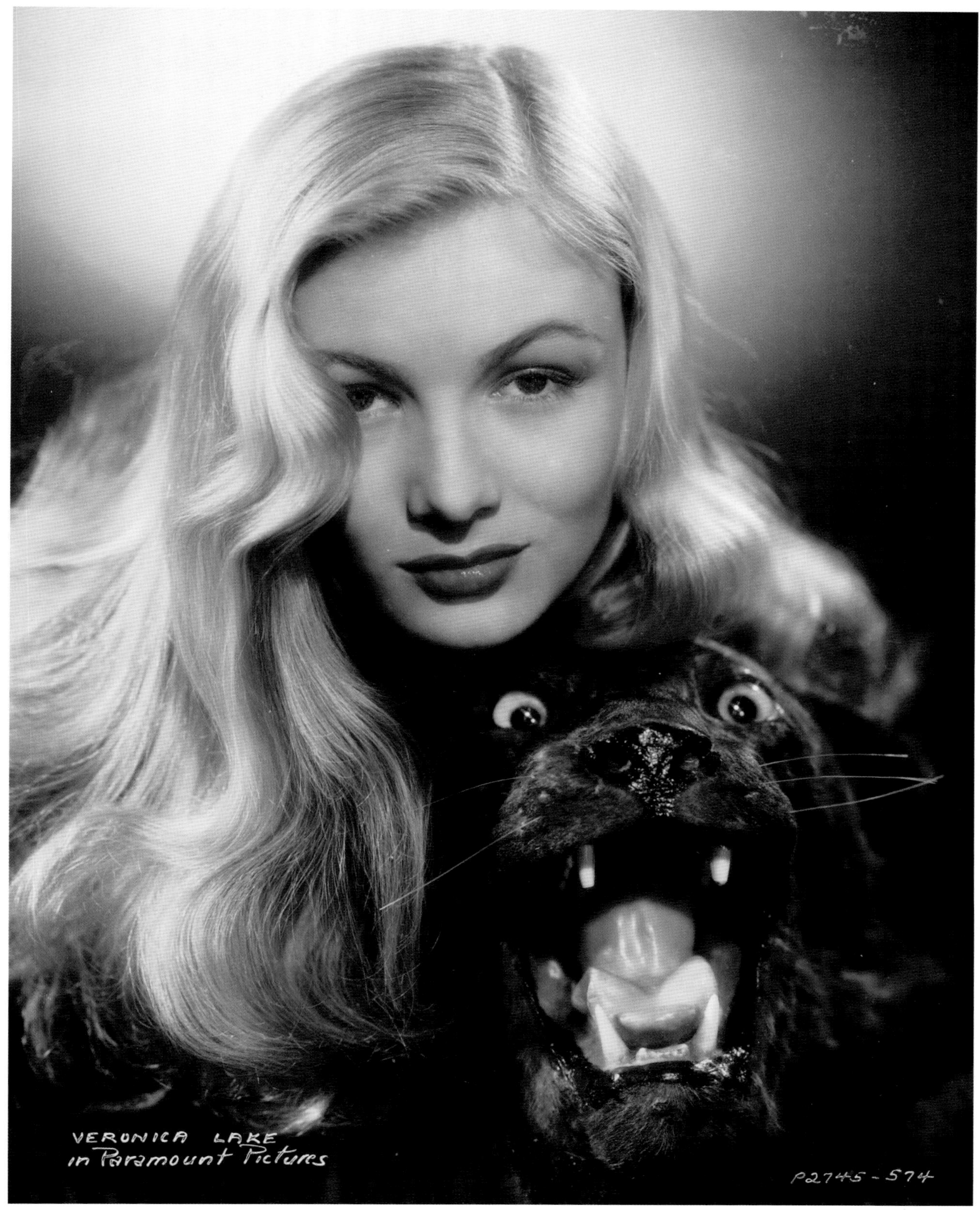

'Beauty and the Beast', Veronica Lake publicity photograph for Paramount Pictures – with her famous 'Witch-Lock' hair-do, 1942

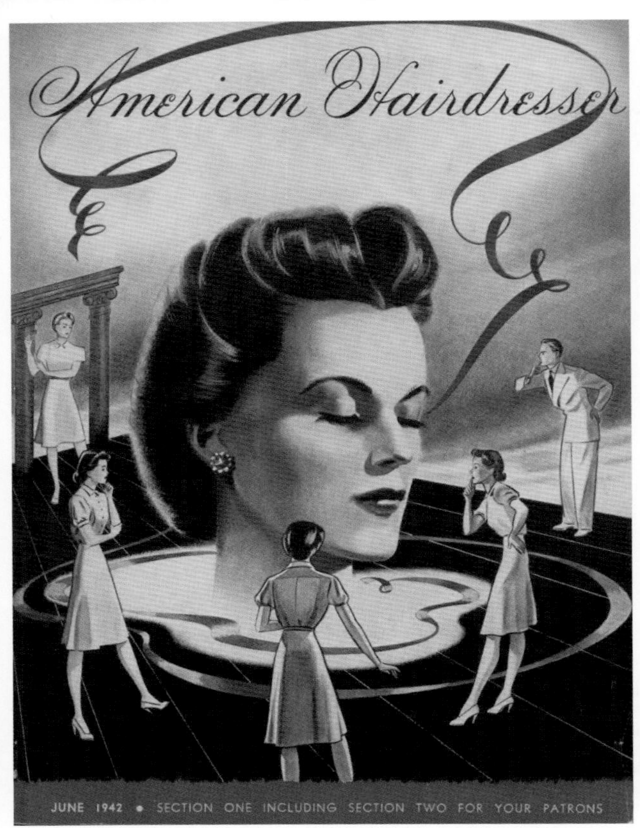

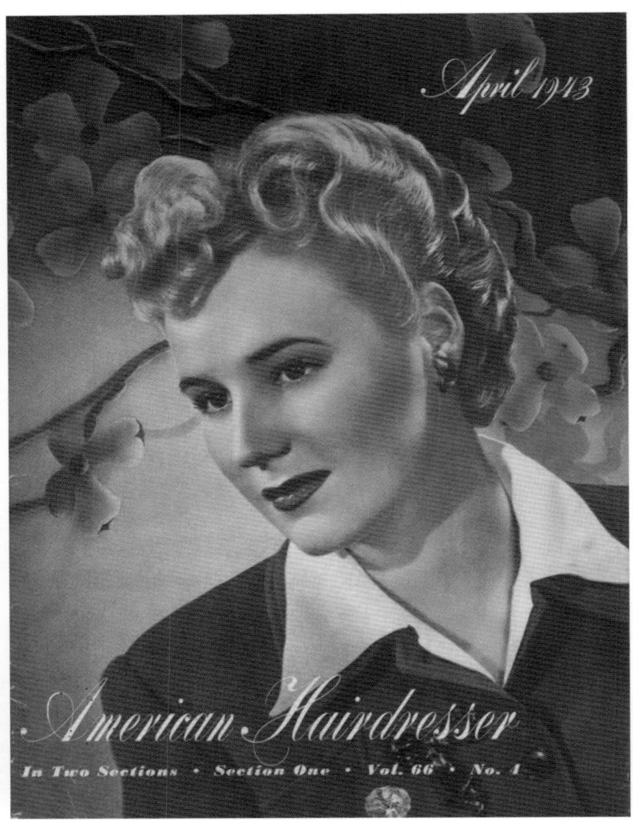

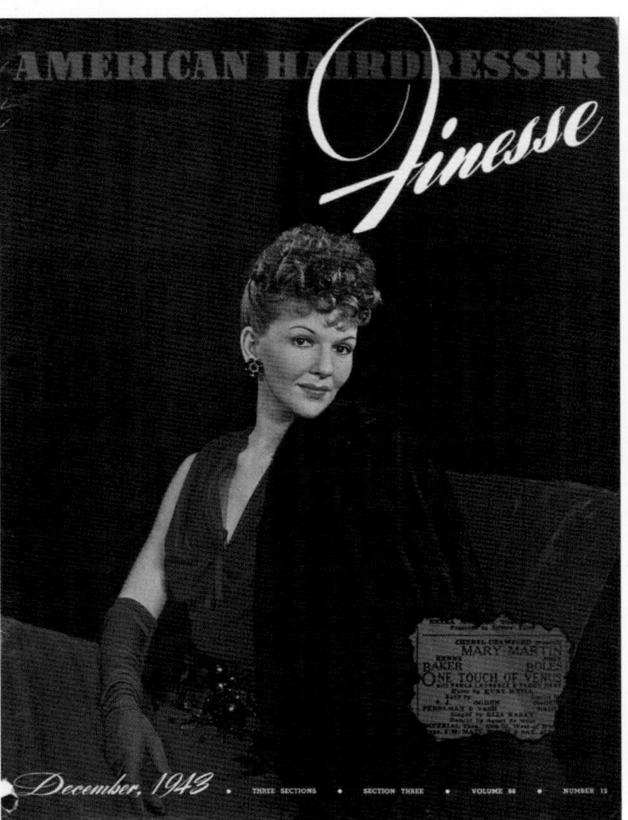

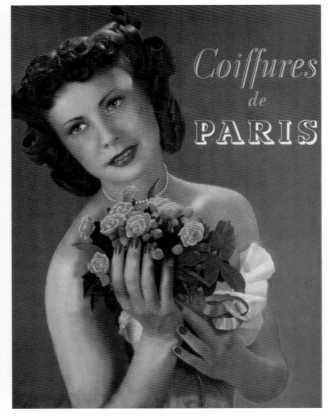

American Hairdresser magazine covers, 1942–43;
Coiffures de Paris magazine cover, 1949

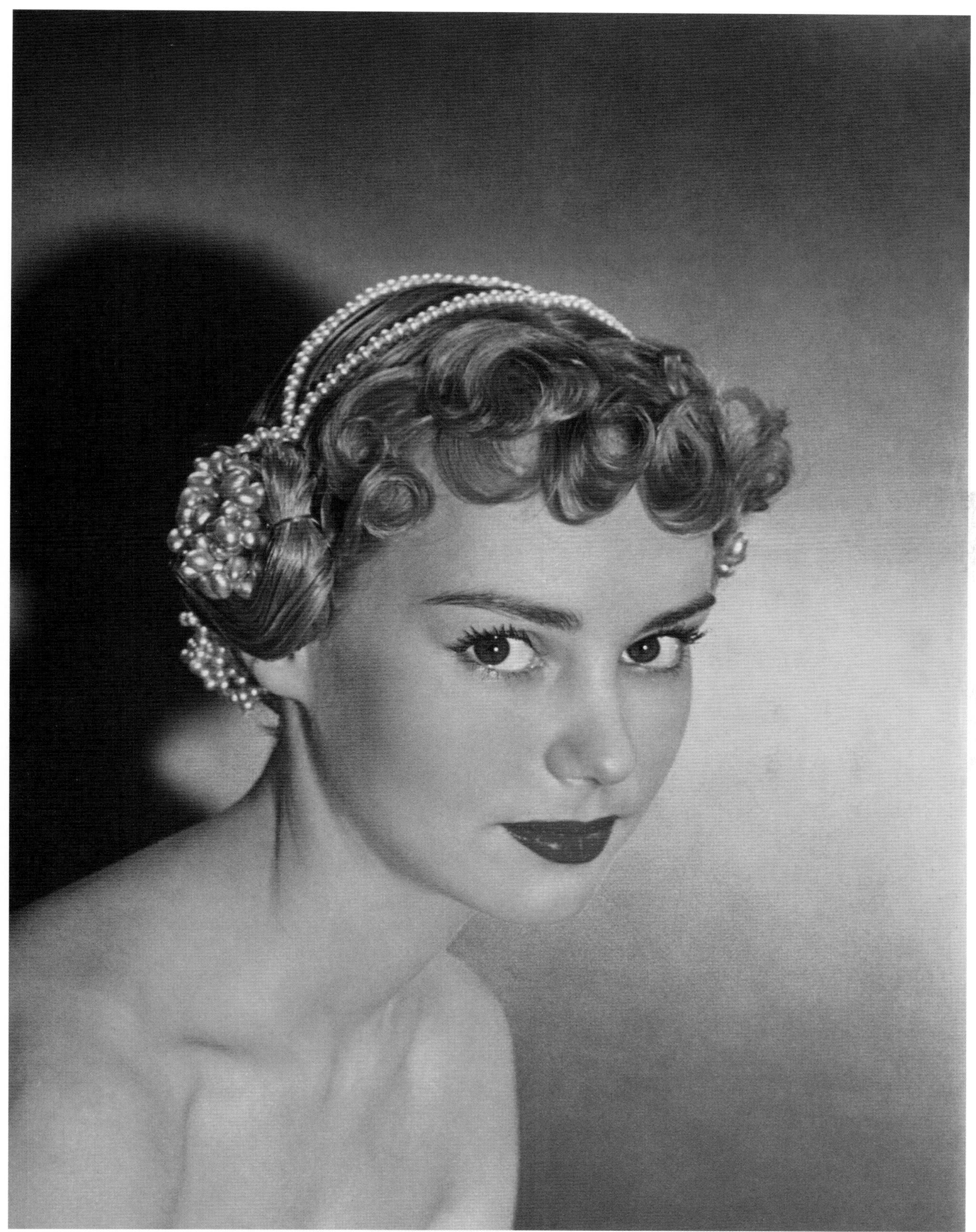

Hairstyle with pearls, 1949,
Coiffures de Paris

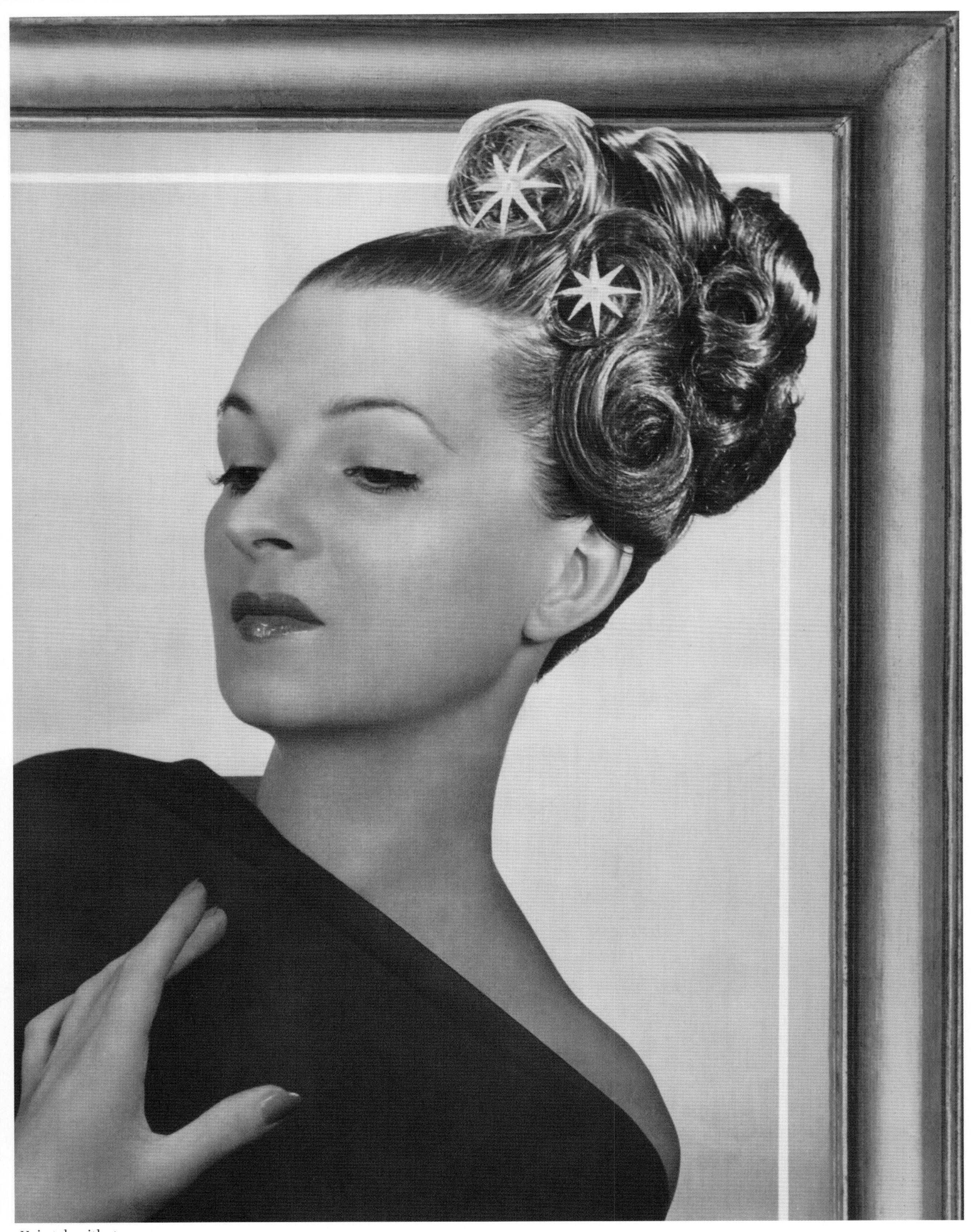

Hairstyle with stars, 1949,
Coiffures de Paris

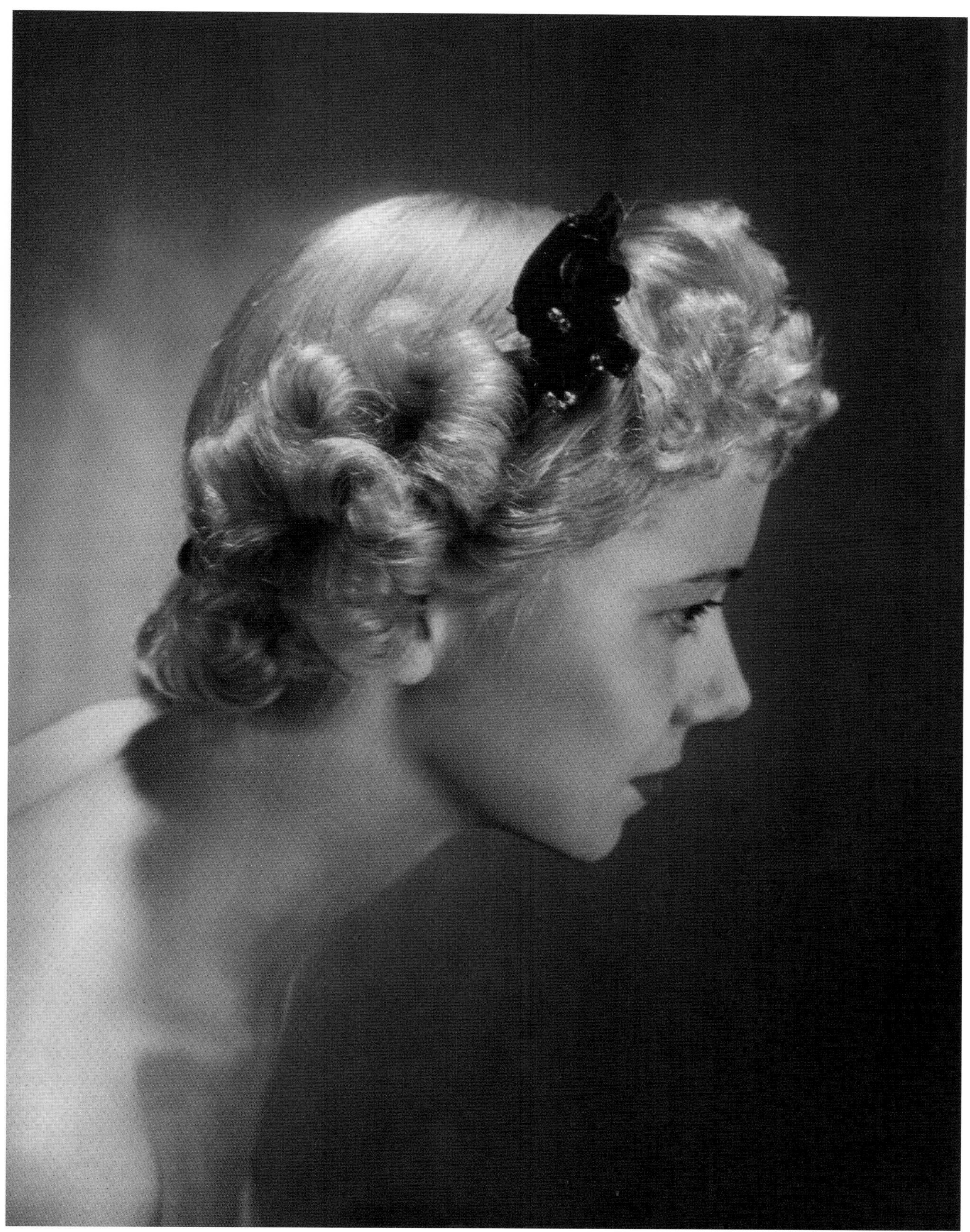

Hairstyle, 1949, *Coiffures de Paris*

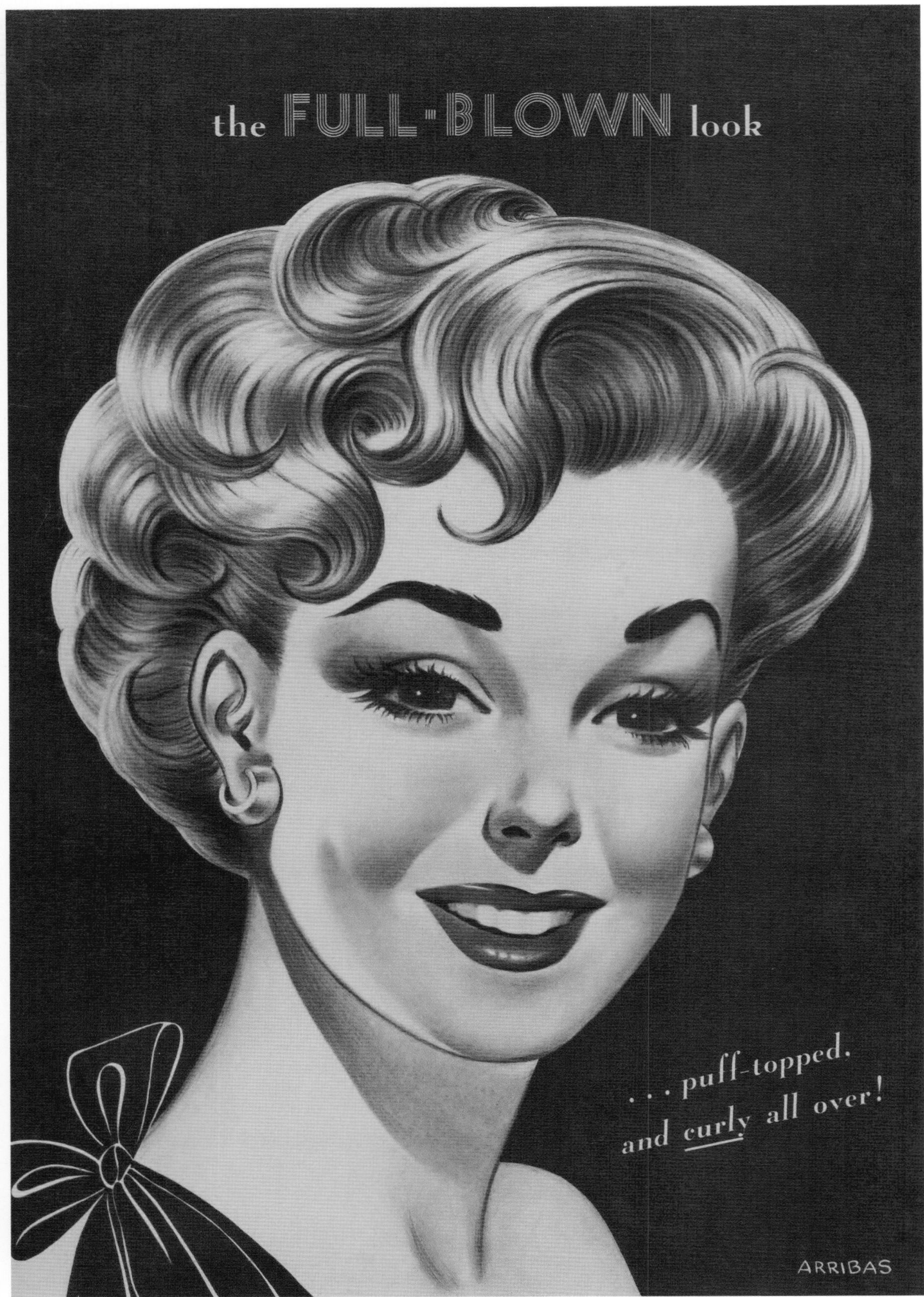

'The Full Blown Look' salon poster by Arribas, c.1959

1950S

n 1950 the vogue was for either exceptionally short shingle uts or slightly longer styles that were swept upwards away rom the forehead and the back of the neck. However, within year there was a new trend for hair to be worn slightly onger at the back and streaked blonde highlights also ecame fashionable. The Coronation of Queen Elizabeth II n 1953 saw many women adopt the young monarch's short ndulating hairstyle with its wispy fringe. Other women referred the more casual shaggy Italian look, which was nspired by the country's film stars who made stylish ophistication look effortless during this "La Dolce Vita" eriod. From 1954 until the decade's end, numerous short tyles gained popularity only to be replaced by the next ew look, with the vogue in hairstyles changing literally very season – from bouffant beehives and oriental-inspired reations to poodle-like cuts and high ponytails.

The 1950s also saw the launch of the first one-step home air colour formula by Clairol which debuted in 1956 with the ow-famous advertising catchphrase, "Does she... or doesn't he? Only her hairdresser knows for sure." Within six years f the "Miss Clairol Hair Color Bath" launch, a staggering 0% of women were colouring their hair and Clairol's sales ad increased by an astounding 413% – not only revealing the ncredible power of advertising, but also the common desire mong women to have hair that is coloured differently from vhat nature intended. It was also during the 1950s, that rma Kusely became the first hairdresser to be credited on elevision for her styling of Lucille Ball's hair in *I Love Lucy*, hereby revealing the increasing status of the professional tylist. In France, another "haut coiffeur", Alexandre de aris, also rose to fame. Initially he had trained under the reat Antoine and then worked as a stylist for among others, he Duchess of Windsor, who took him under her wing nd introduced him to hundreds of new clients. In 1952 he ntered into an association with Maria and Rosy Carita, two sisters who became known as the "magicians of beauty" and who were some of the earliest hairstylists to create their own haircare and beauty products. Five years later, Alexandre opened his own salon on the Rue du Faubourg St-Honoré in Paris and there he styled not only models for all the great fashion houses but also looked after an impressive roster of celebrity clients, including Greta Garbo, Lauren Bacall, Sophia Loren and Elizabeth Taylor, the latter being given by him the memorable wide-fringed hairstyle for 1963 film epic, *Cleopatra*. Importantly Alexandre, who was nicknamed the "Sphinx of Hairstyling" by his friend Jean Cocteau, believed that the key to success was the ability to match the hairstyle to the personality of the client, and certainly he was able achieve this time and again thanks to his formidable talent.

During the 1950s, Britain also boasted its own celebrity hairdresser, Pierre Raymond Bessone, who opened an influential salon in Mayfair with gilt mirrors and chandeliers. Raymond was soon besieged by a host of celebrity clients and became affectionately known as "Mr Teasie Weasie". Raymond's fame further increased in 1956 when the actress Diana Dors flew him to the United States for a £2,500 shampoo and set – then the price of a small house. With his pencil-thin moustache, Mr Teasie Weasie also appeared on a popular television show where every week he would wheel out a glamorous model sporting his latest gravity-defying and often extravagantly coloured creation. Then, with his gold scissors and tortoiseshell comb, he would explain in a faux French accent how to create the (often imaginatively named) hairdo. Known as "The Maestro", Raymond was not only a highly gifted cutter but also a veritable hair impresario, whose influence on the subsequent generation of British hairdressers was immense – he showed that it was possible to be both a well-known and much-loved personality as well as an accomplished stylist who could set trends.

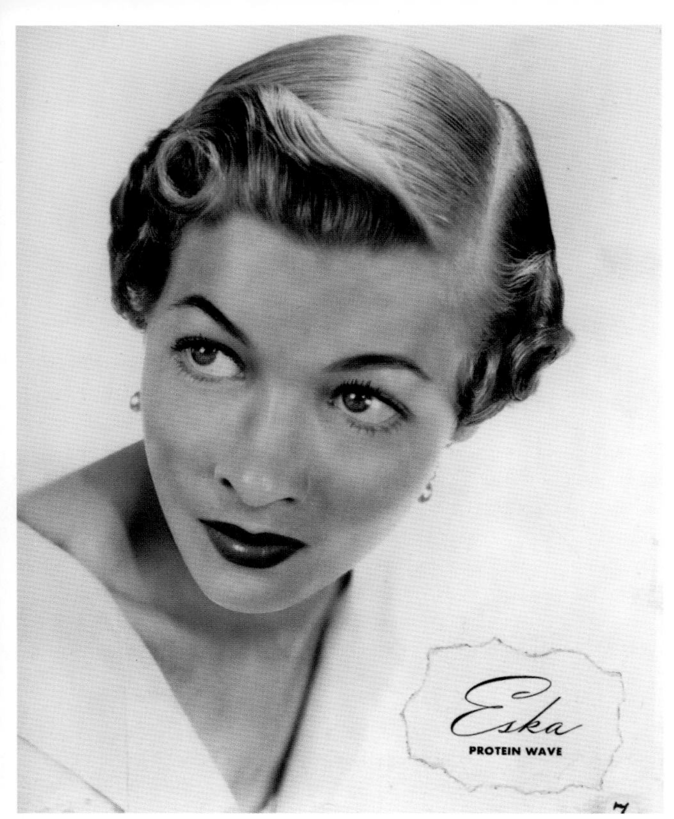

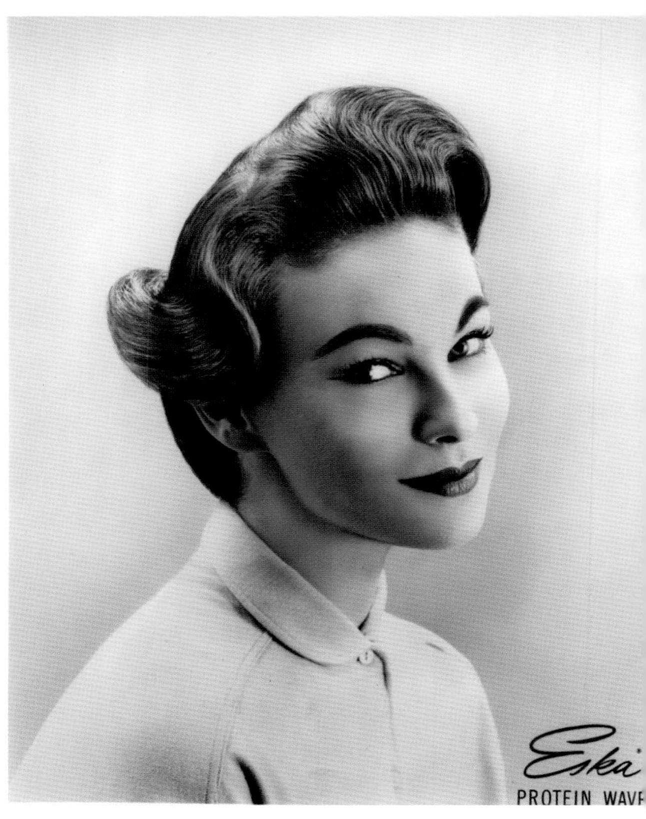

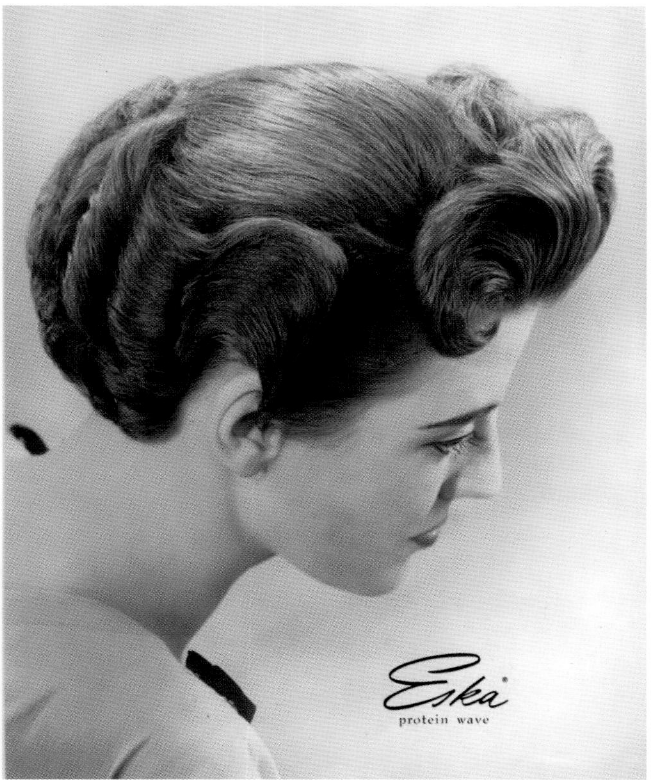

Salon photographs advertising
Eska Protein Wave, 1950s

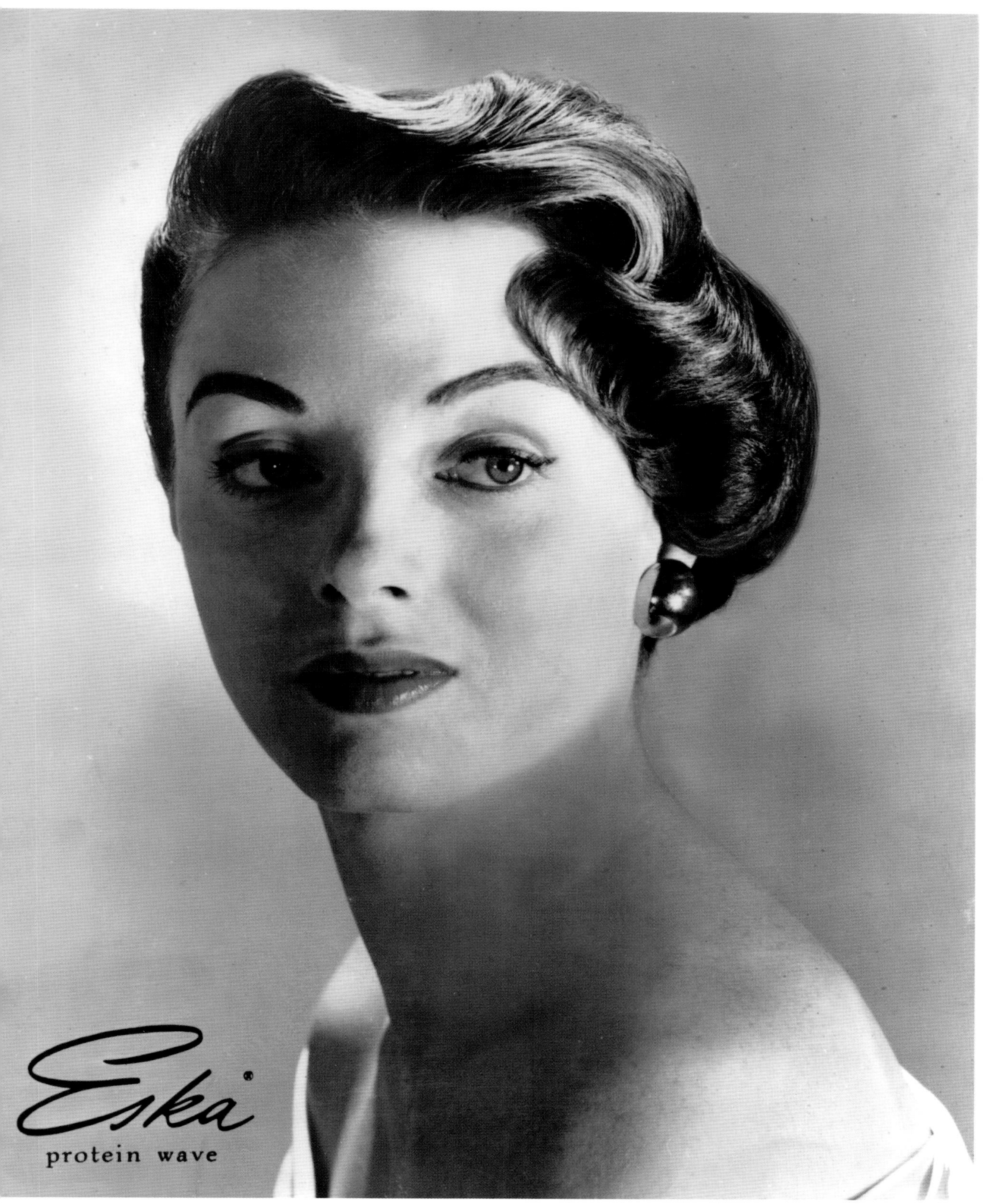
Eska®
protein wave

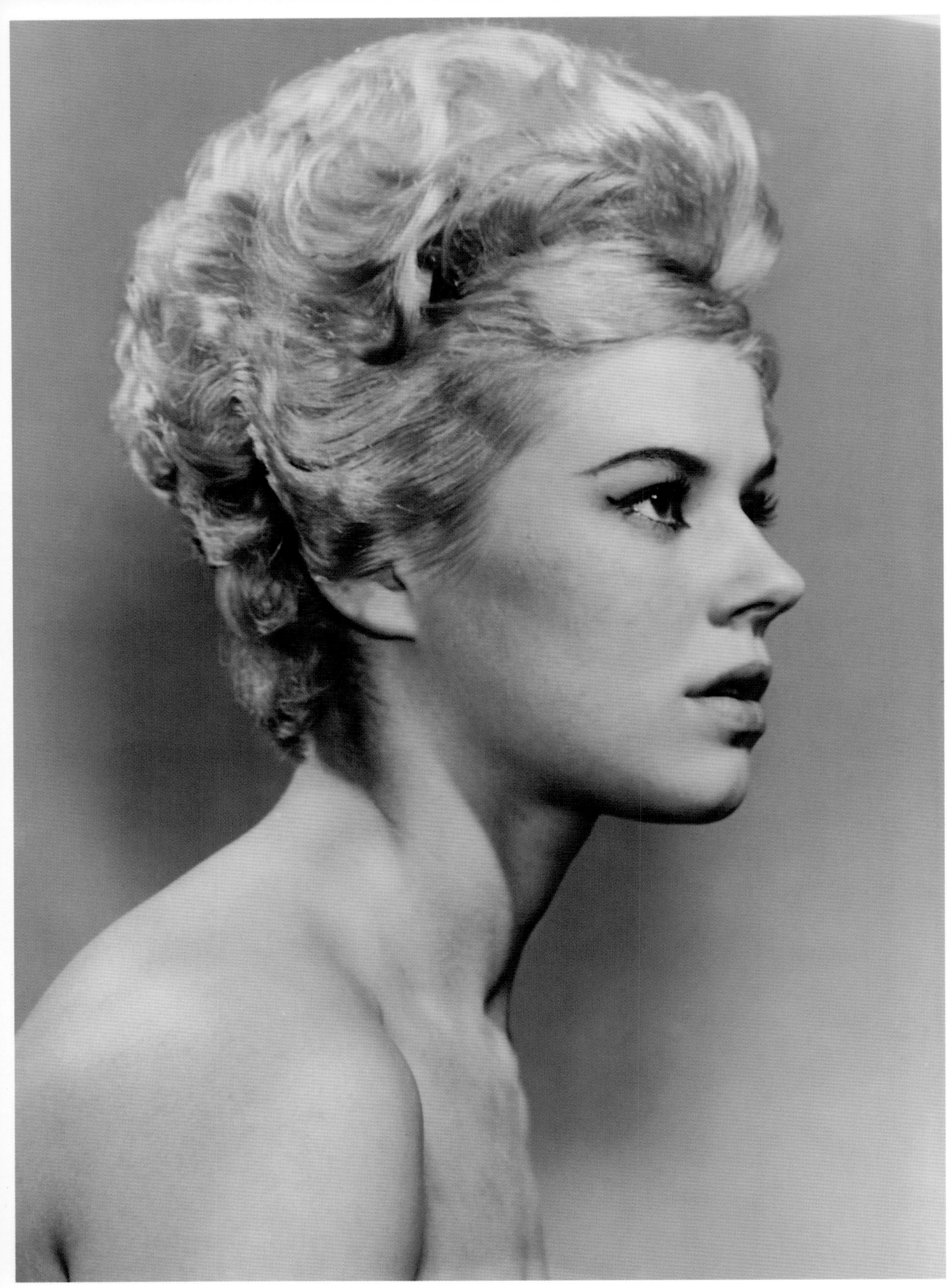

Hairstyle, Berlin, 1950s,
Foto-Linke, Berlin

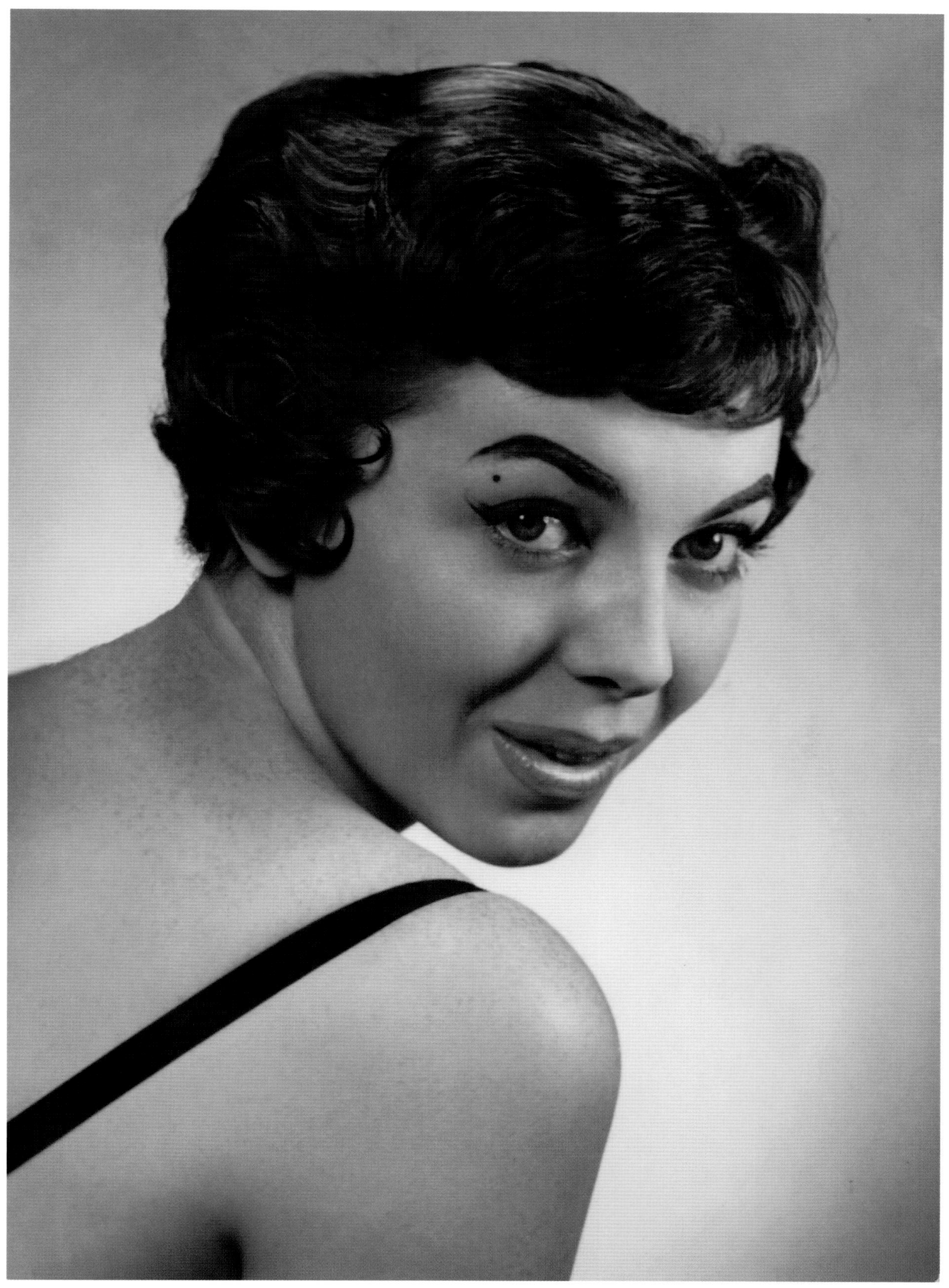

Cropped hairstyle, Berlin, 1950s,
photographed by B. Leidenfrost

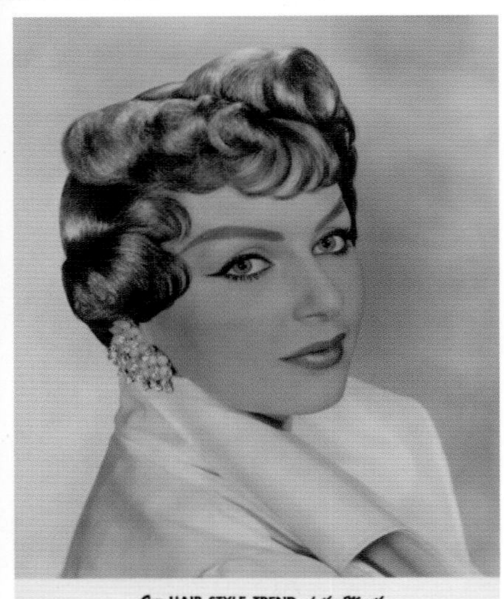

Our HAIR STYLE TREND of the Month

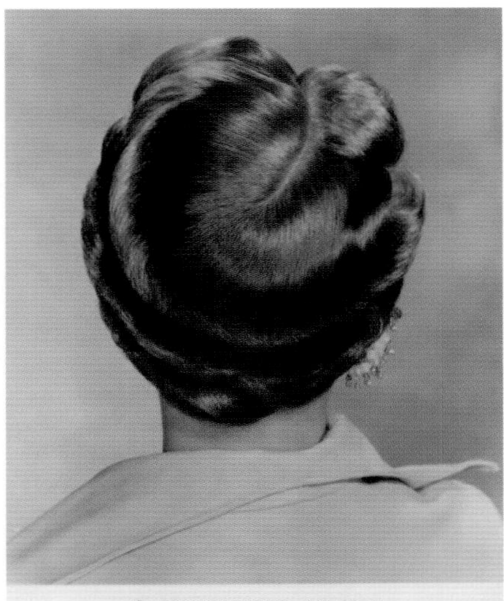

Our HAIR STYLE TREND of the Month

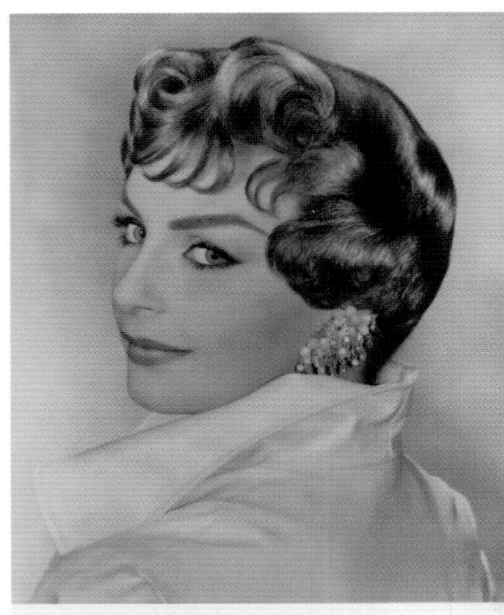

Our HAIR STYLE TREND of the Month

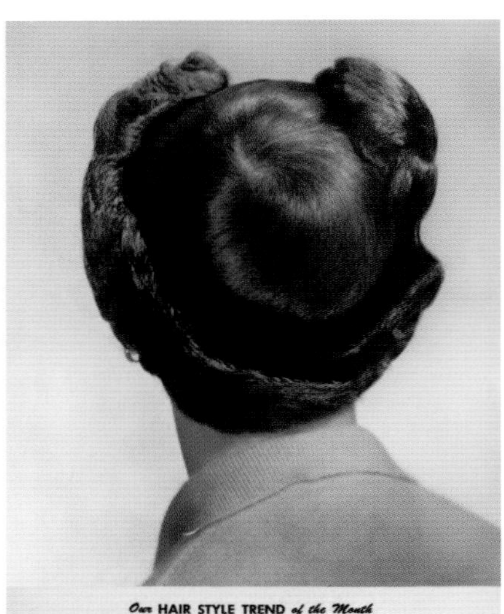

Our HAIR STYLE TREND of the Month

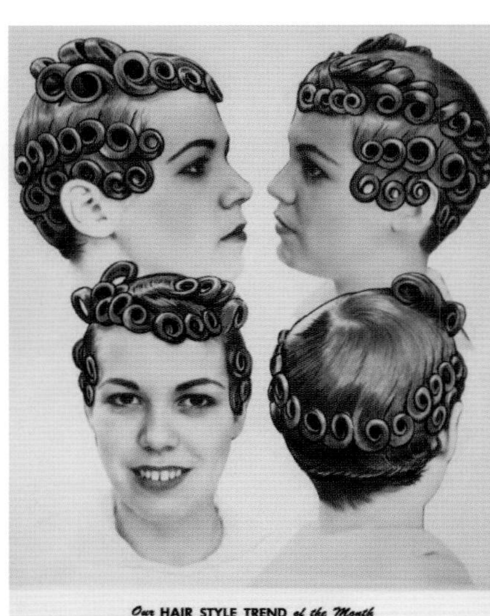

Our HAIR STYLE TREND of the Month

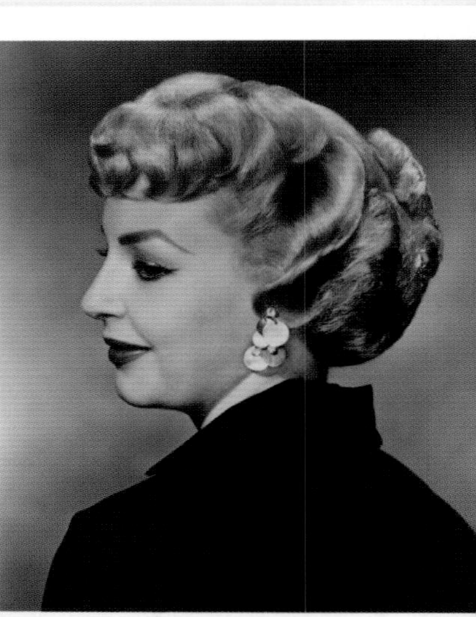

Our HAIR STYLE TREND of the Month

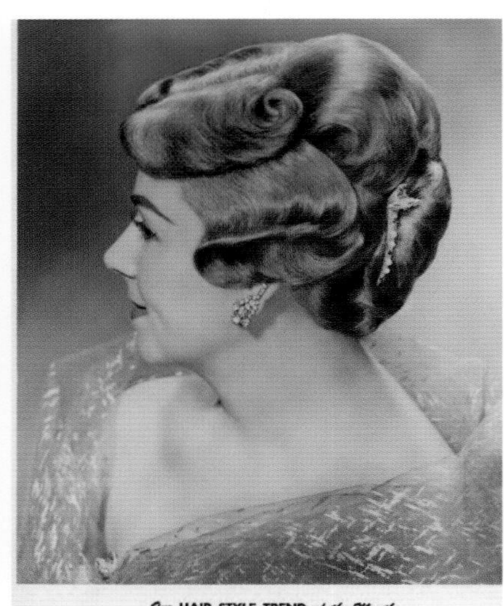

Our HAIR STYLE TREND of the Month

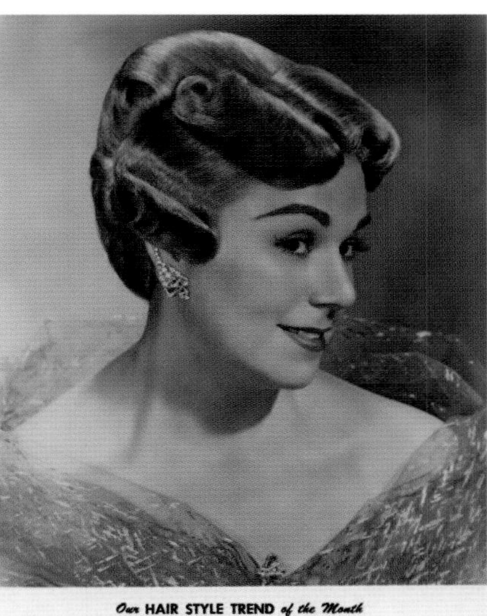

Our HAIR STYLE TREND of the Month

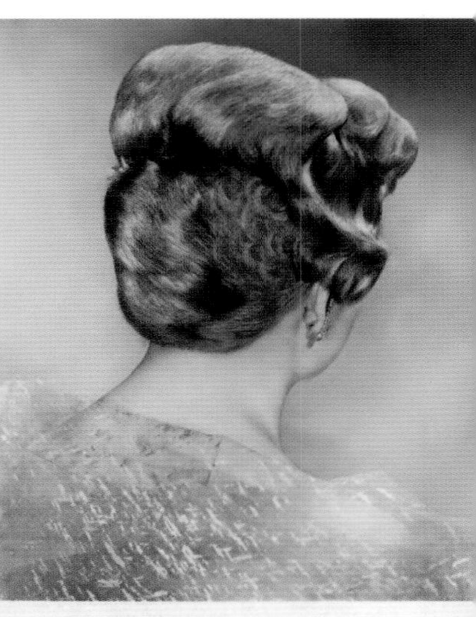

Our HAIR STYLE TREND of the Month

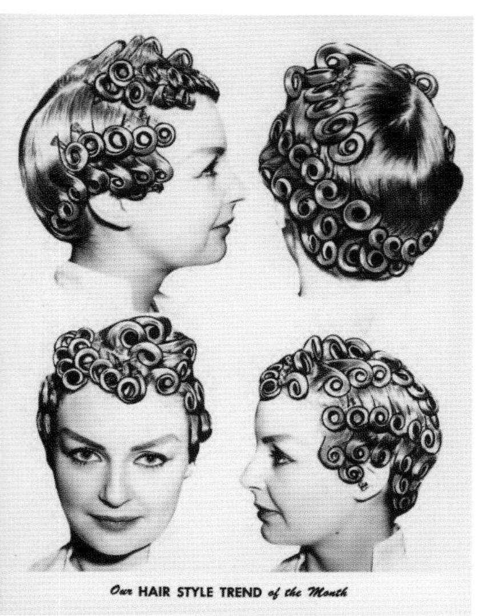

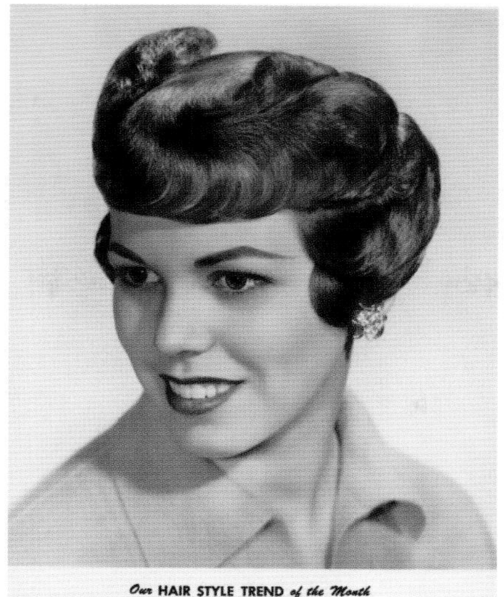

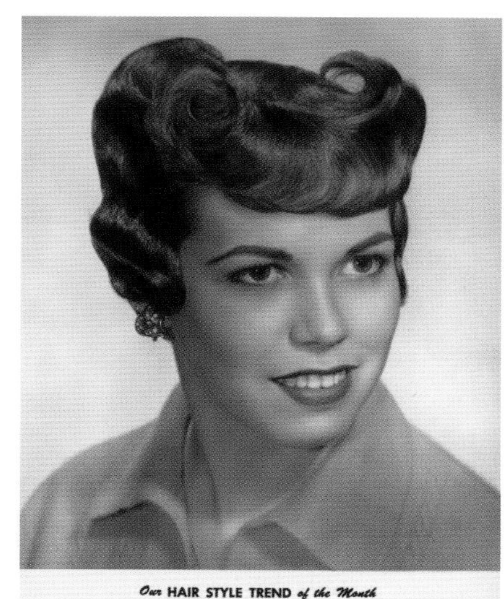

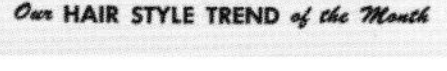

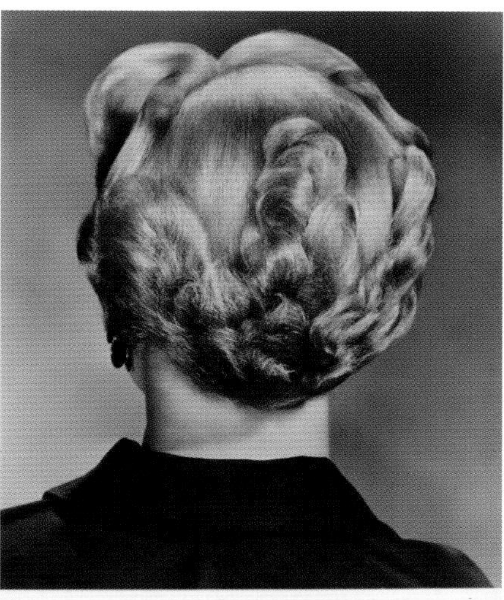

Our HAIR STYLE TREND of the Month

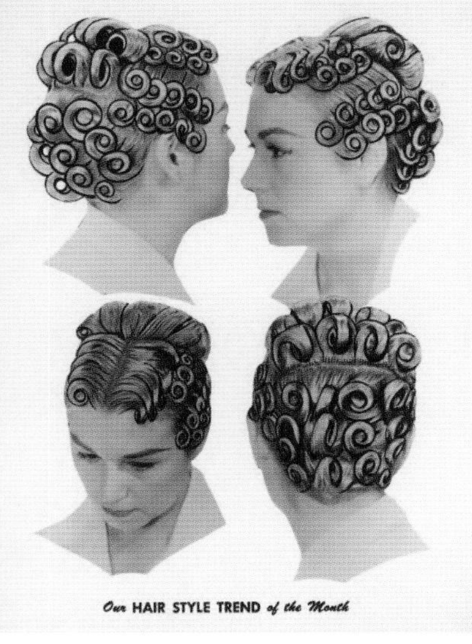

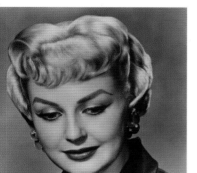

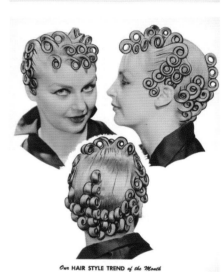

'Our Hair Style Trend of the Month' hair setting instructions and final results, Hollywood Hair Design Council, 1950s

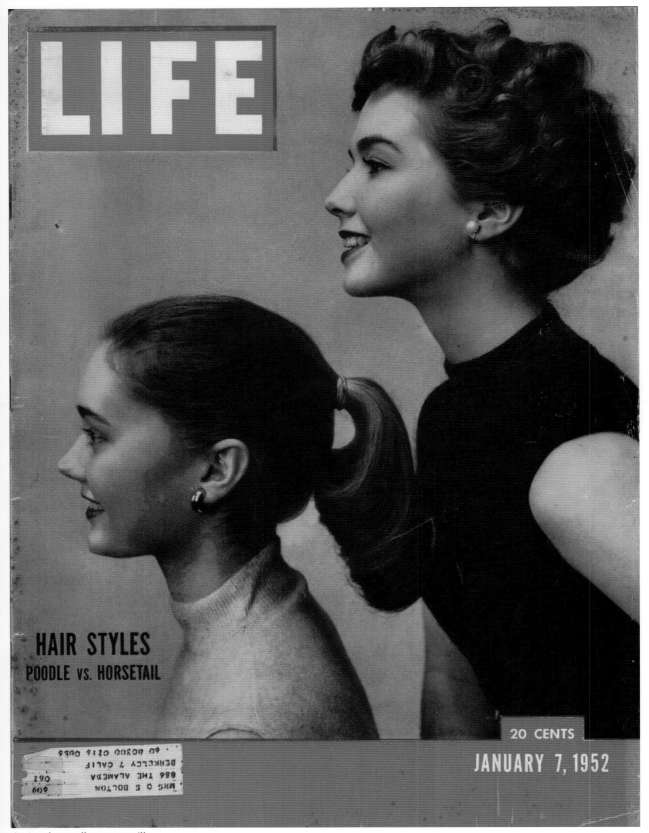

'Hair Styles: Poodle vs. Horsetail',
Life magazine cover, 1952

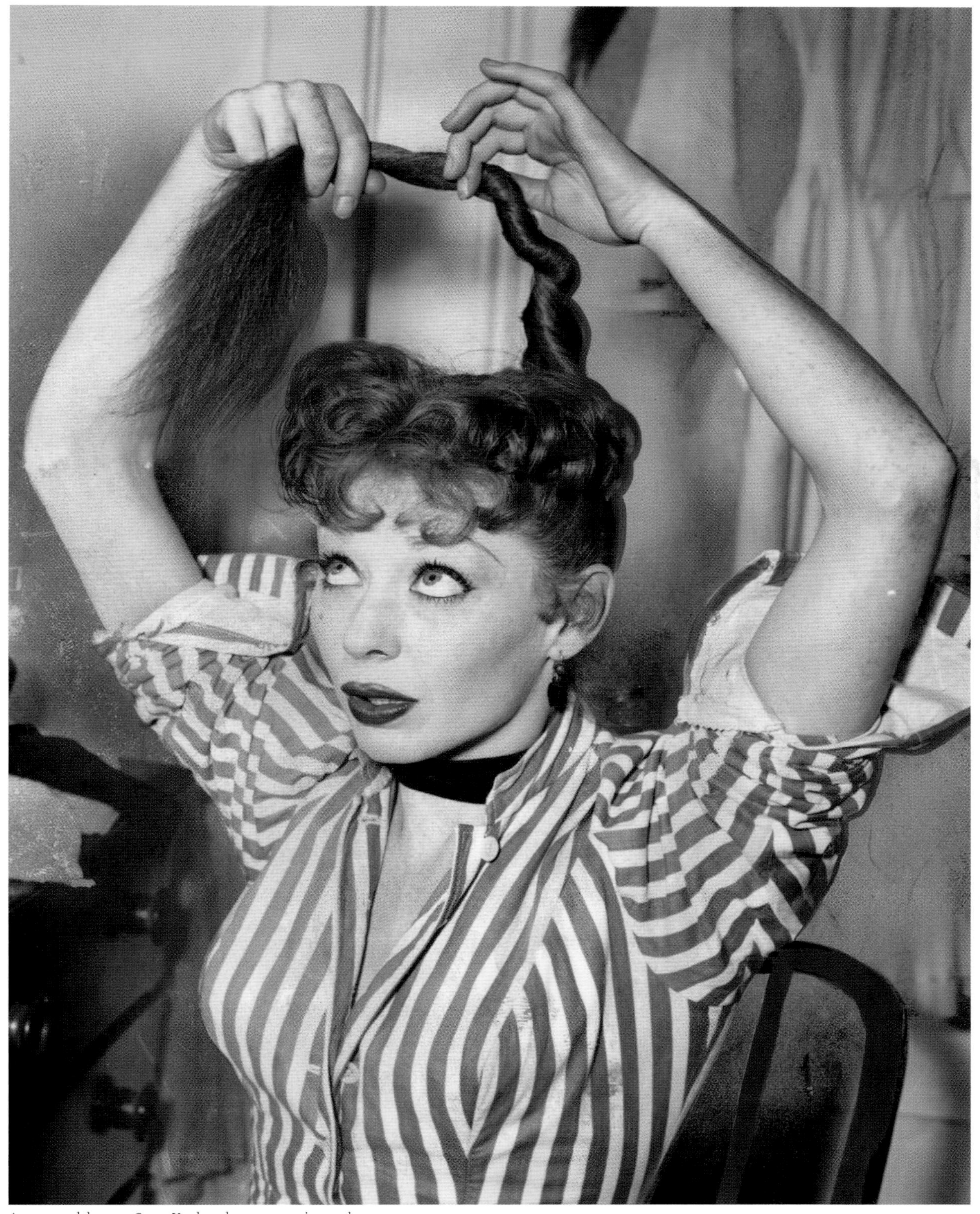

Actress and dancer, Gwen Verdon shown wrapping and twisting her hair into her unique 'Egg-Beater' style, 1953

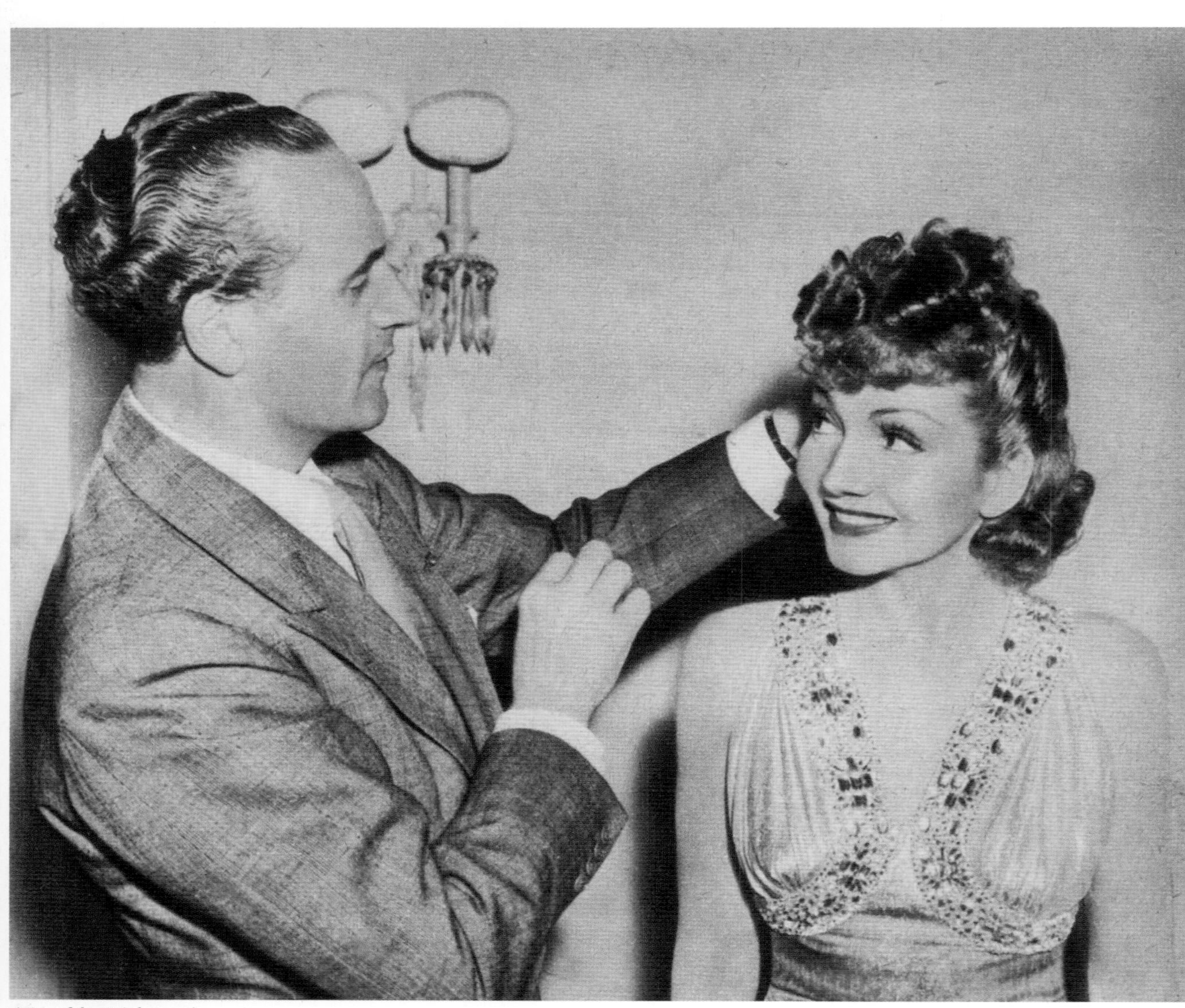

'King of the Hairdressers'
Monsieur Antoine, 1959

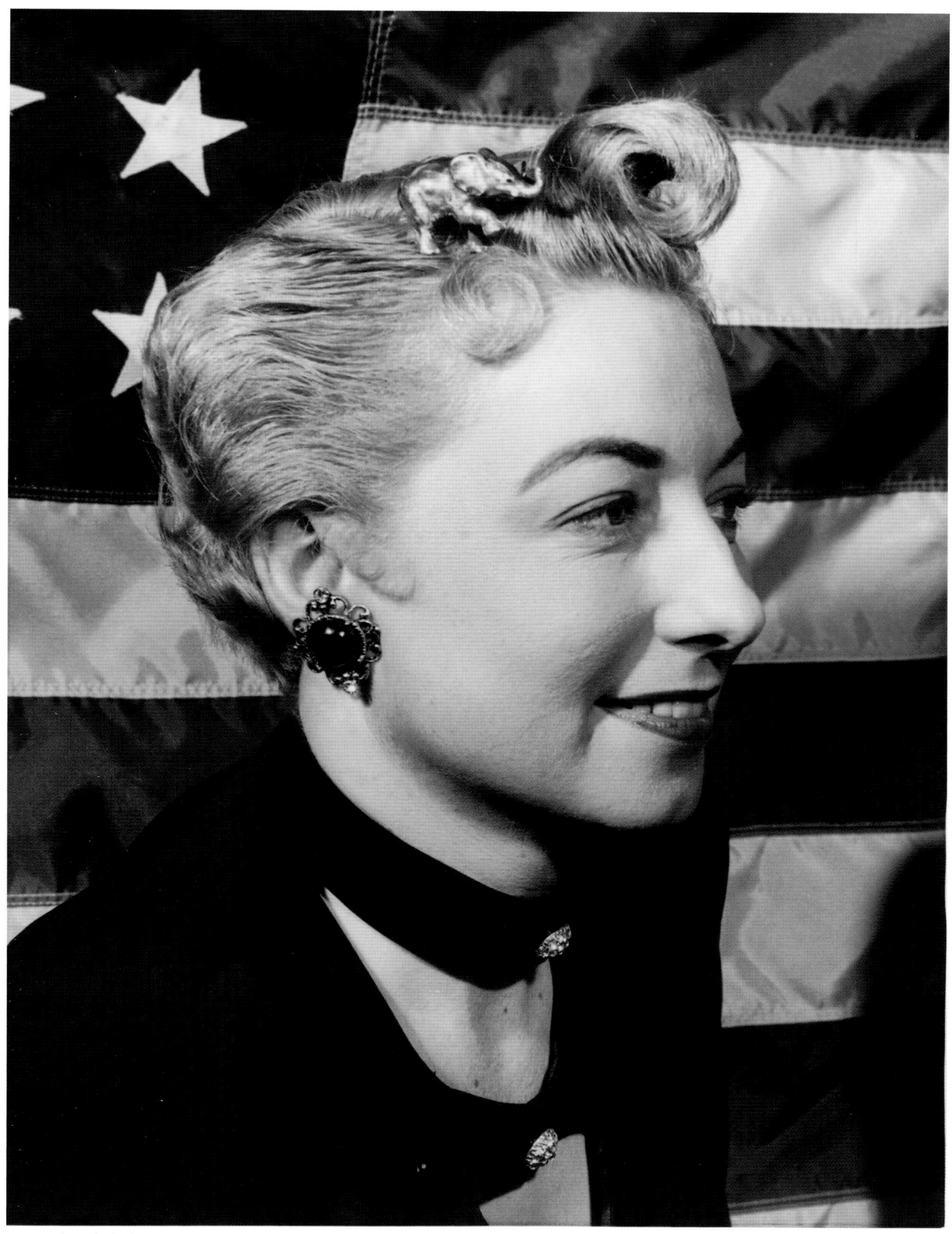

GOP Hairdo with elephant mascott
of the Republican Party, 1956

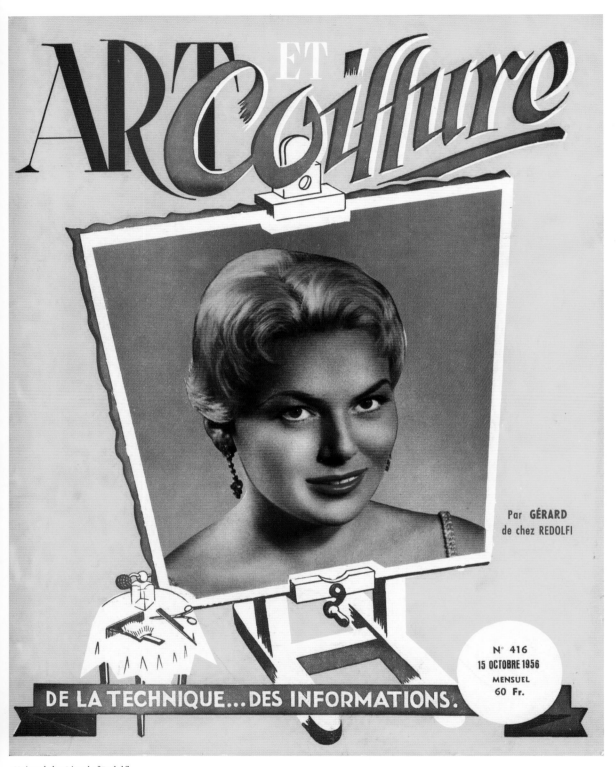

Hairstyle by Gérard of Redolfi, 1956, *Art et Coiffure*

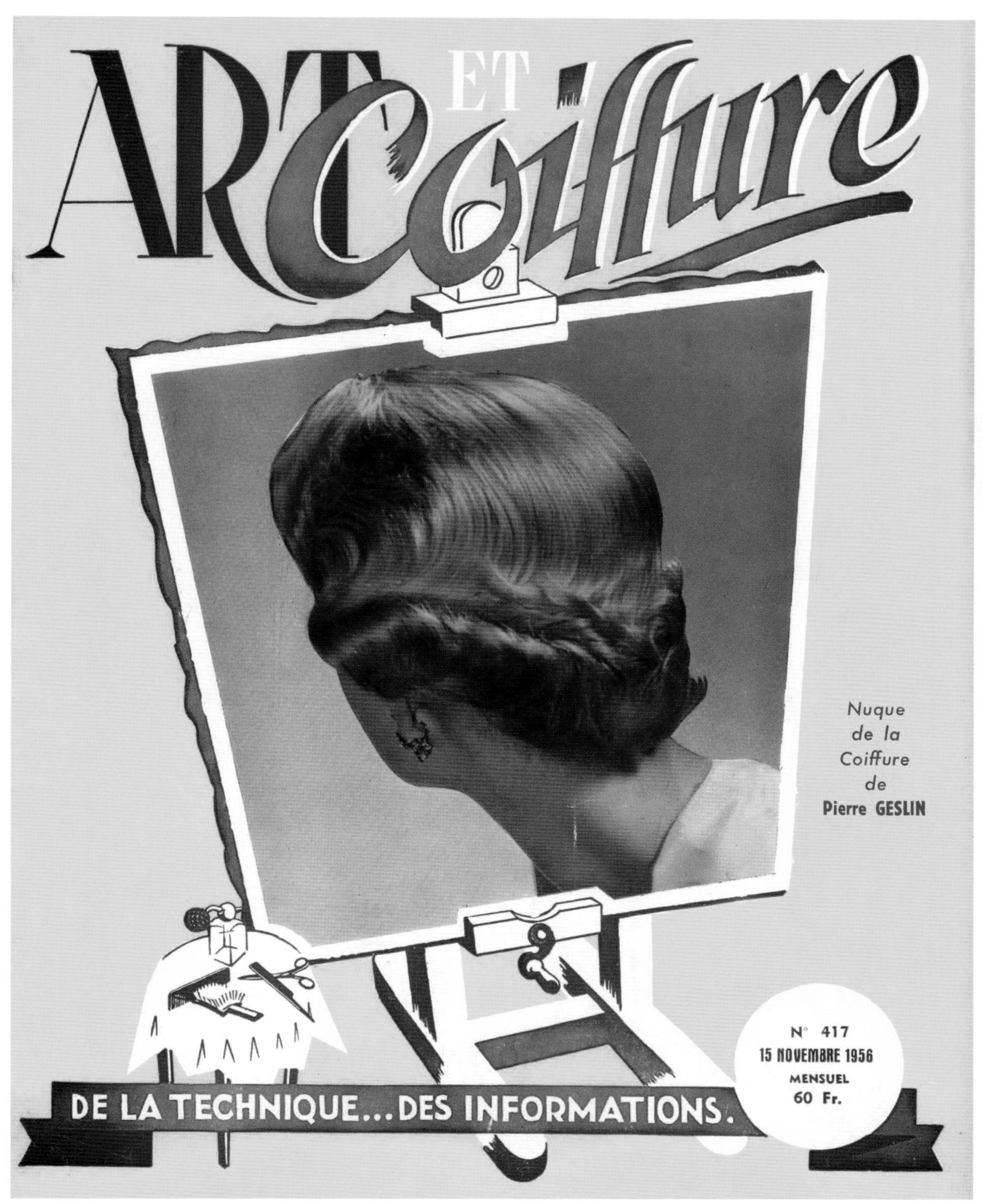

Hairstyle by Pierre Geslin, 1956,
Art et Coiffure

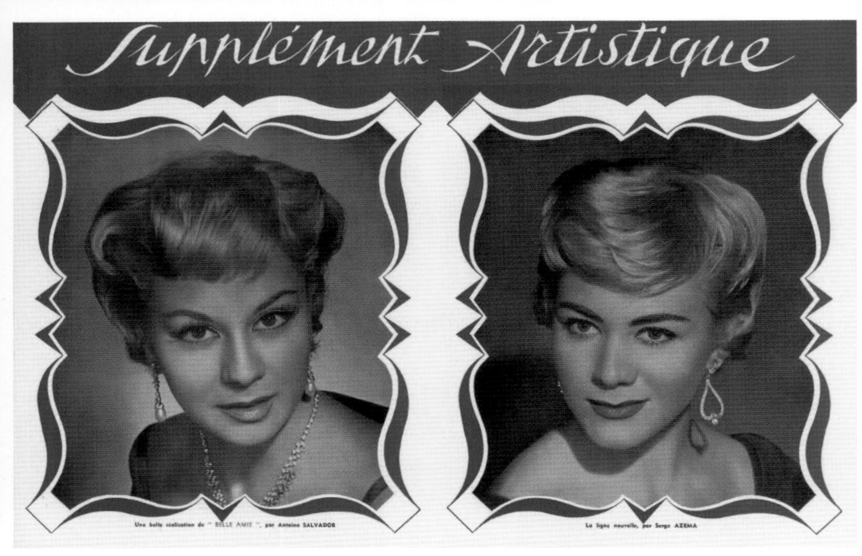
Supplément Artistique
Une belle réalisation de " BELLE AMIE ", par Antoine SALVADOR
La ligne nouvelle, par Serge AZEMA

Supplement showing hairstyles by Antoine Salvador and Serge Azema, 1957, *Art et Coiffure*

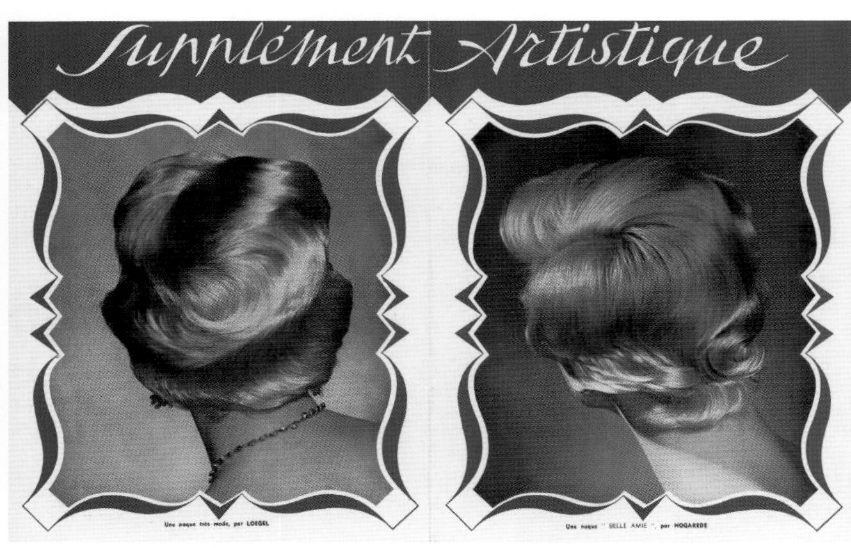

Supplement showing hairstyles by Loegel and Nogarede, 1957, *Art et Coiffure*

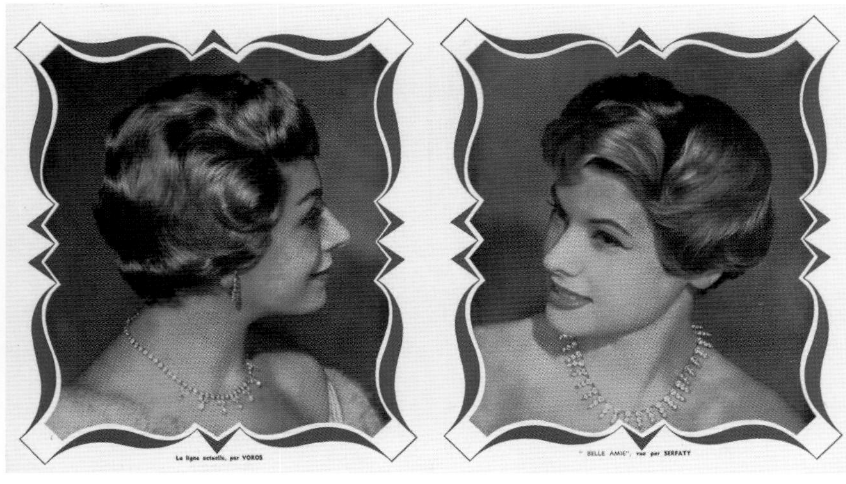

Supplement showing hairstyles by Voros and Serfaty, 1957, *Art et Coiffure*

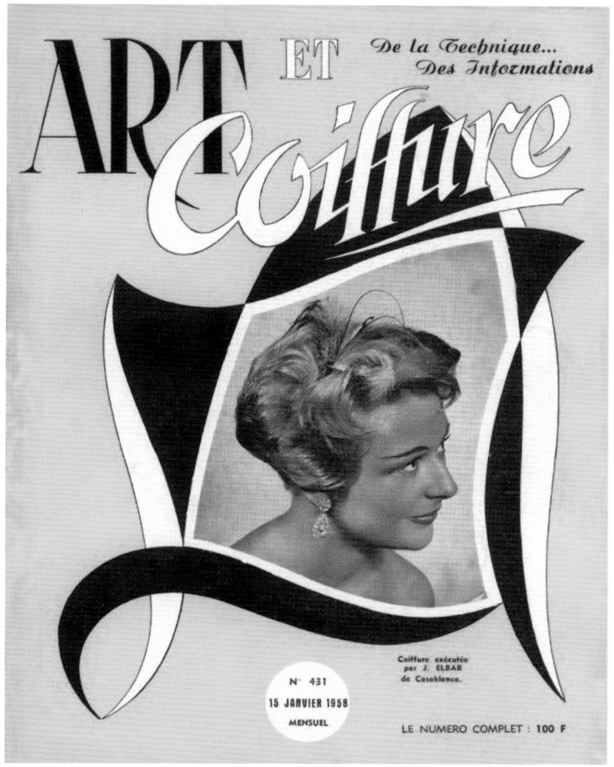

Hairstyle by J. Elbar of Casablanca, 1958, *Art et Coiffure*

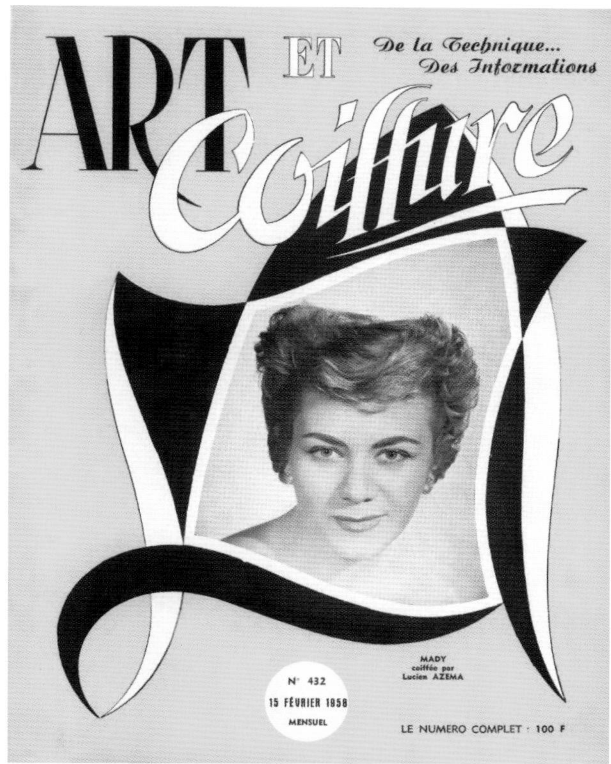

Hairstyle by Lucien Azema, 1958, *Art et Coiffure*

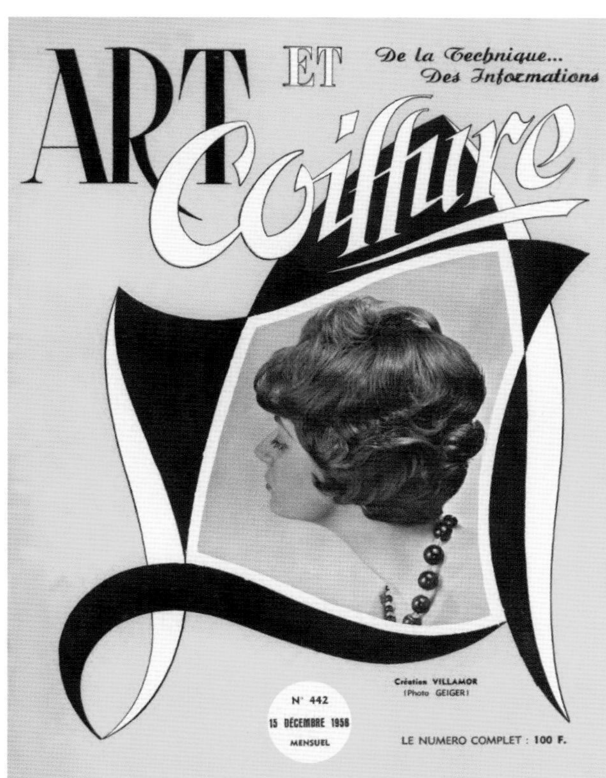

Hairstyle by Villamor, 1958, *Art et Coiffure*

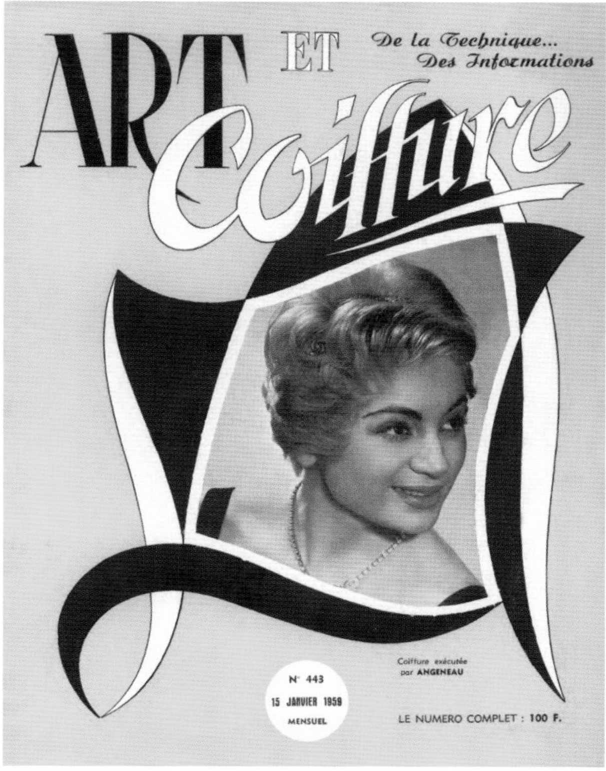

Hairstyle by Angeneau, 1959, *Art et Coiffure*

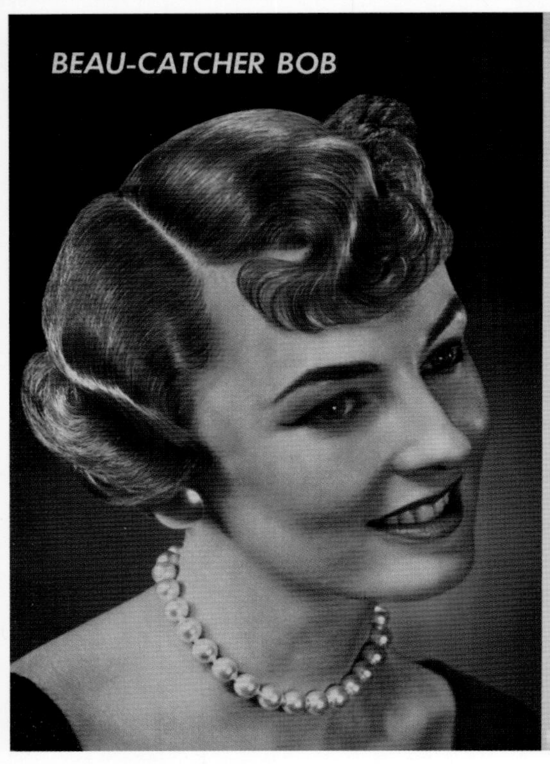

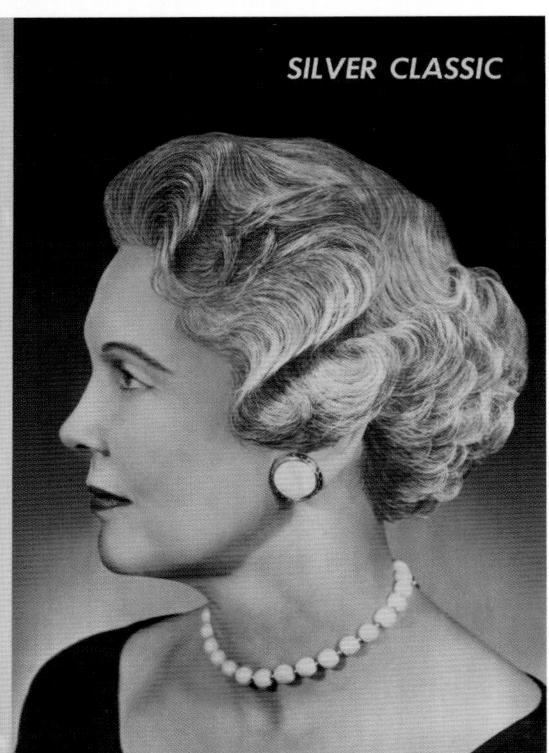

'Beau-Catcher Bob' and 'Silver Classic' hairstyles, 1957, *Modern Beauty Shop*

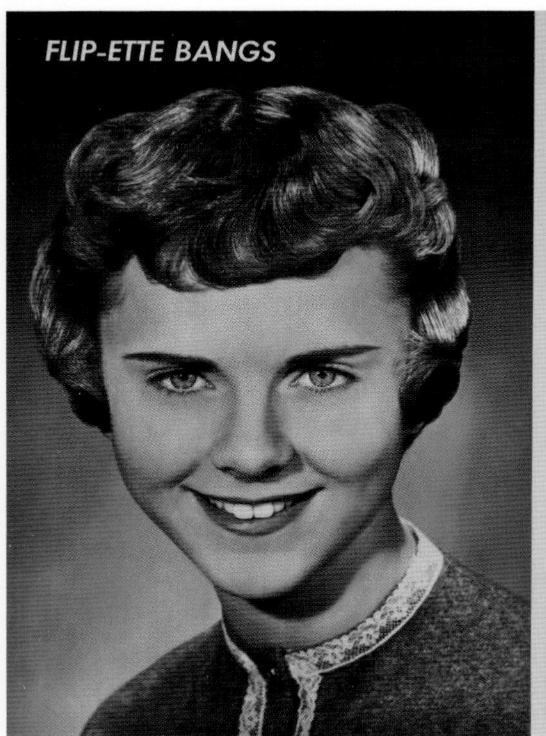

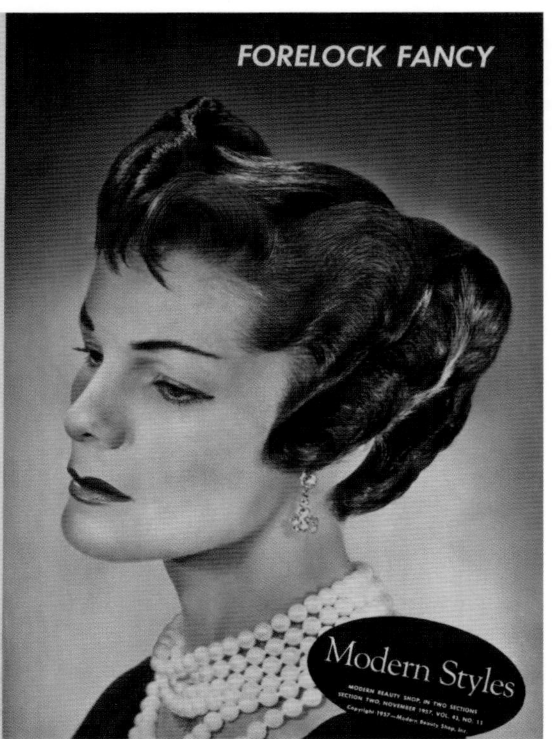

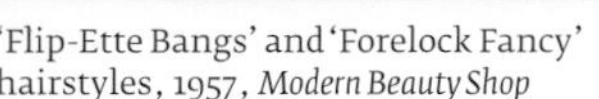
'Flip-Ette Bangs' and 'Forelock Fancy' hairstyles, 1957, *Modern Beauty Shop*

Does she... or doesn't she?

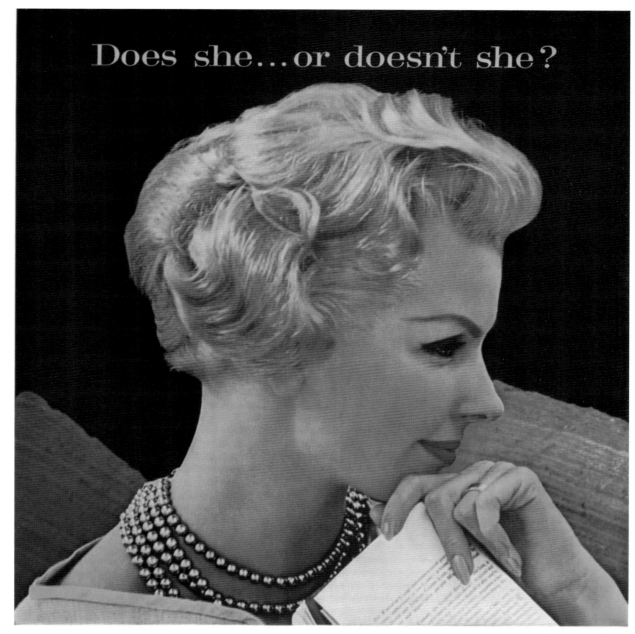

Hair color so natural
only her hairdresser knows for sure!

MISS CLAIROL®

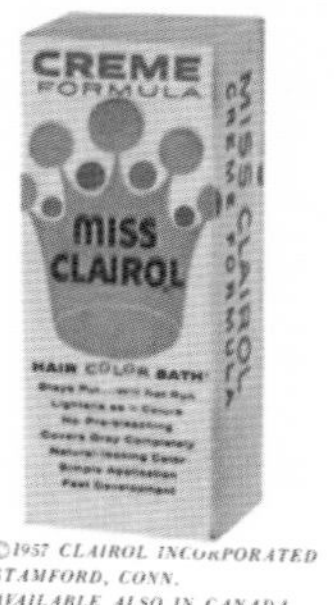

HAIR COLOR BATH®

Advertisement for Miss Clairol
Hair Color Bath, 1950s

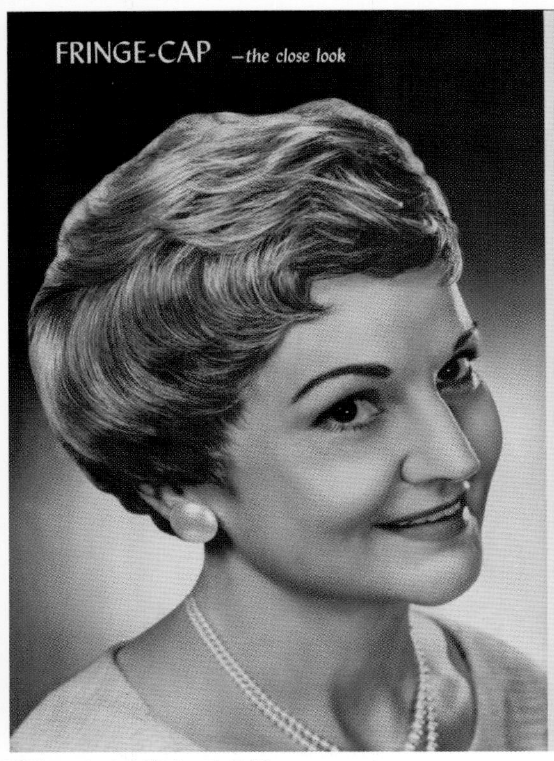

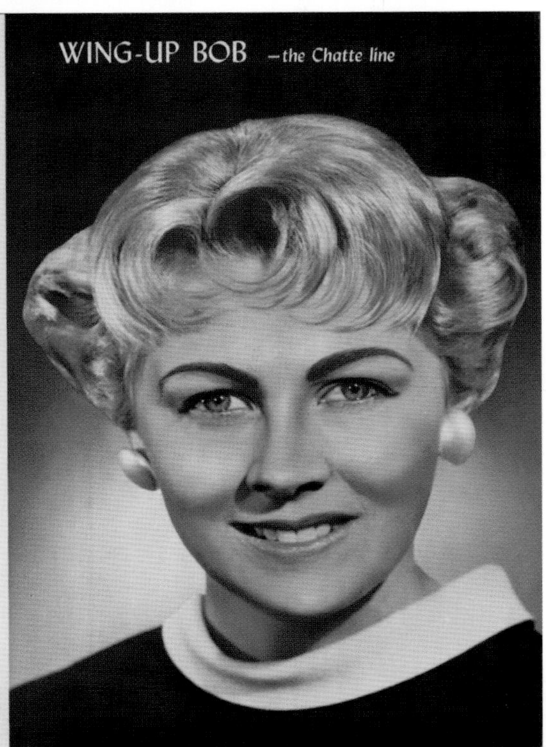

'Fringe-Cap' and 'Wing-Up Bob'
hairstyles, 1959, *Modern Beauty Shop*

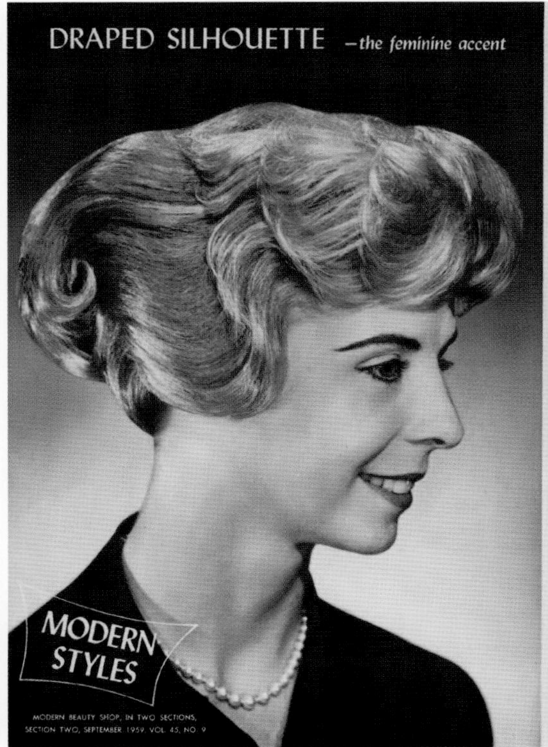

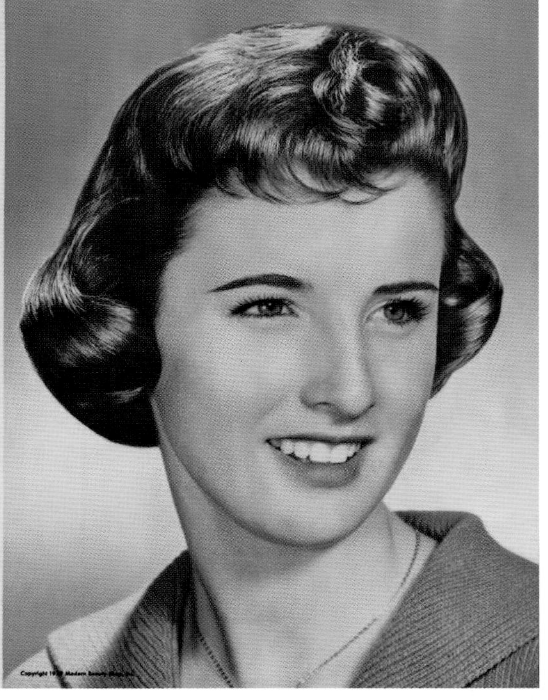

'Draped Silhouette' and 'Teen Queen'
hairstyles, 1959, *Modern Beauty Shop*

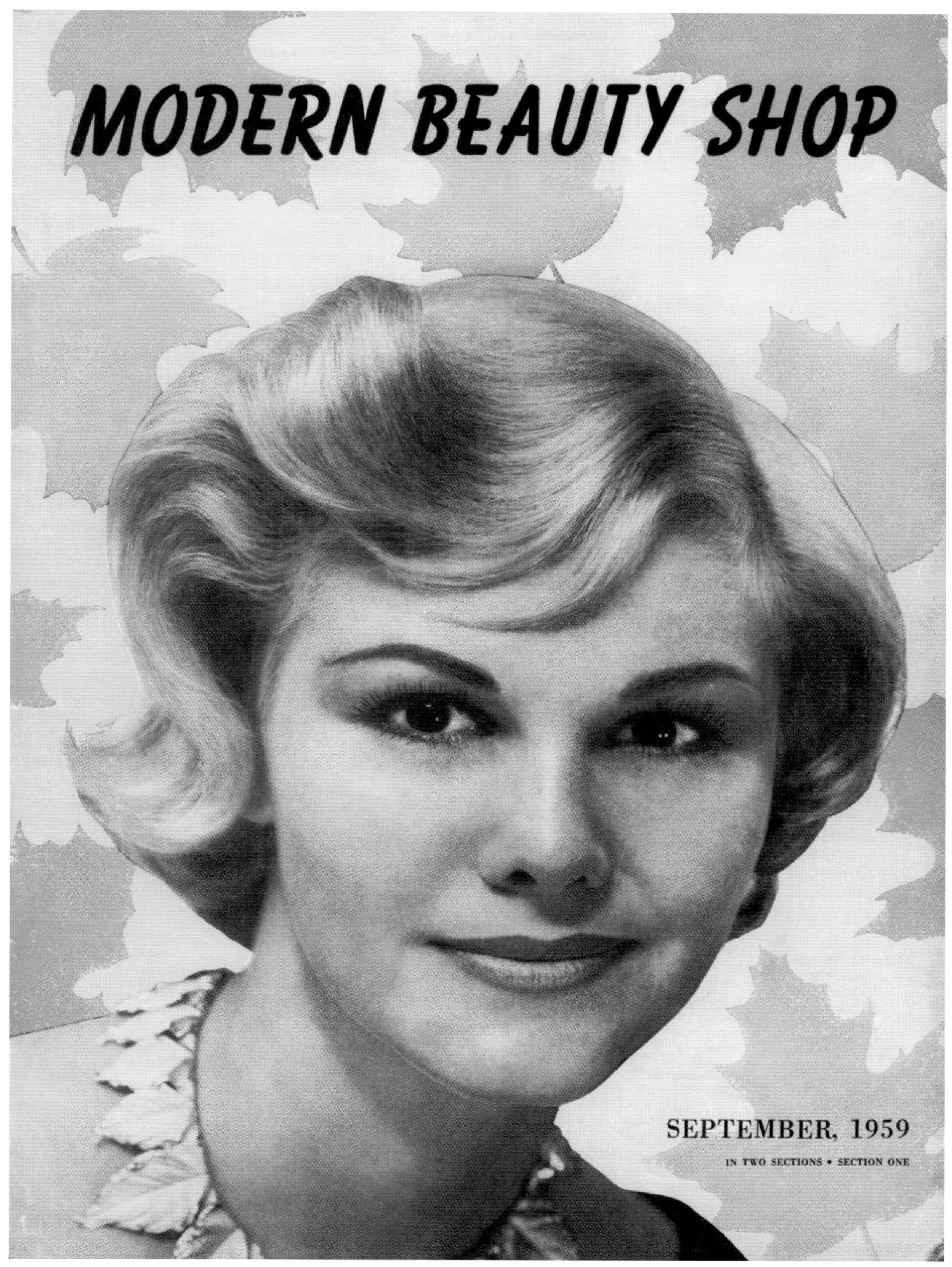

Modern Beauty Shop
magazine cover, 1959

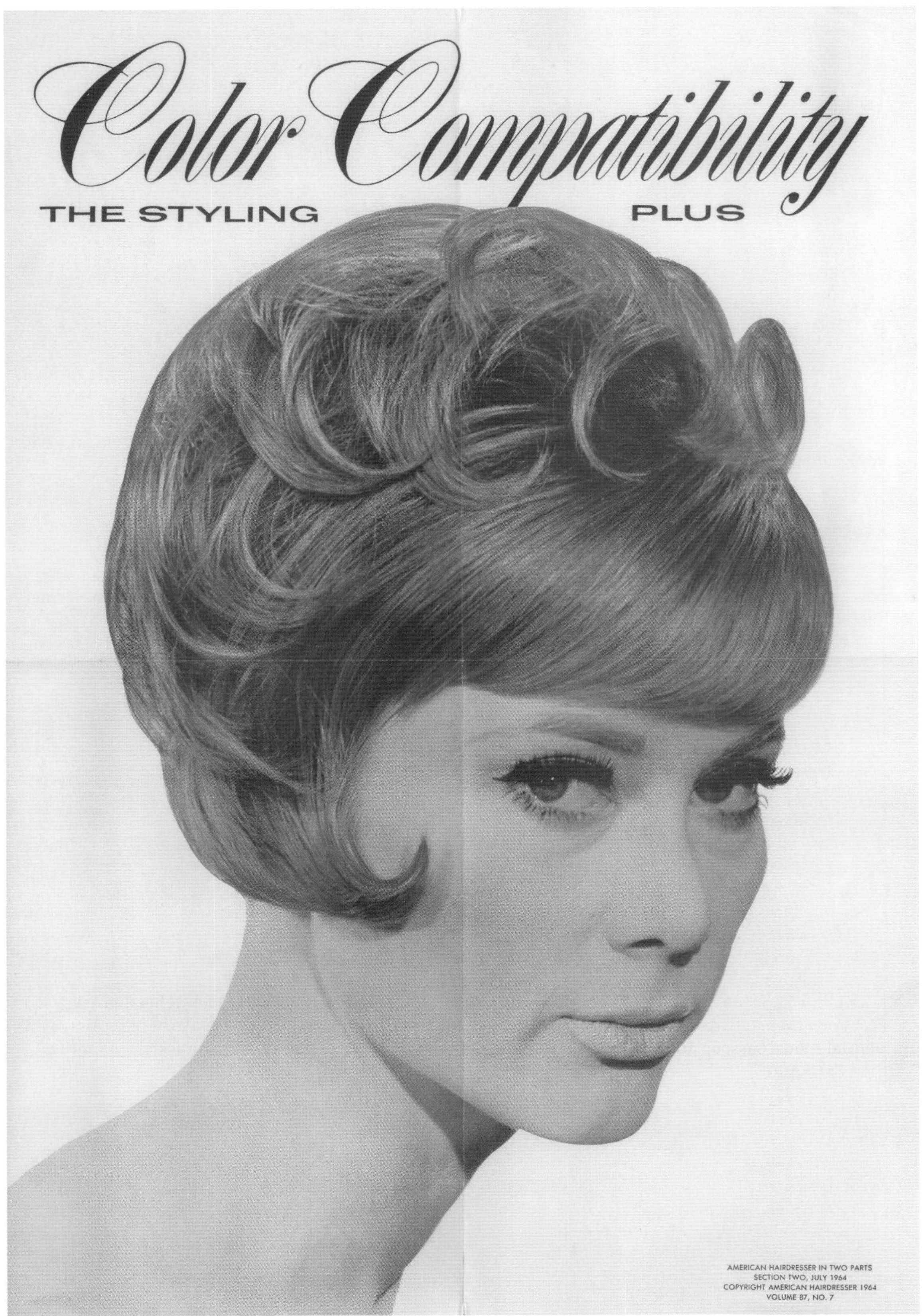

'Color Compatibility' salon poster, 1964, *American Hairdresser*

1960S

'he 1960s was a period of unprecedented social change vhich saw the increasing empowerment of women, and heir newly found sexual liberation was mirrored in their hoices of hairstyles. The early years of the 1960s, however, aw hairstyles that were slightly more extreme versions of uts that had been popular in the late 1950s, and the first ew years of the decade were dominated with "big hair" tyles. For example, the influential bouffant hairdo styled by enneth Batelle aka "Mr Kenneth" for Jaqueline Kennedy for er husband's presidential inauguration in 1961. Mr Kenneth pecialised in, as he put it, "soft, romantic hair – healthy air you'd want to touch" and was a firm believer in what vas described by *Glamour* beauty editor, Karlys Daly as "loose, asy, wash-and-wear hair". He certainly did not subscribe to ashionable fads and instead gave his clients, such as Marilyn Aonroe, Barbara Walters, Diana Vreeland and Goldie Hawn, legant styles that fitted their personalities. As he noted, Crazes come and go: the one factor I feel important is the ut... I realised the cut was important – nobody else did – as he set hid a multitude of sins."

Another hairdresser from the 1960s who similarly achieved elebrity status was the suave Gene Shacove, whose life was he inspiration for the 1975 movie *Shampoo* featuring Warren eatty as the outrageous George Roundy. Based in Beverly Iills, Gene Shacove owned a salon on Rodeo Drive beneath vhich he operated the Candy Store nightclub ensuring he ecame a central figure in LA's social life. As Nancy Griffin and im Masters later recalled, "Shacove was hip and handsome, a tud with a blowdryer." He was, however, also a gifted stylist 'ho preferred using his fingers when blowdrying hair rather han using brushes or combs, thereby creating a more casual nd natural look that was perfectly in tune with the more exually permissive times of the late 1960s.

Across the Atlantic, London also had two celebrity stylists vho were hugely influential – Vidal Sassoon and Leonard ewis – who could perhaps be better described as "hair esigners" than hairdressers. Vidal Sassoon had initially rained with Raymond before opening his first salon in 954. As he later recalled in a film (made by Tony Rizzo and nthony Mascolo), "So there was an evolution before the evolution! It took me a long time to get to the Five-Point cut! Iairdressing wasn't a job, it was a lifestyle." In 1963, Vidal assoon introduced his innovative "Five-Point" hairstyle – a triking asymmetric and easy-to-wear haircut based on a lassic 1920s Bob. Unlike earlier hairdressers, Sassoon did not battle to tame hair into a specific style, but rather expertly cut hair in such a way that it could swing free but remain looking fantastic. He created several other bob-type styles, notably a simple geometric bob worn by Mary Quant, a short and layered cut known as "The Shape" and perhaps best known, the elegant "Nancy Kwan", which was a graduated bob that was longer at the front than the back and was named after the actress who wore it. Vidal Sassoon also created in 1968 a boyish pixie cut for Mia Farrow. Sometimes cited as "the founder of modern hairdressing", Vidal Sassoon created hairstyles that were radical but also practical, stylish yet easy-to-wear, and as such he altered the hairdressing landscape forever... while his Bond Street salon became a magnet for London's trend-seeking youth. Sassoon also fully understood the art of presentation, presumably a lesson well learnt from his former mentor Raymond, and in his later and bigger Old Bond Street salon there was a viewing gallery that allowed the public to come in and watch London's most famous hairstylist at work.

Though less well known than Sassoon, the prodigiously talented Leonard Lewis also helped put the swing into the Swinging Sixties. A hugely influential hairdressing figure during this era, Lewis briefly worked at Vidal Sassoon's salon before establishing his own salon in Duke Street. A few years later he opened the extraordinary "House of Leonard" salon in a six-storey Georgian town house in Upper Grosvenor Street. This luxurious salon decorated in grey and shocking pink was a veritable hair palace that became a mecca for the rich and famous. In this resplendent setting, "Leonard of Mayfair" plied his craft with style and charm, however unlike Sassoon, he did not subscribe to any hair-cutting formula but rather freely experimented. One day his friend, Justin de Villeneuve came in with a teenage girl with very straggly and long bleached hair. Leonard took one look at her and asked his then assistant Keith Wainwright to take her upstairs and give her a treatment. After a while he asked for another treatment because her hair was in such bad condition. He then started cutting her hair and just kept chopping more and more off, until finally she was left with a becoming urchin-like crop – and it was this transformative haircut that turned the young teenager into "Twiggy", the iconic waif-like model of Swinging London. As Twiggy later recalled "Looking in the mirror at the back, I saw all these faces staring at me, in a way that no one had ever done before."

Importantly Leonard had some of the most talented young stylists working for him including Michael Rasser and John

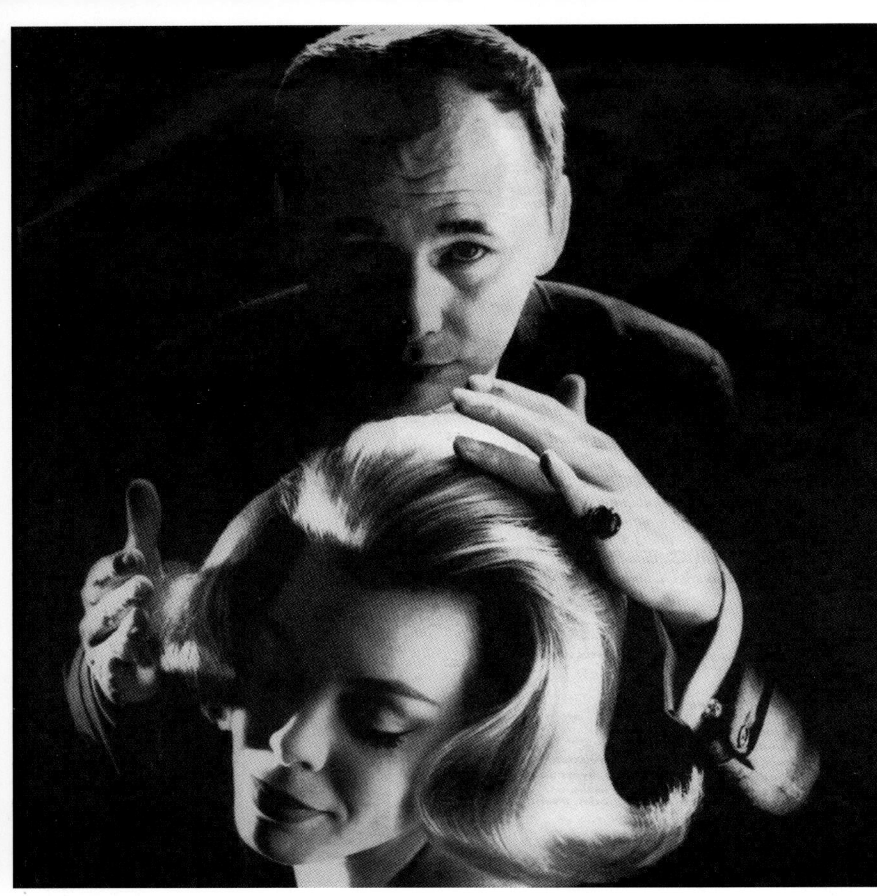

Winged coiffure styled by Mr Kenneth of Lilly Daché salon to advertise Clairol Colorfast Shampoo, 1962

Isaacs who later went on to found Michaeljohn; Keith Wainwright and Leslie Russell who later opened Smile; John Frieda, Daniel Galvin and Nicky Clarke – all of whom went on to achieve success in their given field. Leonard's was also the first salon to cater to both men and women, although the sexes were kept in separate rooms. He also pioneered the use of colour photography for hairstyles; before Leonard, most hairdressers had preferred to use black and white photographs because it focused attention on the fundamentals of the cut. However, in around 1968, Leonard began experimenting with "Crazy Colours" at the suggestion of the fashion designer Zandra Rhodes. For one of her collections he coloured the models' hair shocking hues with the same silk dyes used to make Rhodes' quirky clothes, and, of course, monochrome prints could not do this new trend in hair fashion any justice. As Keith Wainwright and Leslie Russell recall, "Leonard could just do it… he was the best hairdresser we have ever known." While Vidal Sassoon remembers him as "a brilliant individualist" whose "hair-house in Mayfair had great style which personified the man" and whose work "gave to our craft a credence."

The 1960s also saw the advent of the hairdressing session stylist – a practitioner who specialises in hairstyles specifically created for hair shows, advertising campaigns and magazine editorial shoots. One of the first and greatest of this new breed of hairdressers was Ara Gallant, who worked extensively with the fashion photographers Richard Avedon and Irving Penn. Gallant's work continuously graced the pages of American *Vogue* during the late 60s, and it was Gallant who was the first hairstylist to ever receive a credit in the magazine. Using hairpieces, he created extraordinary hairstyles for various models, most notably Jean Shrimpton, Twiggy and Penelope Tree, that were eye-catching extravaganzas – fantasy dos that were the hair equivalent of haute couture fashion. The flip-side of this was the emerging hippy movement, which was to also have a huge influence on the styling of hair with its anything-goes attitude… which was perhaps best summed up by the Mamas and Papas' memorable 1967 lyrics: "If you're going to San Francisco, Be sure to wear some flowers in your hair." The hippy look was long and unkempt, and reflected the movement's desire for a more natural *modus operandi* that rejected outright the need for fastidious grooming. Around the same time, the dome-like Afro became fashionable among the African-American community who saw it as a symbol of black pride and liberation… essentially an overt celebration of the Civil Rights Act that had finally been legislated in 1964. And finally, opening on Broadway and in the West End in 1968, the rock musical "Hair" was a bold declaration of anti-Vietnam War sentiment that graphically portrayed hair as a political statement. It is not an understatement to say the Sixties rocked the hair profession in more ways than one, and there was definitely no looking back…

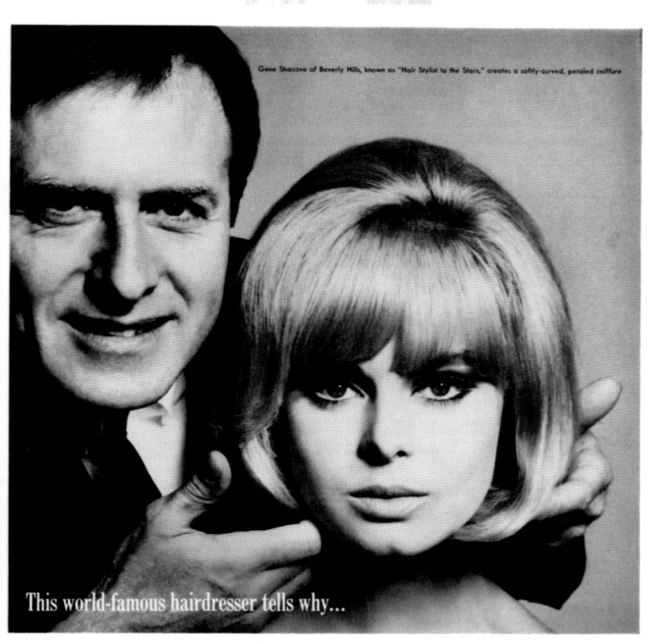

Gene Shacove of Beverly Hills, known as "Hair Stylist to the Stars," creates a softly-curved, petaled coiffure

This world-famous hairdresser tells why...

why you should use a special colorfast shampoo if you color or lighten your hair

"Because you want beautiful haircoloring to *stay* beautiful—fresh and lively! Not be dulled or clouded by the wrong shampoo," says Gene Shacove. "To *keep* enjoying the flattery of haircoloring chosen just for you, you should insist on this special colorfast shampoo by Clairol, which won't change hair color." Very different from other leading shampoos, this colorfast shampoo by Clairol was specifically created for women who color or lighten their hair. In two unique formulas: Clairol Blue for all light delicate blonde shades of lightened and toned hair. Clairol Green for all red, brown and black shades of tints and lasting rinses. At beauty salons and cosmetic counters.

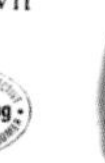

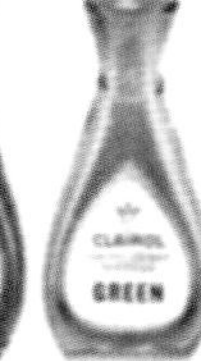

BLUE – for blondes and lightest tones

GREEN – for tint and lasting rinse users

CLAIROL® SHAMPOO the colorfast shampoo

©Clairol Inc. 1964

irol shampoo advertisement
turing Gene Shacove, 1964

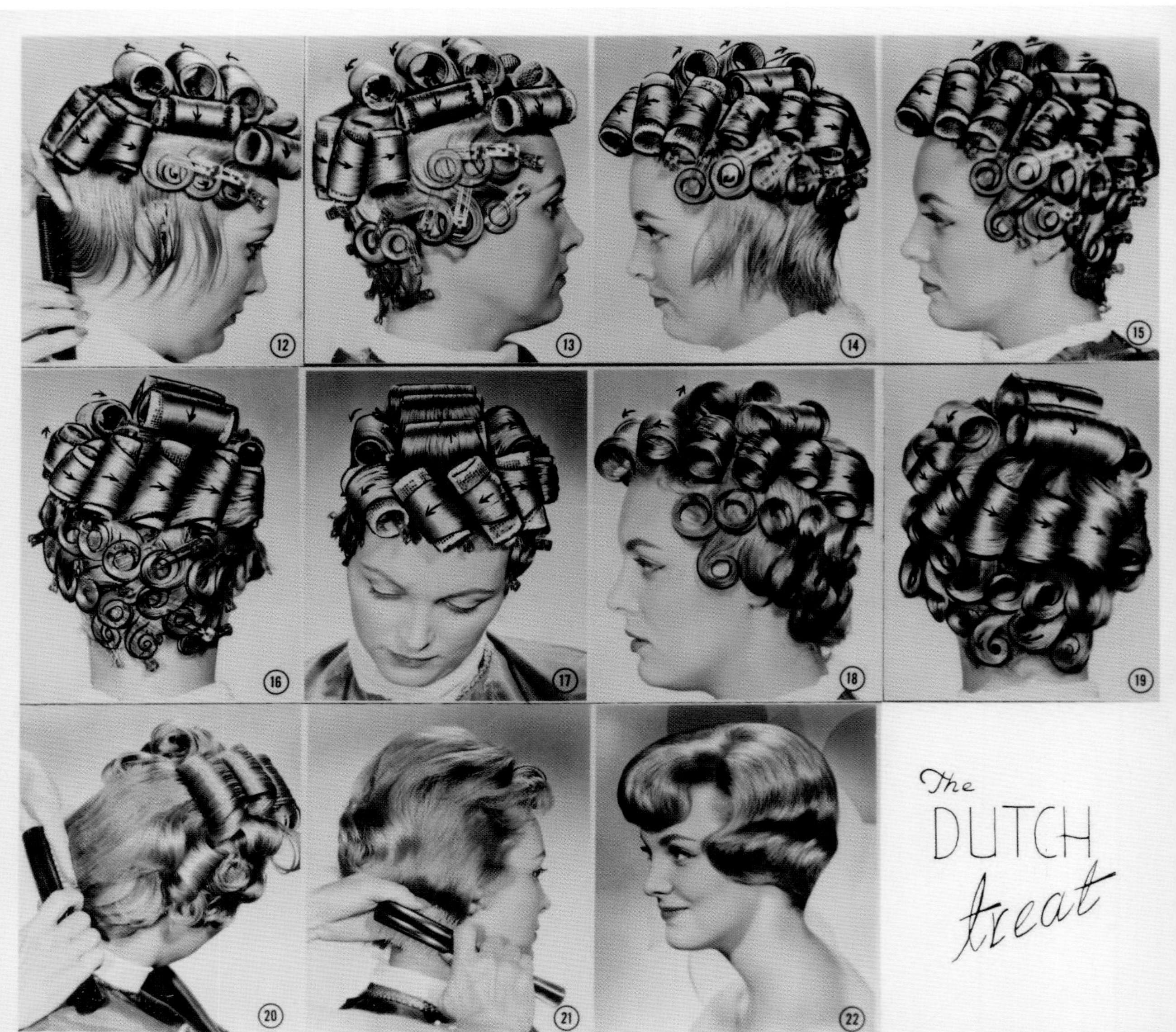

'The Dutch Treat' hair setting instructions steps 12 to 22 and the final result, USA, 1960, Hollywood Hair Design Council

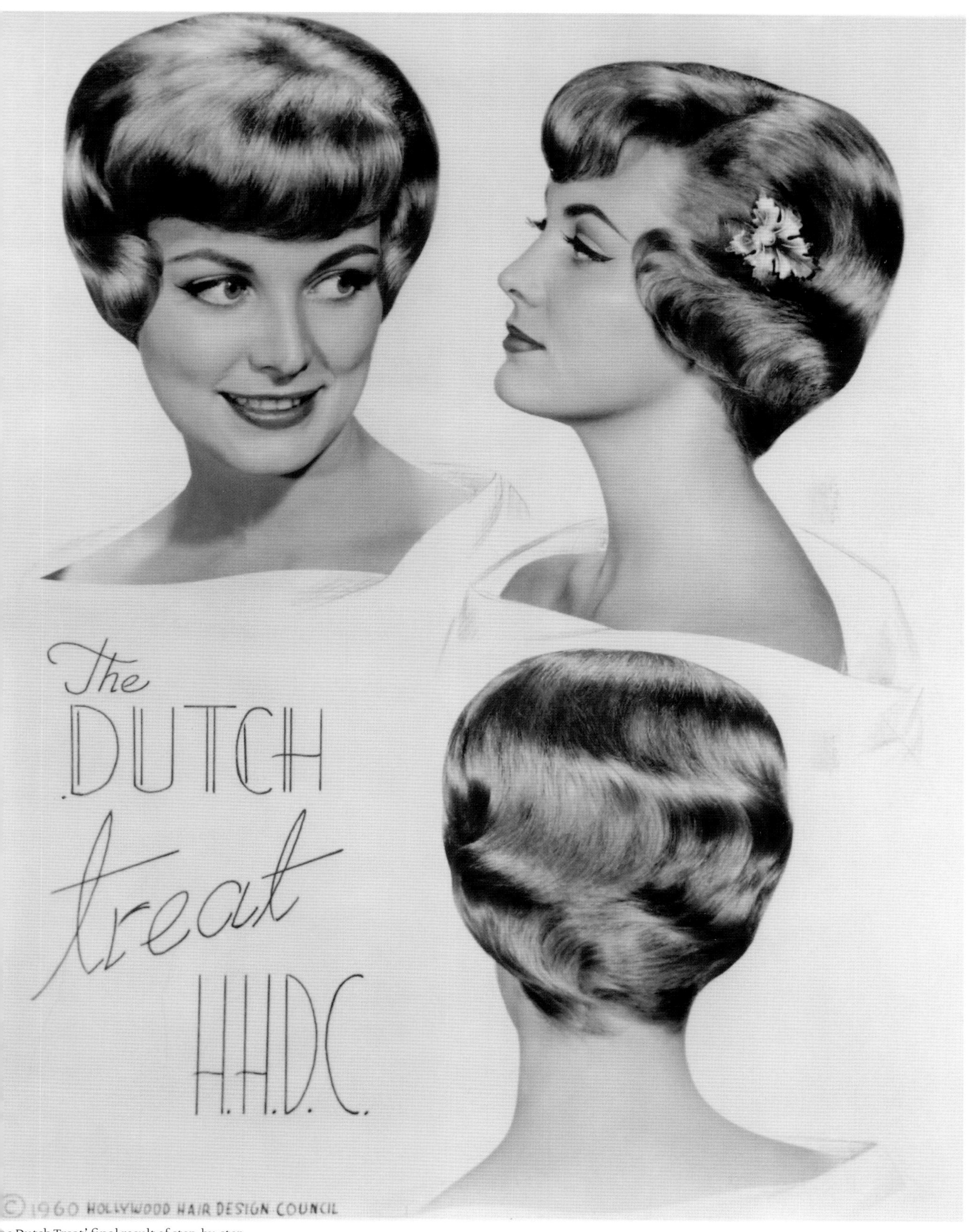

ıe Dutch Treat' final result of step-by-step
ıstructions, 1960, Hollywood Hair Design Council

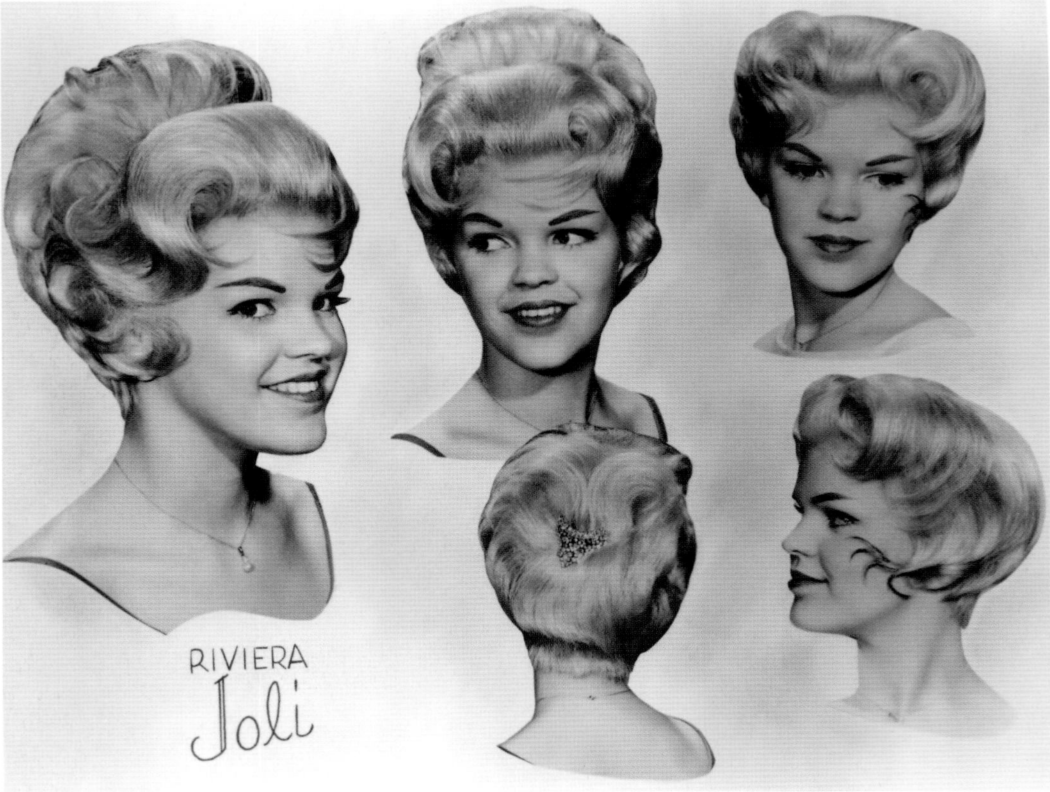

RIVIERA
Joli

'Riviera Joli' hairstyle shown from different angles, USA, 1960, Hollywood Hair Design Council

RIVIERA
Caprice

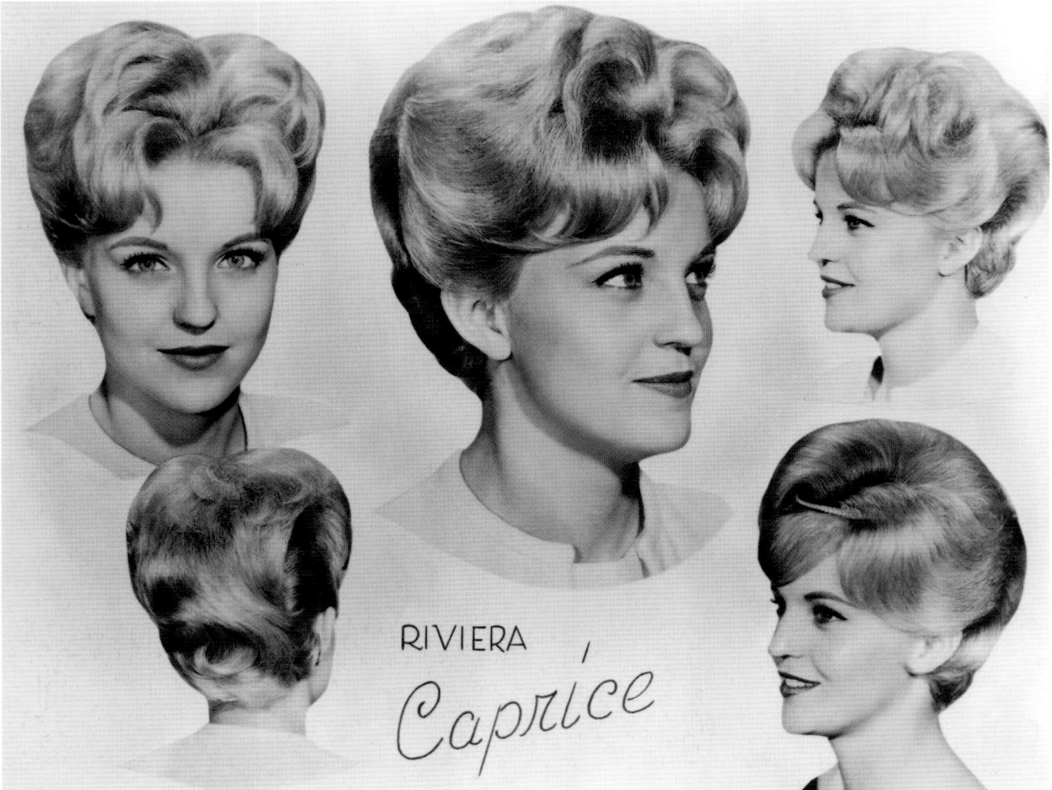

'Riviera Caprice' hairstyle shown from different angles, USA, 1960, Hollywood Hair Design Council

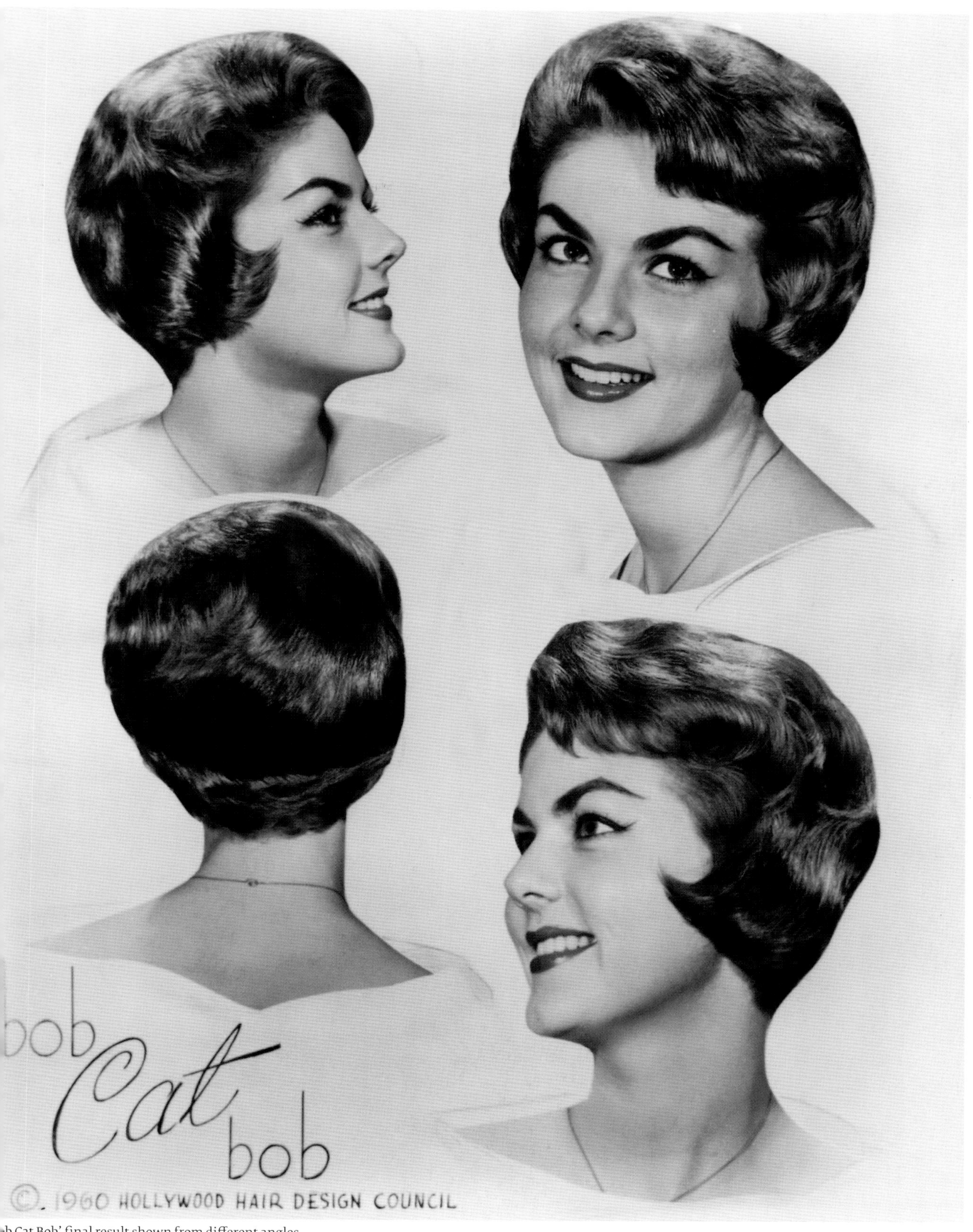

b Cat Bob' final result shown from different angles,
, 1960, Hollywood Hair Design Council

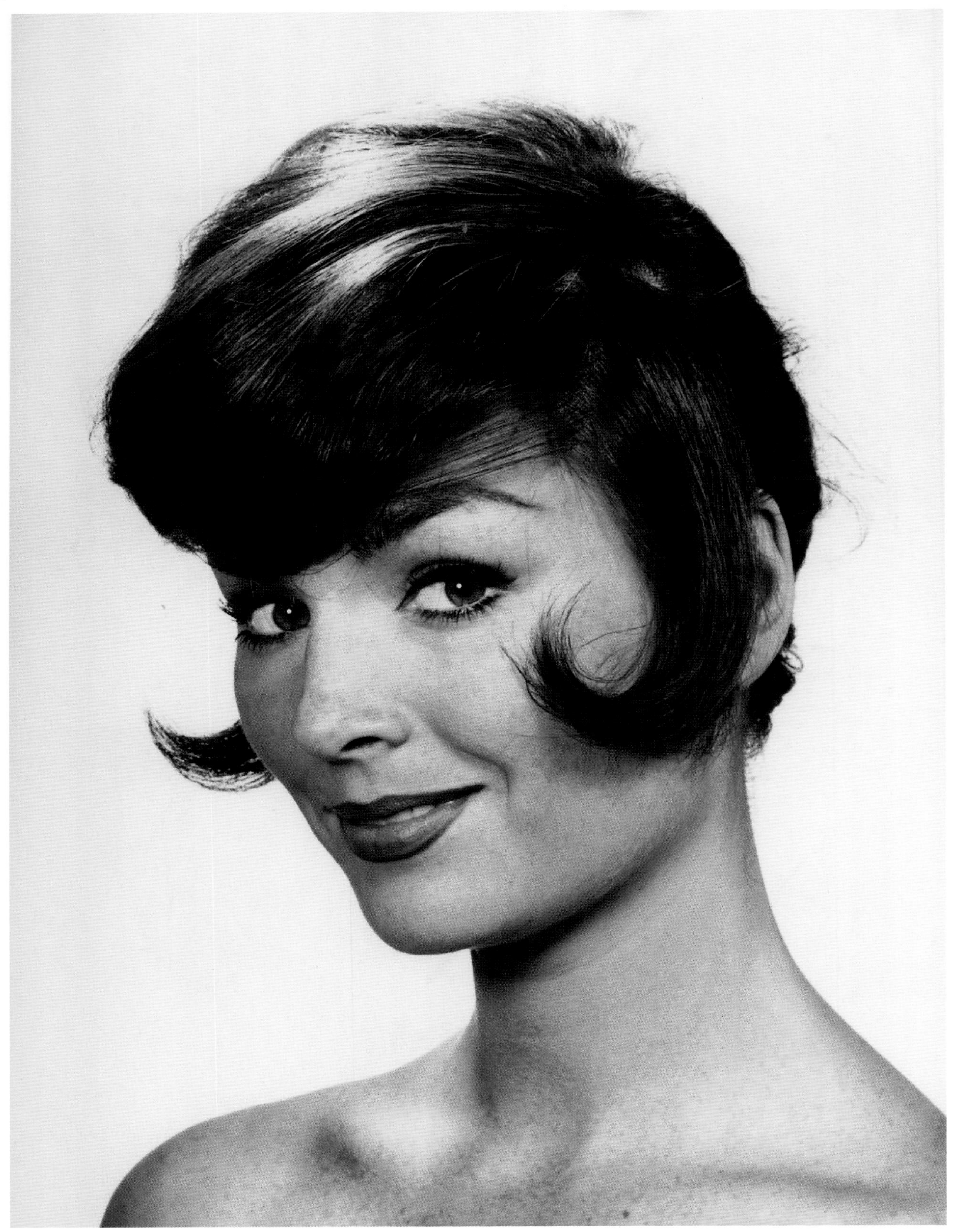

Early 1960s hairstyle

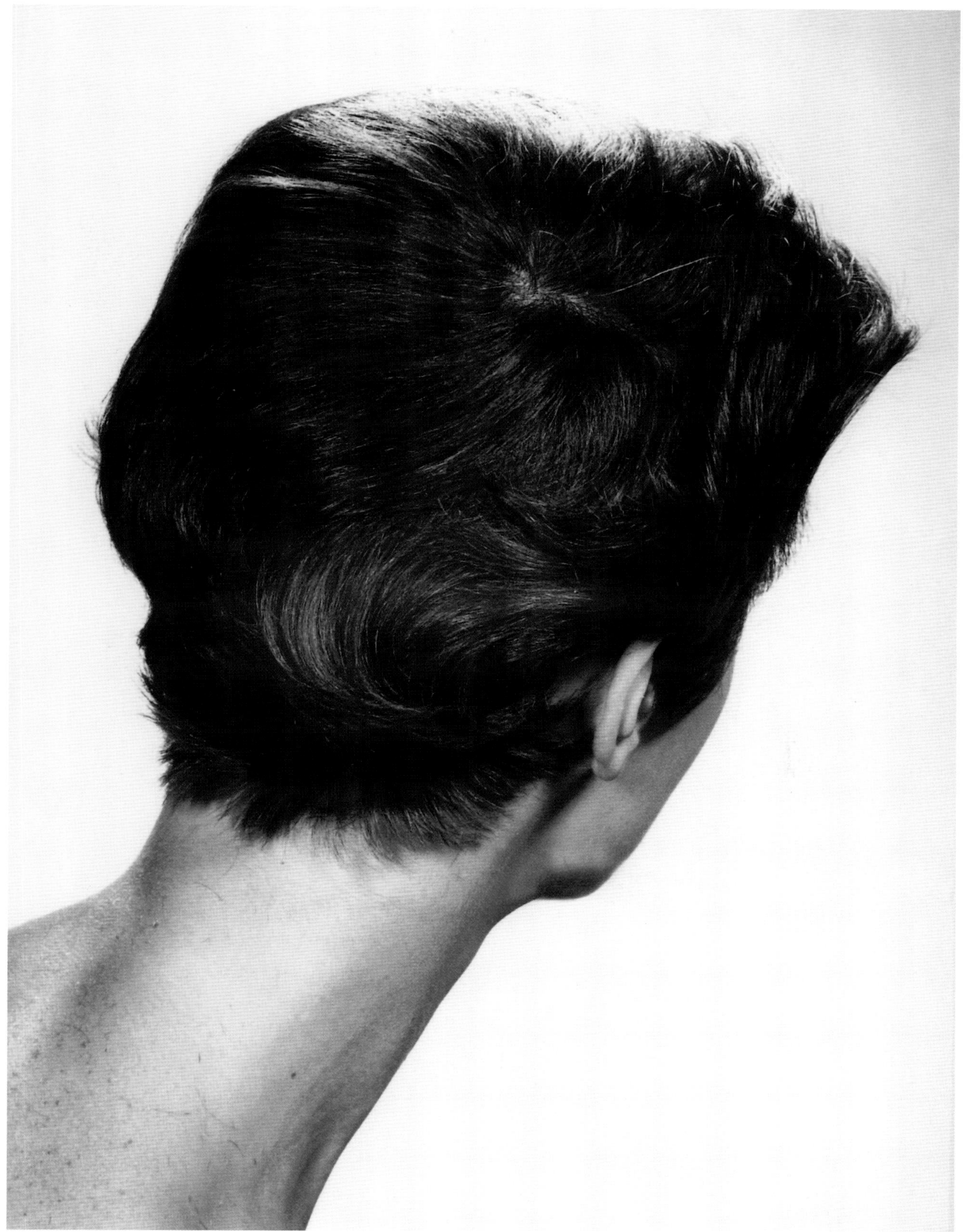
Early 1960s hairstyle

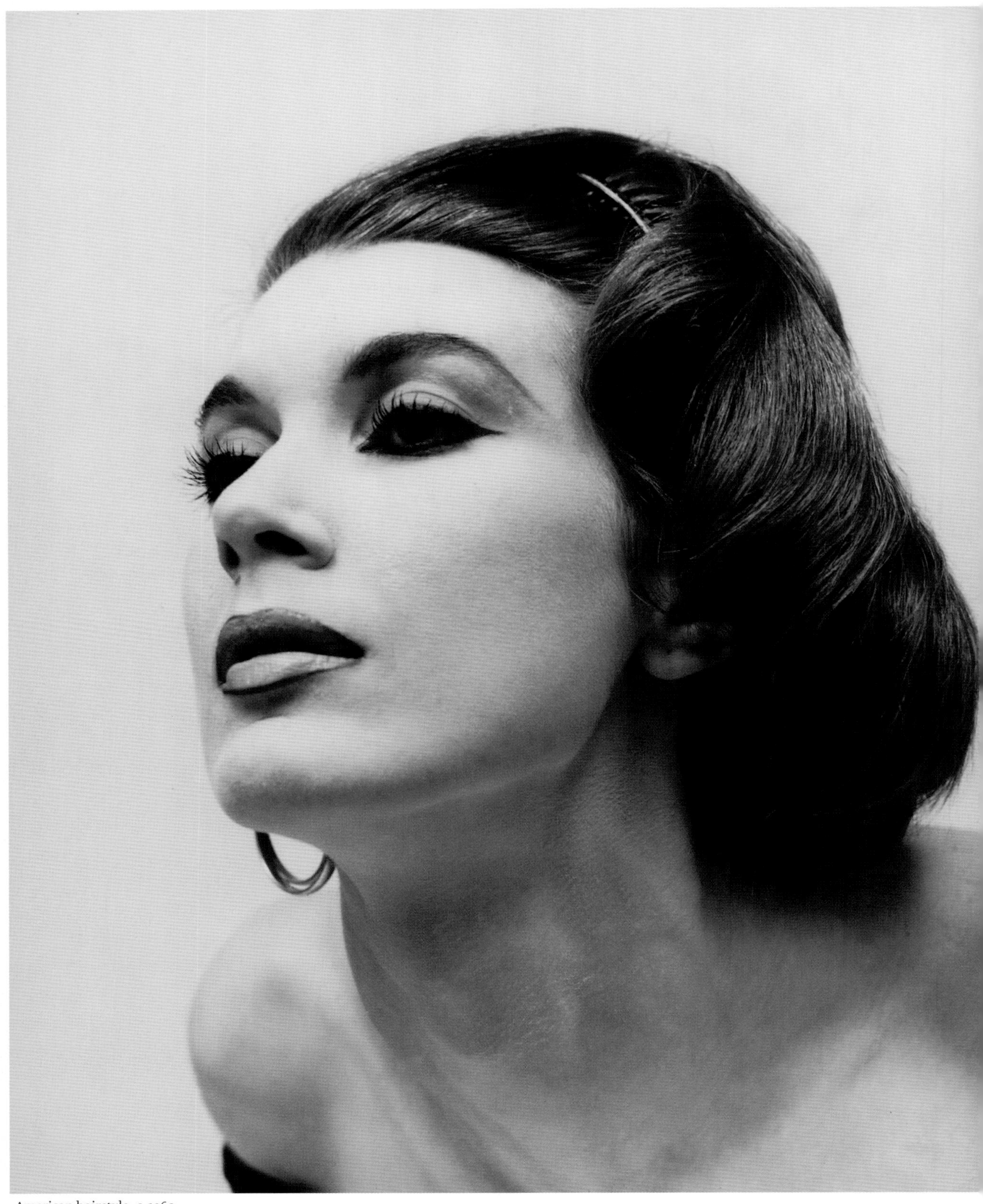

American hairstyle, c.1960,
photographed by Ref Sanchez

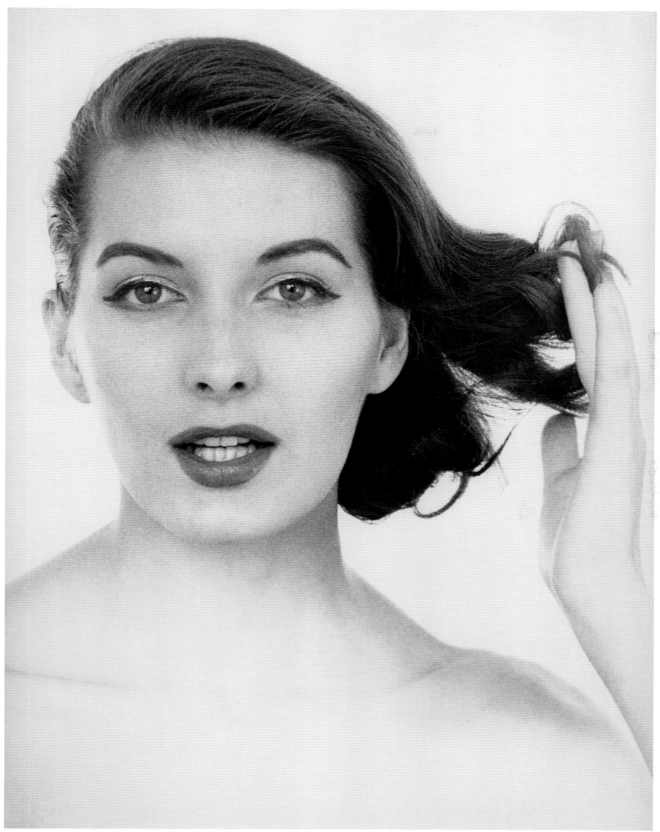

American hairstyle, c. 1960,
photographed by Ref Sanchez

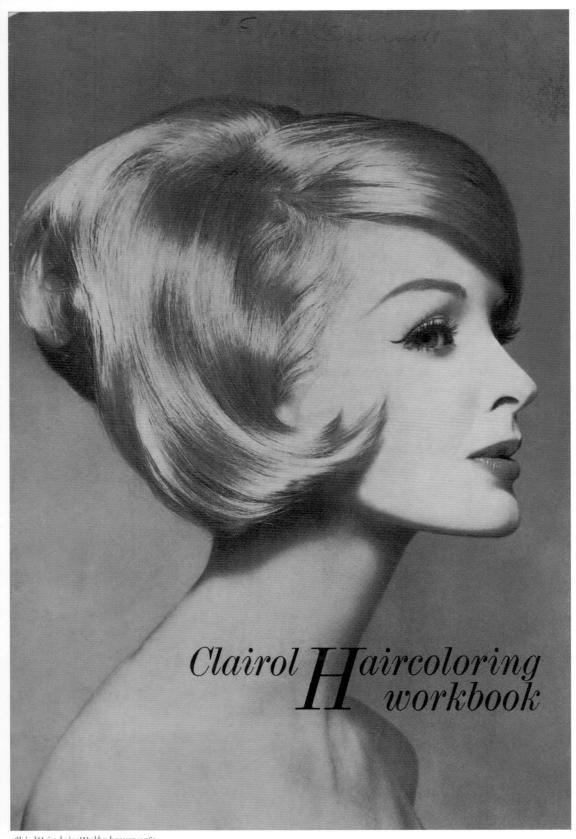

Clairol Haircoloring Workbook cover, 1961

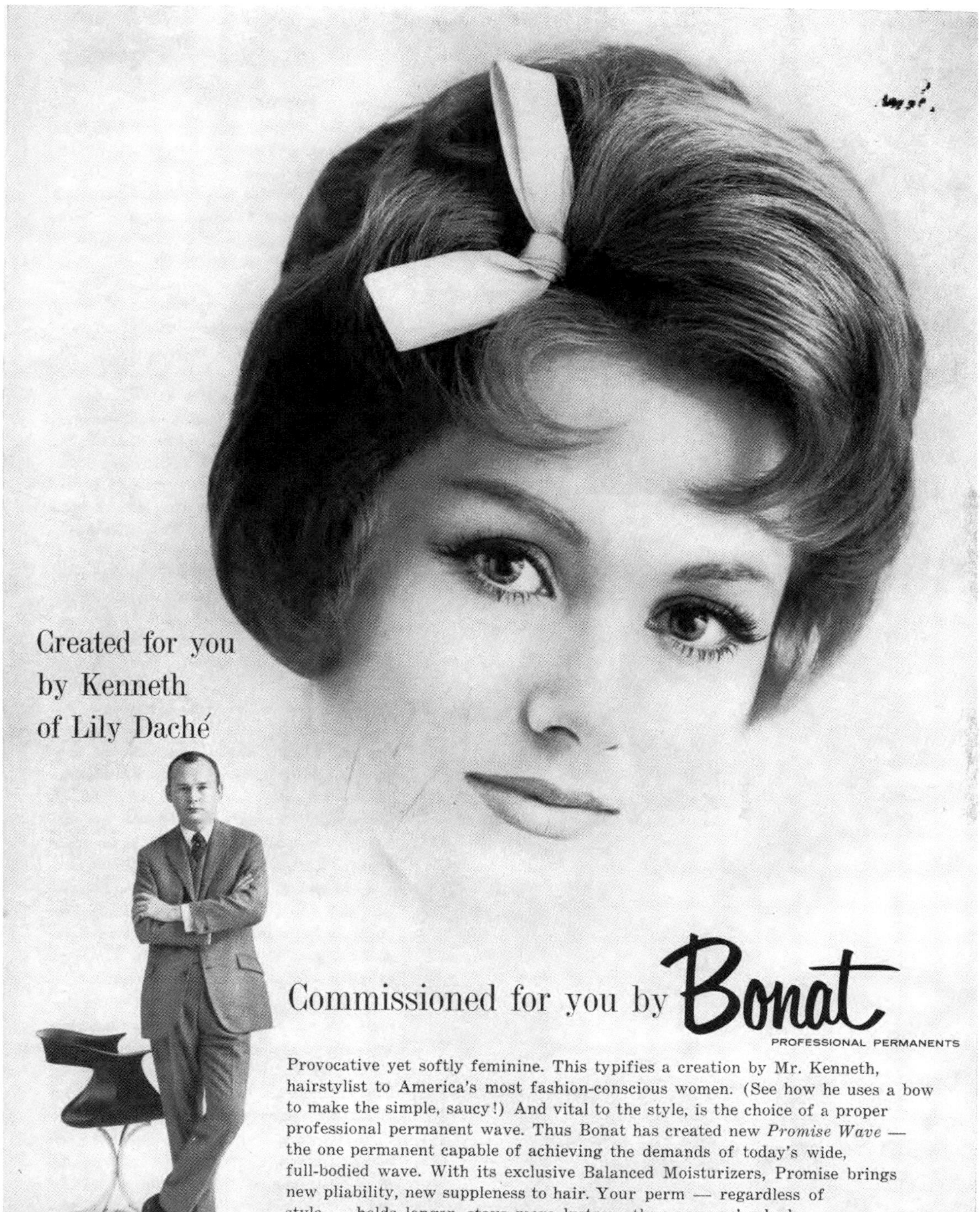

Created for you
by Kenneth
of Lily Daché
Commissioned for you by Bonat
PROFESSIONAL PERMANENTS
Provocative yet softly feminine. This typifies a creation by Mr. Kenneth, hairstylist to America's most fashion-conscious women. (See how he uses a bow to make the simple, saucy!) And vital to the style, is the choice of a proper professional permanent wave. Thus Bonat has created new Promise Wave — the one permanent capable of achieving the demands of today's wide, full-bodied wave. With its exclusive Balanced Moisturizers, Promise brings new pliability, new suppleness to hair. Your perm — regardless of style — holds longer, stays more lustrous than any you've had. Try Promise Wave — ask for it next time you visit your beauty salon.
HAIRSTYLISTS ARE A GIRL'S BEST FRIEND!

Hairstyle by Mr Kenneth of Lilly Daché salon to advertise Bonat perms, 1961

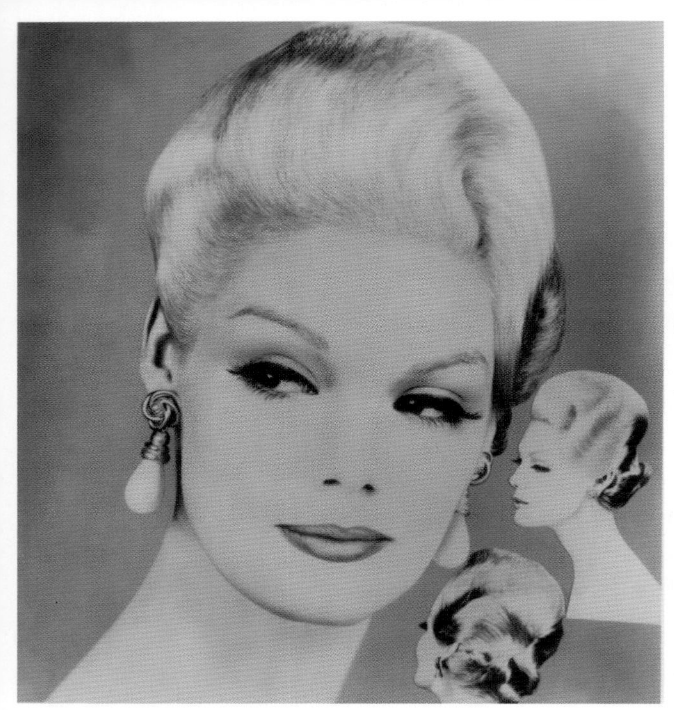

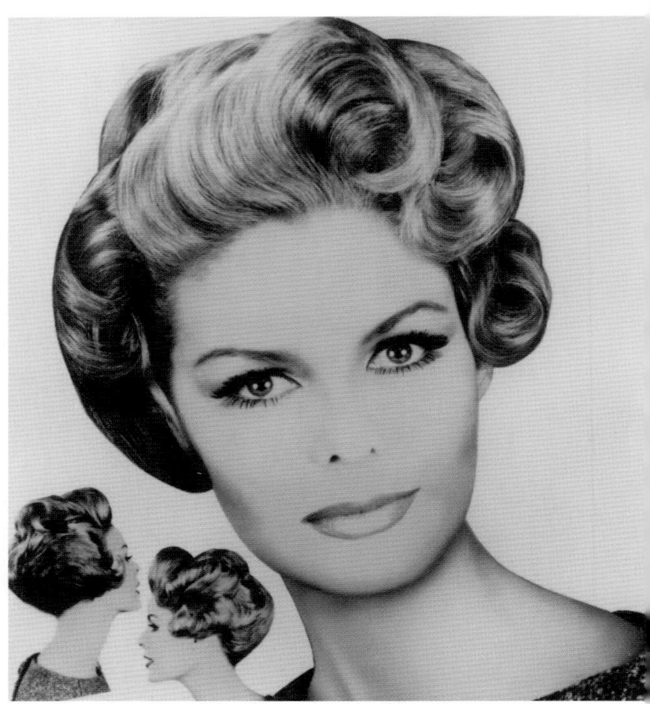

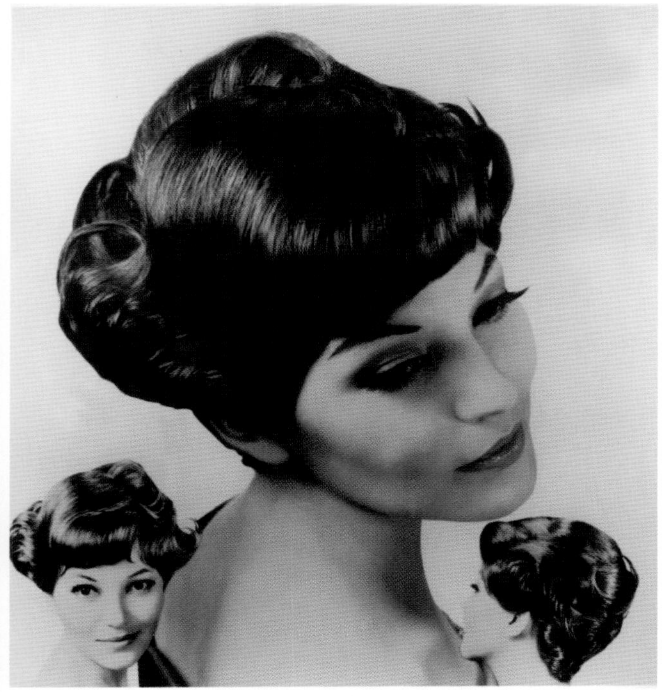

'Spellbound Coiffure', 'Casual Elegance Coiffure' and 'Enchanted Elegance Coiffure', part of Dancing Waves Hair Fashion Collection, USA, 1962, National Hairdressers and Cosmetologists Association Inc.

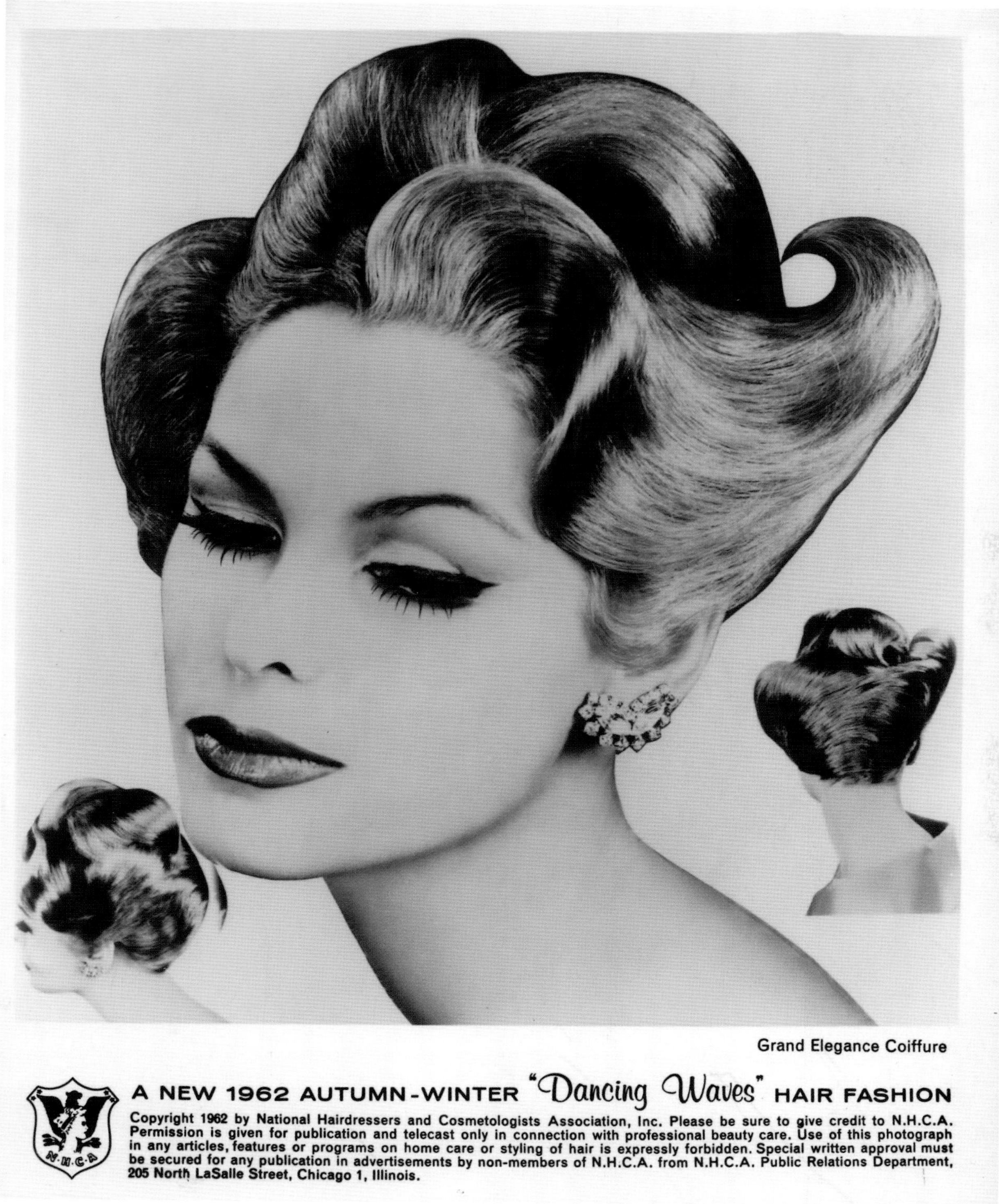

Grand Elegance Coiffure

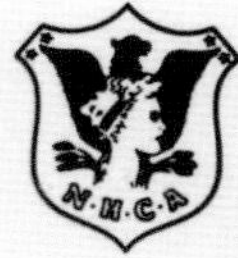

A NEW 1962 AUTUMN-WINTER "Dancing Waves" HAIR FASHION

'Grand Elegance Coiffure', part of Dancing Waves Hair Fashion Collection, USA, 1962, National Hairdressers and Cosmetologists Association Inc.

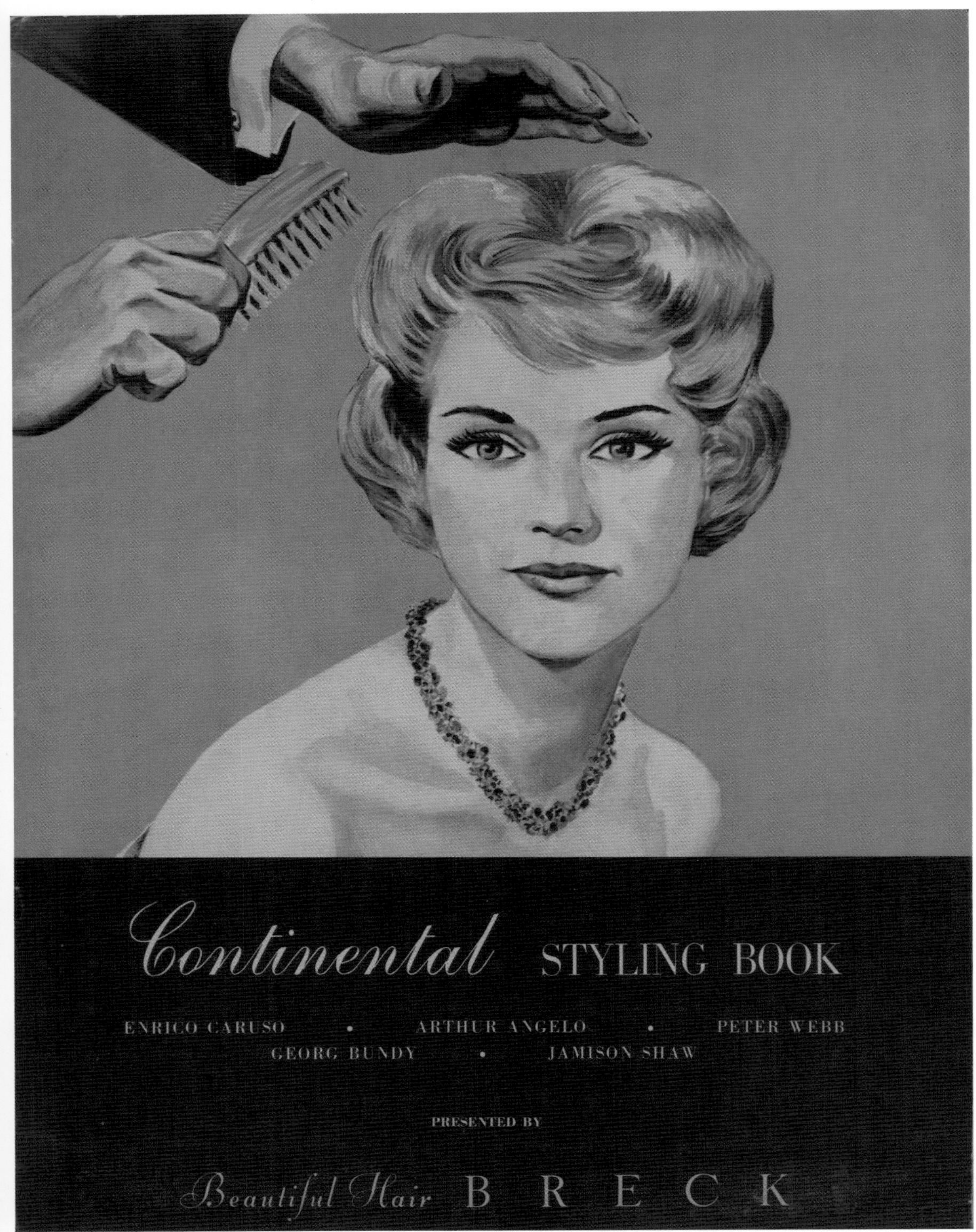

Continental Styling Book
for Breck, 1963

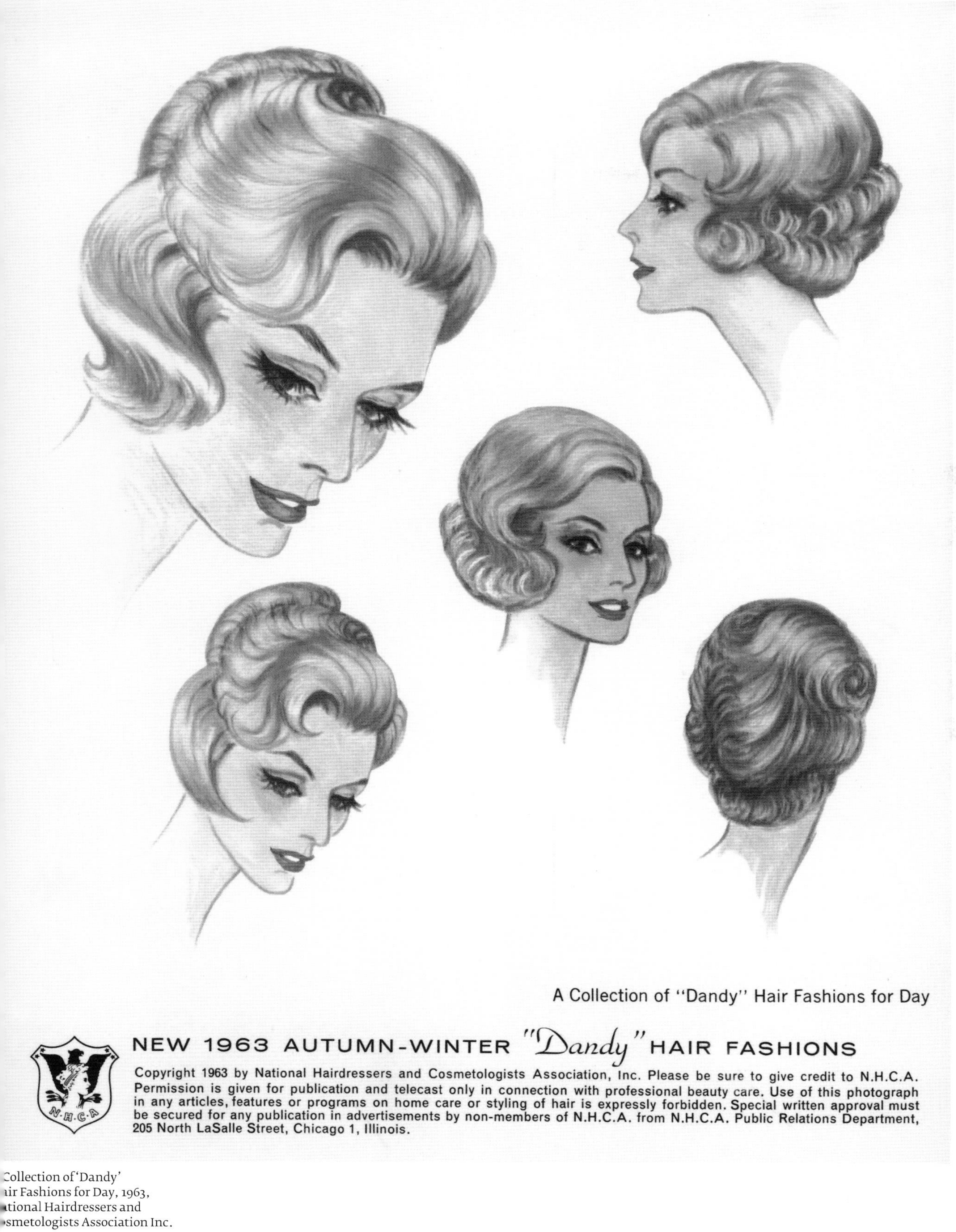

A Collection of "Dandy" Hair Fashions for Day
NEW 1963 AUTUMN-WINTER "Dandy" HAIR FASHIONS
N·H·C·A
Copyright 1963 by National Hairdressers and Cosmetologists Association, Inc. Please be sure to give credit to N.H.C.A. Permission is given for publication and telecast only in connection with professional beauty care. Use of this photograph in any articles, features or programs on home care or styling of hair is expressly forbidden. Special written approval must be secured for any publication in advertisements by non-members of N.H.C.A. from N.H.C.A. Public Relations Department, 205 North LaSalle Street, Chicago 1, Illinois.

Collection of 'Dandy'
air Fashions for Day, 1963,
tional Hairdressers and
smetologists Association Inc.

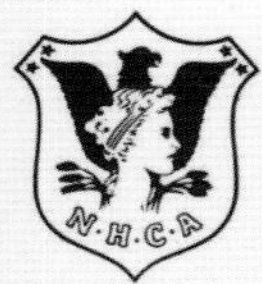

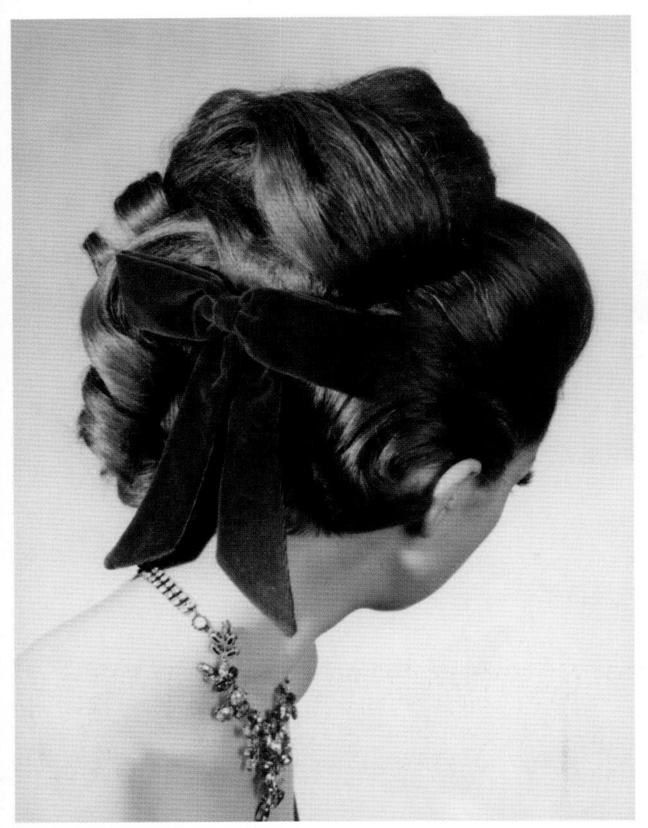

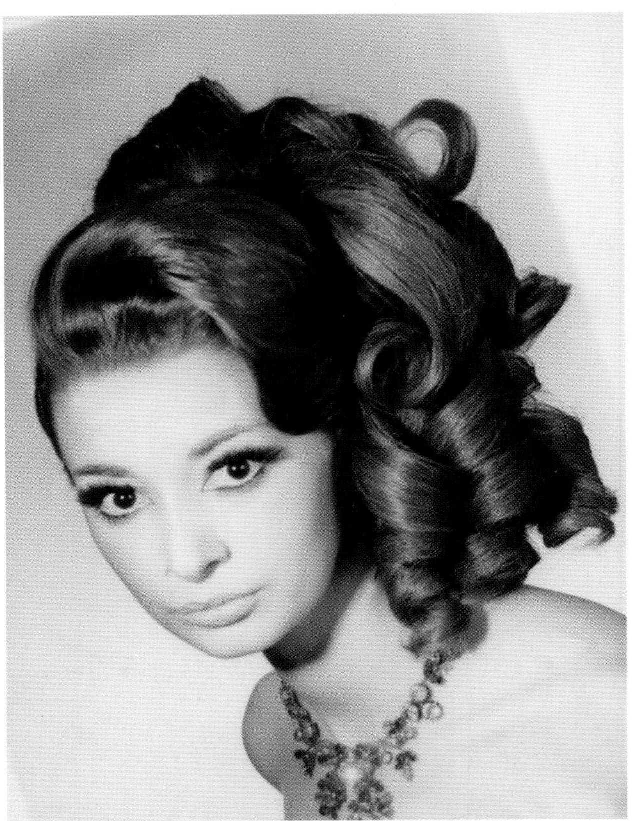

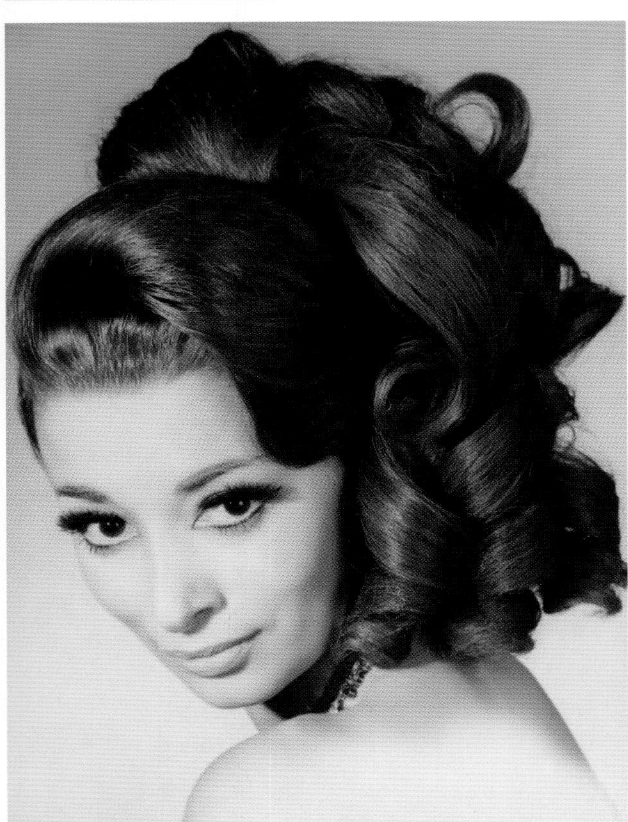

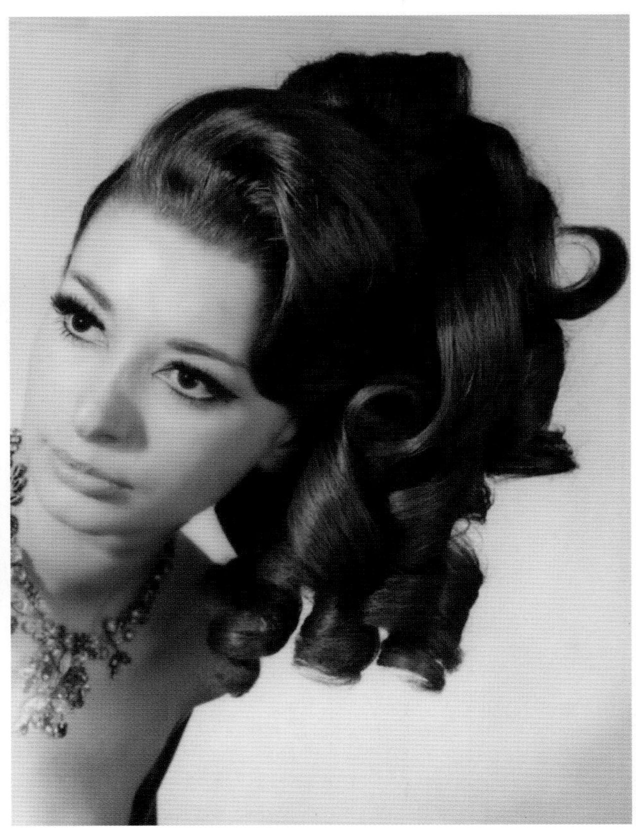

French Curled Up-Do
hairstyle, 1960s

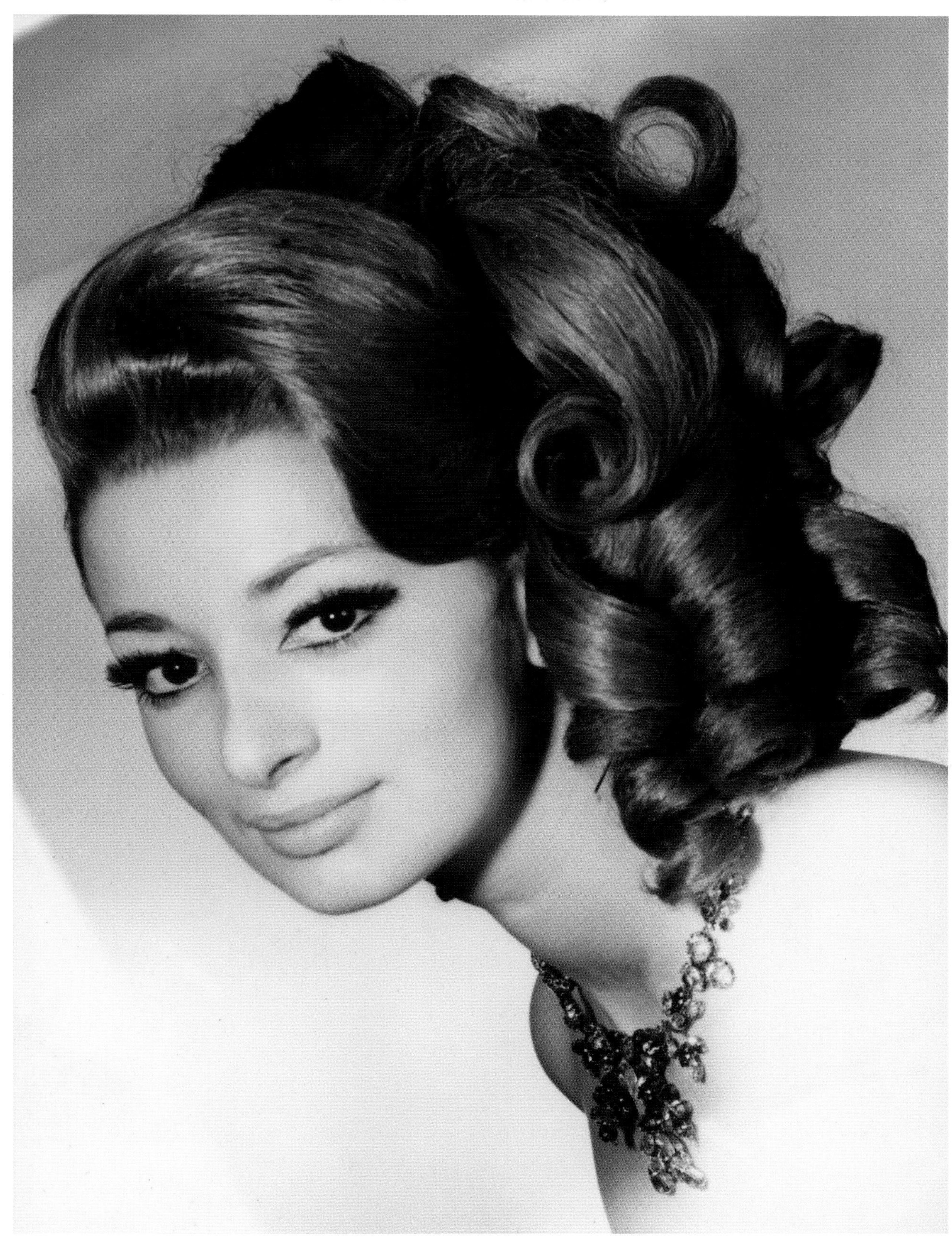

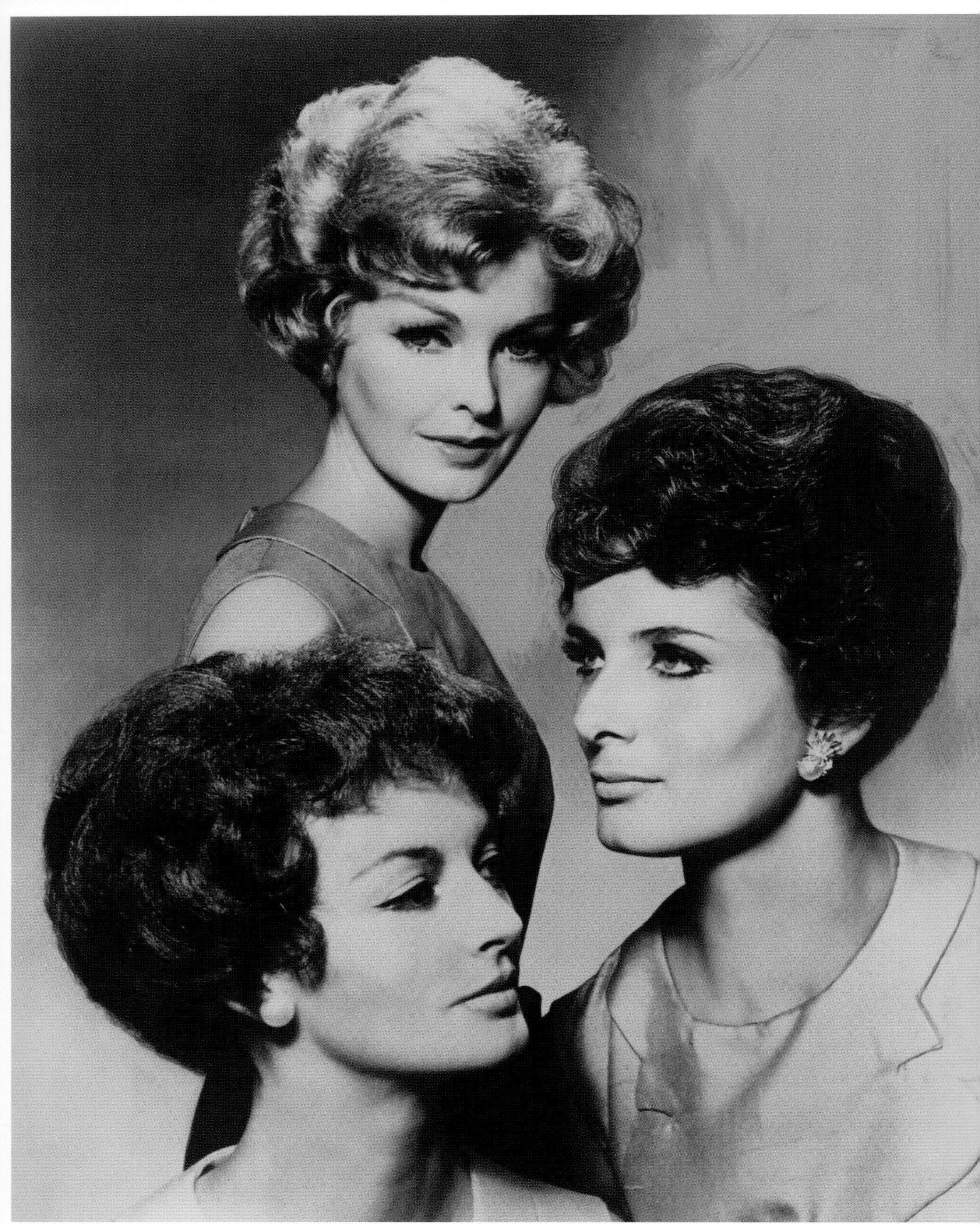

Wash & Wear Wigs, USA, 1963

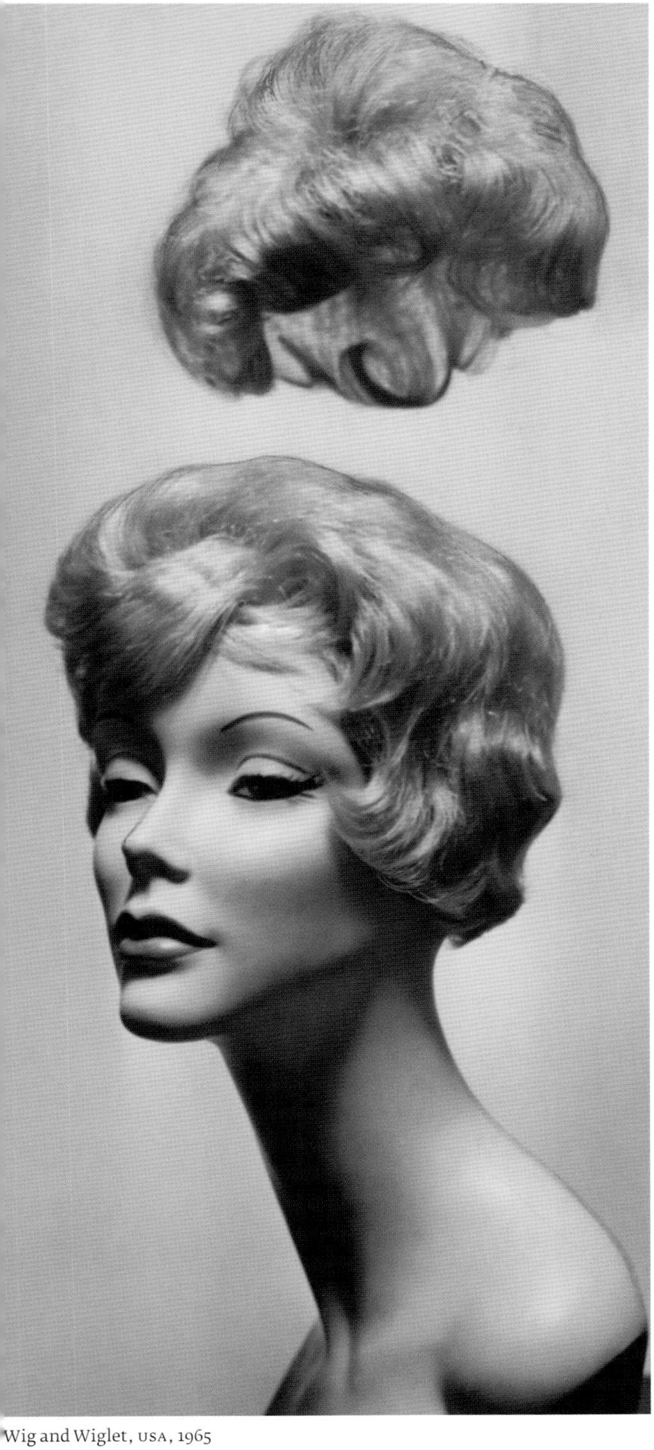

Wig and Wiglet, USA, 1965

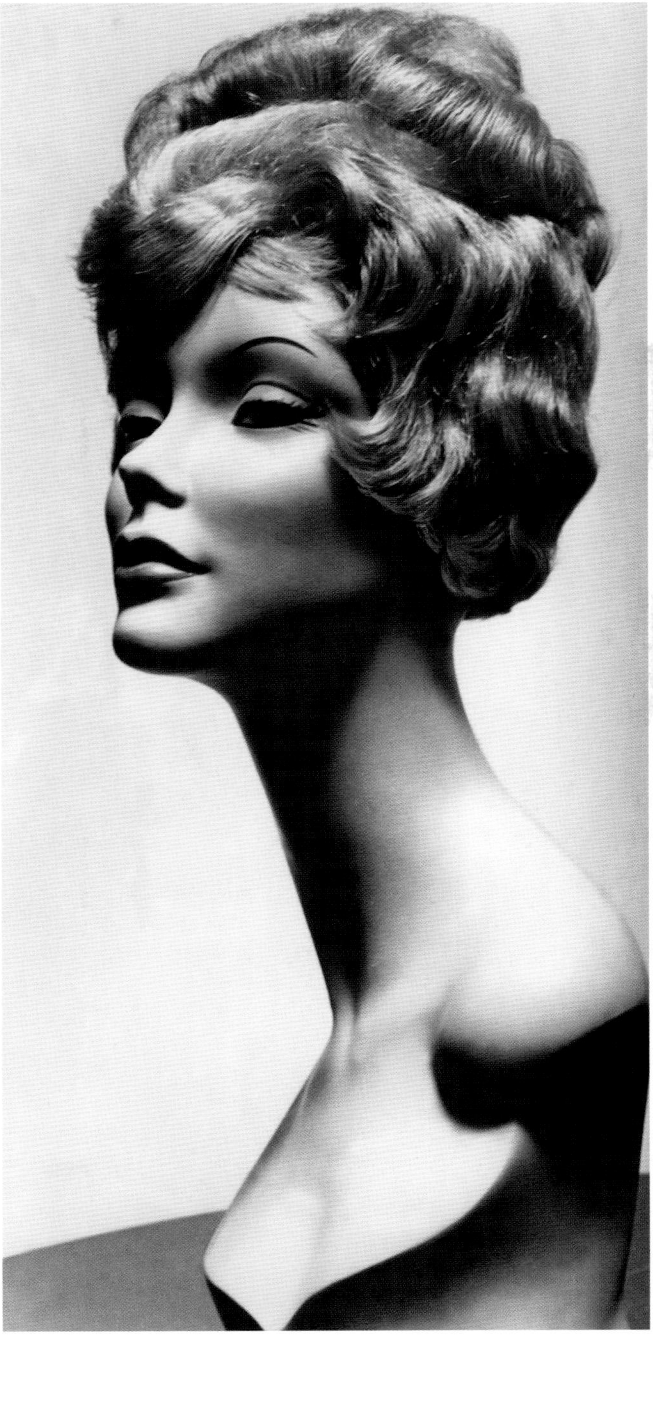

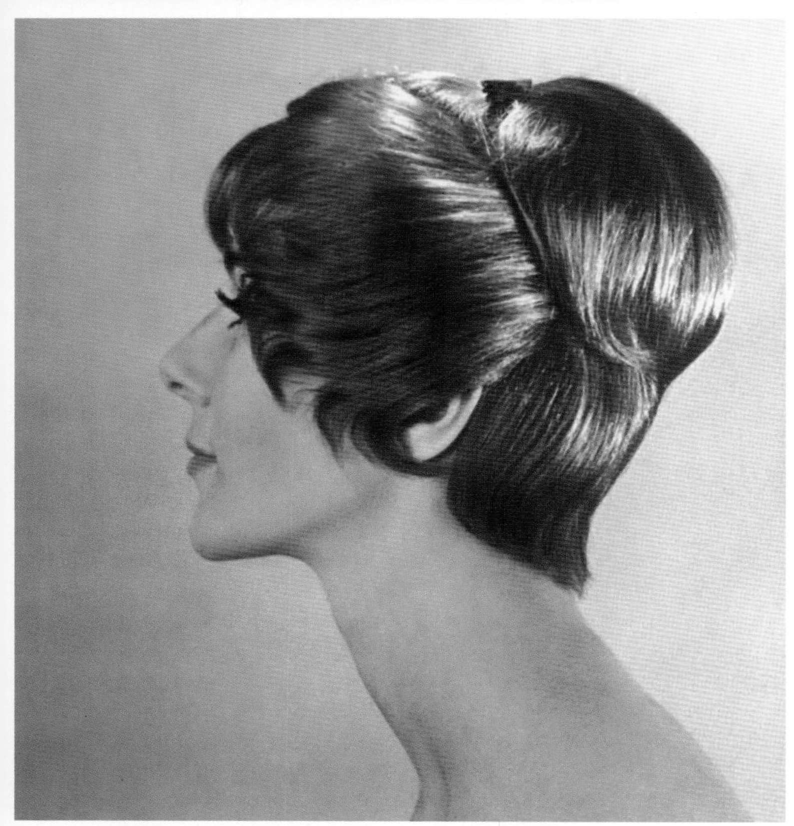

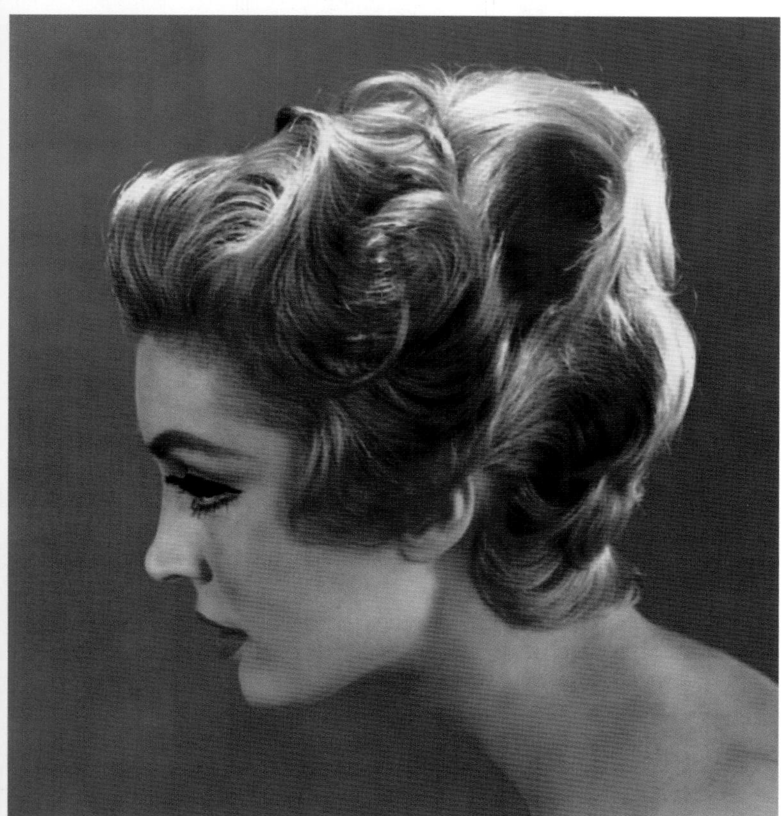

'Dandy Coiffure' and 'Dandy Overture Coiffure', 1963,
National Hairdressers and Cosmetologists Association Inc.

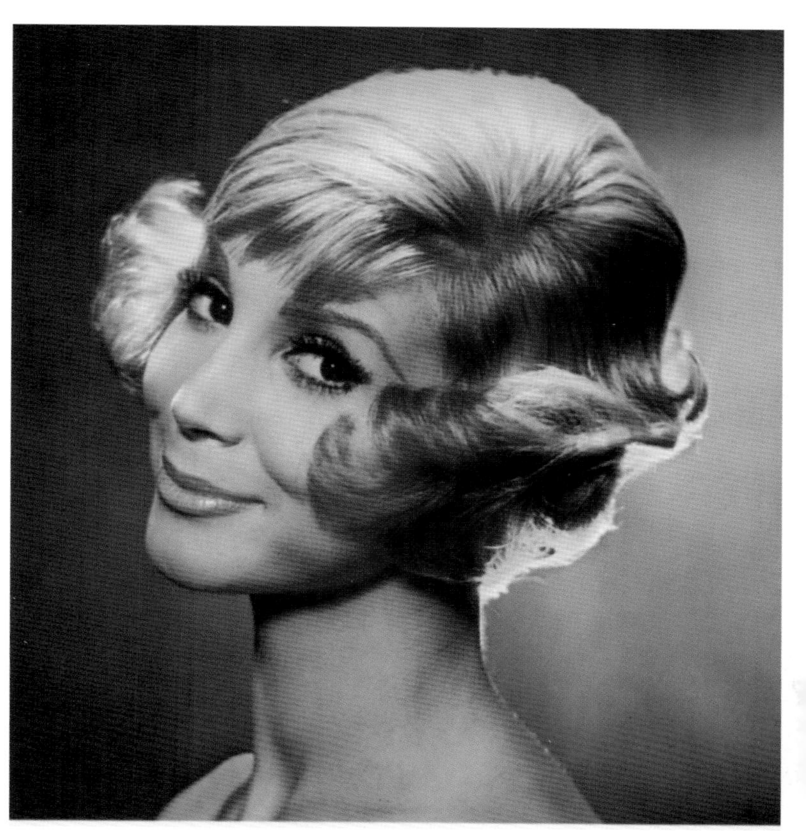

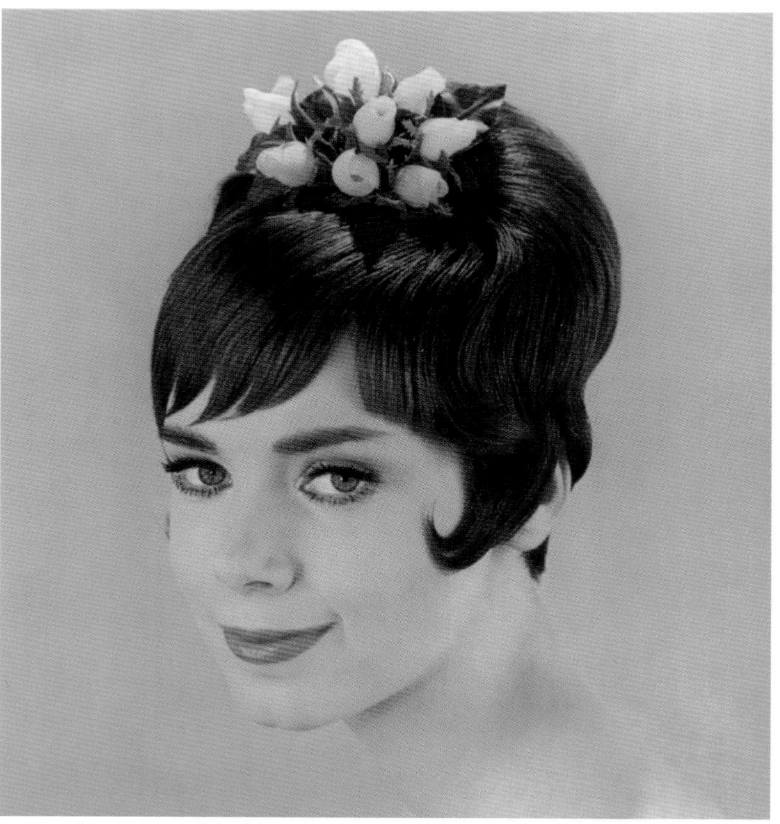

'Just Dandy Coiffure' and 'Fine 'n' Dandy Overture Coiffure', 1963, National Hairdressers and Cosmetologists Association Inc.

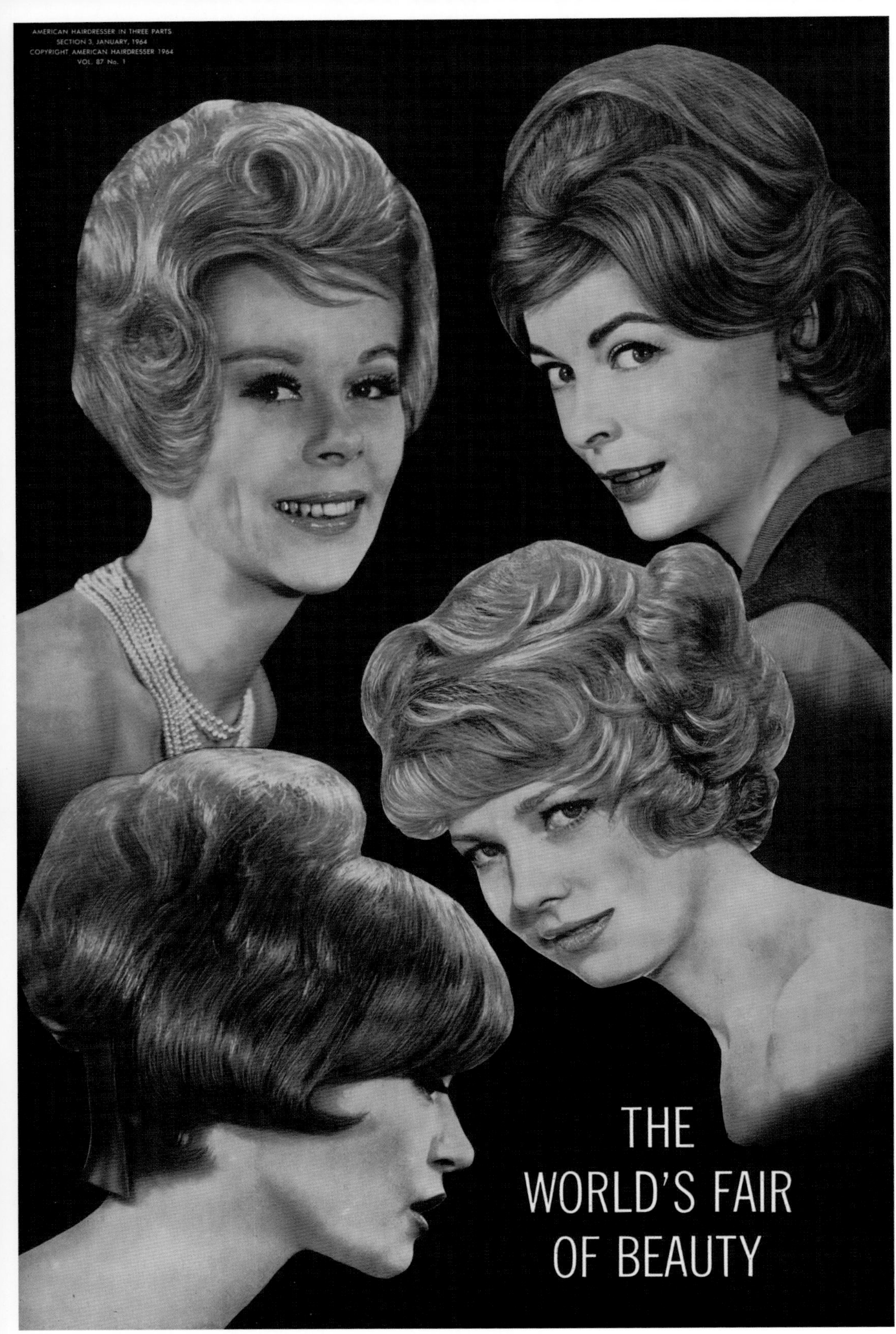

'The World's Fair of Beauty' poster, 1964, *American Hairdresser*

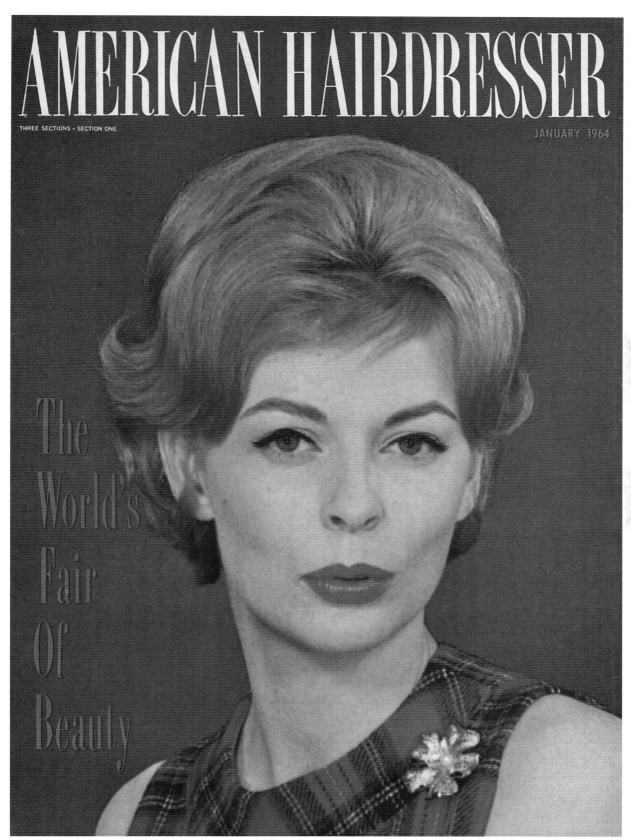

'The World's Fair of Beauty' issue, 1964, *American Hairdresser*

In the magic world of movies where lovely hair is so important, top movie stars use Lustre-Creme...

A shampoo so rich you only need to "lather once"!

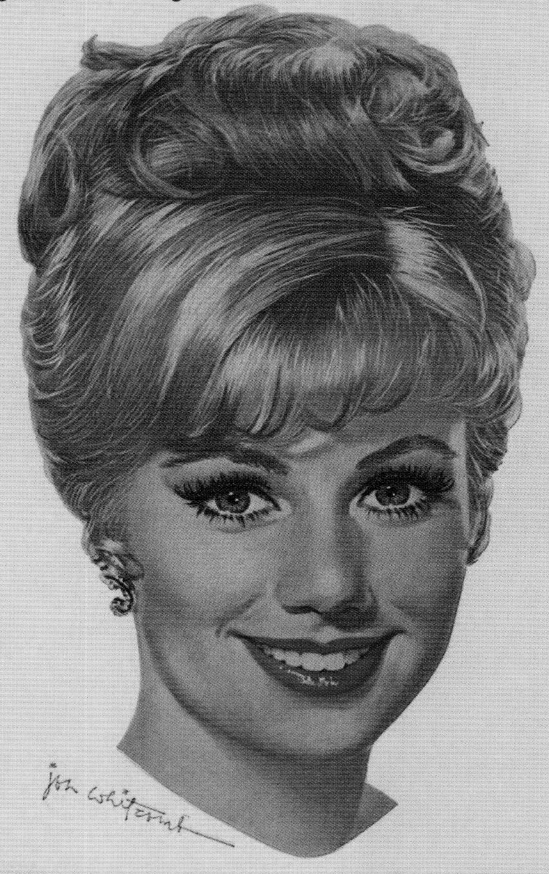

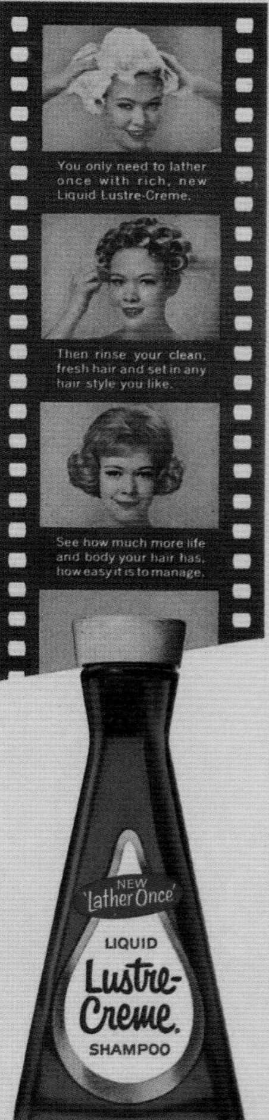

SHIRLEY JONES, starring in "Dark Purpose" a Universal release, uses new "Lather Once" Lustre-Creme and her hair behaves beautifully! Yours will, too, because—instead of over-washing your hair, stripping away the oils, leaving it dry and hard to manage—you only need to lather once with rich, instant-foaming Lustre-Creme shampoo. Then your hair has more life and body; any hair style behaves beautifully. Try it and see!

OTHER FAMOUS LUSTRE-CREME PRODUCTS

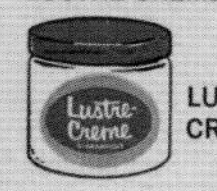
LUSTRE-CREME CREAM SHAMPOO

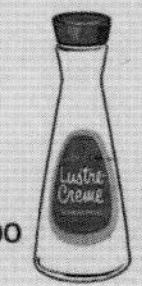
LUSTRE-CREME LOTION SHAMPOO

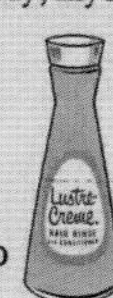
LUSTRE-CREME RINSE

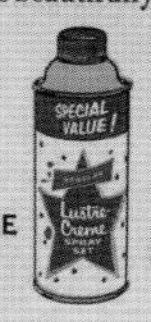

LUSTRE-CREME SPRAY SET

Advertisement for Lather Once Lustre-Crème Shampoo, 1964

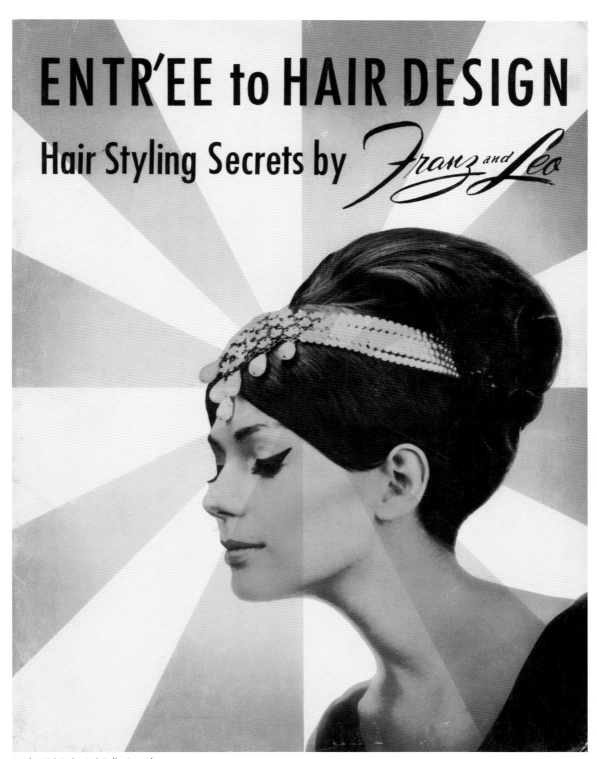

Entrée to Hair Design: Hair Styling Secrets by Franz and Leo magazine cover, 1964

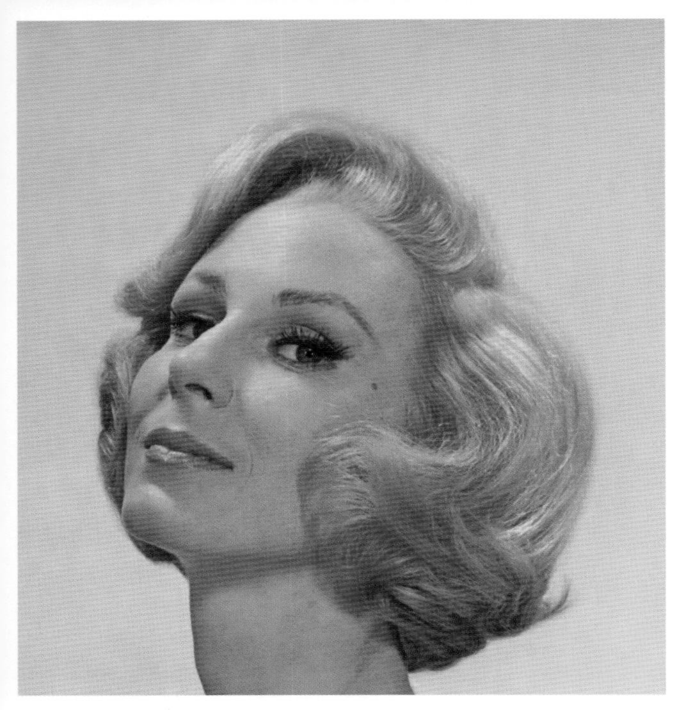

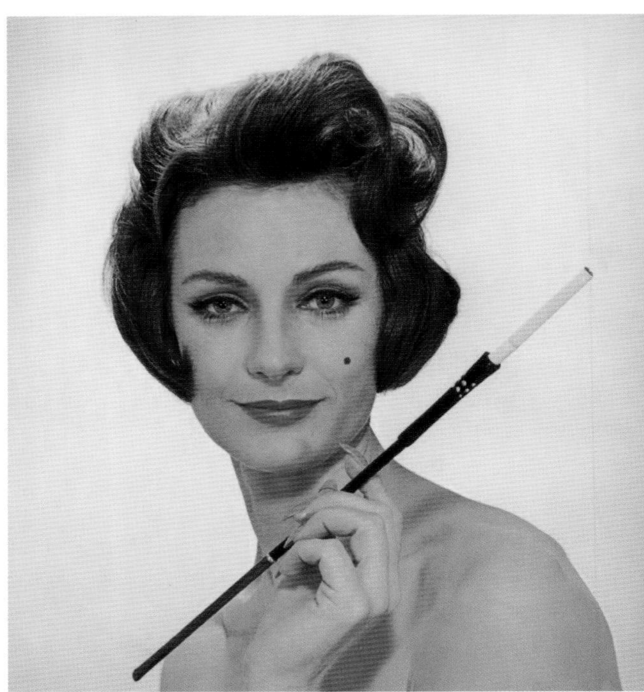

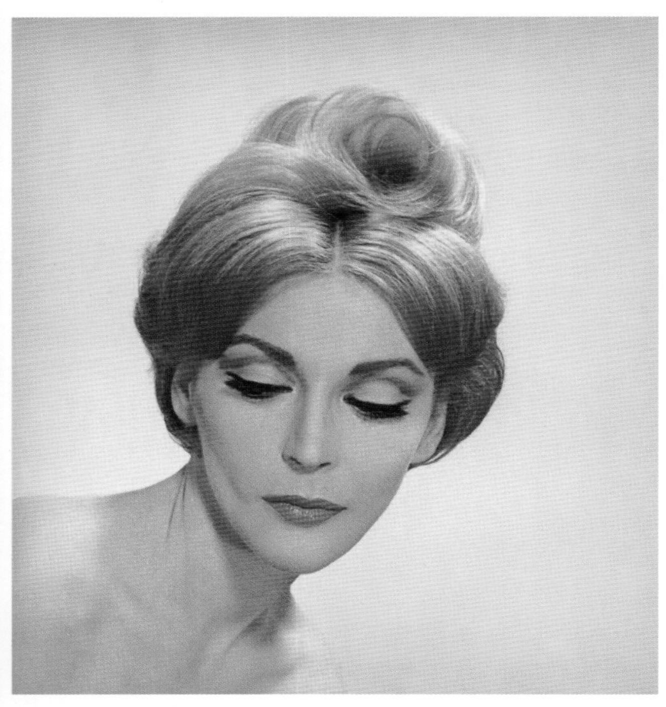

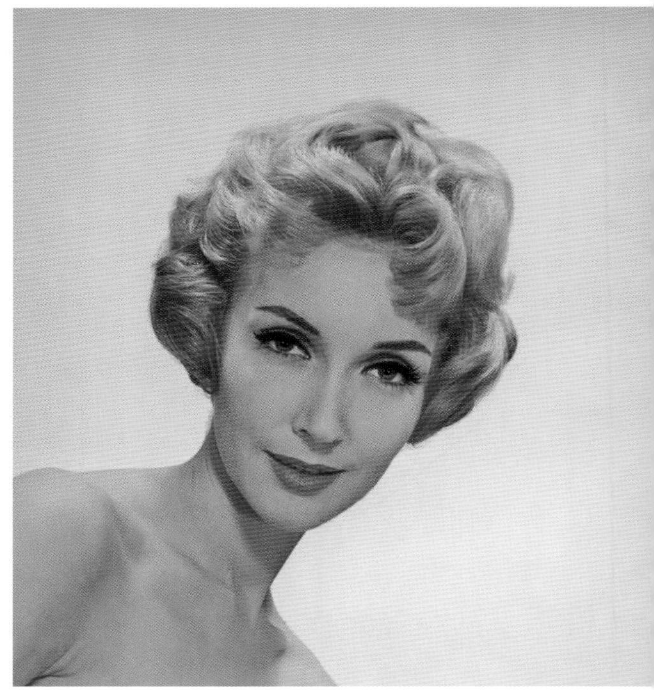

'Young Natural Coiffure', 'Vamp Coiffure', 'Romance Coiffure', 'Marlene Coiffure' from the Leap Year Coiffure Collection, 1964, National Hairdressers and Cosmetologists Association Inc.

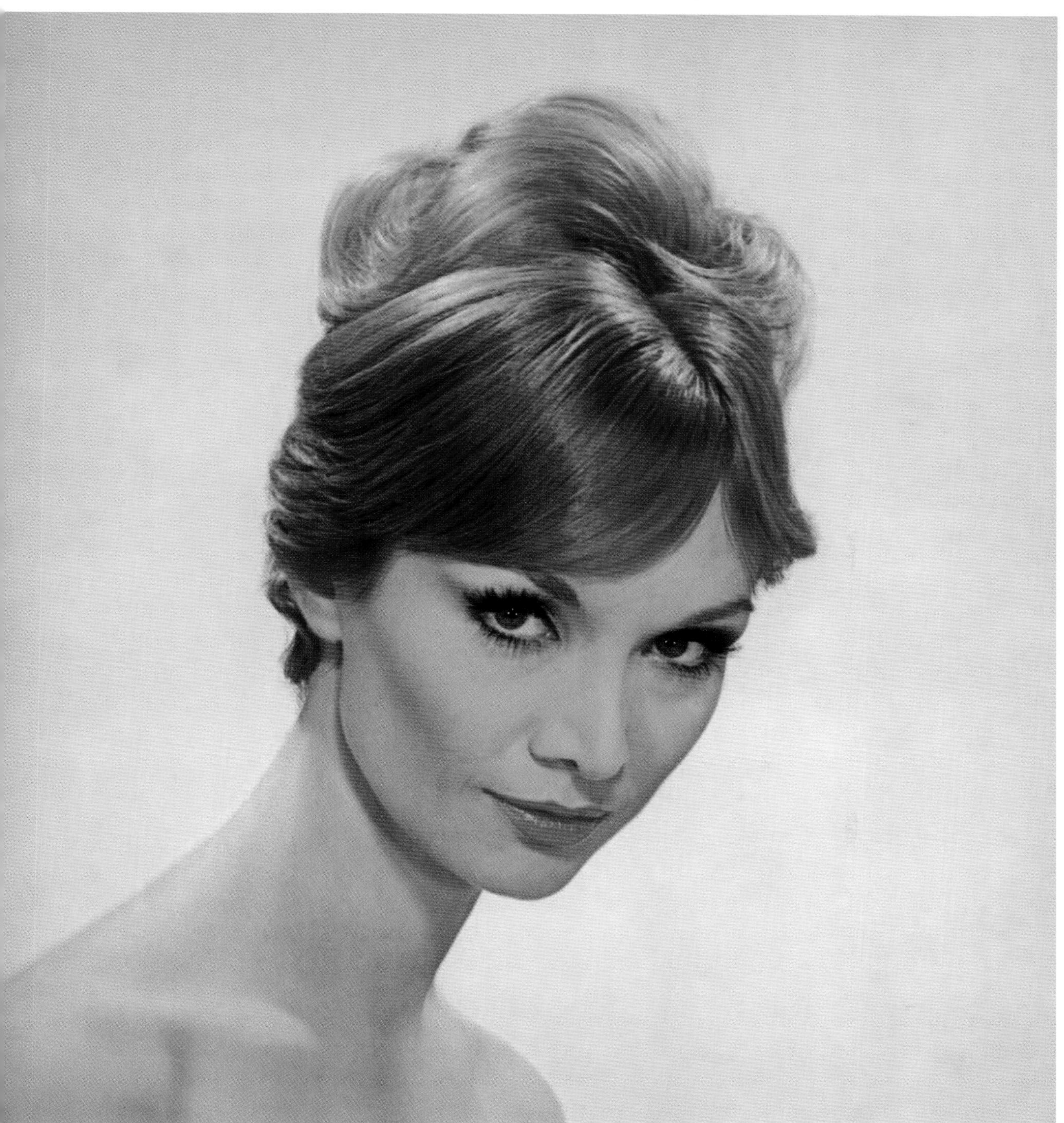

mp Coiffure' from the Leap
ear Coiffure Collection, 1964,
ational Hairdressers and
osmetologists Association Inc.

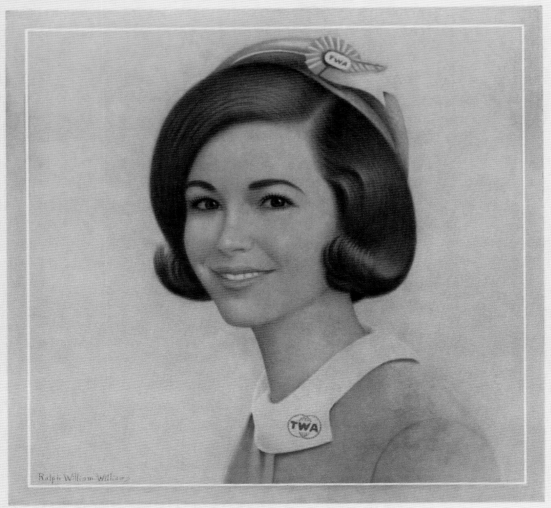

Ralph William Williams

TWA Hostess Judy Neumann was voted "The girl in the air with the most beautiful hair."

With changes of climate, windy airports and busy schedules, it isn't easy for an airline hostess to keep her hair always lovely. But Judy manages beautifully with Breck Shampoo.

Breck leaves hair shining clean, yet manageable, because it's the only leading shampoo that does not have a synthetic detergent base. It never makes hair dry, dull or flyaway as harsh shampoos can.

And Breck comes in three special formulas: for dry, normal or oily hair.

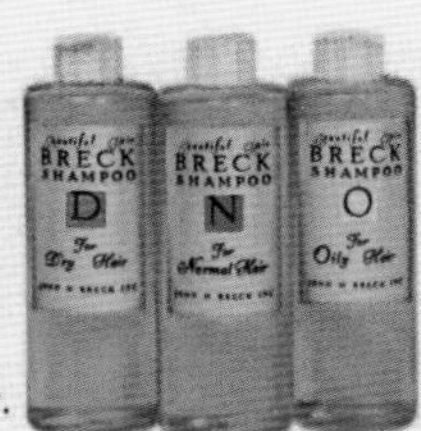

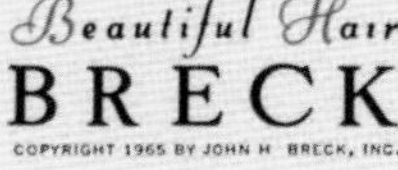

Breck Shampoo advertisement, 1965

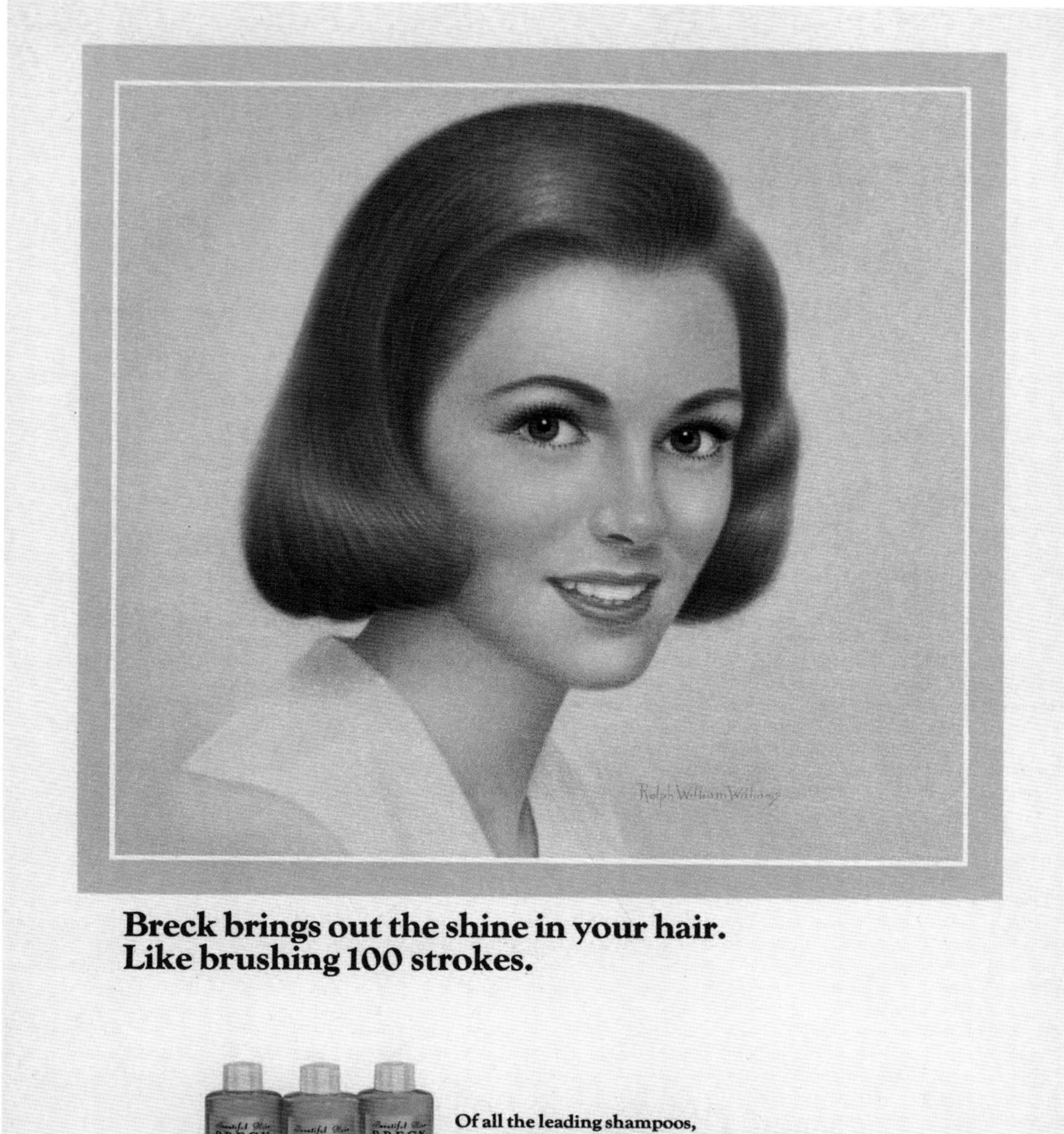

Breck brings out the shine in your hair.
Like brushing 100 strokes.

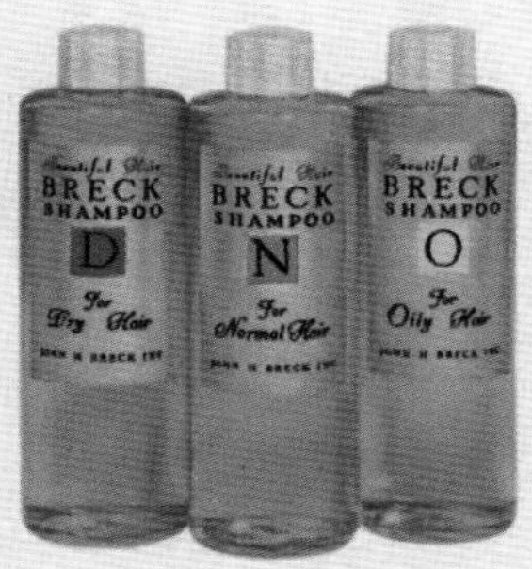

Of all the leading shampoos, only Breck does not have a synthetic detergent base.

While other shampoos can dry away shine, Breck's natural formula uncovers your natural shine. It brings hair to life, the way brushing can. Breck leaves hair smoother, more manageable, too. Choose the formula that was made just for you—Dry, Normal or Oily.

Beautiful Hair
BRECK

COPYRIGHT 1966 BY JOHN H. BRECK, INC.

32 WOMAN'S DAY

Breck Shampoo advertisement, 1966

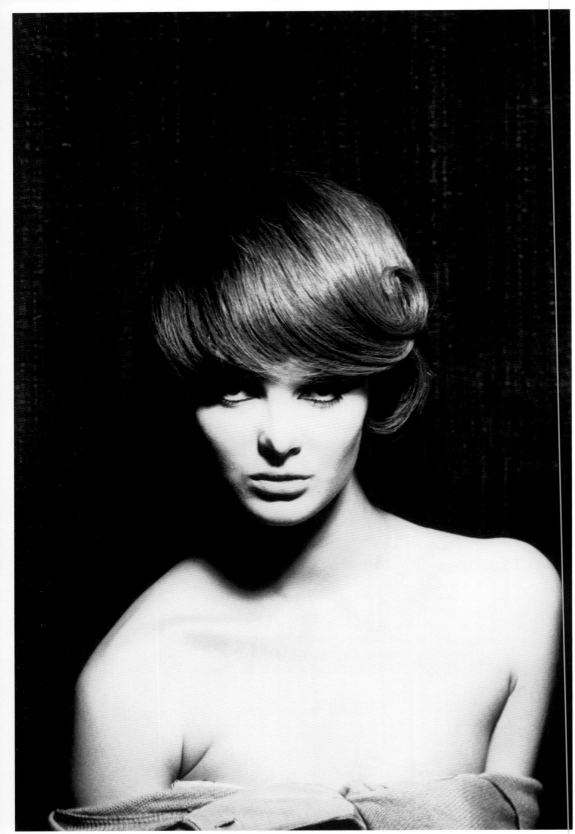

Grace Coddington with haircut by Vidal Sassoon, 1961, photographed by Terence Donovan

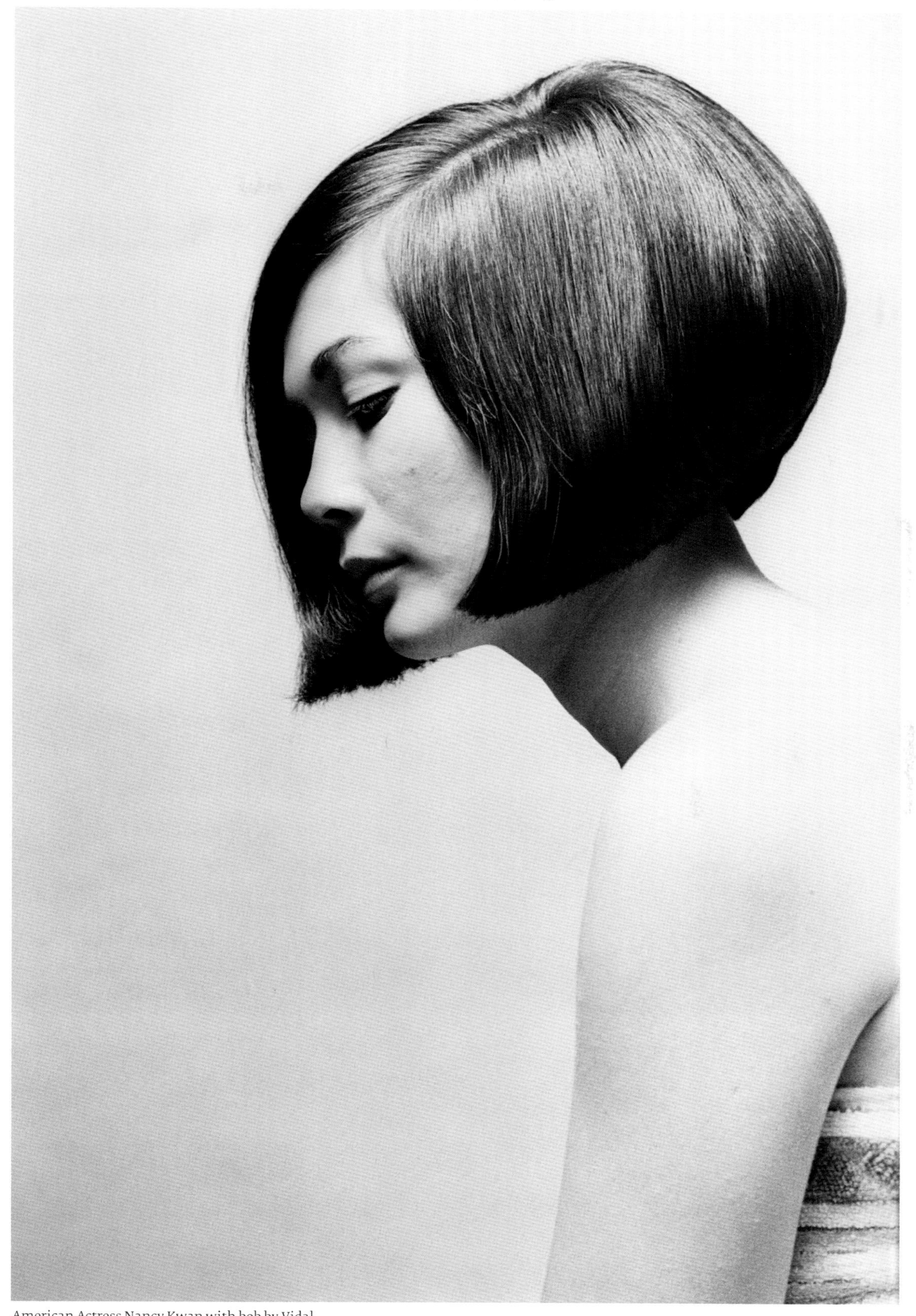

American Actress Nancy Kwan with bob by Vidal Sassoon, 1963, photographed by Terence Donovan

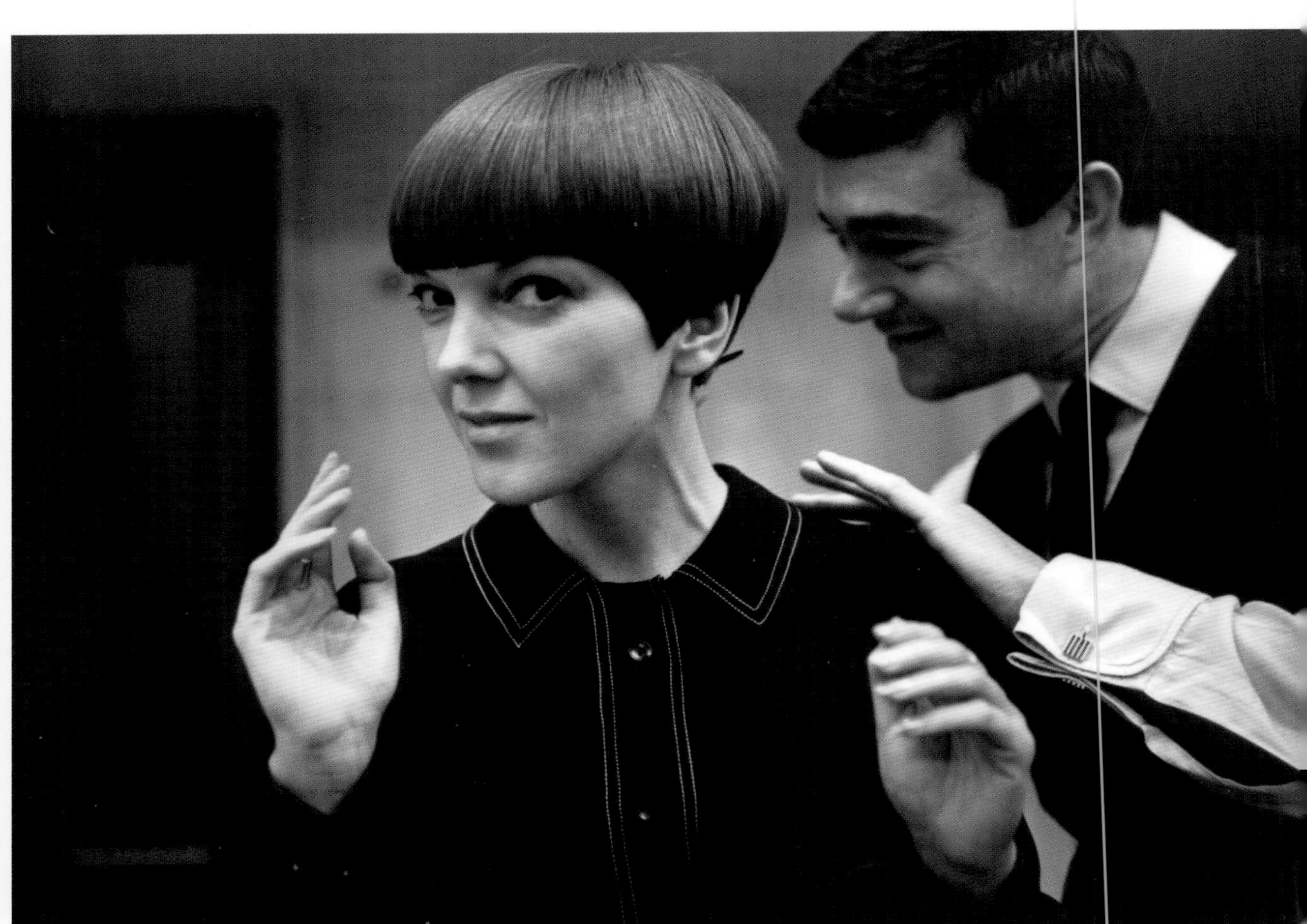

Mary Quant having her hair cut by Vidal Sassoon, 1964, photographed by Ronald Dumont

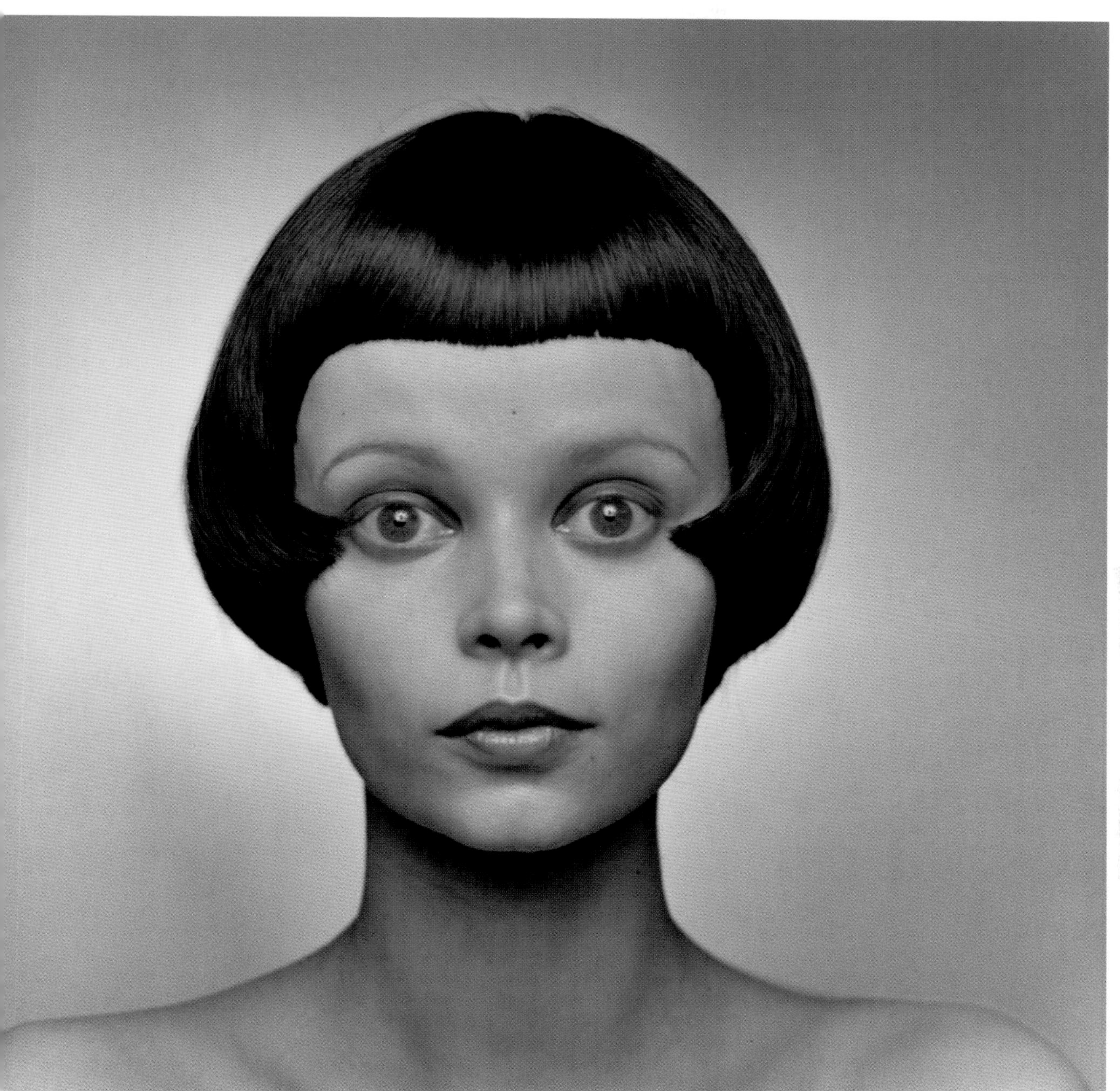

airstyle by Vidal Sassoon, 1960s,
otographed by Barry Lategan

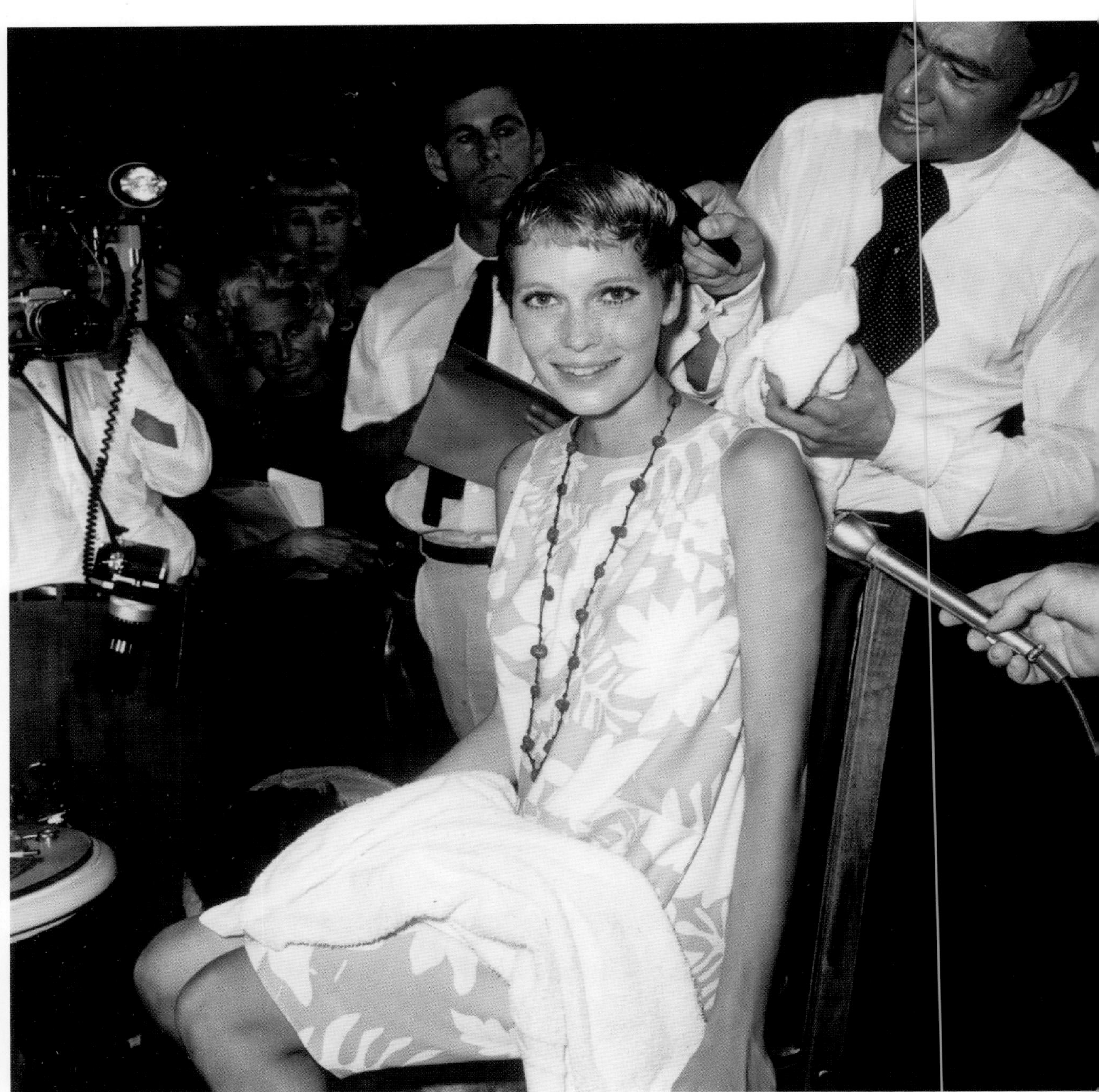

Mia Farrow having her blonde hair cut short by Vidal Sassoon, 1967

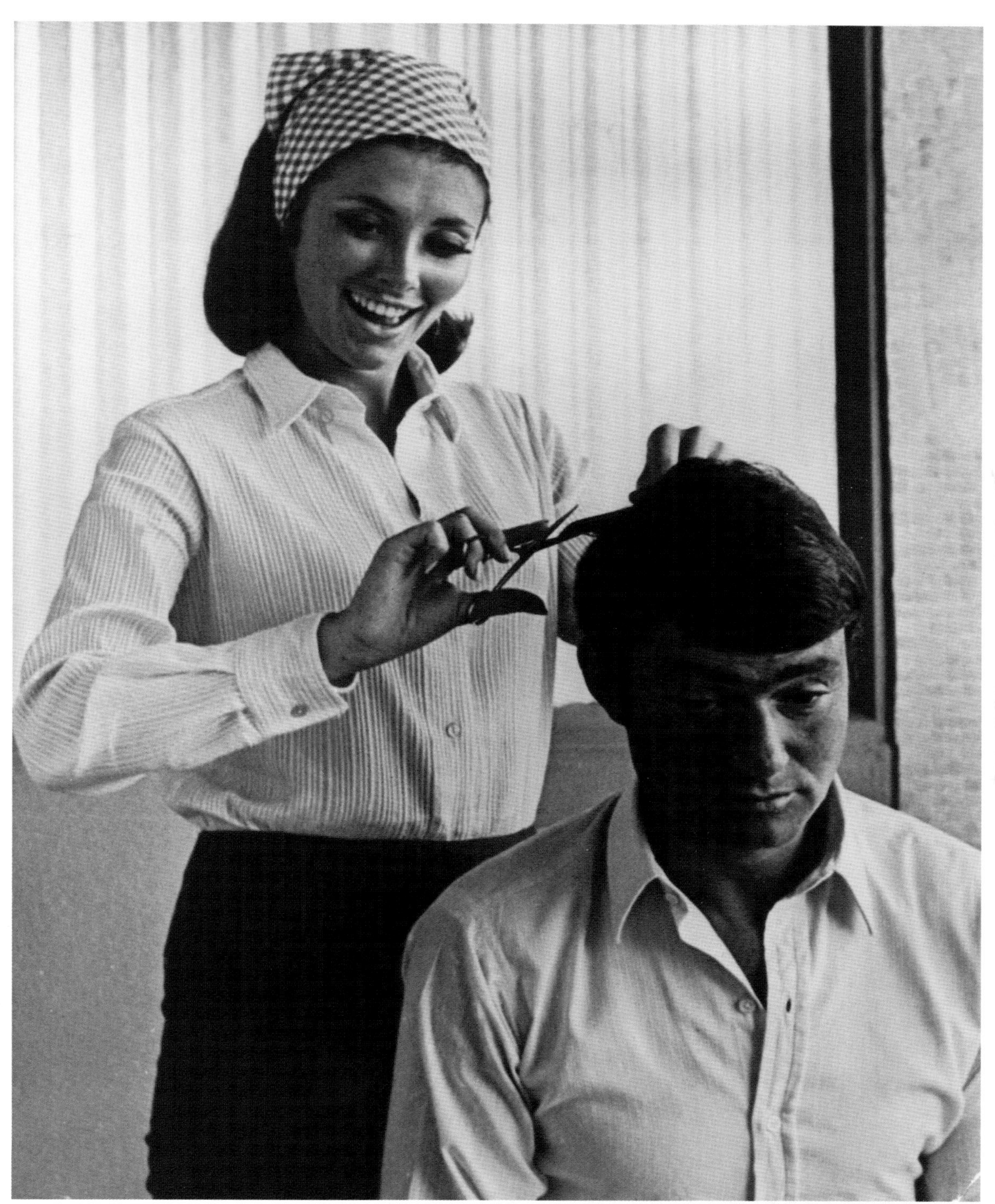

Vidal Sassoon & his wife,
actress Beverly Adams, 1967

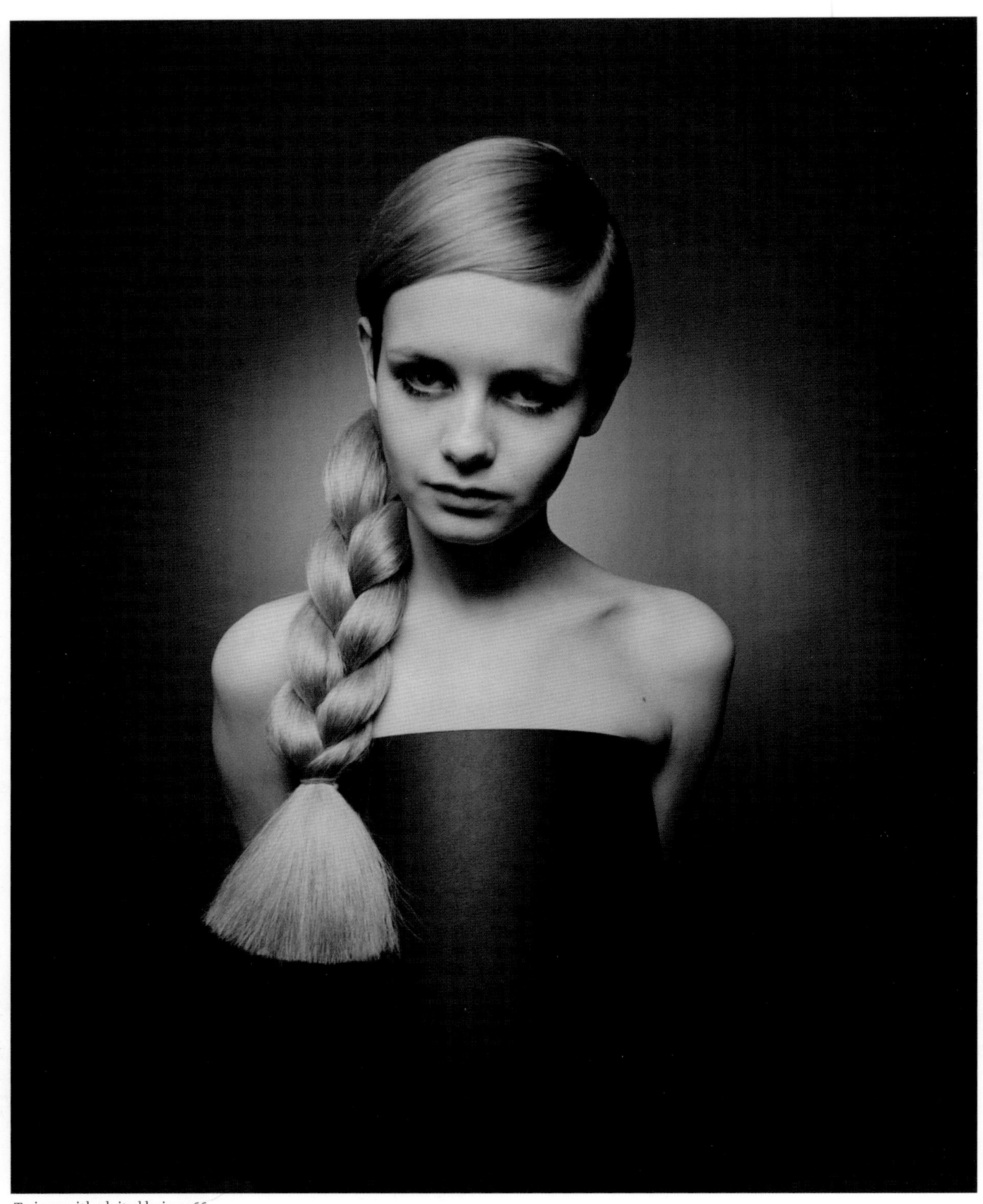

Twiggy with plaited hair, 1966,
photographed by Barry Lategan

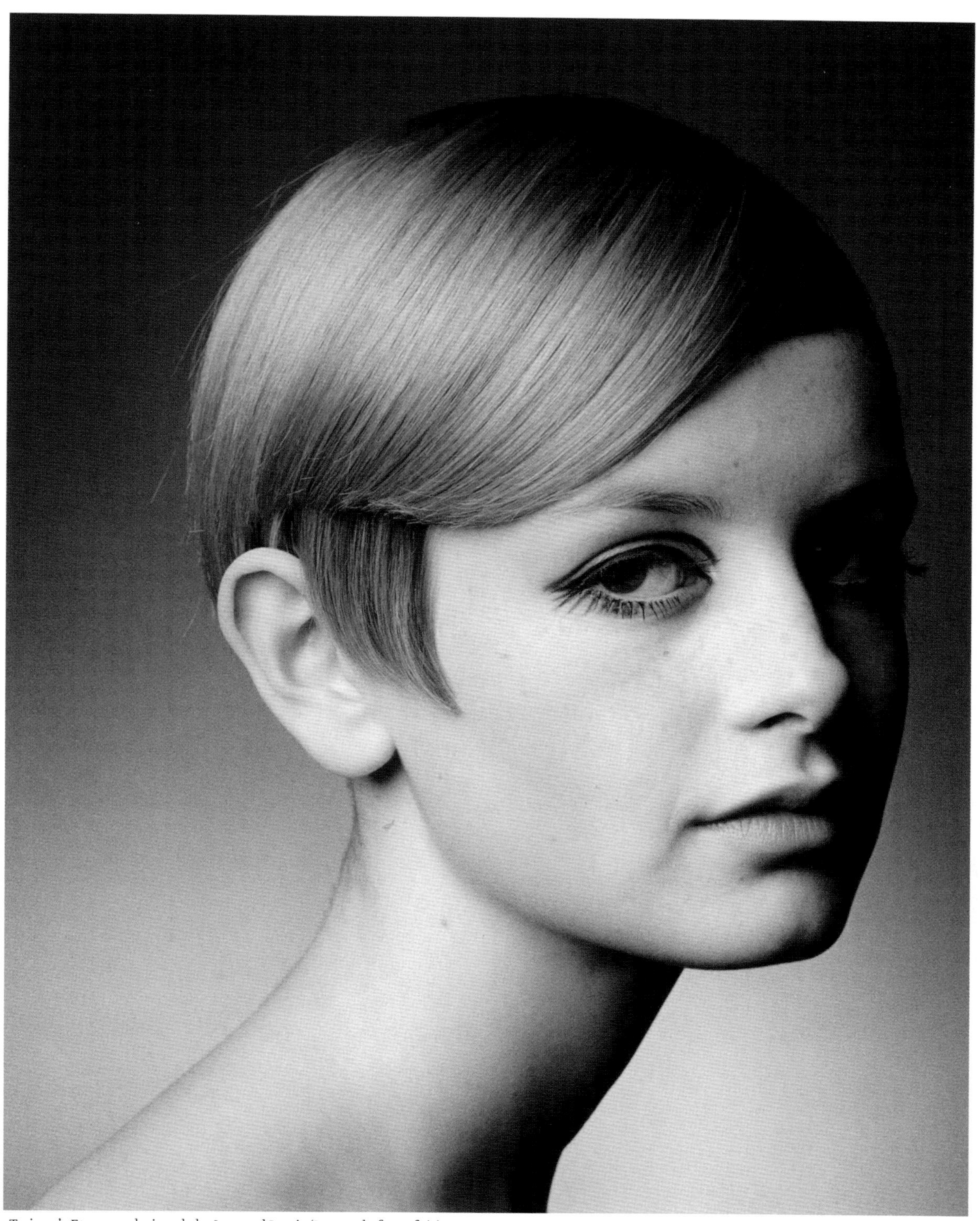

Twiggy's Eton crop hairstyle by Leonard Lewis (Leonard of Mayfair), 1966, photographed by Barry Lategan

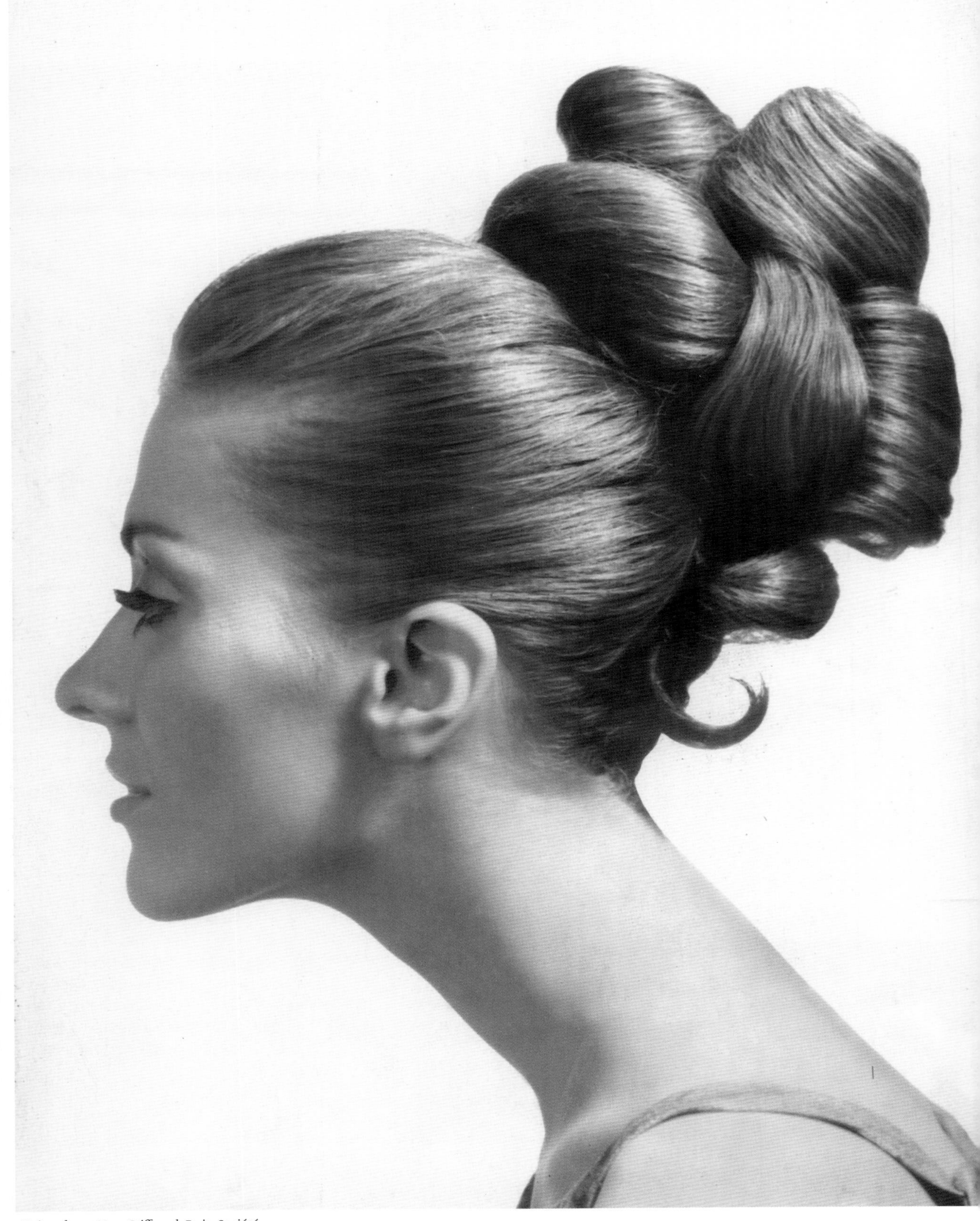

Hairstyle, 1966, *30 Coiffures de Paris*, Société d'Editions Modernes Parisiennes

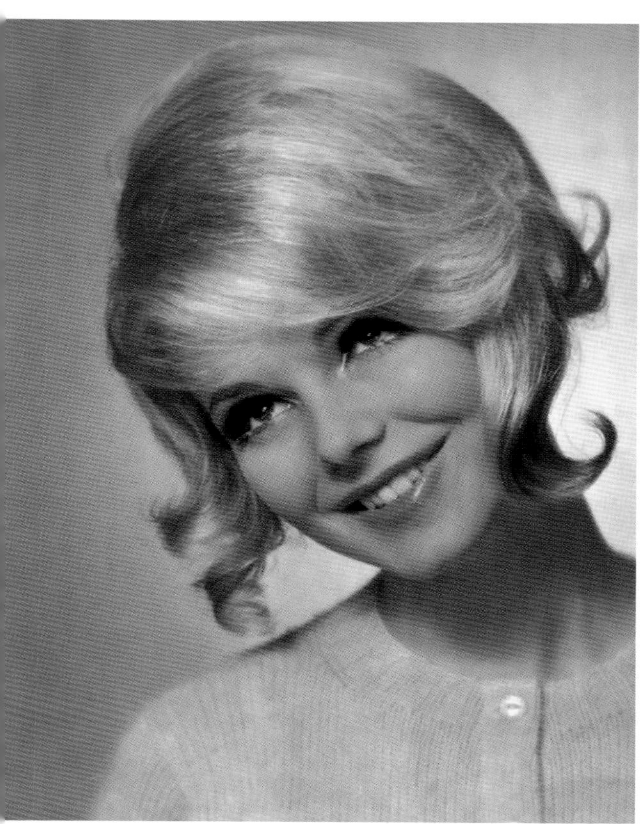

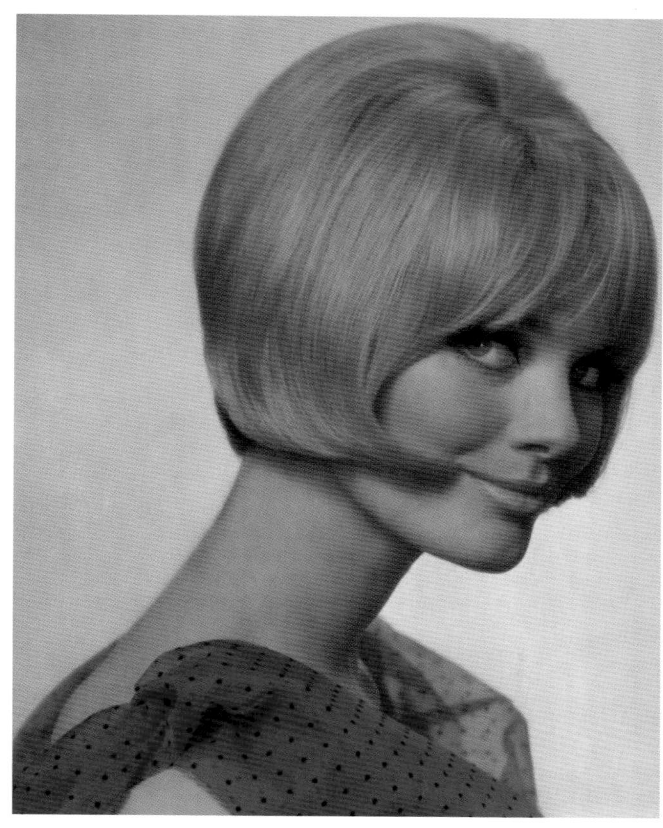

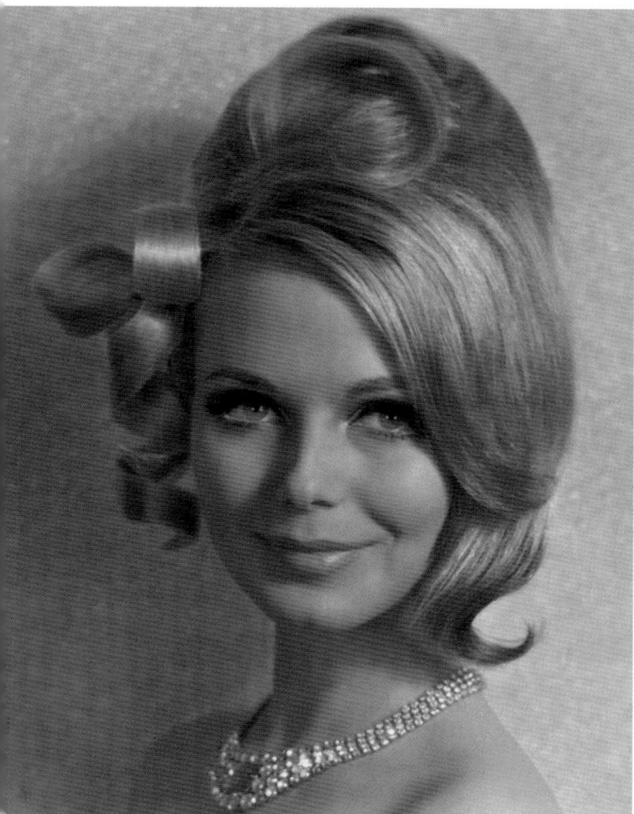

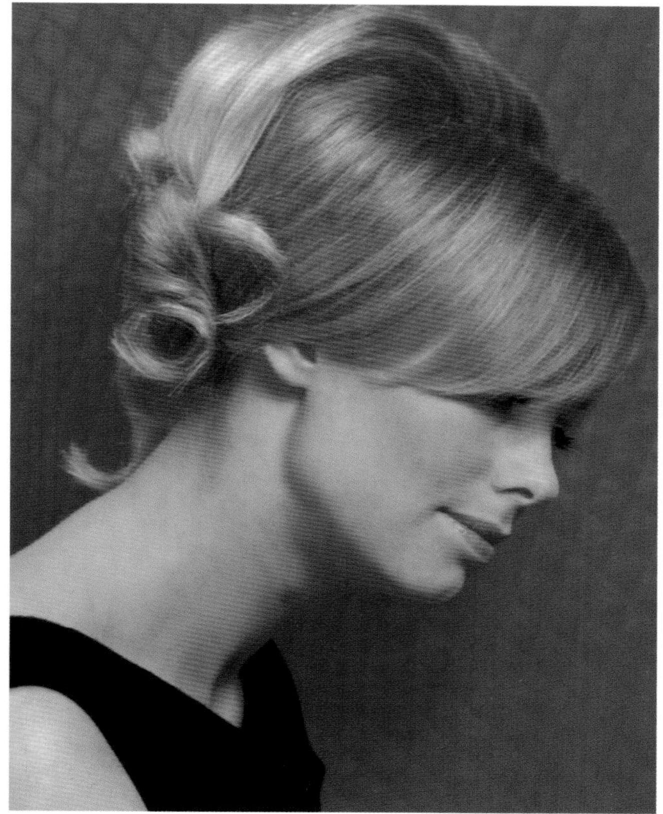

irstyles, 1966, *30 Coiffures de Paris*, Société
Éditions Modernes Parisiennes

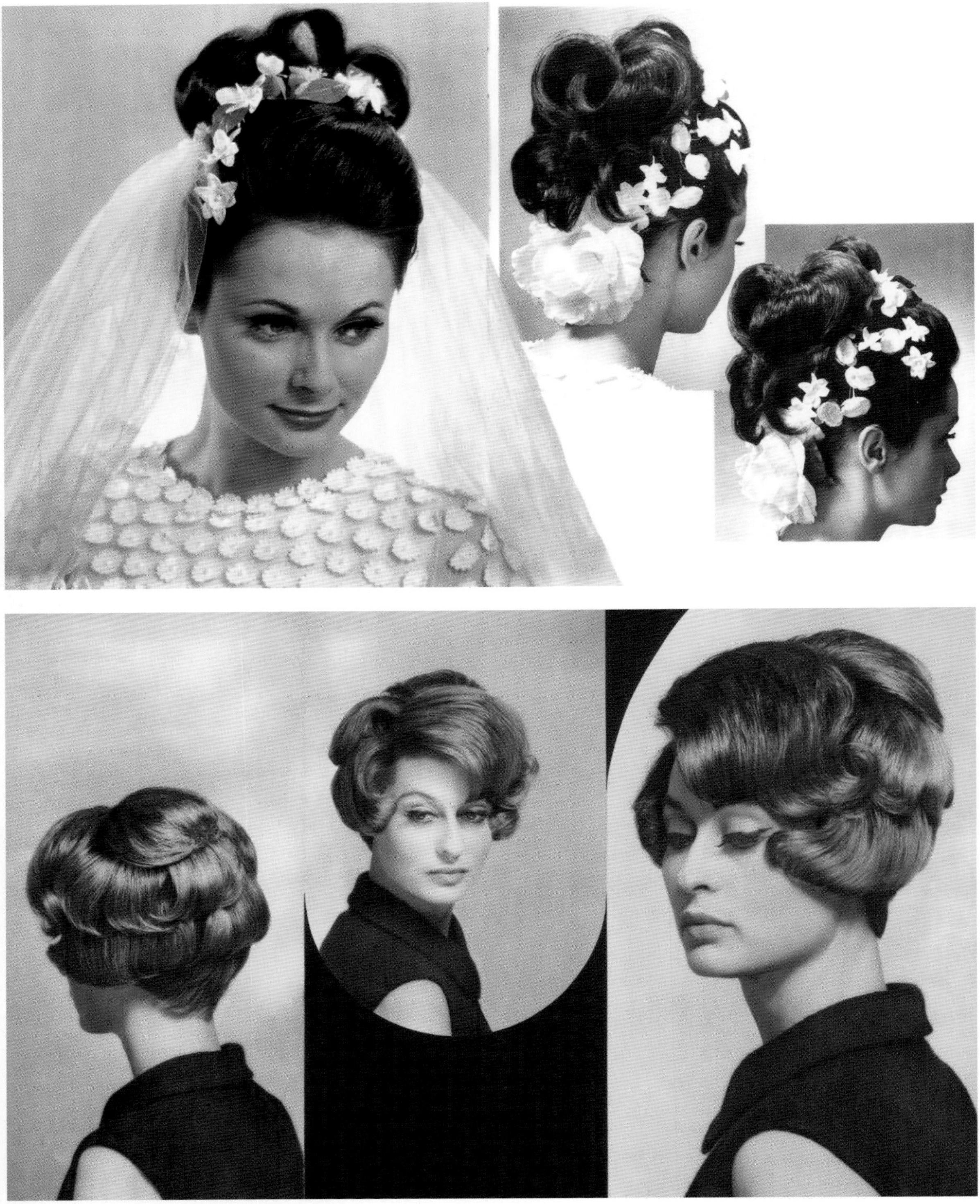

Hairstyles, 1966, *30 Coiffures de Paris*, Société d'Editions Modernes Parisiennes

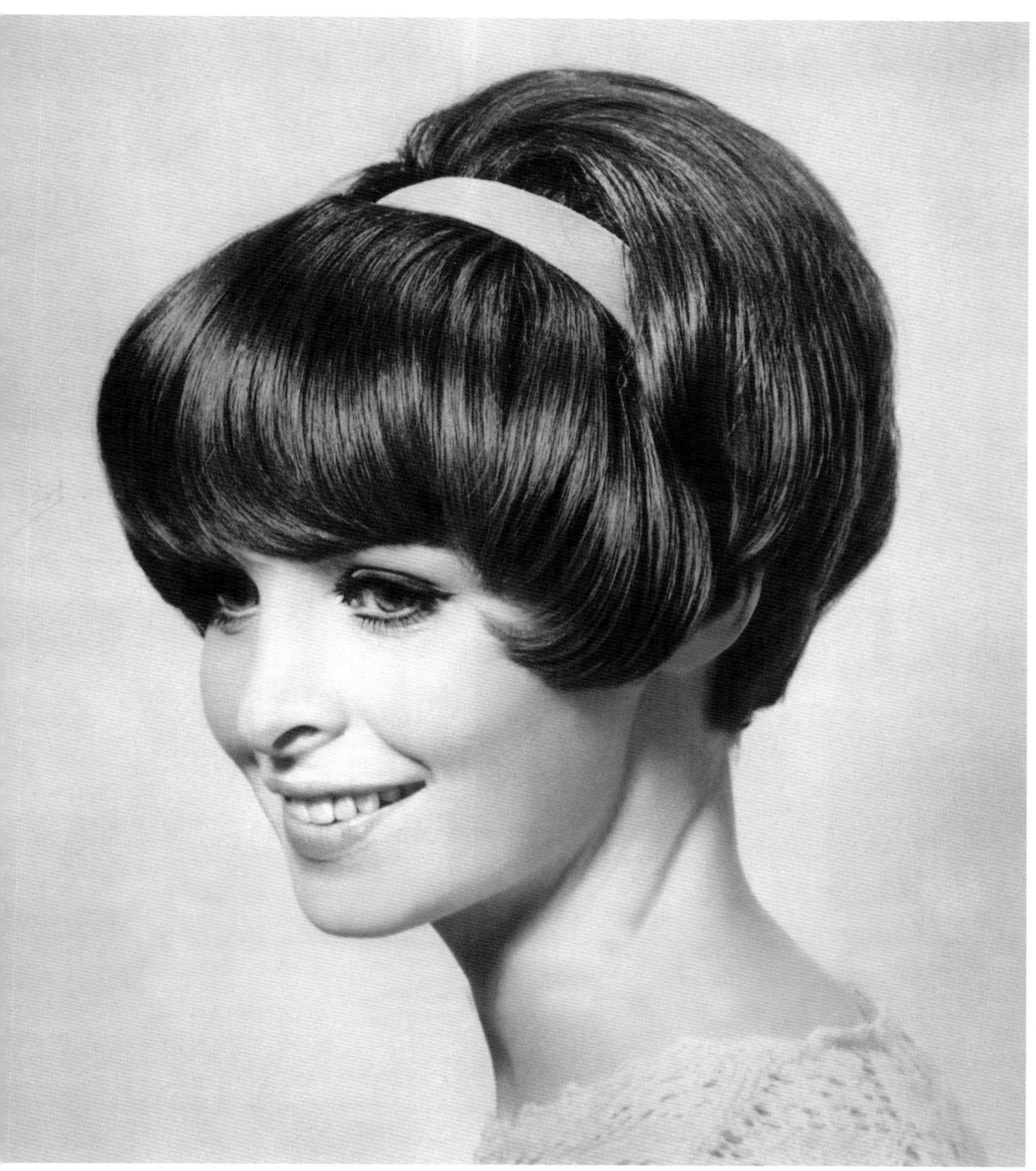

Hairstyle, 1966, *30 Coiffures de Paris*, Société d'Editions Modernes Parisiennes

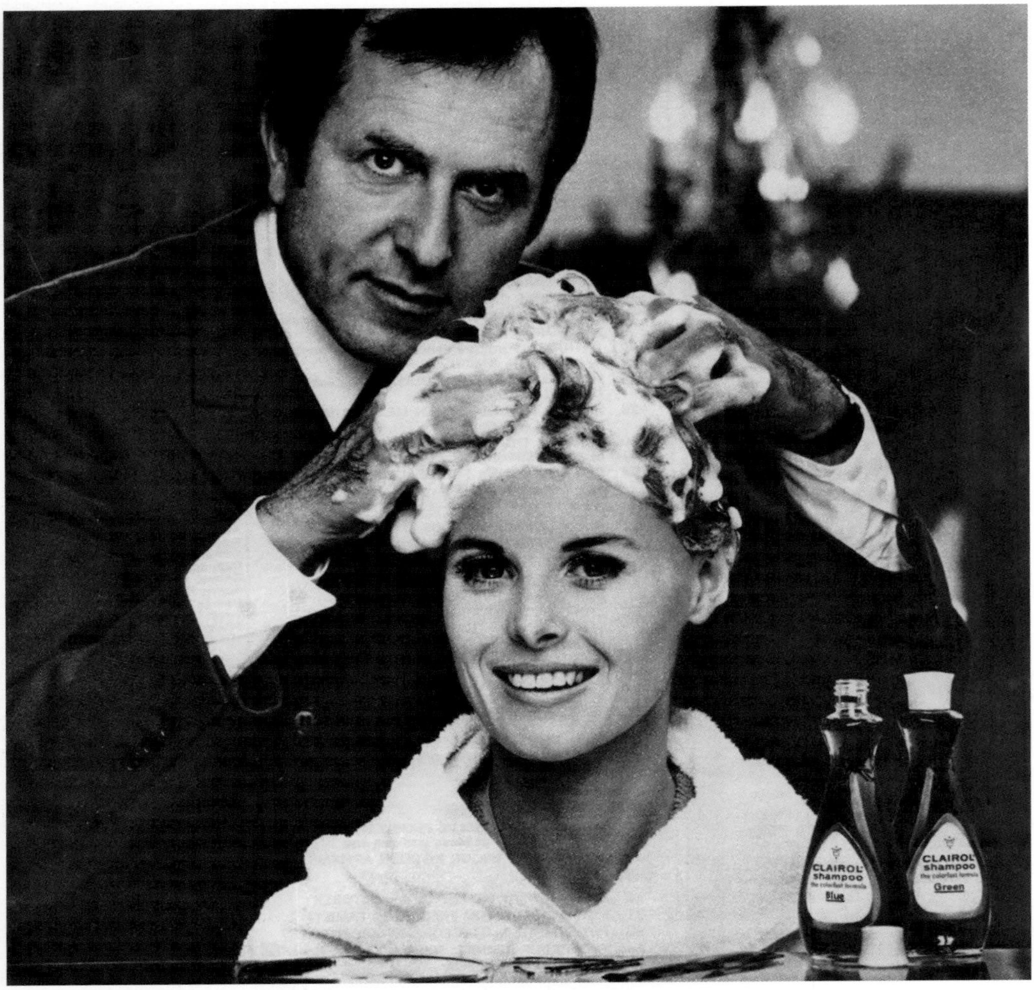

Hairstylist Gene Shacove advertising Clairol Shampoo, 1967

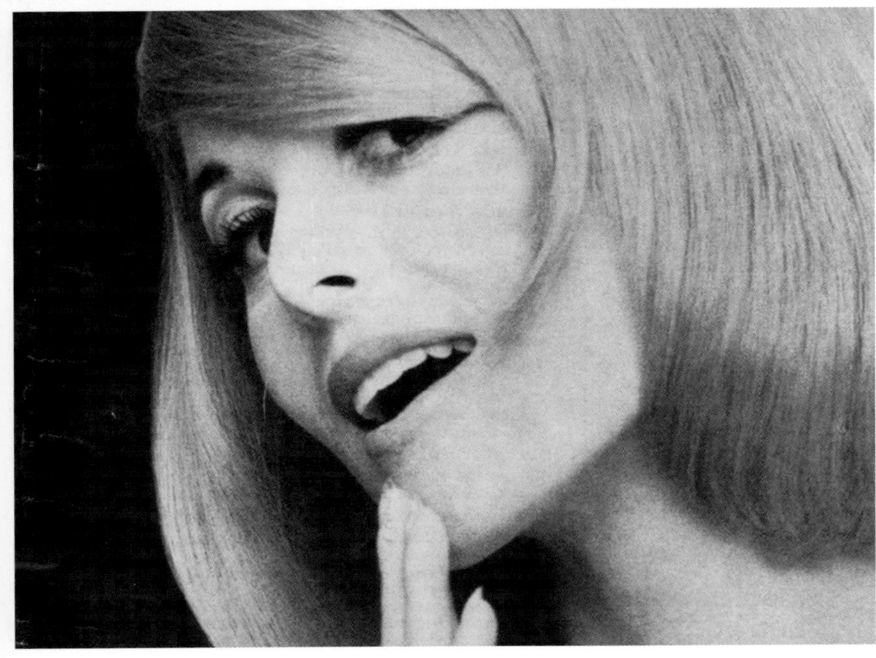

Hairstyle by Gene Shacove (the inspiration for actor Warren Beatty's character in 1975 film 'Shampoo') to advertise Clairol Colorfast Shampoo, 1965

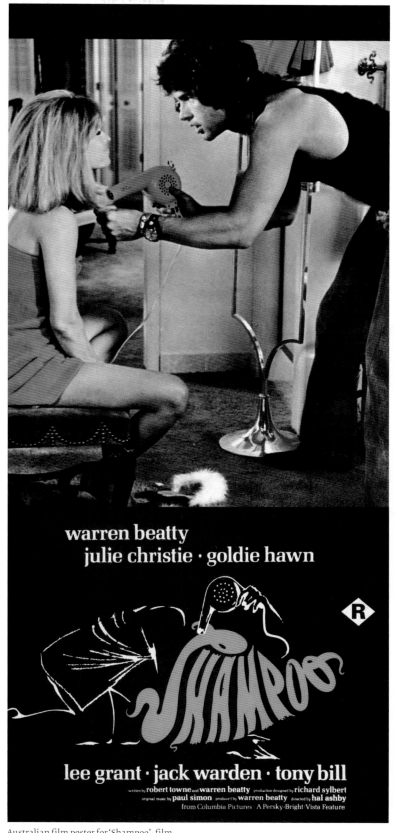

Australian film poster for 'Shampoo', film starring Warren Beatty, released 1975

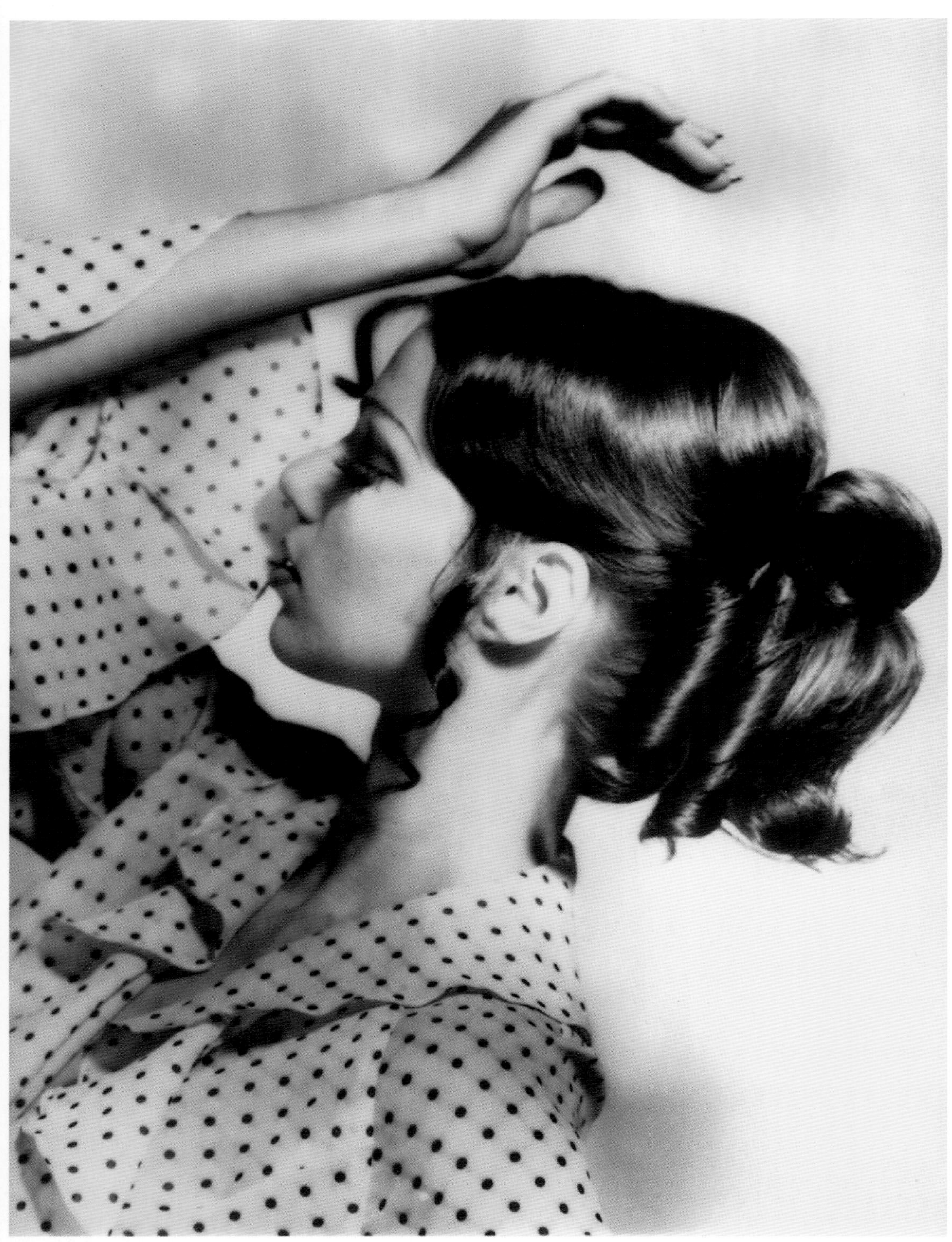

French Up-Do Inspired by
Mexican Chignons, 1968

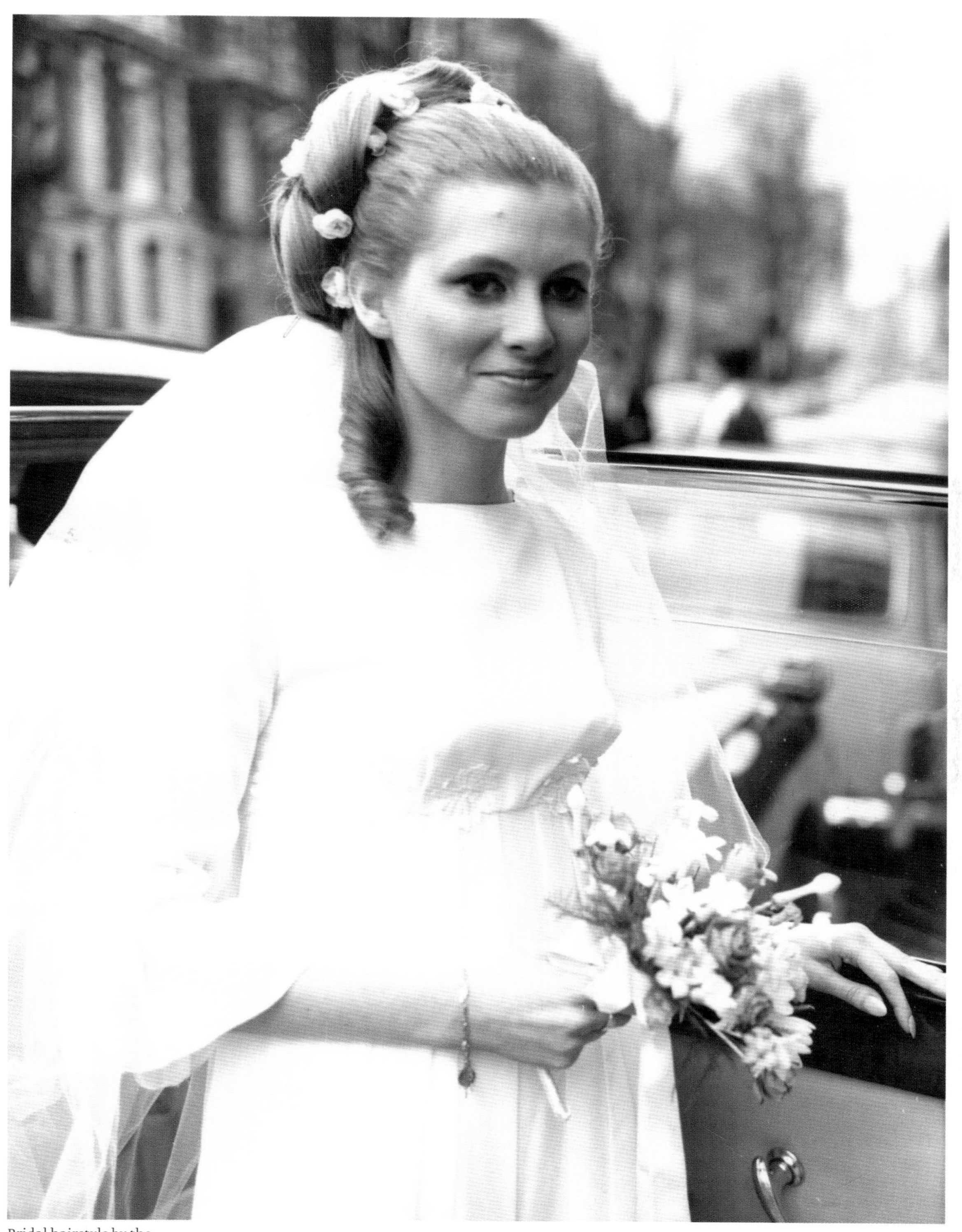

Bridal hairstyle by the Ginger Group, 1967

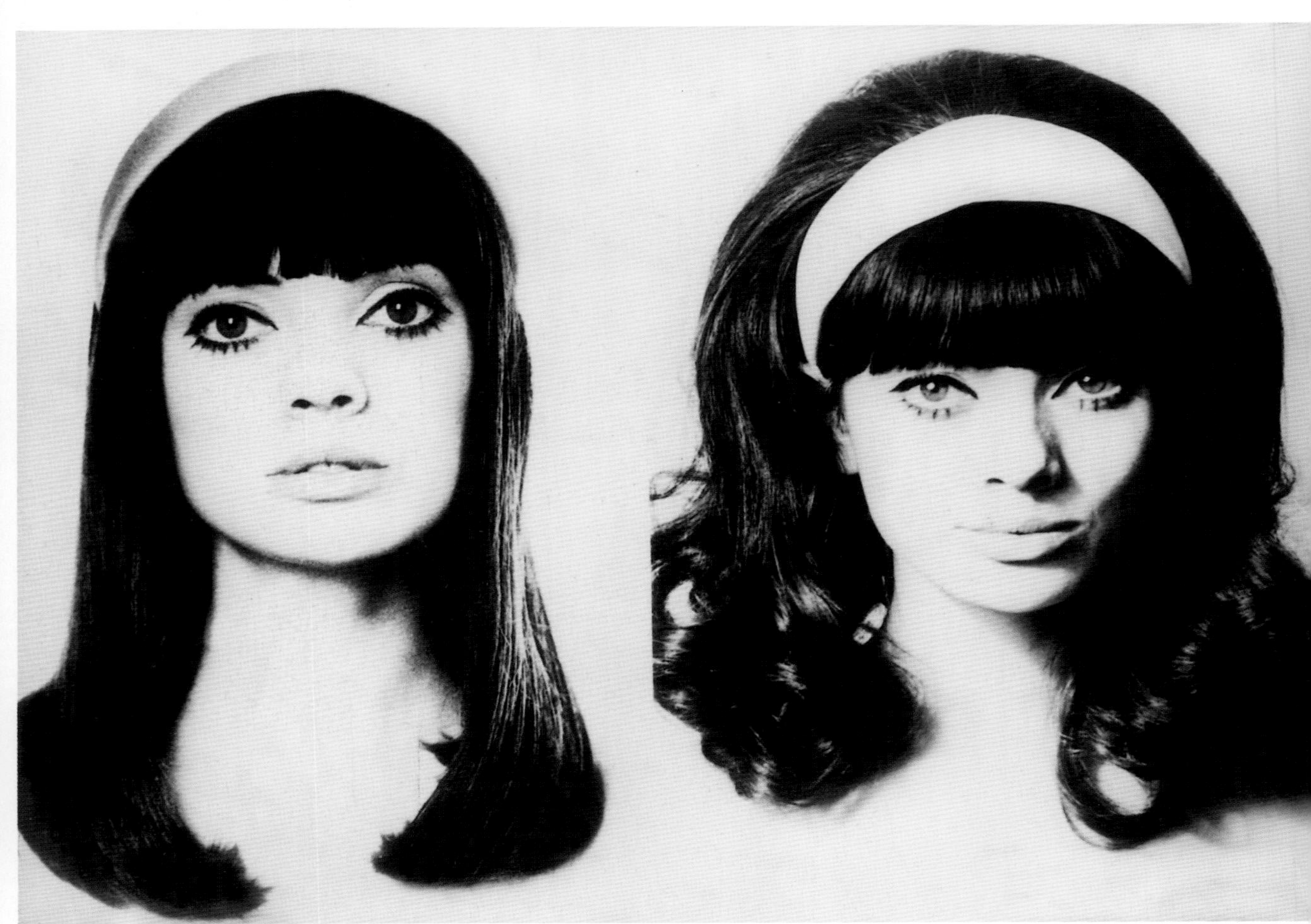

Two hairstyles created by Jean-Louis Saint-Roch to complement the autumn collection of the fashion designer, Ted Lapidus, with the hairbands matching the clothes, 1968

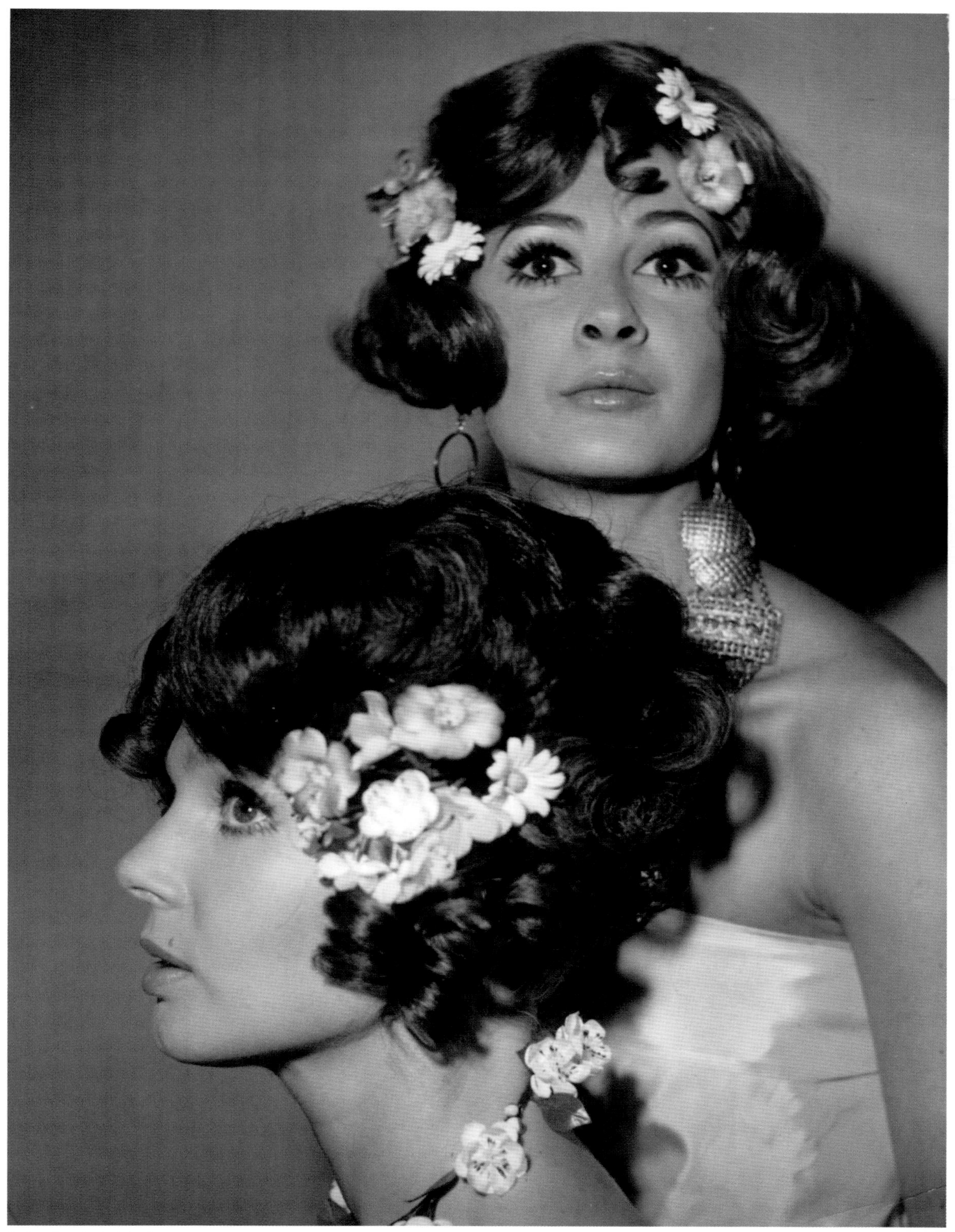

Springtime hairstyles by
Molinaro, Paris, 1968

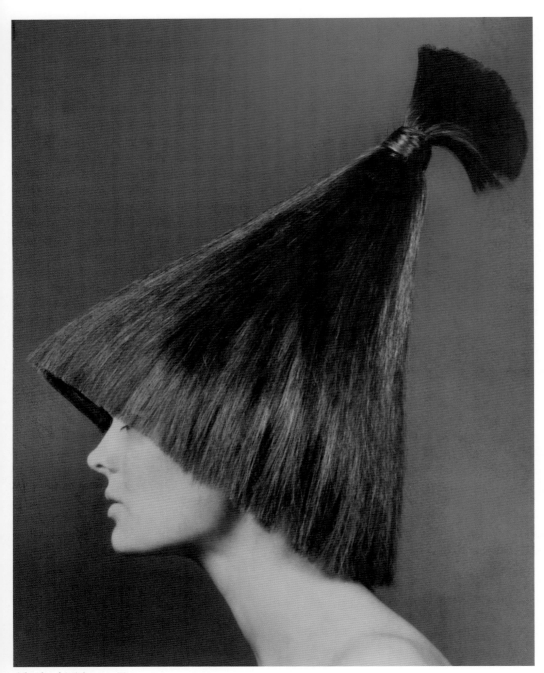

'The Thatch Wig', USA, 1968

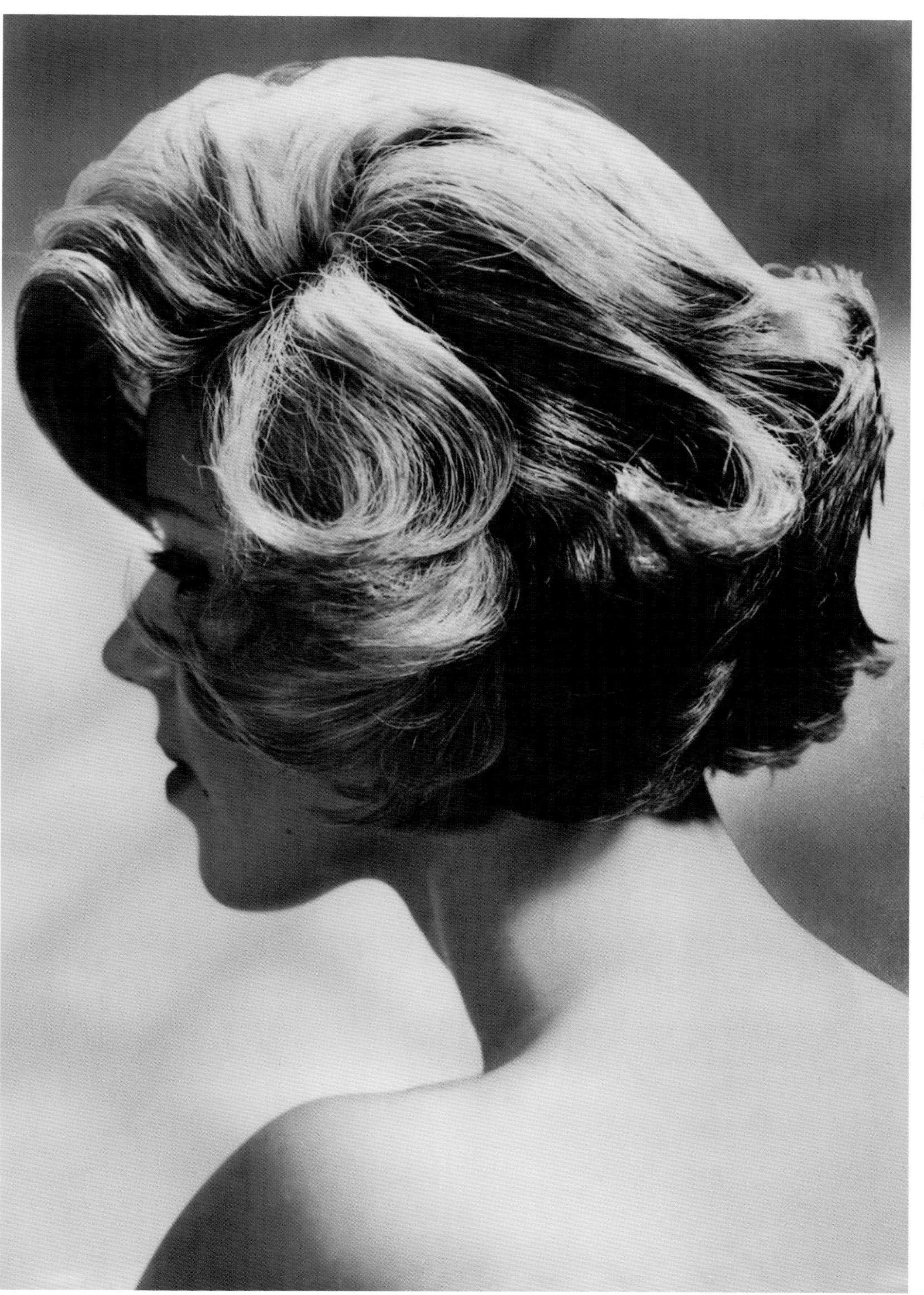

'Natural-Hair' wig, USA, 1969

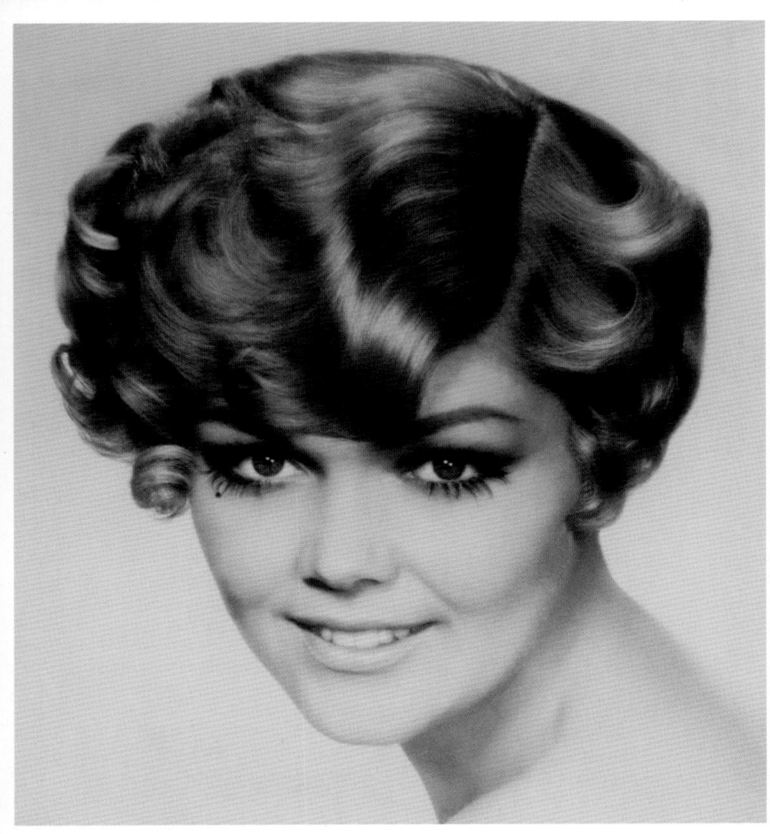

'The Ripple Wave Coiffure: A Natural Wave Look Hair Fashion for Summer', 1969, National Hairdressers and Cosmetologists Association Inc.

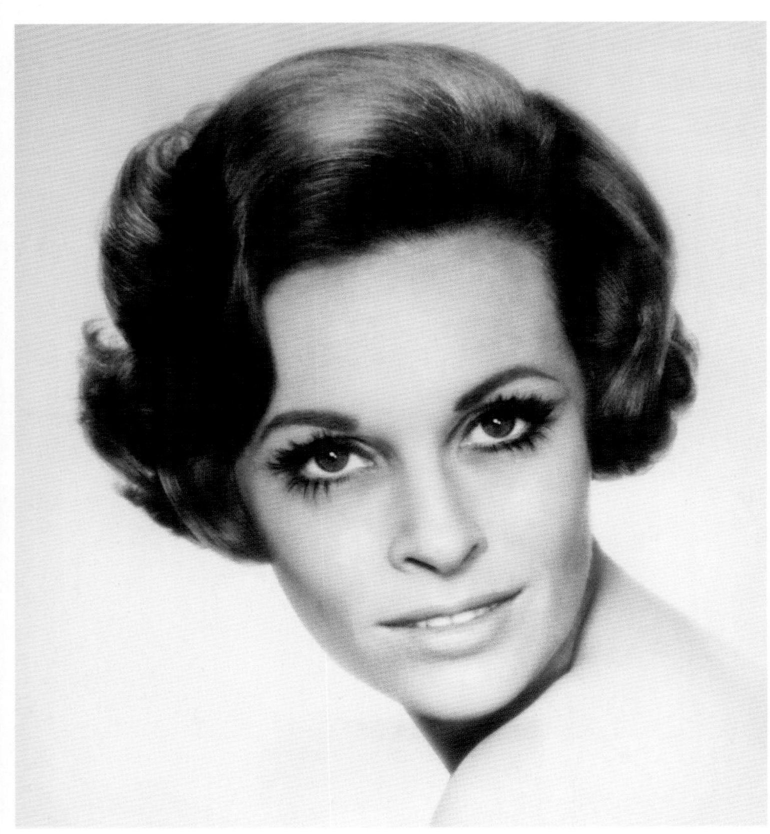

'The Flowing Wave Coiffure: A Natural Wave Look Hair Fashion for Summer', 1969, National Hairdressers and Cosmetologists Association Inc.

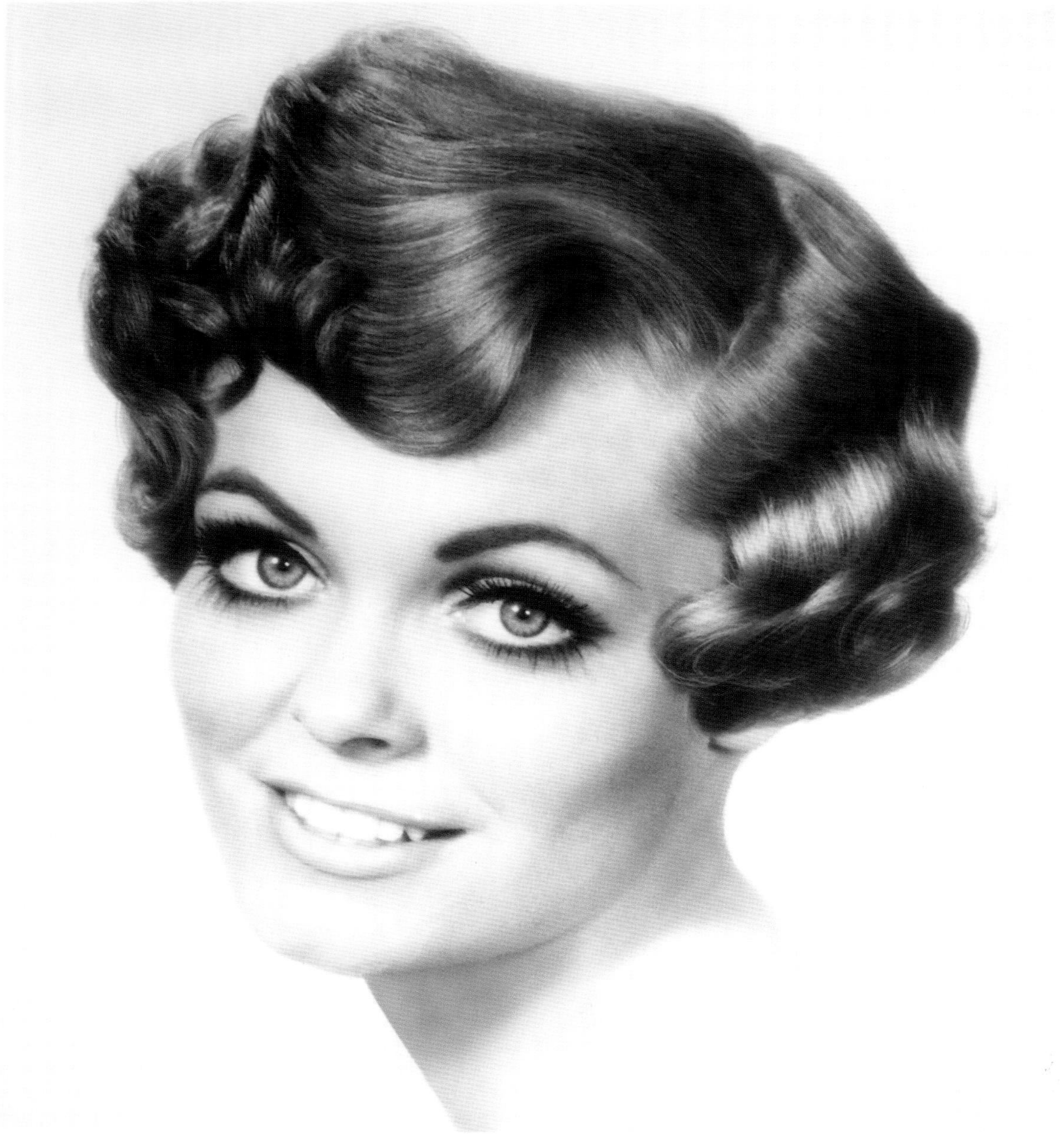

THE NATURAL WAVE LOOK IN HAIR FASHIONS FOR SUMMER, 1969 The Flip Wave Coiffure

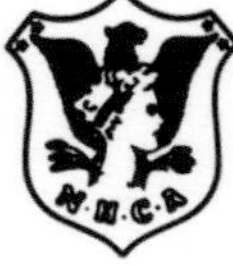

'The Flip Wave Coiffure: A Natural Wave Look Hair Fashion for Summer', 1969, National Hairdressers and Cosmetologists Association Inc.

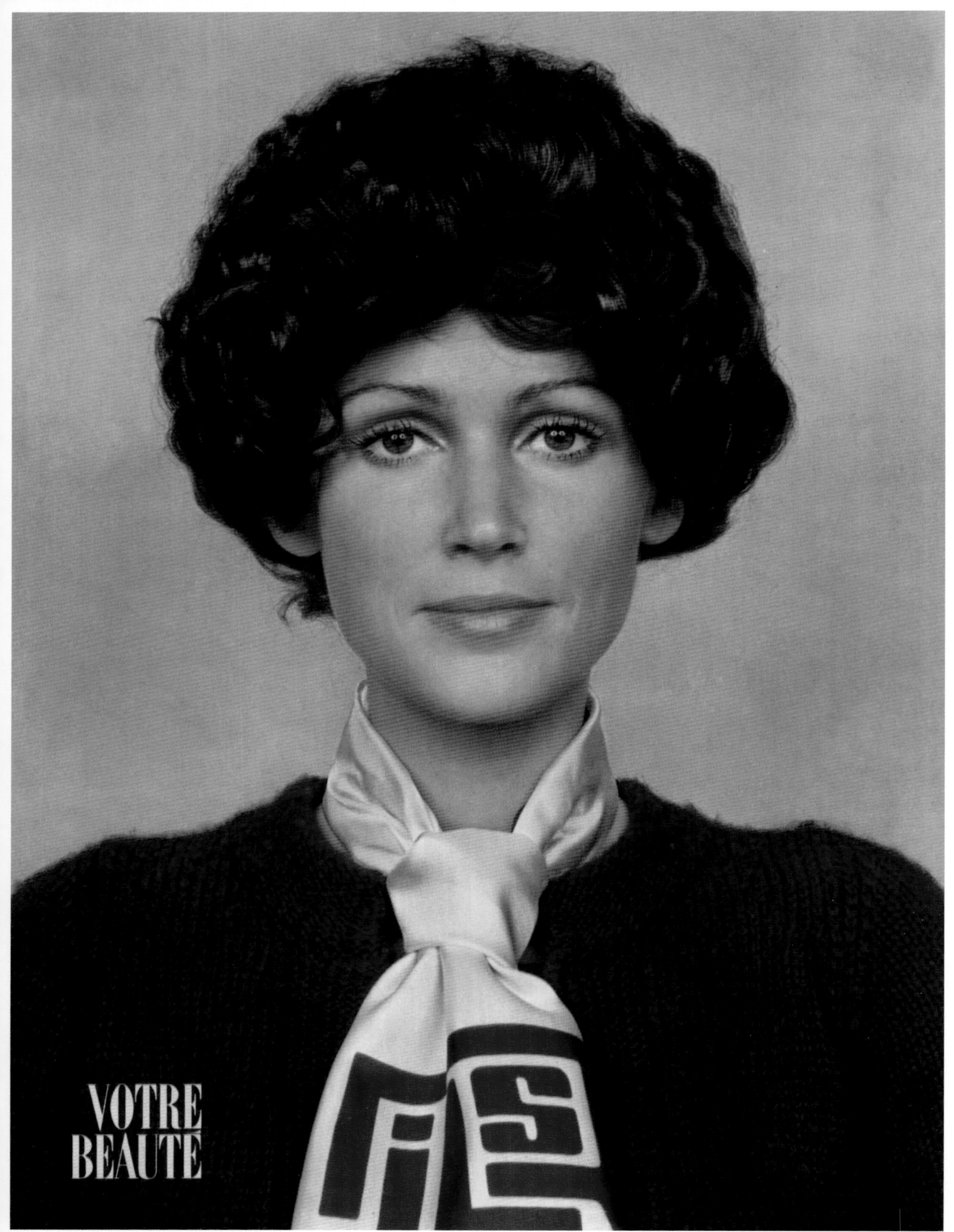

Hairstyle, 1969, *Votre Beauté*

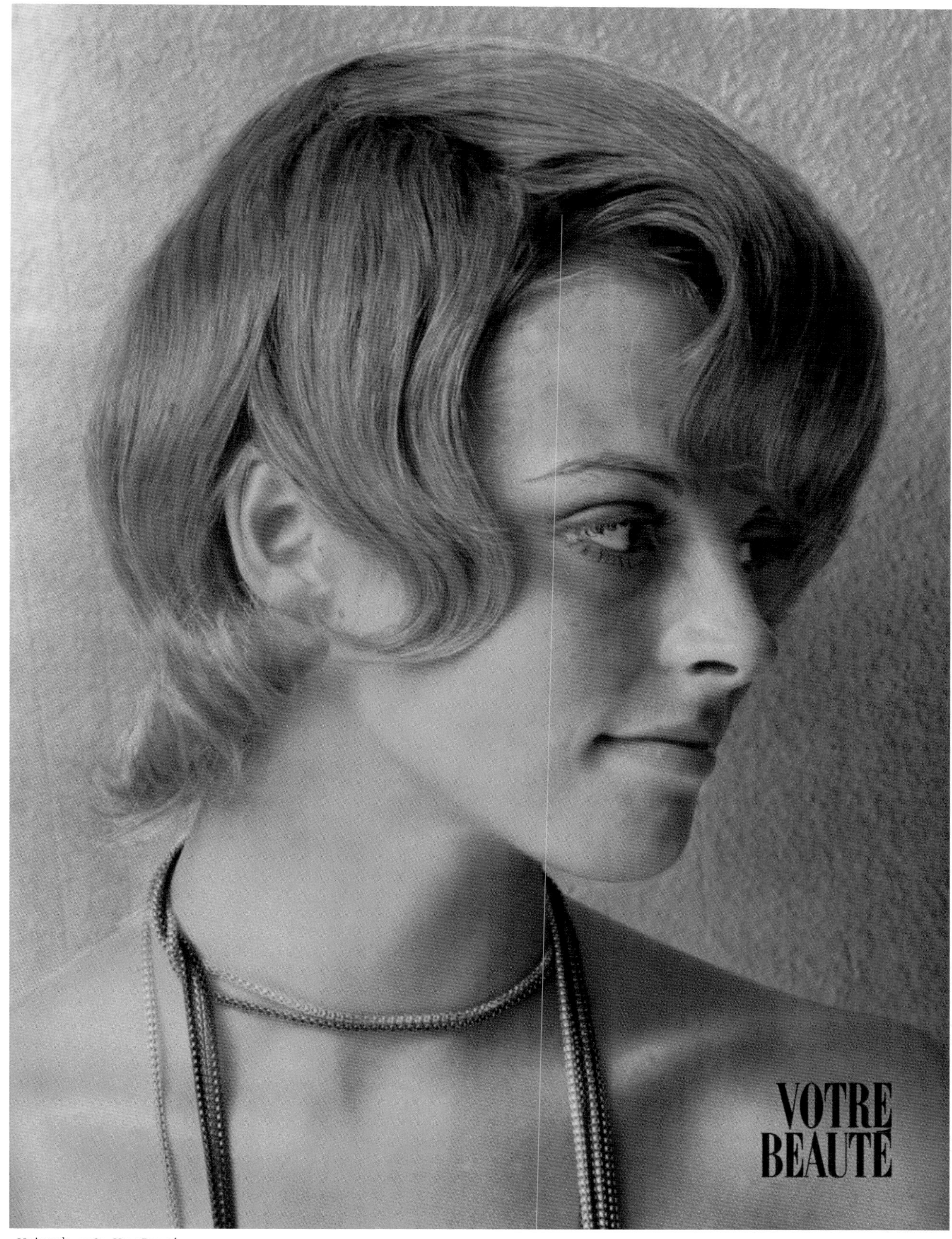

Hairstyle, 1969, *Votre Beauté*

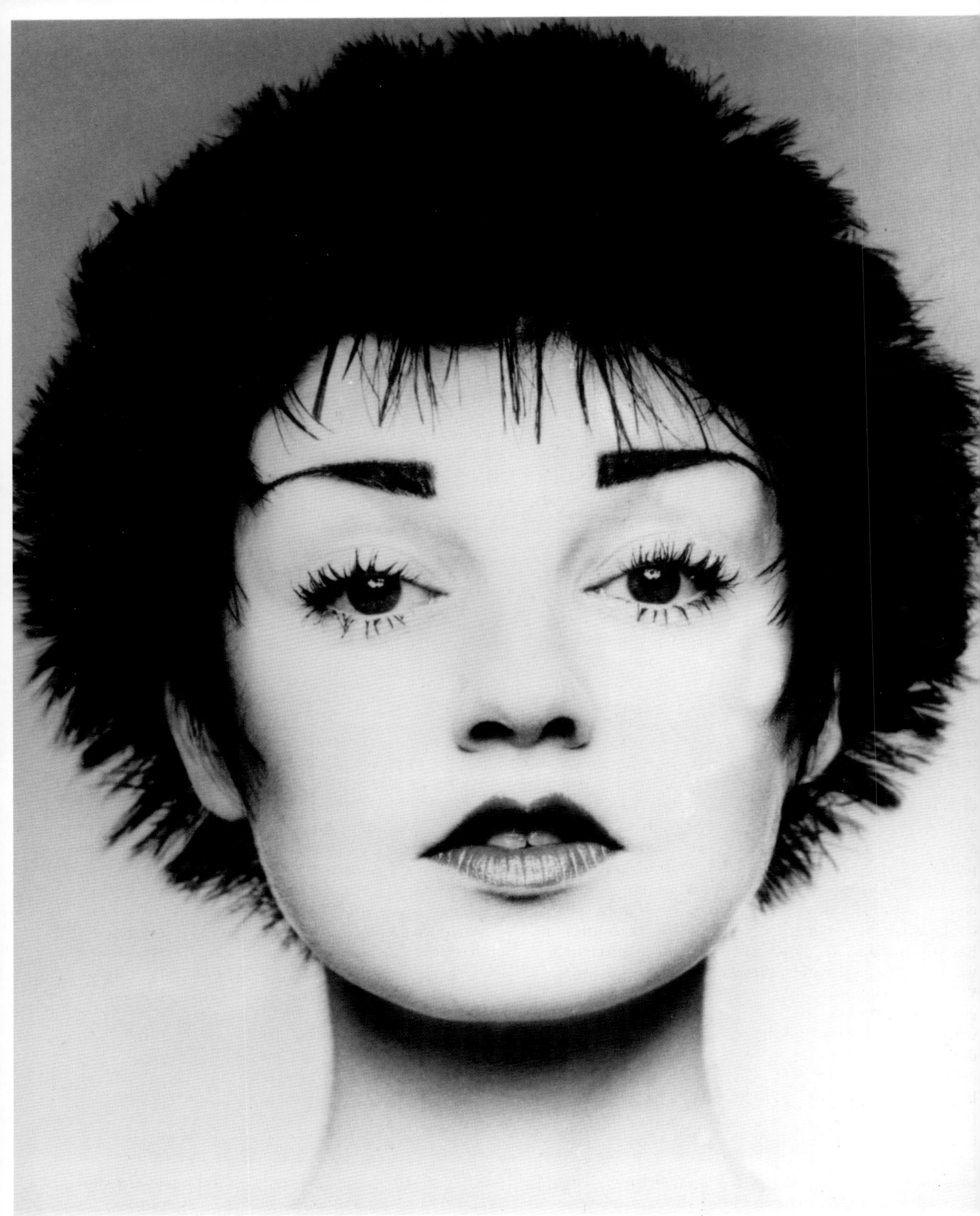

'The Brush' hairstyle by Christopher Brooker, International Creative Director, Vidal Sassoon, photographed by Barry Lategan, 1972

1970S

The early 1970s saw the continuing influence of the "Age of Aquarius", with many "weekend hippies" donning wigs for festivals. The main thing if you were a flower child was to grow your hair as long as possible, and the age-old symbolism connecting hair with power was a recurrent theme. The early Seventies also saw the advent of unisex salons, where men and women were seated alongside each other. The first was the Chelsea salon, Smile, opened in 1969 by Keith Wainwright and Leslie Russell. Throughout the early 1970s, Smile catered to a much younger clientele than either Vidal Sassoon or Leonard of Mayfair which were, in comparison, still purveyors of "haute coiffure". It was really the first salon that was all about youth street culture and as such it attracted youthful pop celebrities. These included the rock broadcaster, Cathy McGowan who became a Mod style icon, and singing sensations Sandy Shaw and Cilla Black. Significantly, in Britain a generational and class shift had occurred in music, fashion and the media, and the young up-and-coming stars of the early 1970s felt much more at home in arty Chelsea than in the well-heeled stomping grounds of Mayfair or Bond Street.

Although the oil crisis of 1973 put an end to the carefree optimism of the hippy era and replaced it with a new age of austerity, women still continued to experiment with innovative hairstyles that reflected the changing times. During the 1970s, Vidal Sassoon continued to offer clients his distinctive and fashionable look, and also had a hairdressing school in Knightsbridge that taught students his simple step-by-step approach that was based on Modernist design principles derived from the Bauhaus. Working for Vidal Sassoon during this period, the stylist Christopher Brooker created some highly progressive styles, including a spiky cut known as "The Brush" in 1972, which presaged the Punk hairstyles of the late 70s. Another highly influential haircut was "The Wedge" created in 1974 by Trevor Sorbie, also for Vidal Sassoon. Importantly during the 1970s, Vidal Sassoon sustained his cutting-edge credentials in the hair world, whilst also becoming a key force in the increasing commercial direction of hairstyling.

The early to mid 1970s also saw a resurgence of progressive hairdressing in France, with hairdressers such as Jacques Dessanges creating hairstyles with a structured modernity. One of the most eye-catching French coiffures from this period was the "Sphinx" which reflected the 70s "Tut-Mania" inspired by the world-touring "Treasures of Tutankhamun" exhibition (1976–1979). The mid 1970s also saw the increasing popularity of the swept-back bangs and big hair look of the "Farrah Do" made popular by the actress, Farrah Fawcett, when she played the role of a sexy private investigator on "Charlie's Angels" in 1976. She also featured in a number of hair product advertisements at the time, which further promoted this all-American mane-like look.

Around this time, in recession-strapped Britain there were rebellious stirrings of an altogether different direction in hairstyling. Instead of big lacquered hair, the new Punk generation wanted something more individualistic, authentic and different. The Smile salon became a leading pioneer of Punk hairstyles, creating luridly dyed crops for women that signalled a new anarchic direction in ladies hairdressing. Toyah Wilcox, Soo Catwoman (Soo Lucas), Jordan (Pamela Rooke) and other Punk luminaries got their revolutionary haircuts at Smile, while the singer Siouxsie Sioux of "Siouxsie and the Banshees" created her own longer spiked hairdo. There was also a tiny salon in the Great Gear Market along King's Road that also produced rough-and-ready razor-spiked punk hairstyles during this period. One favourite cutting method was to take small sections of hair and, twist and then roughly razor or scissor them to produce a jagged crop which could be spiked using gunk-like gel. What started as a small yet potent anarchic explosion soon rippled through the hair industry, and Punk's daring anything-goes attitude had a profound effect on the future course of hairstyling.

Another hairdressing company that began to make serious creative waves in the late 1970s was Toni&Guy, a London-based salon business run by five brothers, whose father had been a barber in a small town near Pompeii. The youngest sibling, Anthony Mascolo soon proved himself to be the creative genius of the family when he started using intricate weaving methods around 1978 to create astonishing hairstyles that were both progressive and experimental. Significantly Anthony Mascolo's creations were more like hair sculptures than pedestrian haircuts, and revealed a mastery of his craft. These elaborate constructions of hair were done using wigs and were creative "hair show" statements. Importantly, Anthony Mascolo demonstrated through example that the art of coiffure was still a highly relevant art form and that exciting new styles could be pioneered – you just needed the imagination, skill and patience. Whether it was the anarchic punk spikes of King's Road or experimental hair sculptures created by Toni&Guy, the progressive hairstyles of the late 1970s had a huge influence on the next generation of young hairdressers, who were to go on to create extraordinary boundary-pushing coiffures for a new Eighties post-punk generation.

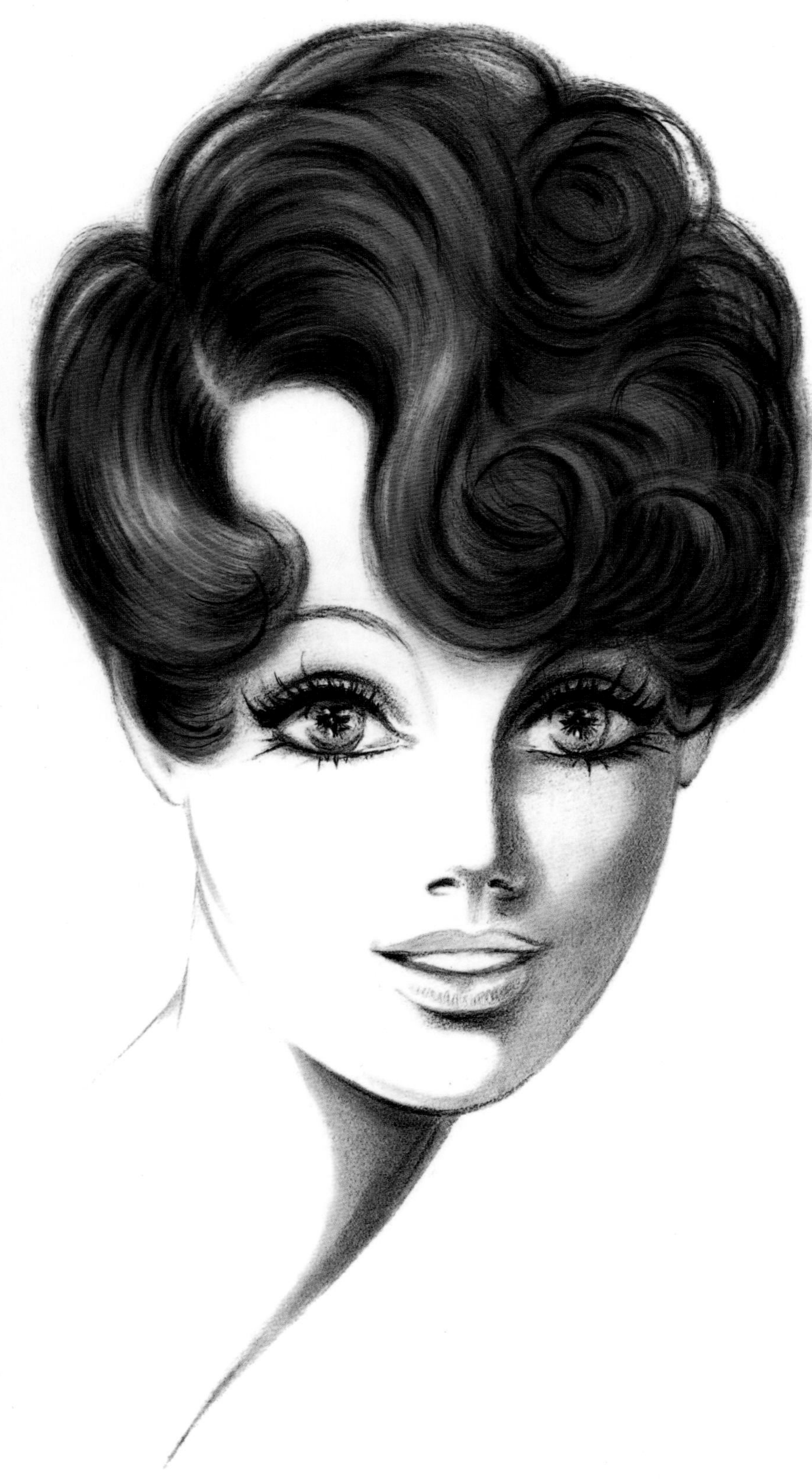

Hairstyle illustration by Martin Matagne for *30 Coiffures de Paris*, 1970

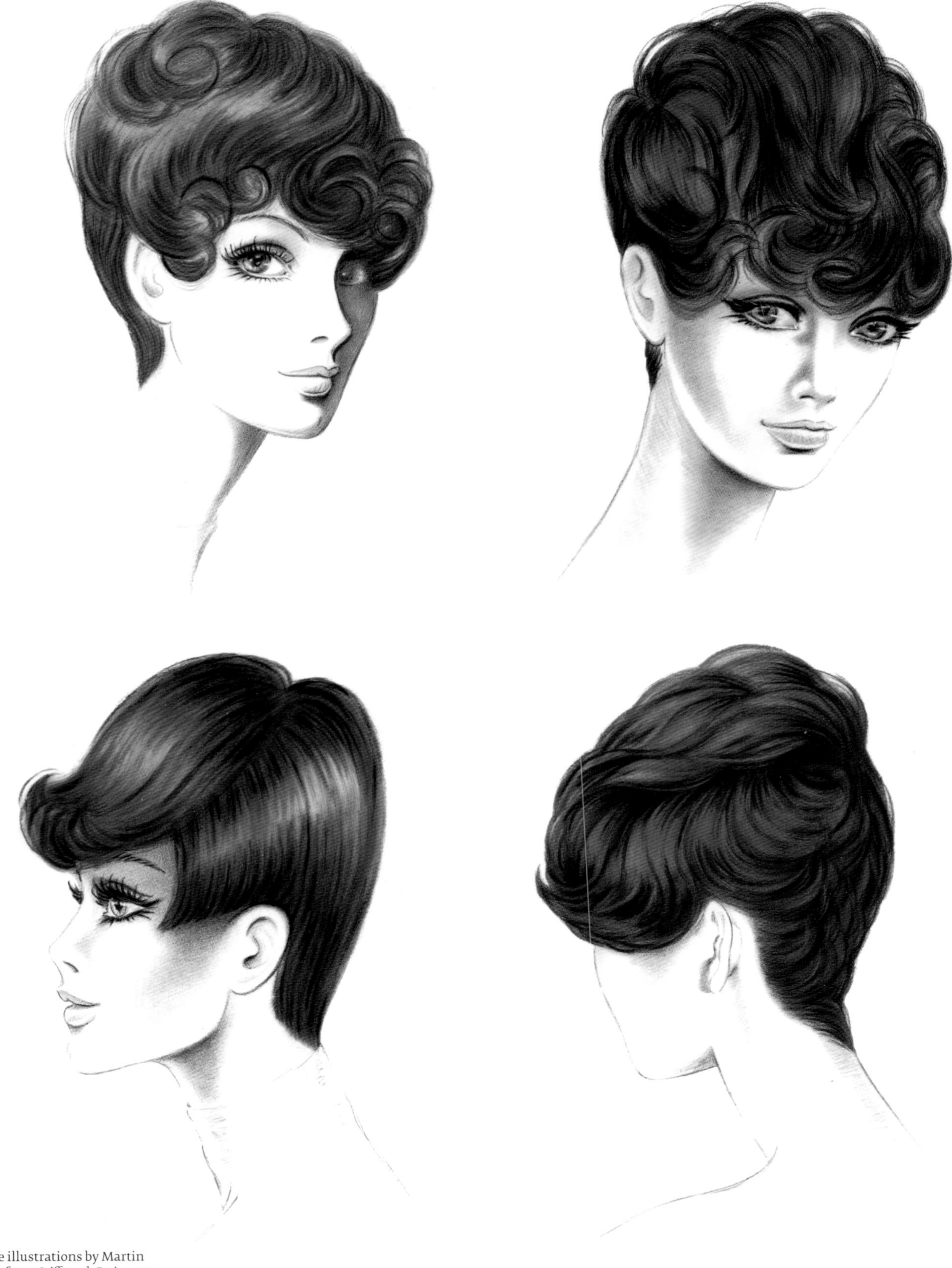

Hairstyle illustrations by Martin Matagne for *30 Coiffures de Paris*, 1970

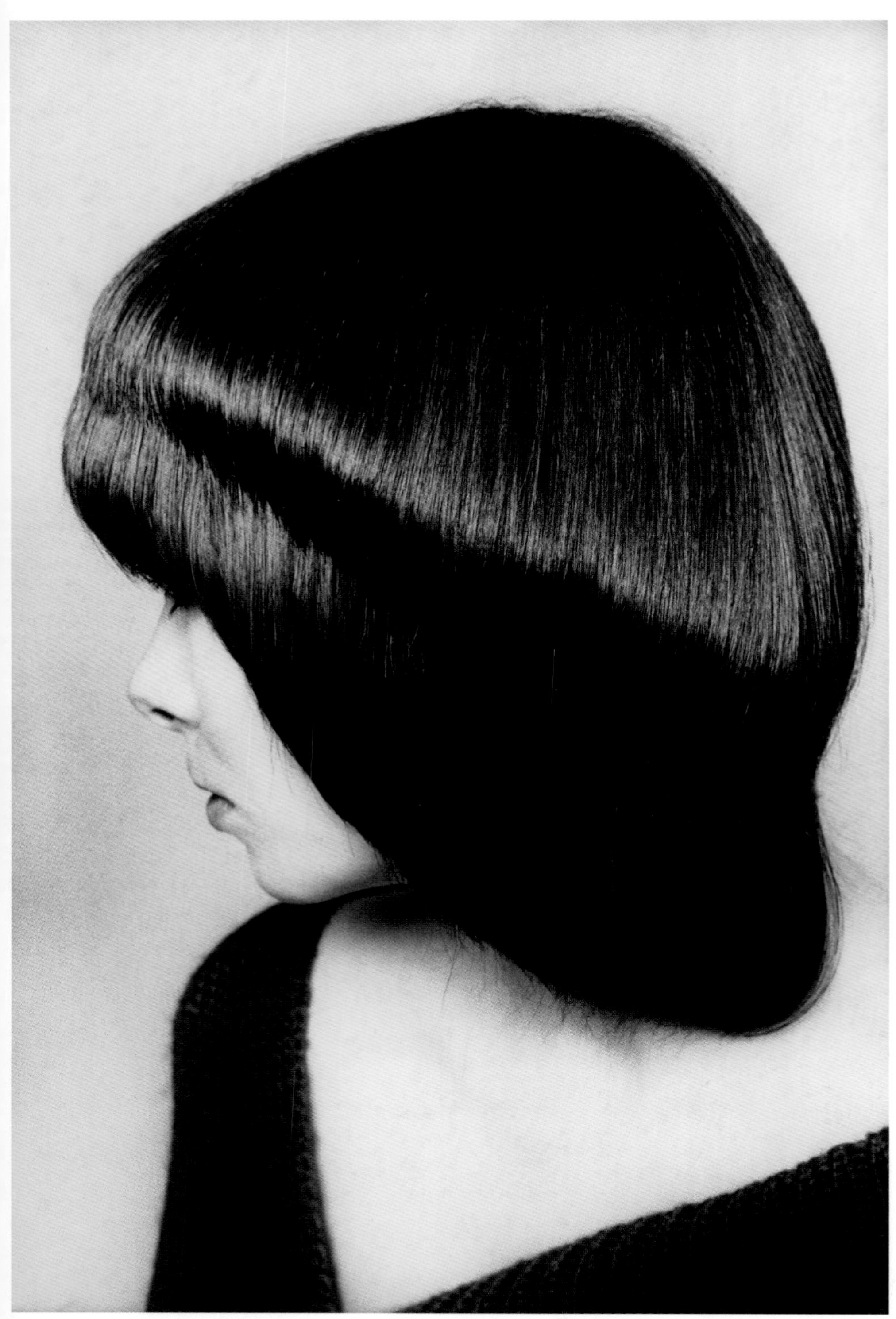

Anna Wintour, hairstyle by Leslie Russell of Smile, 1970, photographed by Steve Hiatt

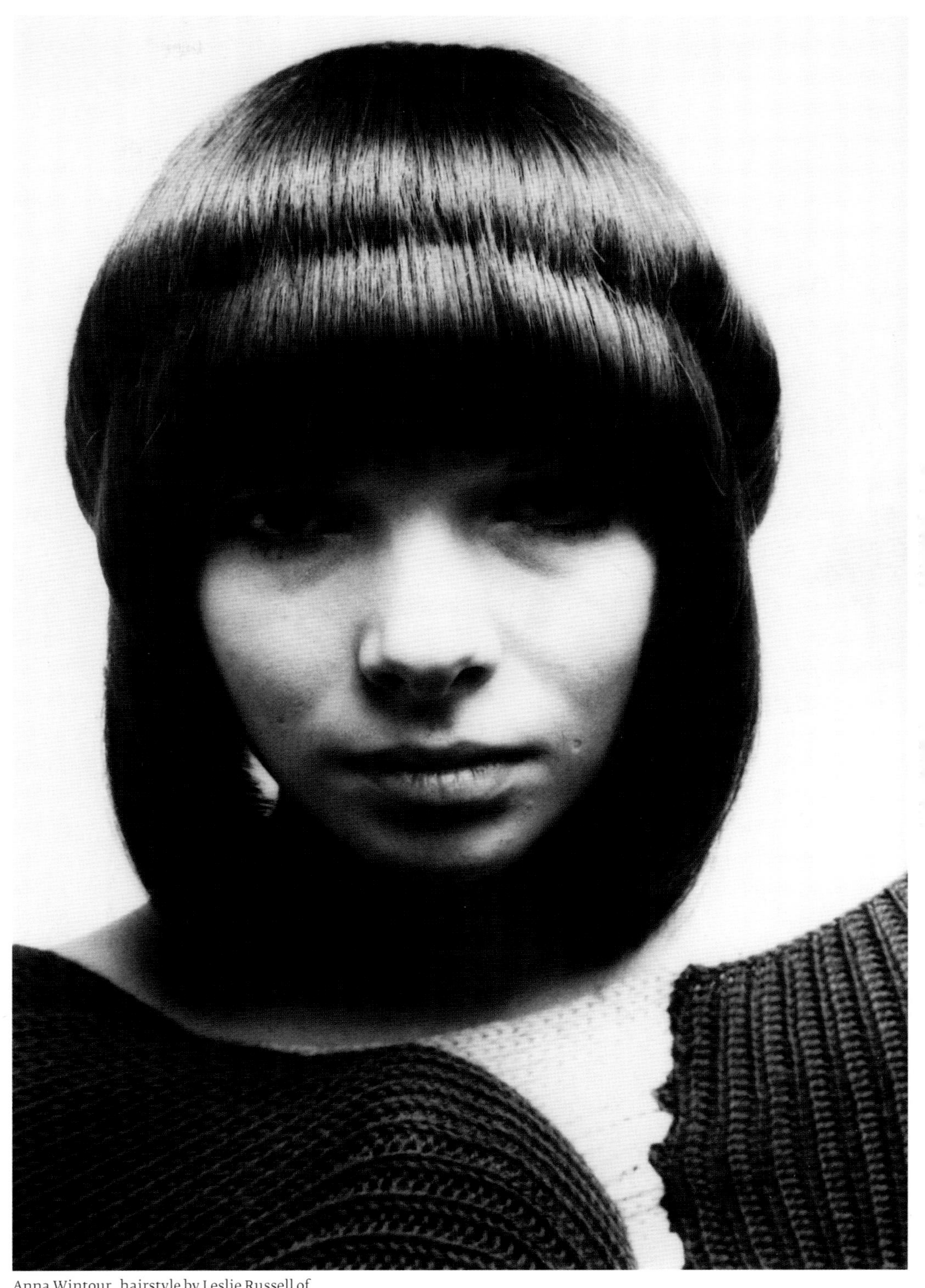

Anna Wintour, hairstyle by Leslie Russell of Smile, 1970, photographed by Steve Hiatt

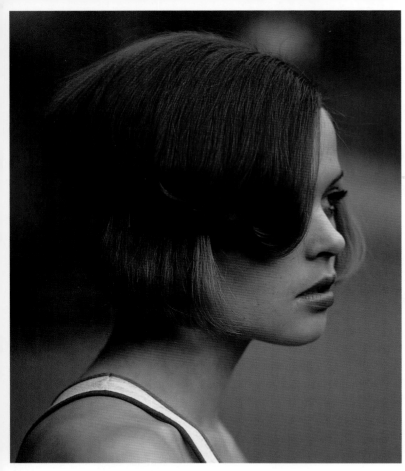

Two-tone hairstyle by Keith Wainwright and Leslie Russell of Smile, 1971, photographed by Steve Hiatt

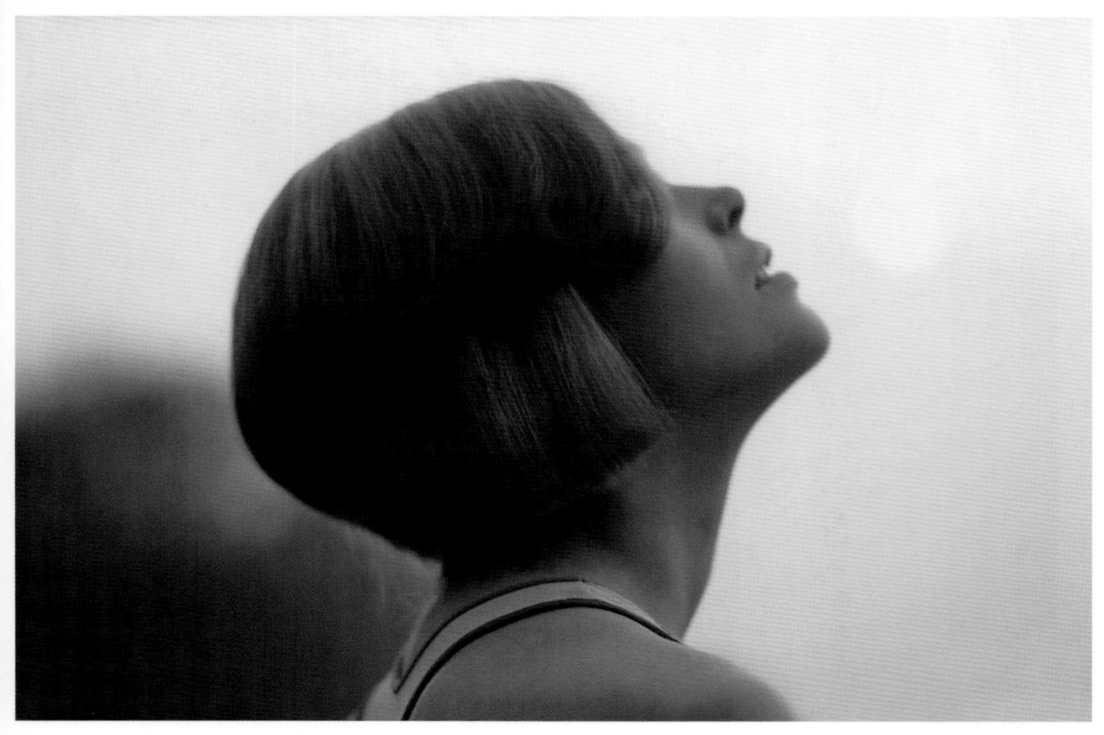

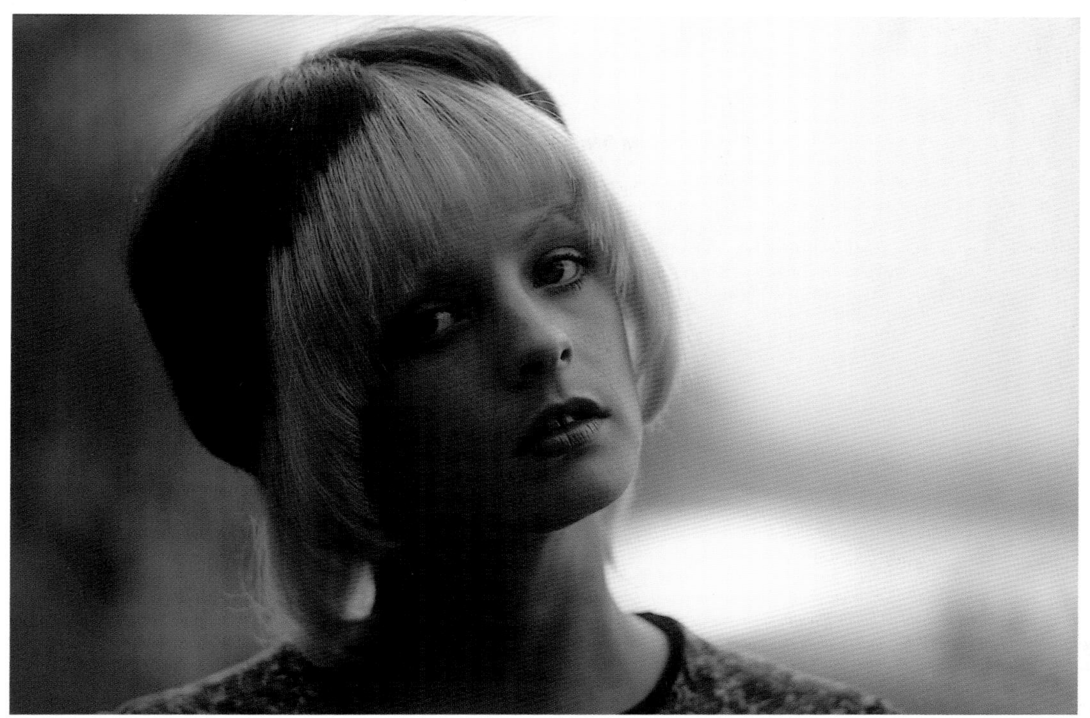

Two-tone hairstyle by Keith Wainwright and Leslie Russell of Smile, 1971, photographed by Steve Hiatt

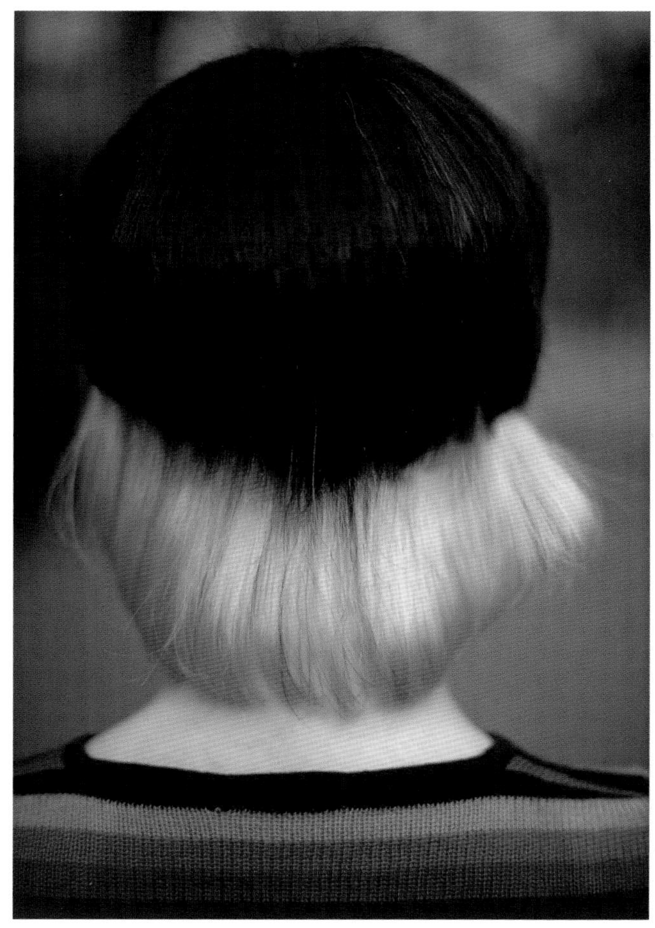

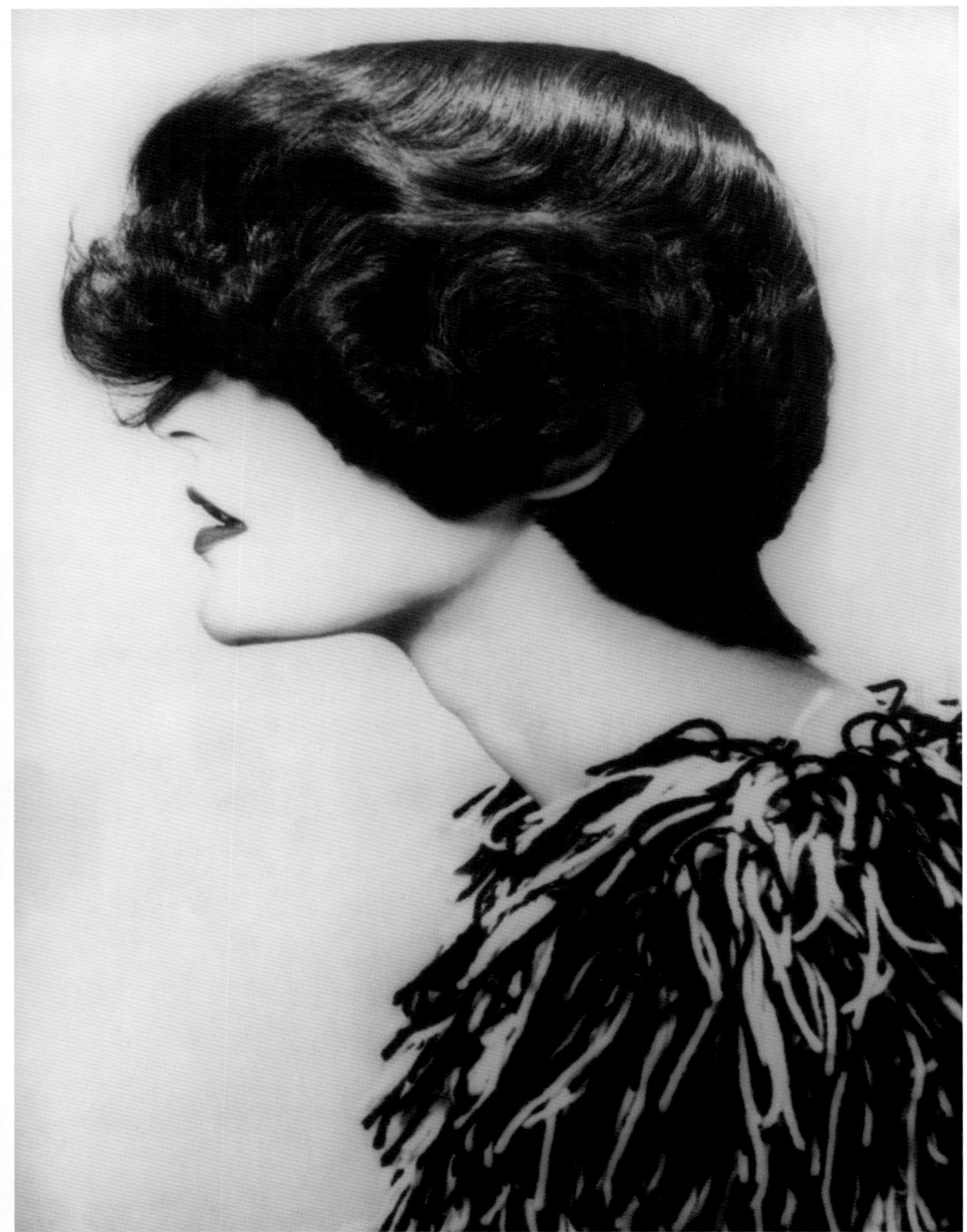

'New Chic' hairstyle, Paris, 1971

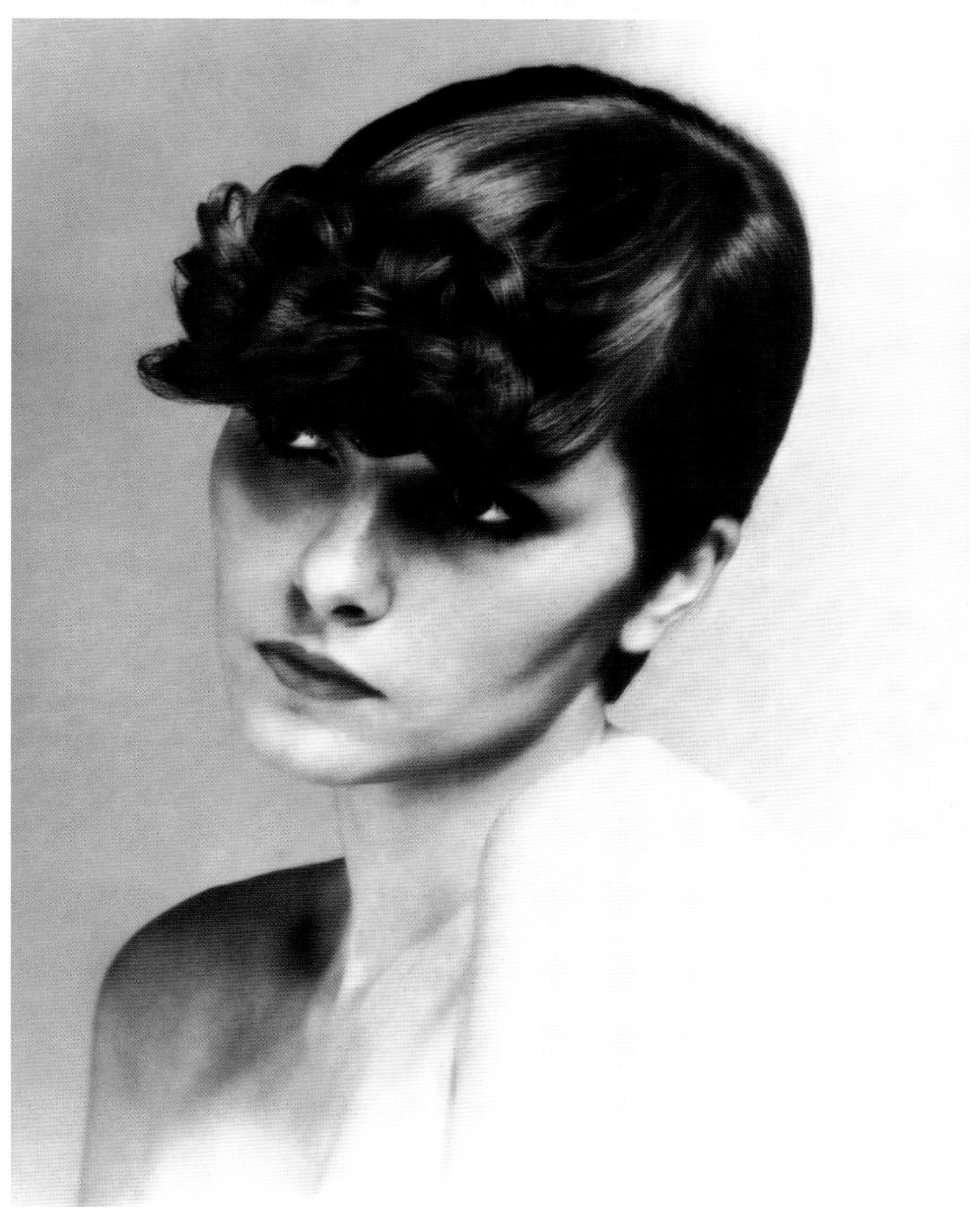

Hairstyle by Leslie Russell of Smile, 1972, photographed by James Wedge

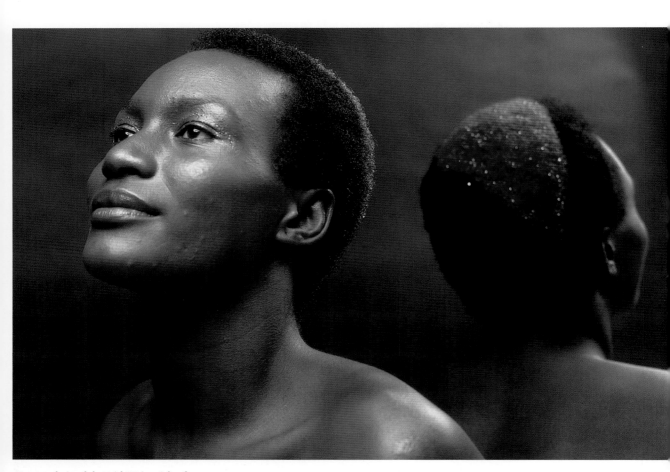

Two-tone hairstyle by Keith Wainwright of Smile, 1972, photographed by Steve Hiatt

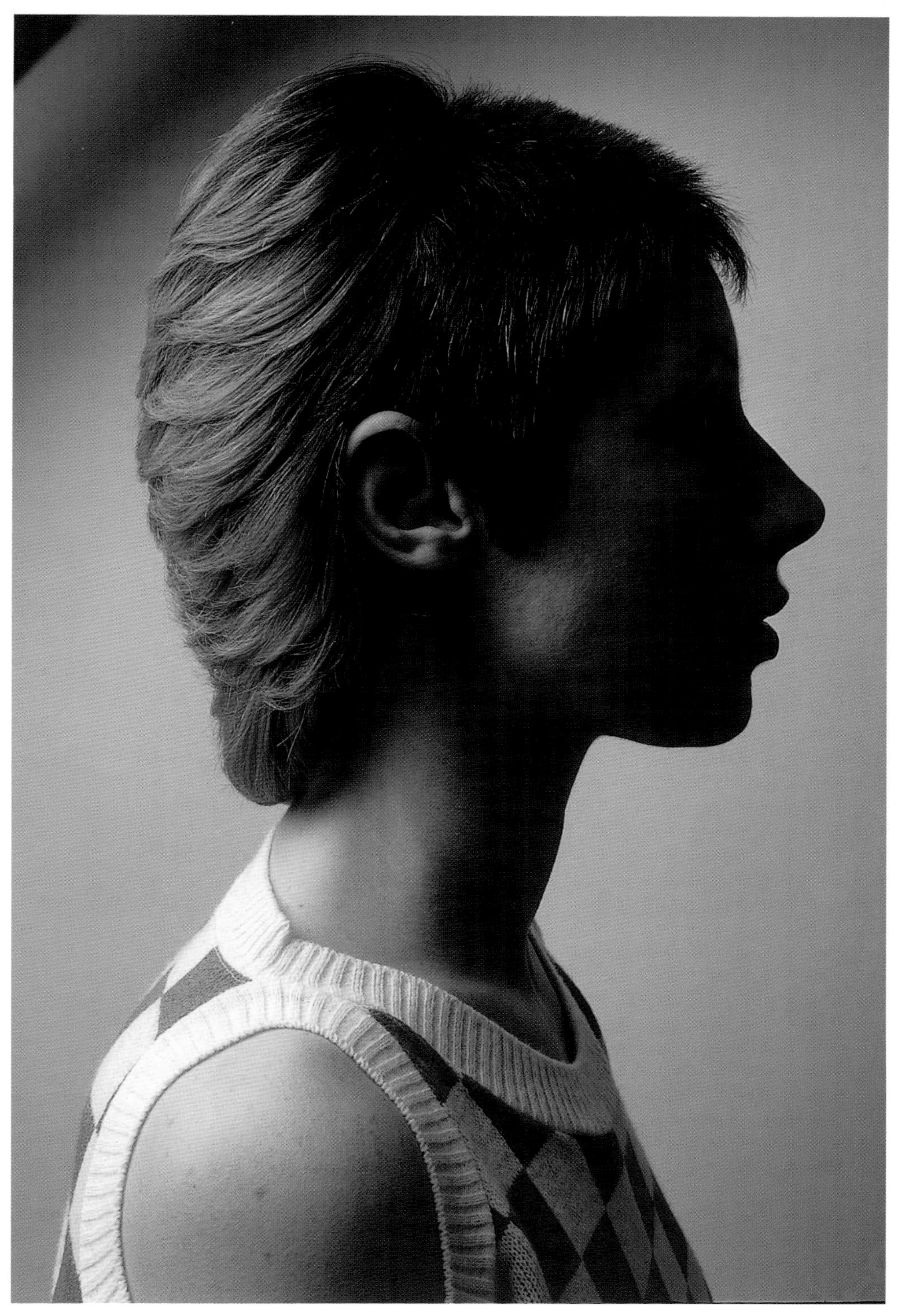

Hairstyle by Keith Wainwright of Smile, 1972,
photographed by Steve Hiatt

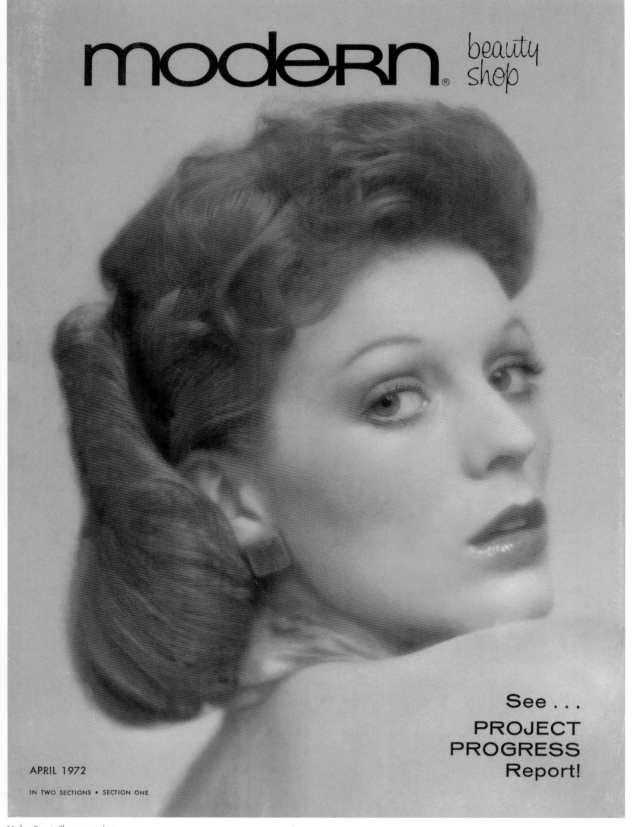

Modern Beauty Shop magazine cover, 1972

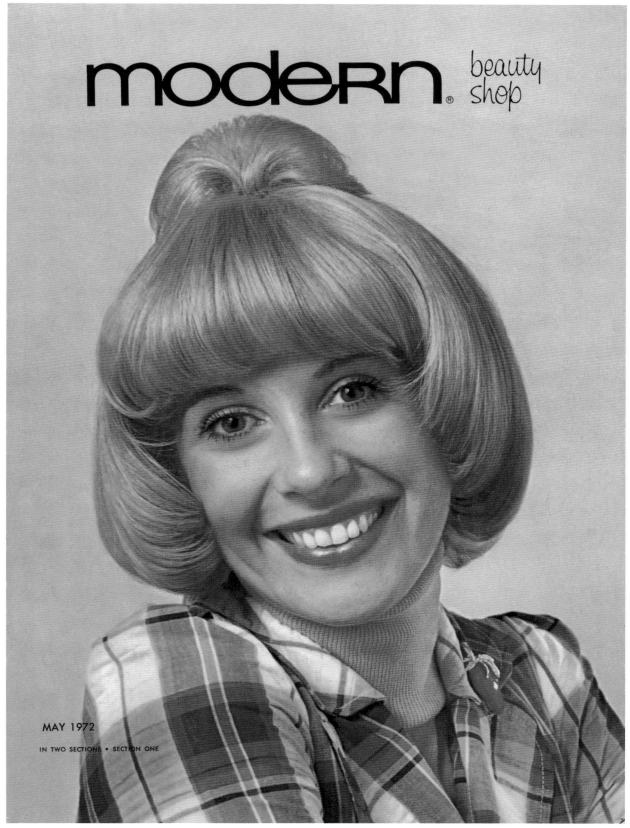

Modern Beauty Shop magazine cover, 1972

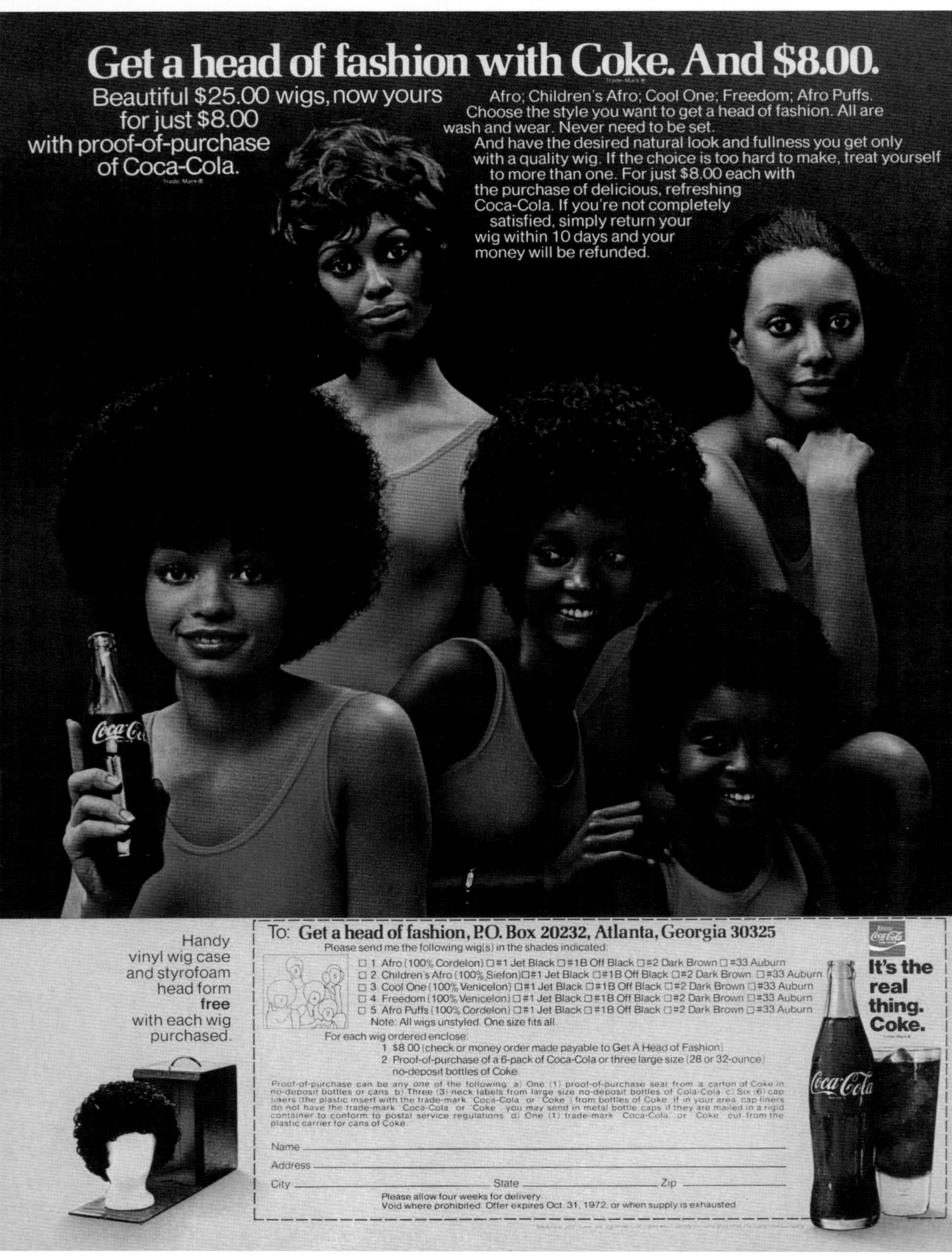

Advertisement for Coca Cola and Afro wig Offer, 1972, *Ebony*

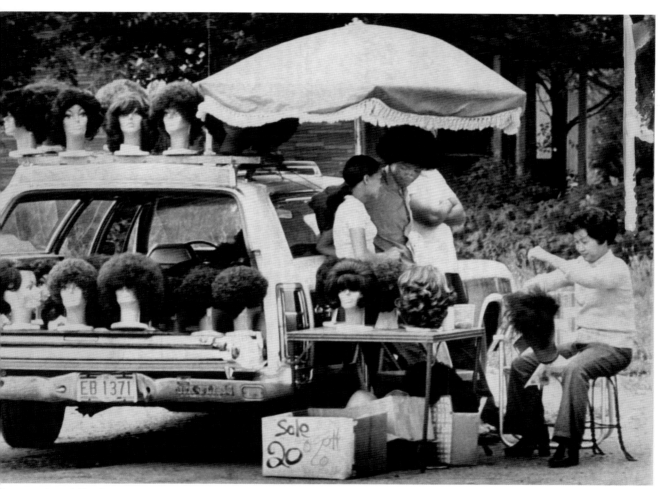

hwa Maxey's Roadside Wig
nd, St. Louis, USA, 1976

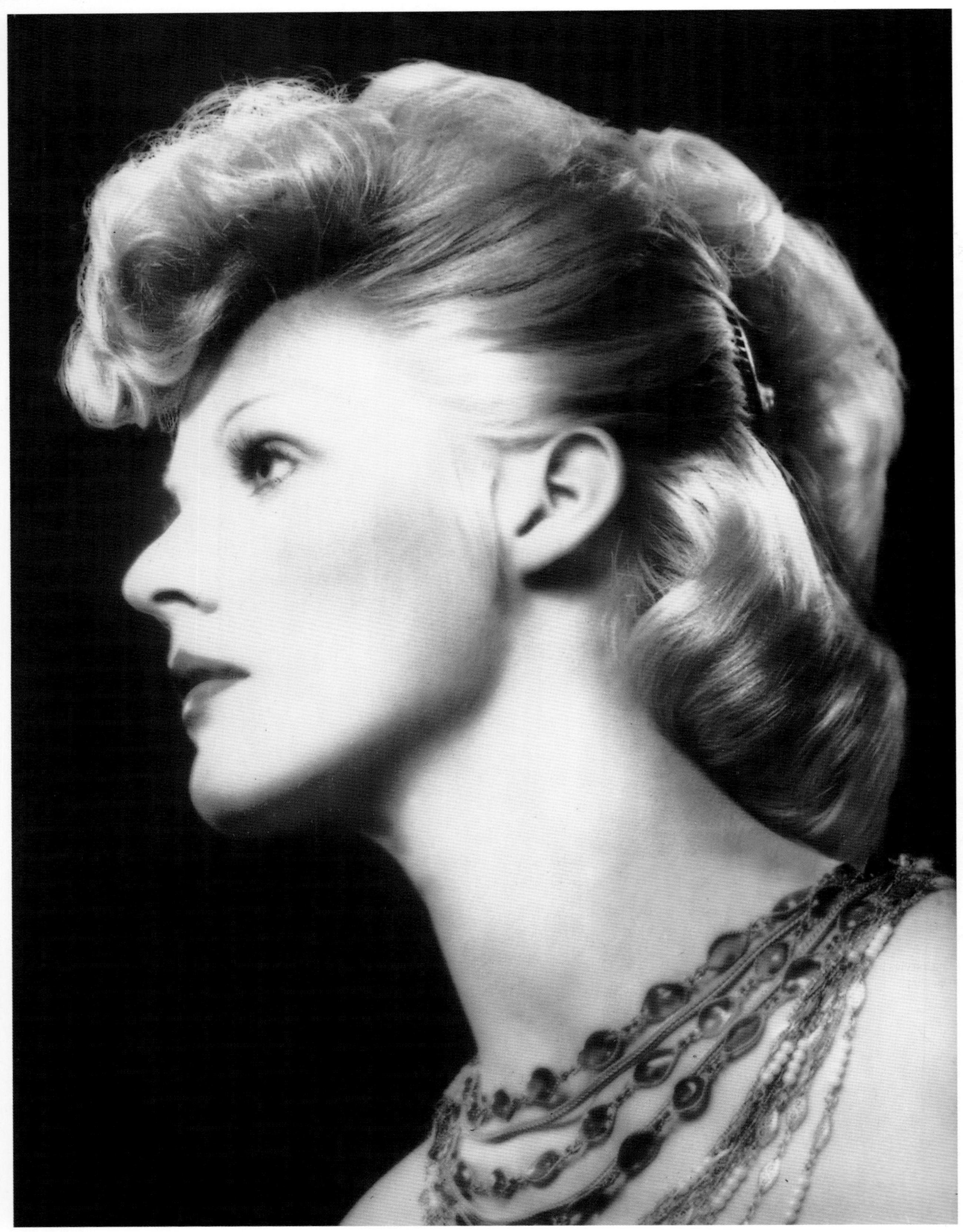

Hairstyle created by La Saint
Sylvestre (Paris), 1972

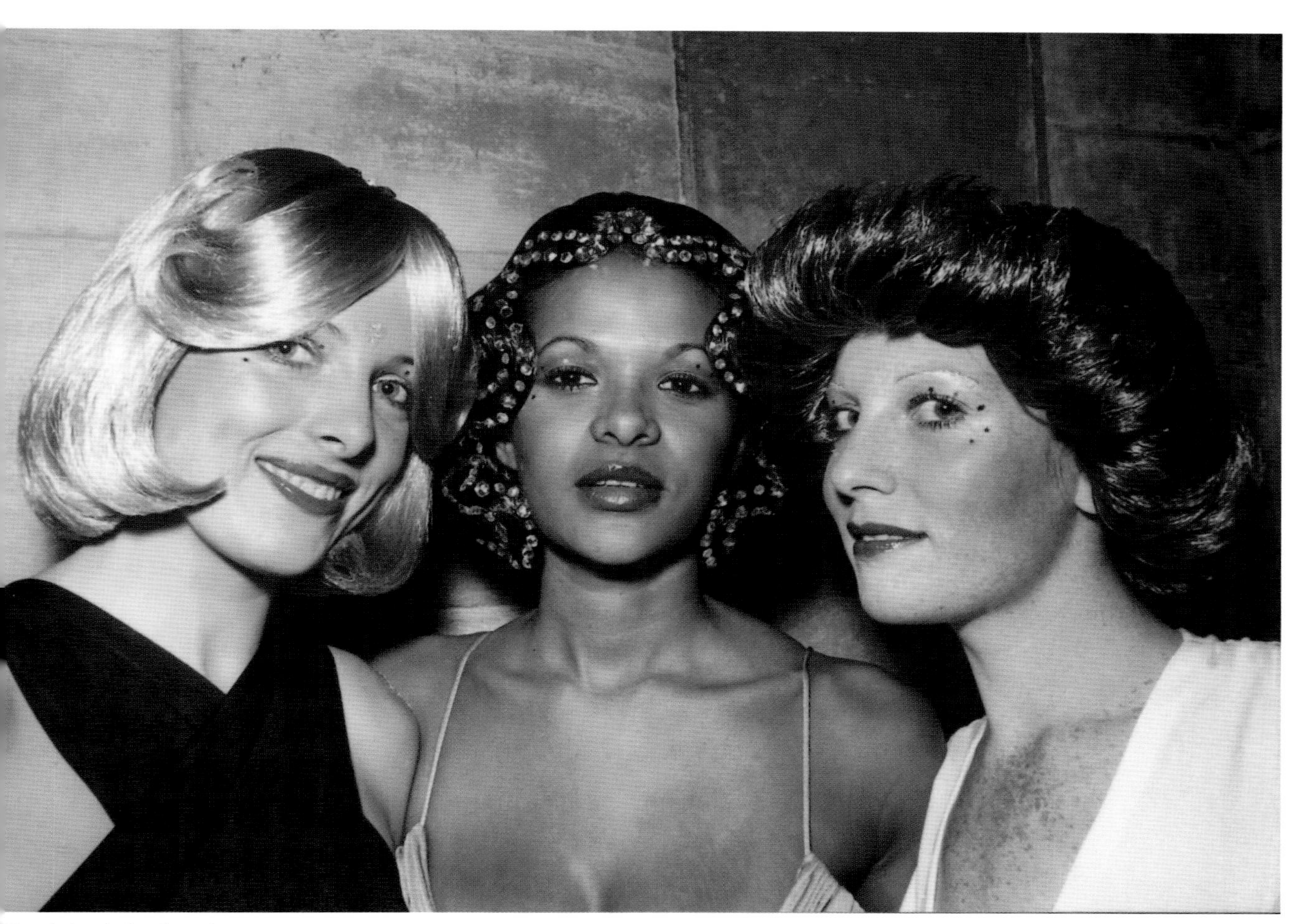

Three hairstyles by Alexandre de Paris, 1974

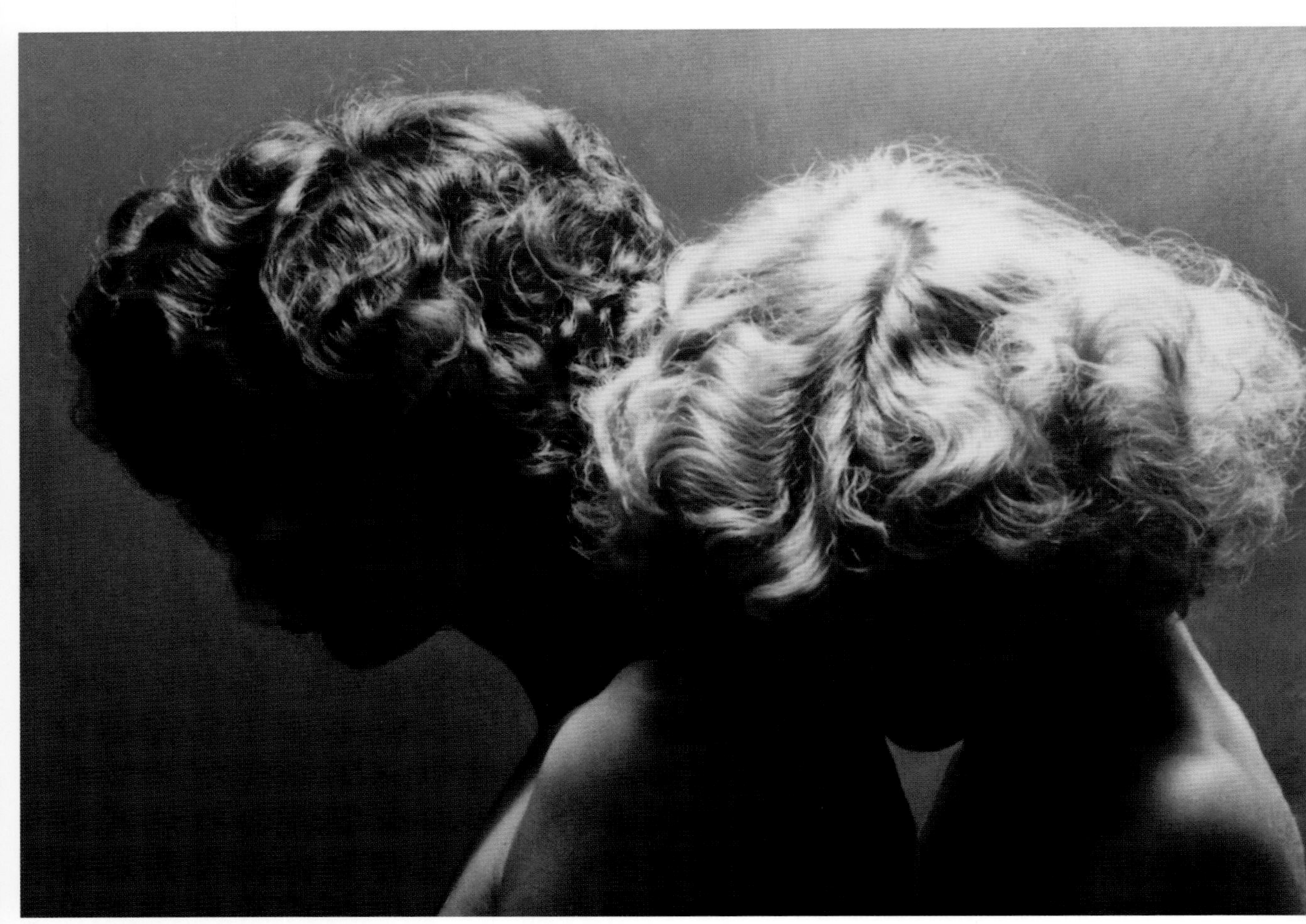

Two hairstyles for autumn/
winter by Jacques Dessange, 1974

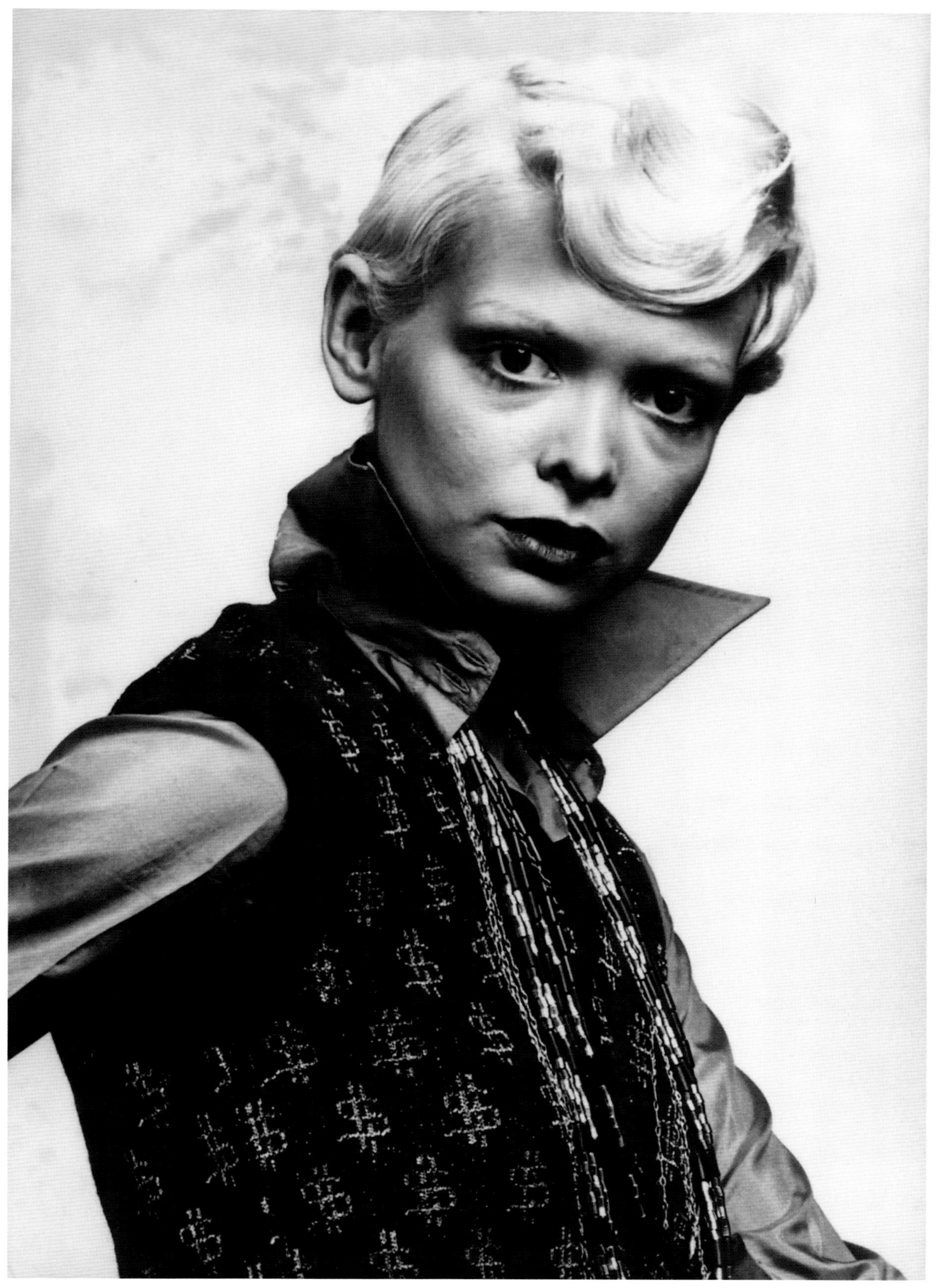

'Crans' hairstyle for the Spring
by Jean-Louis Saint Roch, 1974

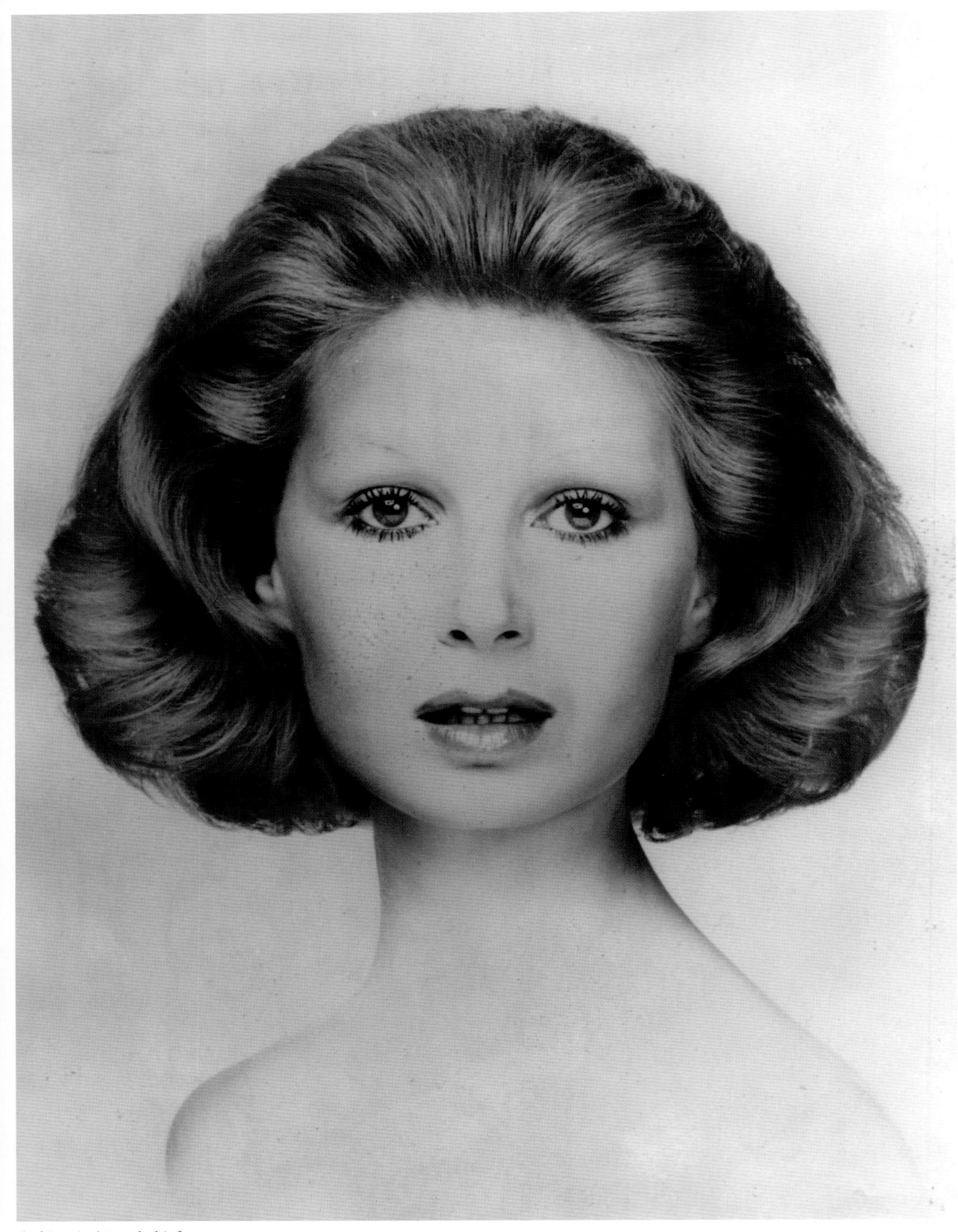

'Sphinx Line', French chic for your autumn locks, Paris, 1974

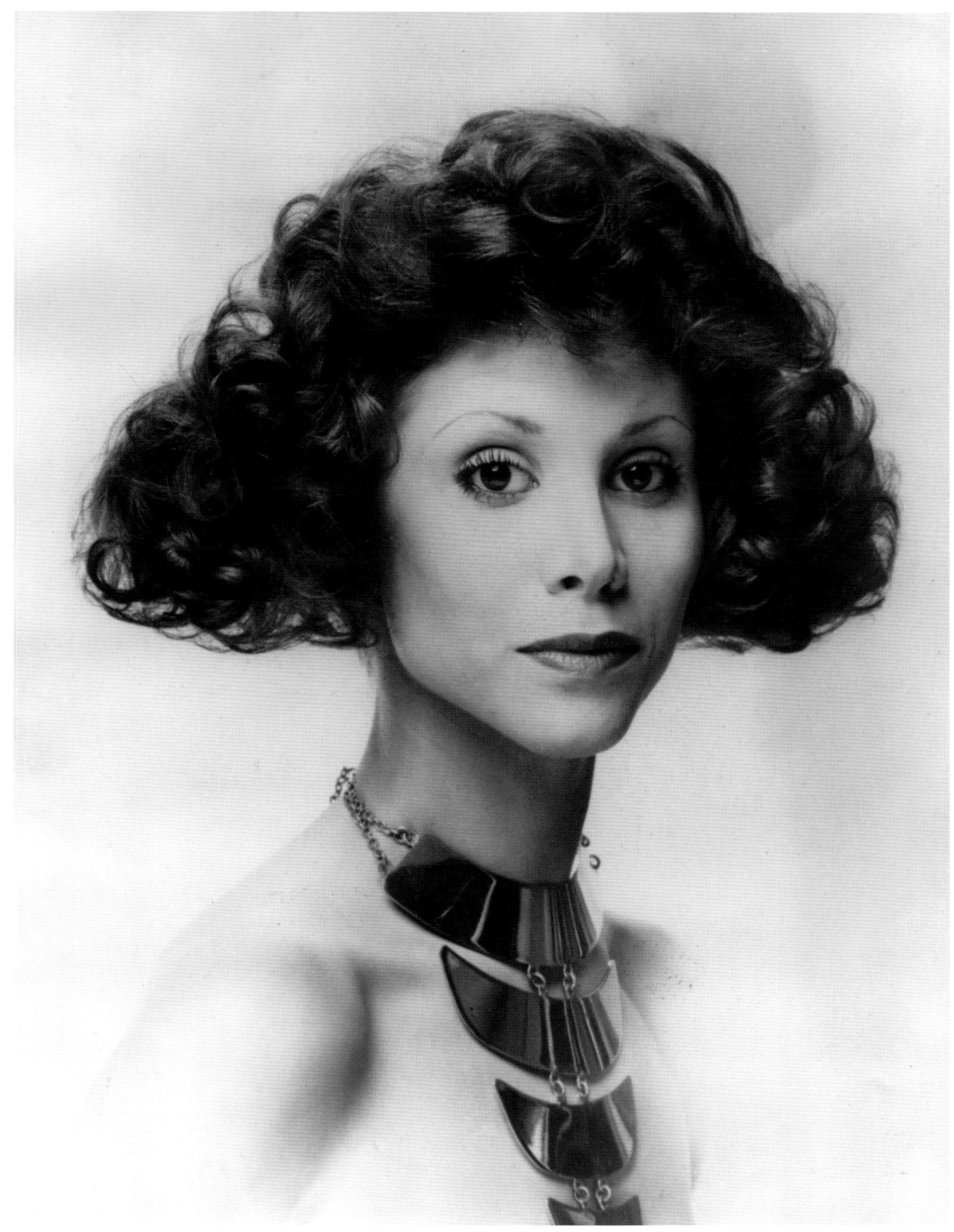

'Sphinx Line', French chic for your autumn locks, Paris, 1974

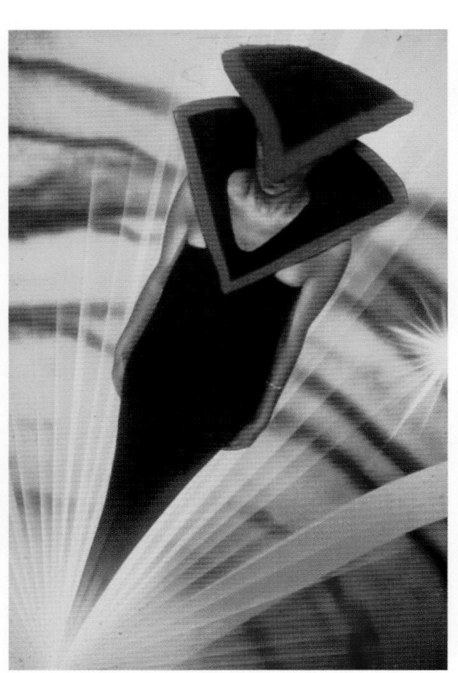

'The Concorde' by Trevor Sorbie at Vidal Sassoon, 1974

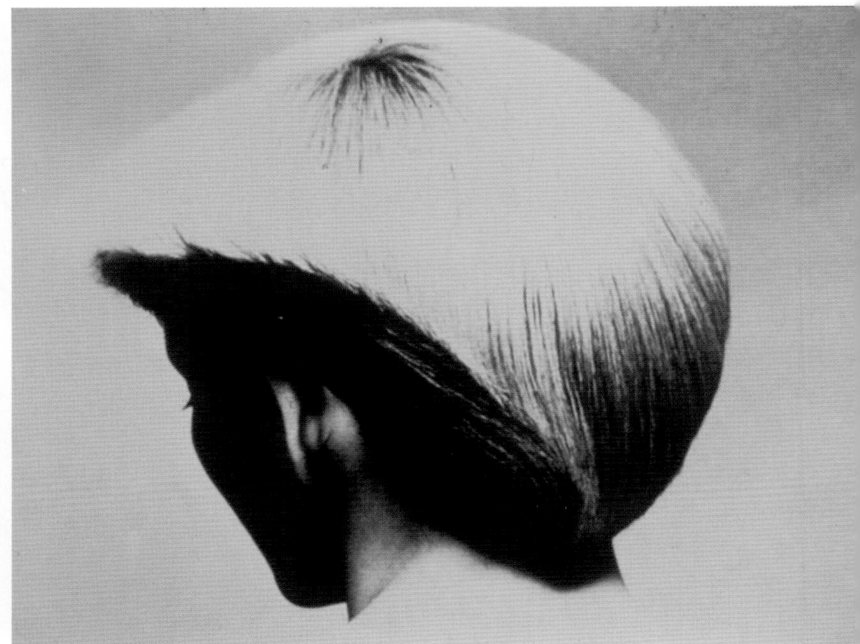

'The Wedge' by Trevor Sorbie at Vidal Sassoon, 1974

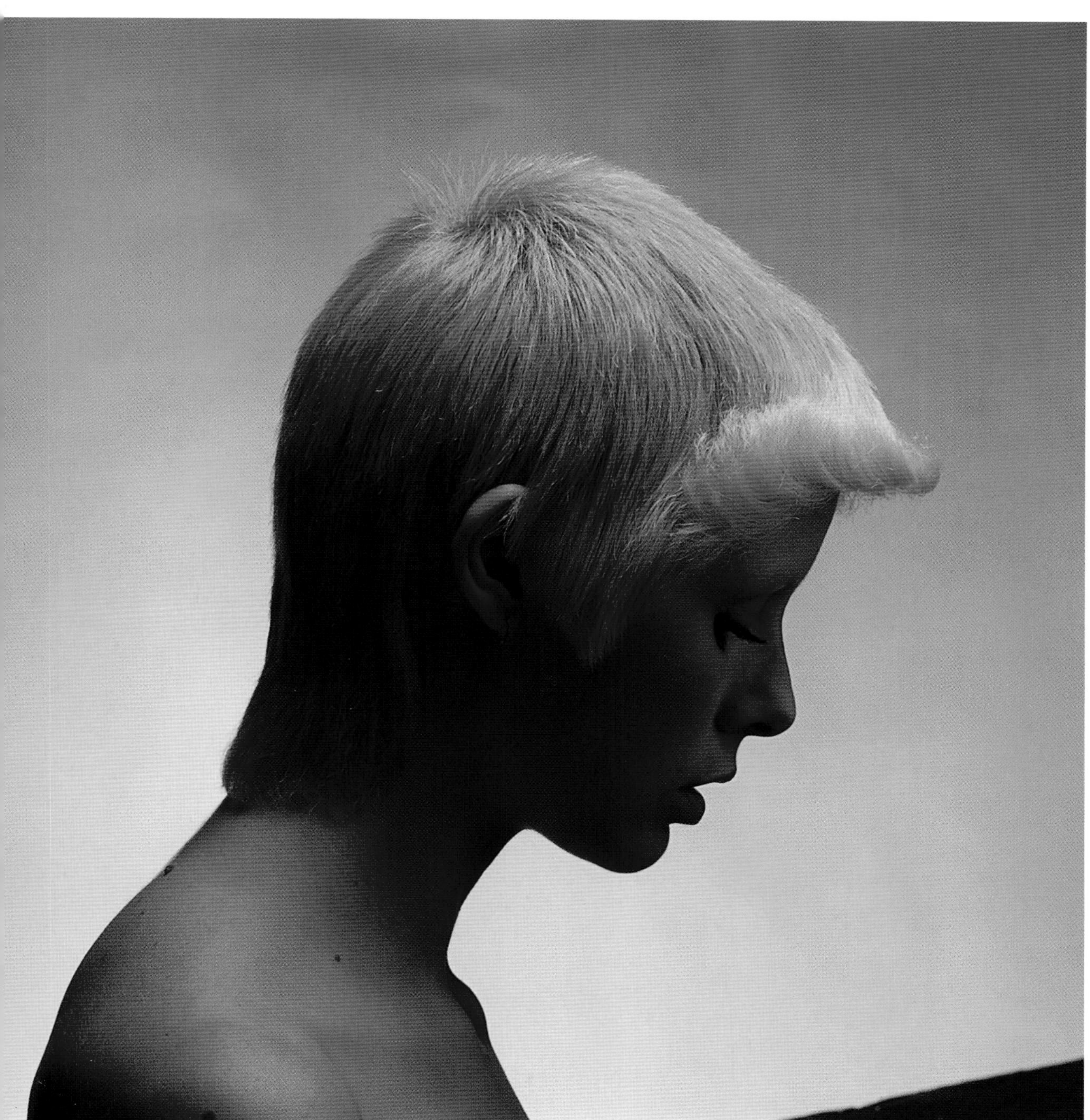

airstyle by Leslie Russell of Smile, c. 1974,
notographed by Steve Hiatt

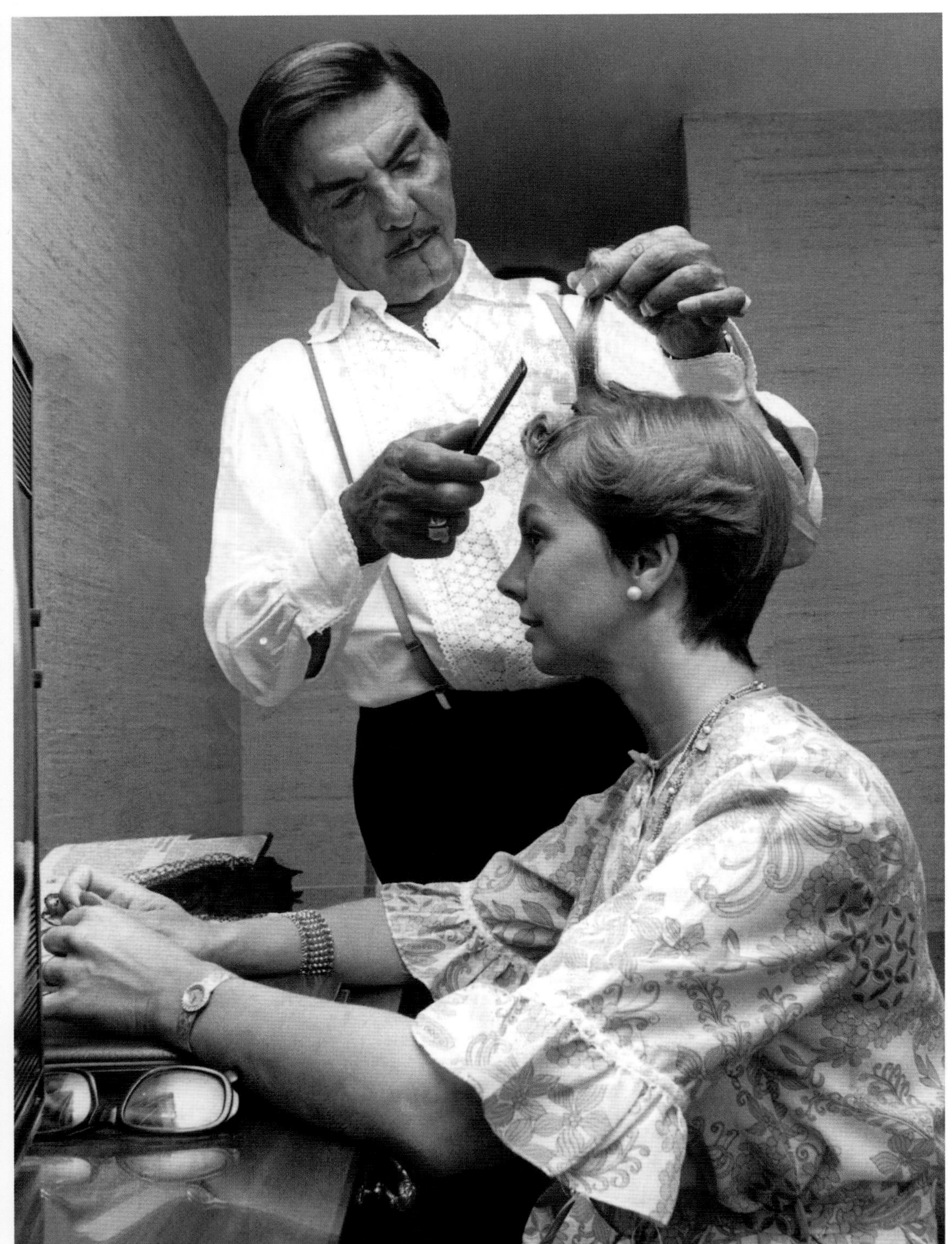

'Putting on the Style', hairdresser Raymond "Teasie Weasie" Bessone, 1975

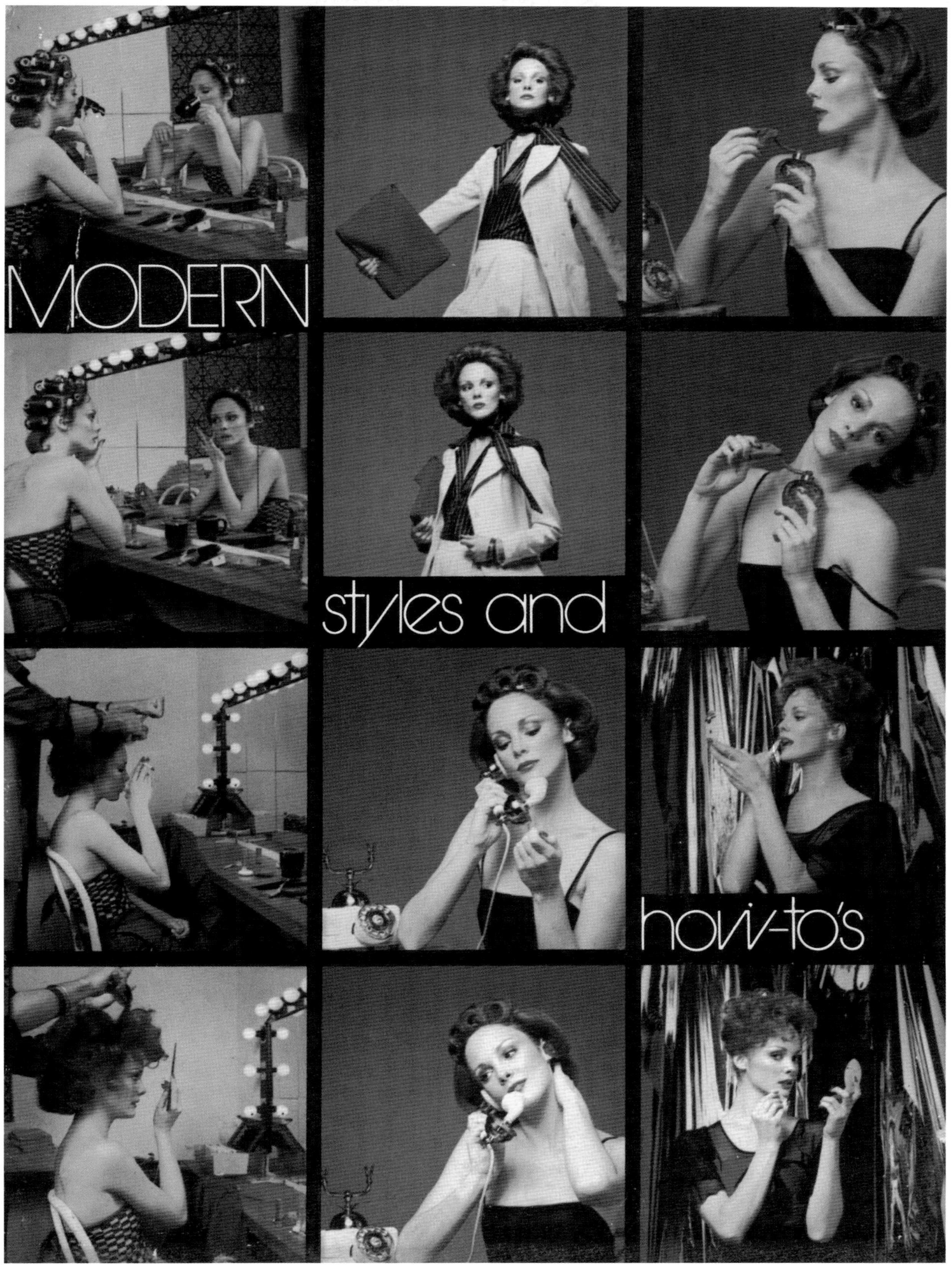

Modern Styles and How-To's magazine cover, 1975

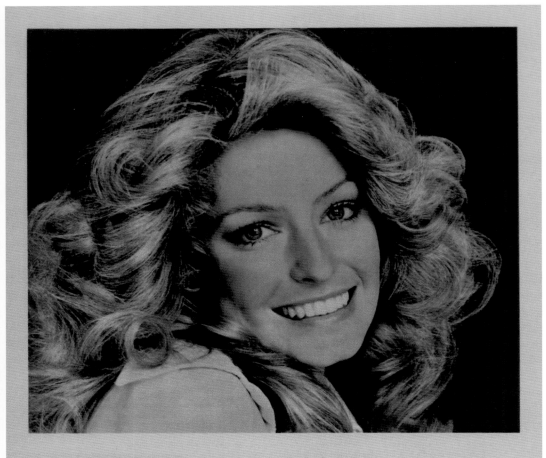

Wella Balsam will make your hair more beautiful than any of its imitators can.

Let your hair convince you.

When Wella created the first balsam conditioner, it started a revolution. Nothing else can make your hair so beautiful, so shiny, so easy to comb, in so short a time. Today there are lots of imitators around, but none surpasses Wella Balsam for making your hair gleam with fresh natural beauty. Even damaged hair!

In just one minute, Wella Balsam strengthens each hair where it is weak, fills in porosity and smooths split ends, leaving your hair tangle-free, lustrous and lusciously beautiful. Get the original balsam and see for yourself. Your hair will show you the difference.

Wella Balsam. Available in Regular and Extra Body formulations, and in Wella Balsam Conditioning Shampoo, the shampoo that conditions *while* you shampoo.

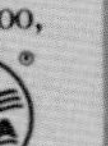

©1975 The Wella Corp.

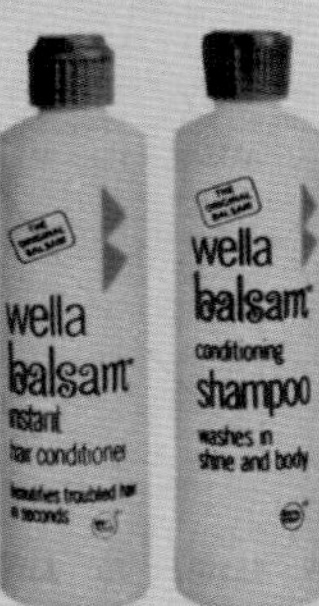

220 NOVEMBER, 1975

Wella shampoo advertisement featuring Farrah Fawcett, 1975

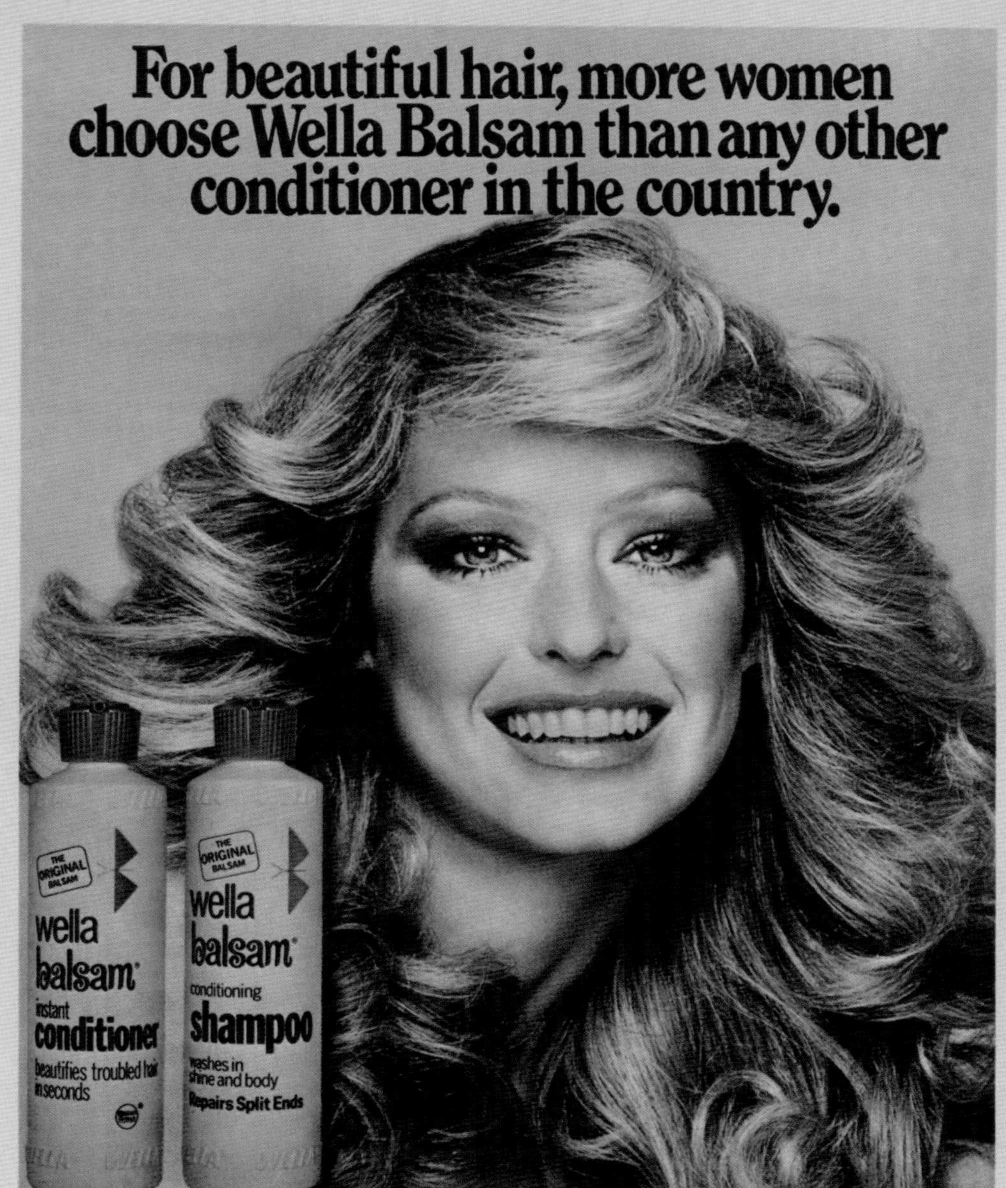

For beautiful hair, more women choose Wella Balsam than any other conditioner in the country.
THE ORIGINAL BALSAM
wella balsam
instant conditioner
beautifies troubled hair in seconds
THE ORIGINAL BALSAM
wella balsam
conditioning shampoo
washes in shine and body
Repairs Split Ends
Here's why.
Wella Balsam is the original balsam conditioner. Whether your hair is long or short, Wella Balsam can make it silky soft, shiny, and easy to comb, all in one minute.
It only takes a half-ounce of Wella Balsam to make your hair gloriously beautiful, so it's more economical, too.
Our imitators tried to fool you by copying our bottle and our name, but they couldn't copy Wella Balsam's performance. So they can't fool the millions of American women who choose Wella Balsam over all other hair conditioners.
For long hair or short hair, get Wella Balsam, America's favorite conditioner. And to get your hair beautifully clean, try Wella Balsam Shampoo, the conditioning shampoo that repairs split ends.
WELLA
©1976 The Wella Corp.
160
WOMAN'S DAY/JUNE 1976

Wella shampoo advertisement featuring Farrah Fawcett, 1976

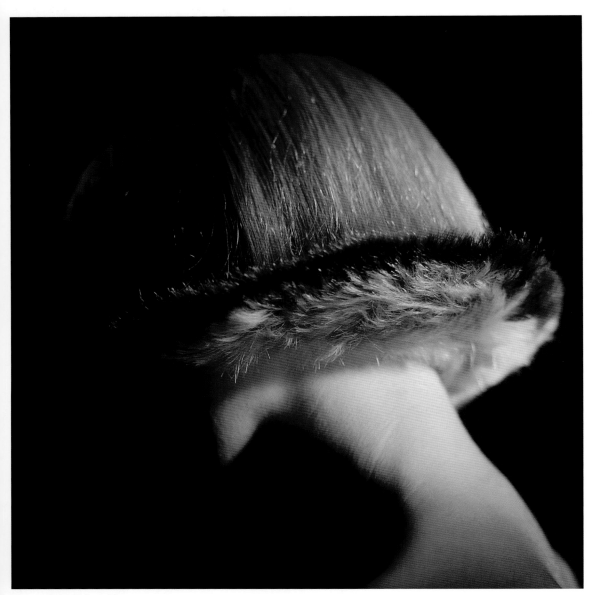

Two-tone hairstyle by Keith Wainwright and Leslie Russell, c.1975

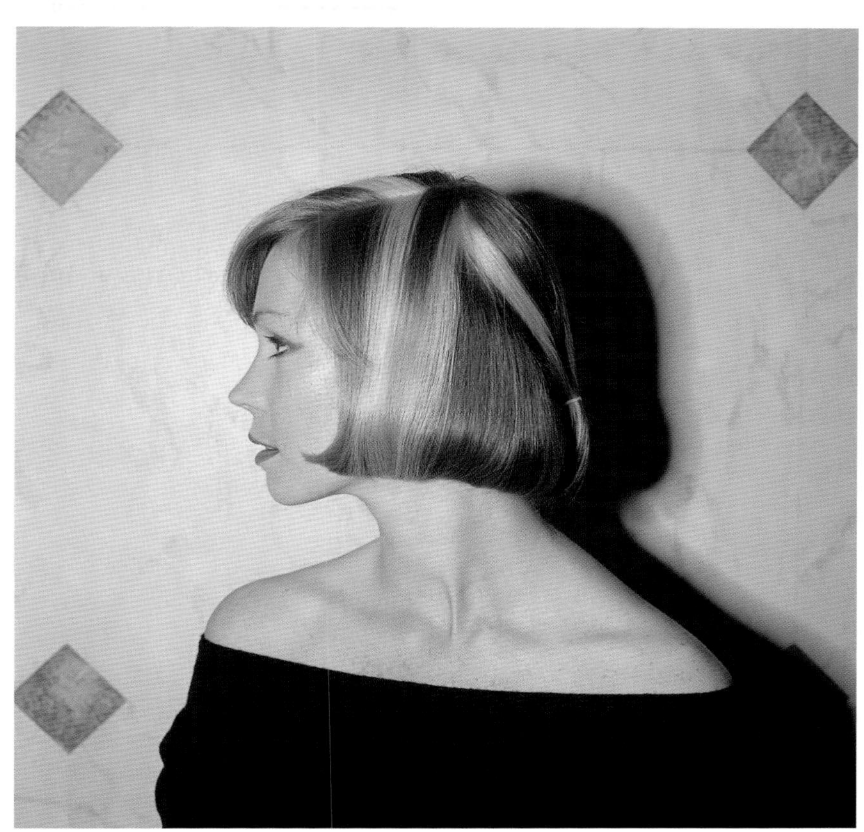

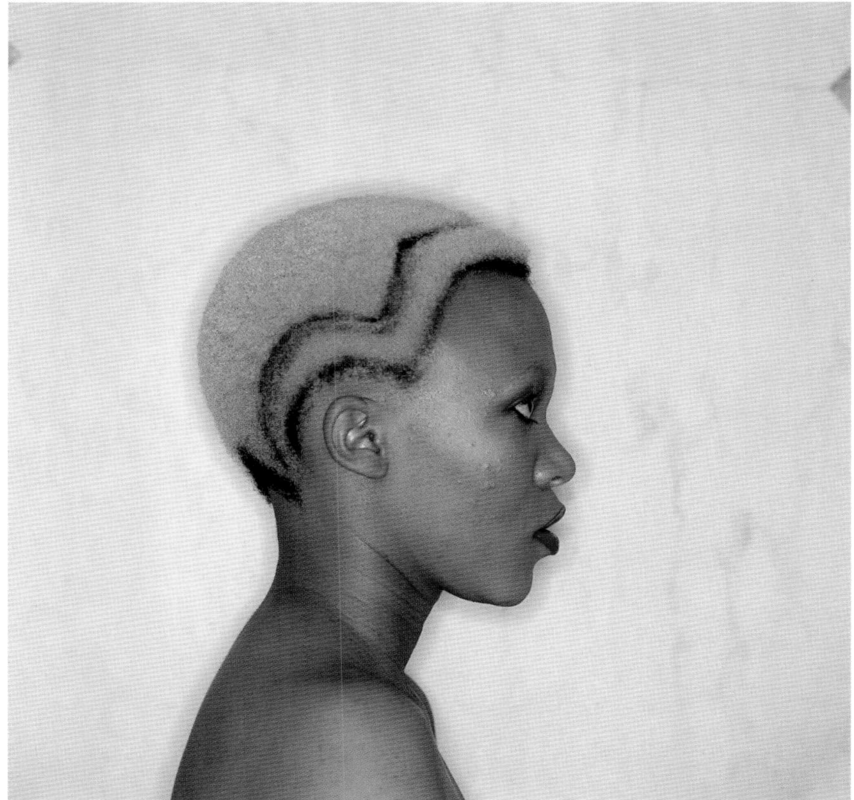

airstyles by Keith Wainwright
f Smile, 1976, photographed by
im Street-Porter

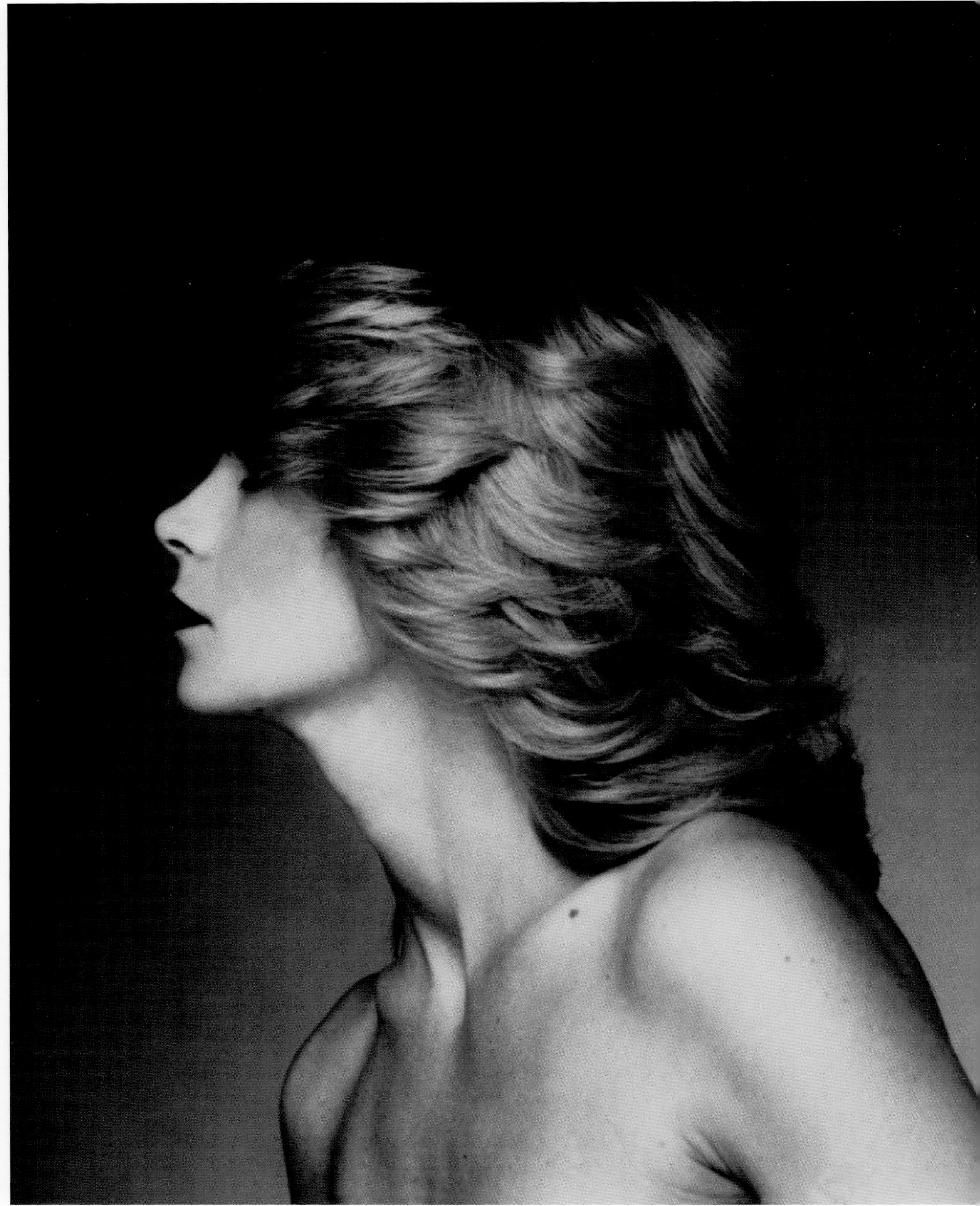

'Chunky' hairstyle by Anthony Mascolo for TONI&GUY, 1976

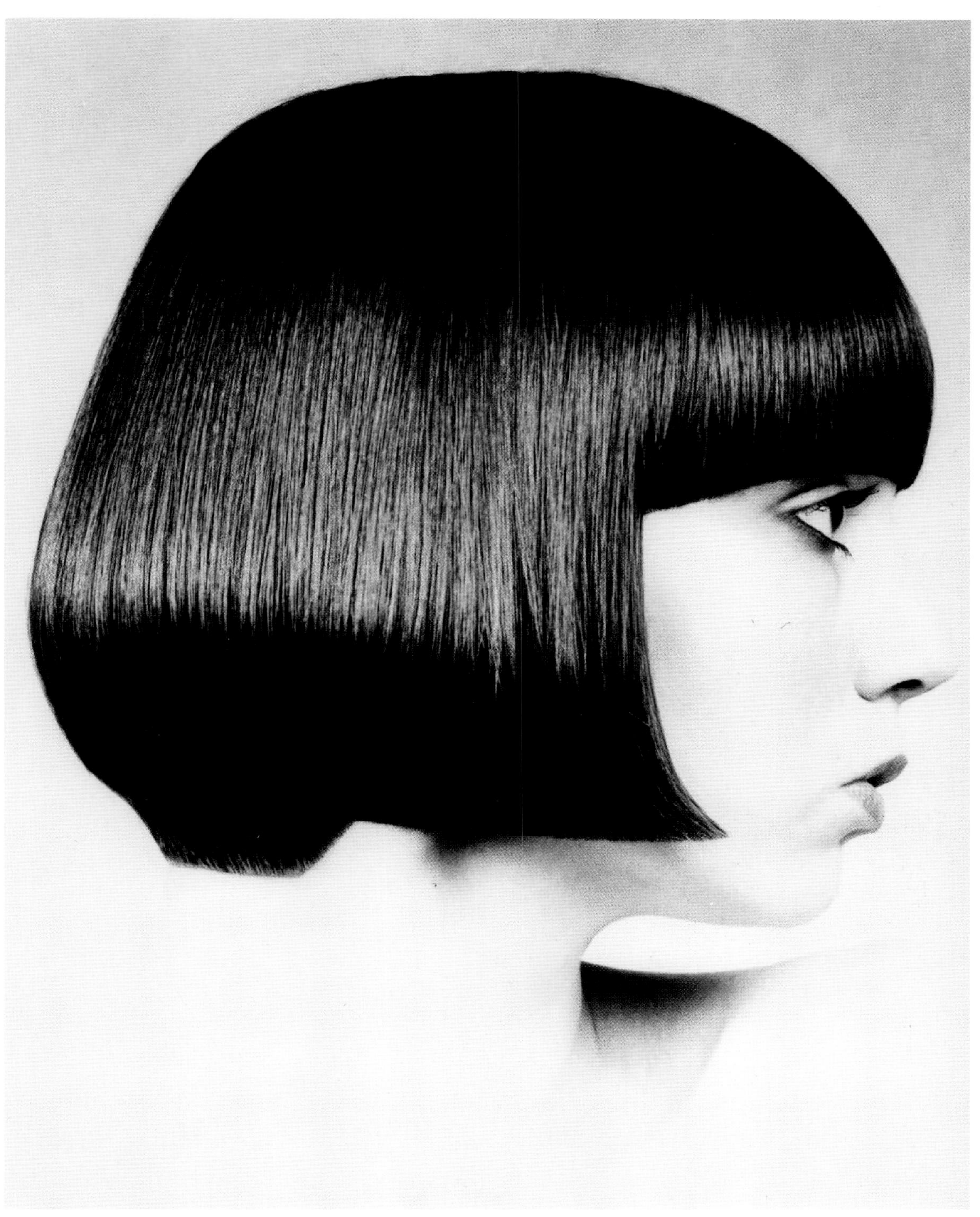

'Bob' hairstyle by Anthony Mascolo for TONI&GUY, 1976

Hairstyle by Keith Wainwright
of Smile, 1976

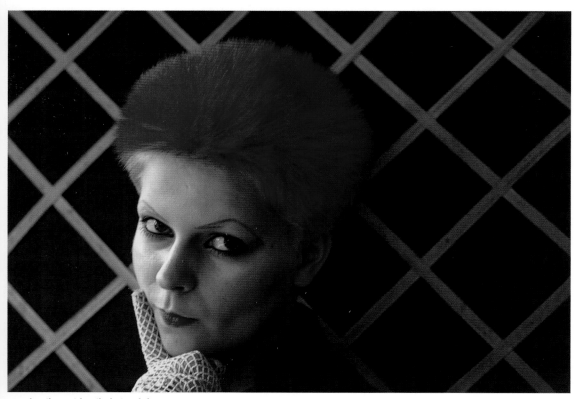

Toyah Wilcox with spiky hairstyle by
Keith Wainwright of Smile, 1977

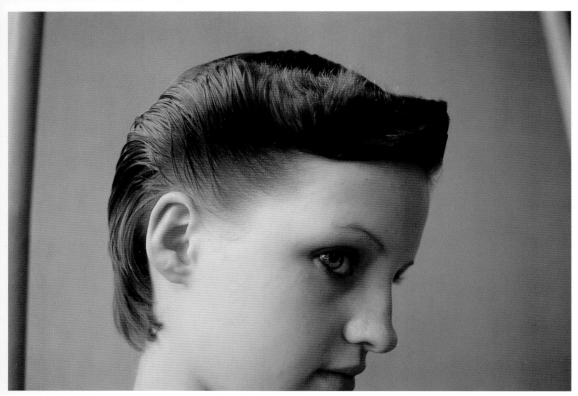

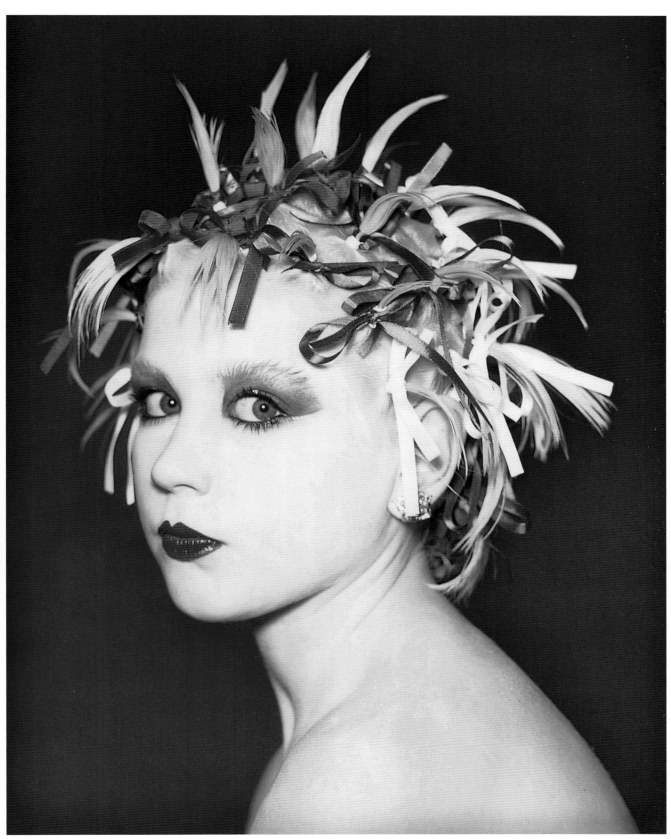

Debbie Juvenile (aka Debbie Wilson),
hairstyle by Keith Wainwright of Smile, 1977

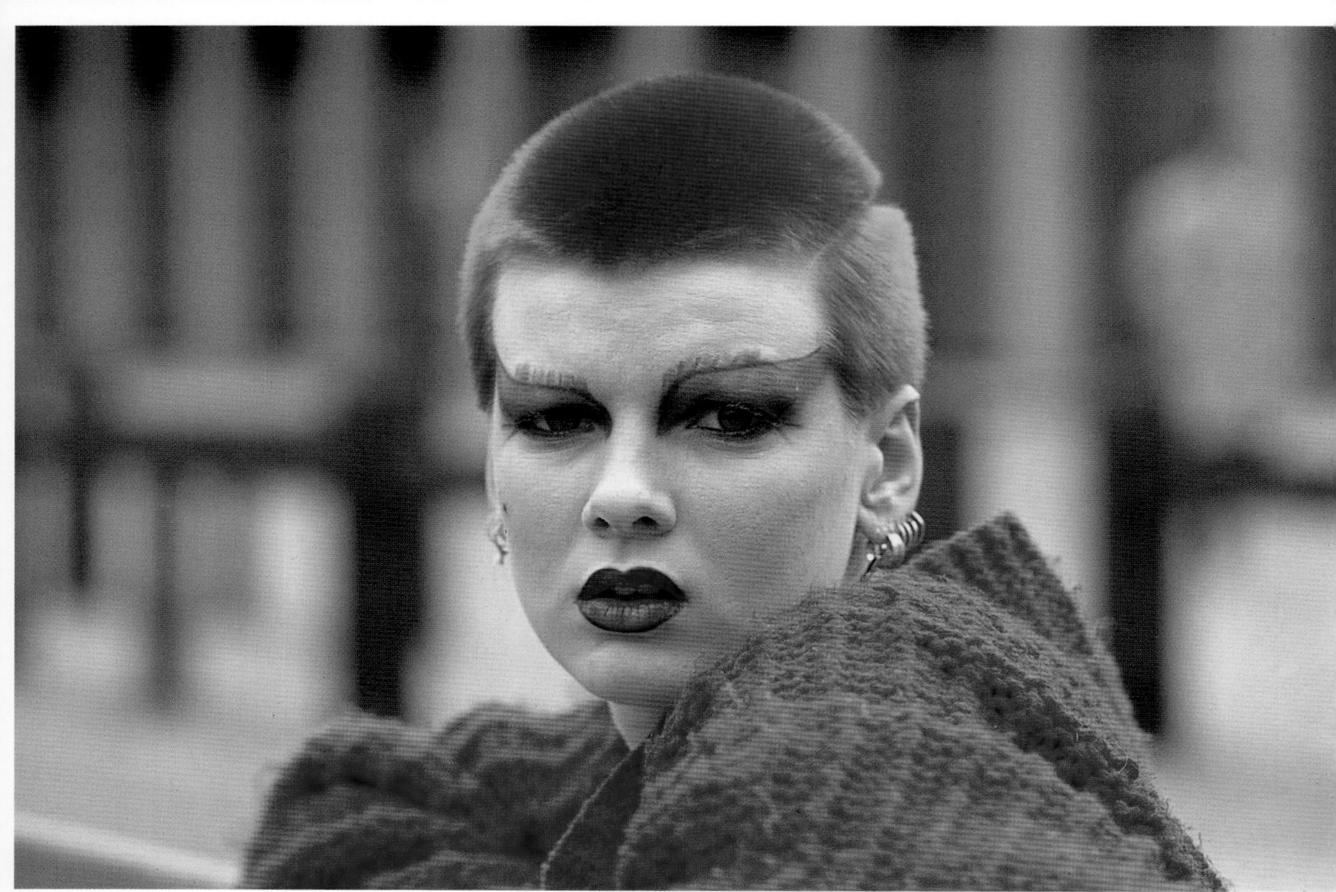

Soo Catwoman with 'Jubilee' hairstyle,
by Keith Wainwright of Smile, 1977

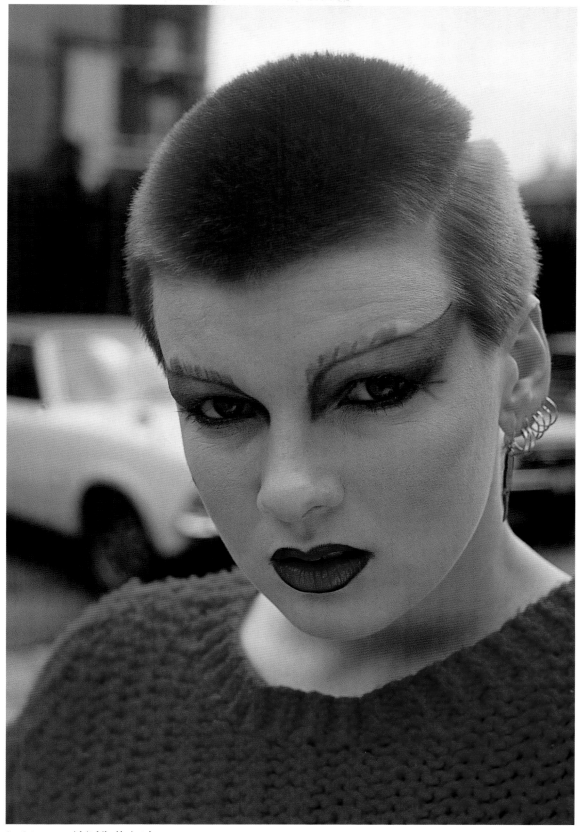

Soo Catwoman with 'Jubilee' hairstyle,
by Keith Wainwright of Smile, 1977

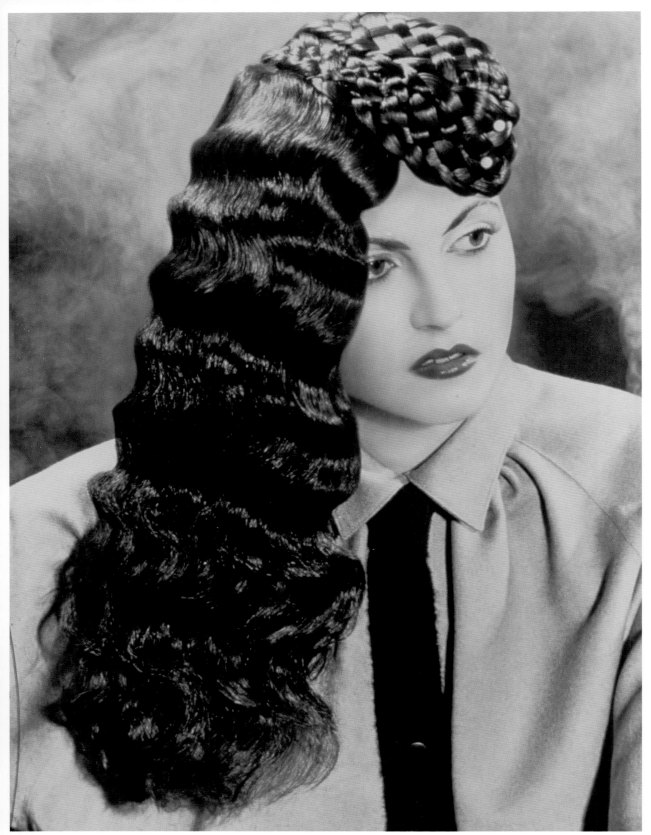

Plaited hairstyle by Andrew Collinge, 1977, photographed by Bill Ling

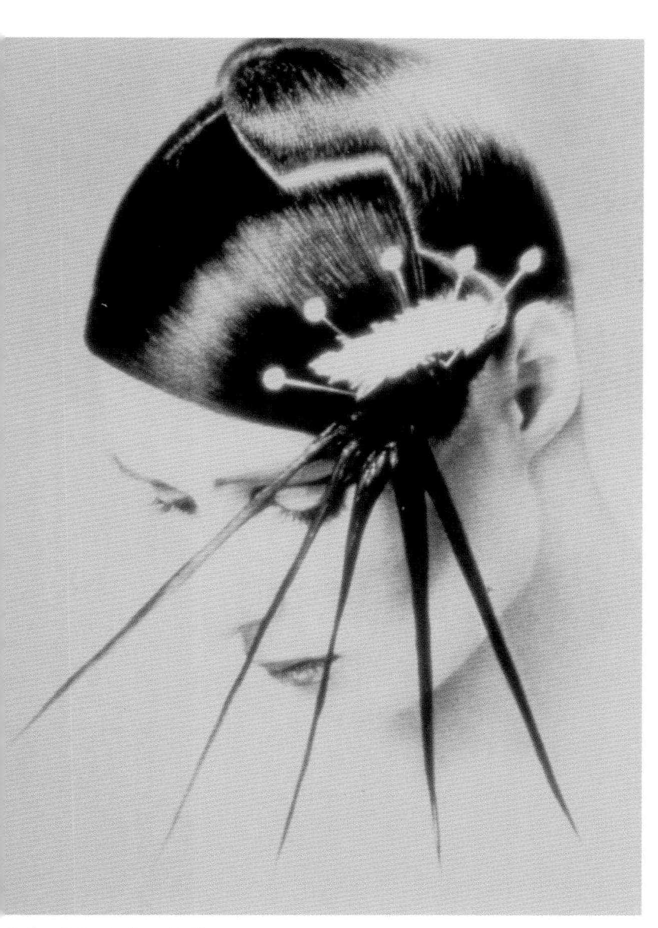

Hairstyle by Andrew Collinge, 1978, photographed by Bill Ling

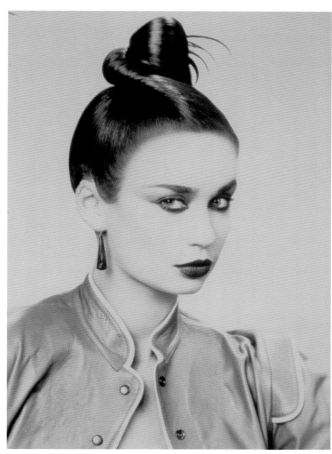

'Topknot' hairstyle by Andrew Collinge, 1978, photographed by Mike Balfre

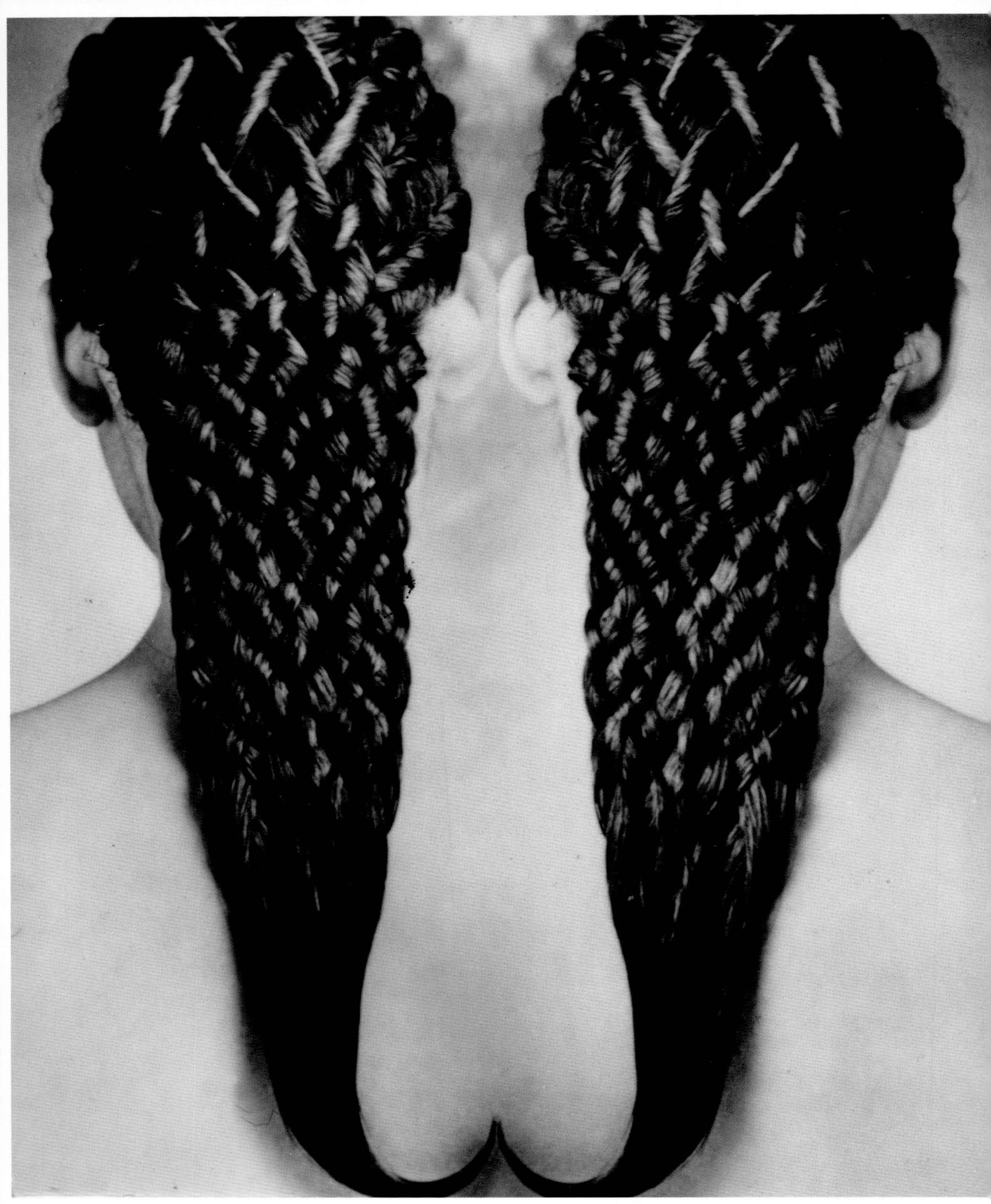

'Weaves' hairstyle by Anthony
Mascolo for TONI&GUY, 1978

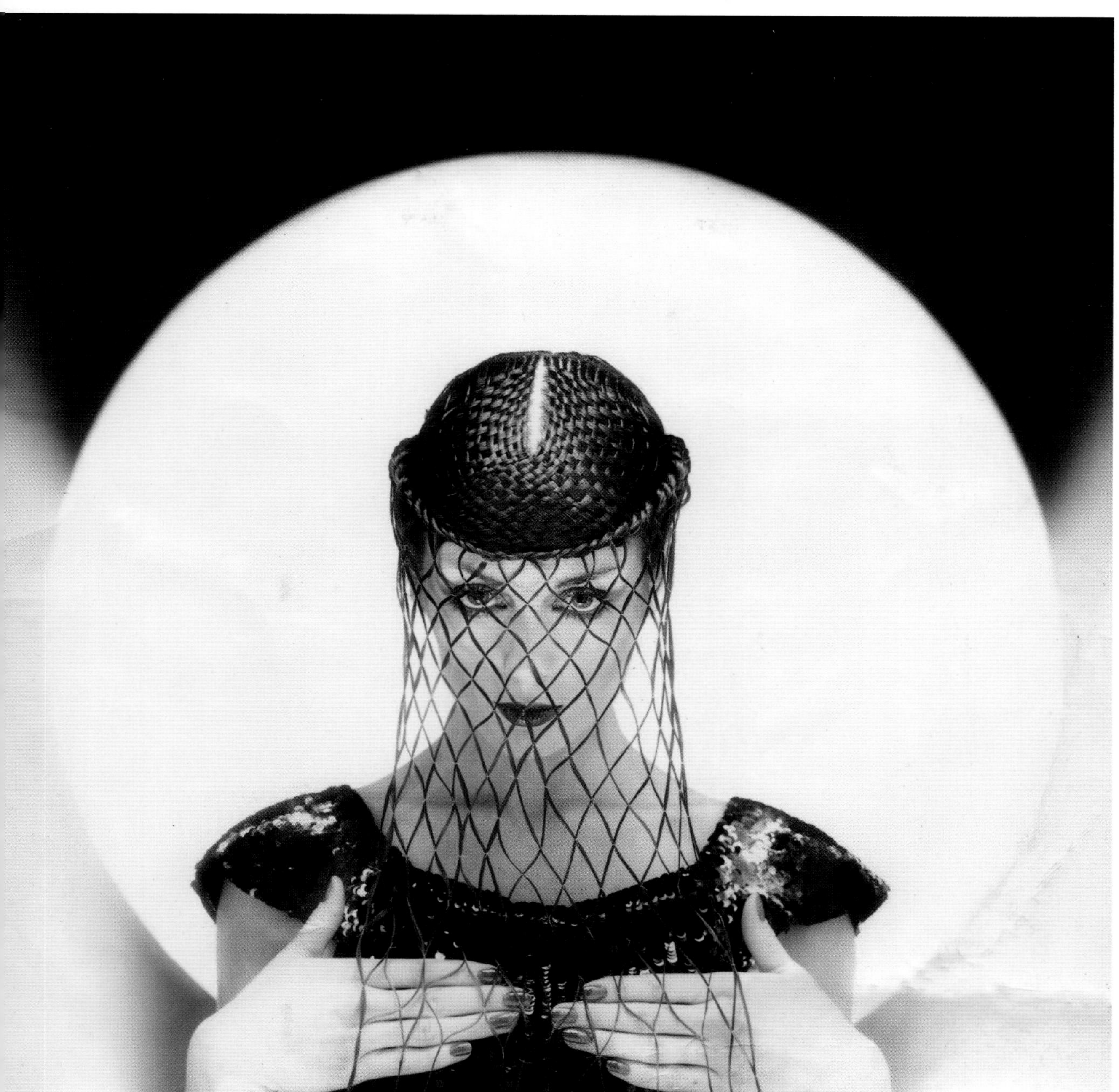

'Veil' hairstyle by Anthony Mascolo for TONI&GUY, 1978

Overleaf: Hairstyle by Anthony Mascolo for TONI&GUY, 1979

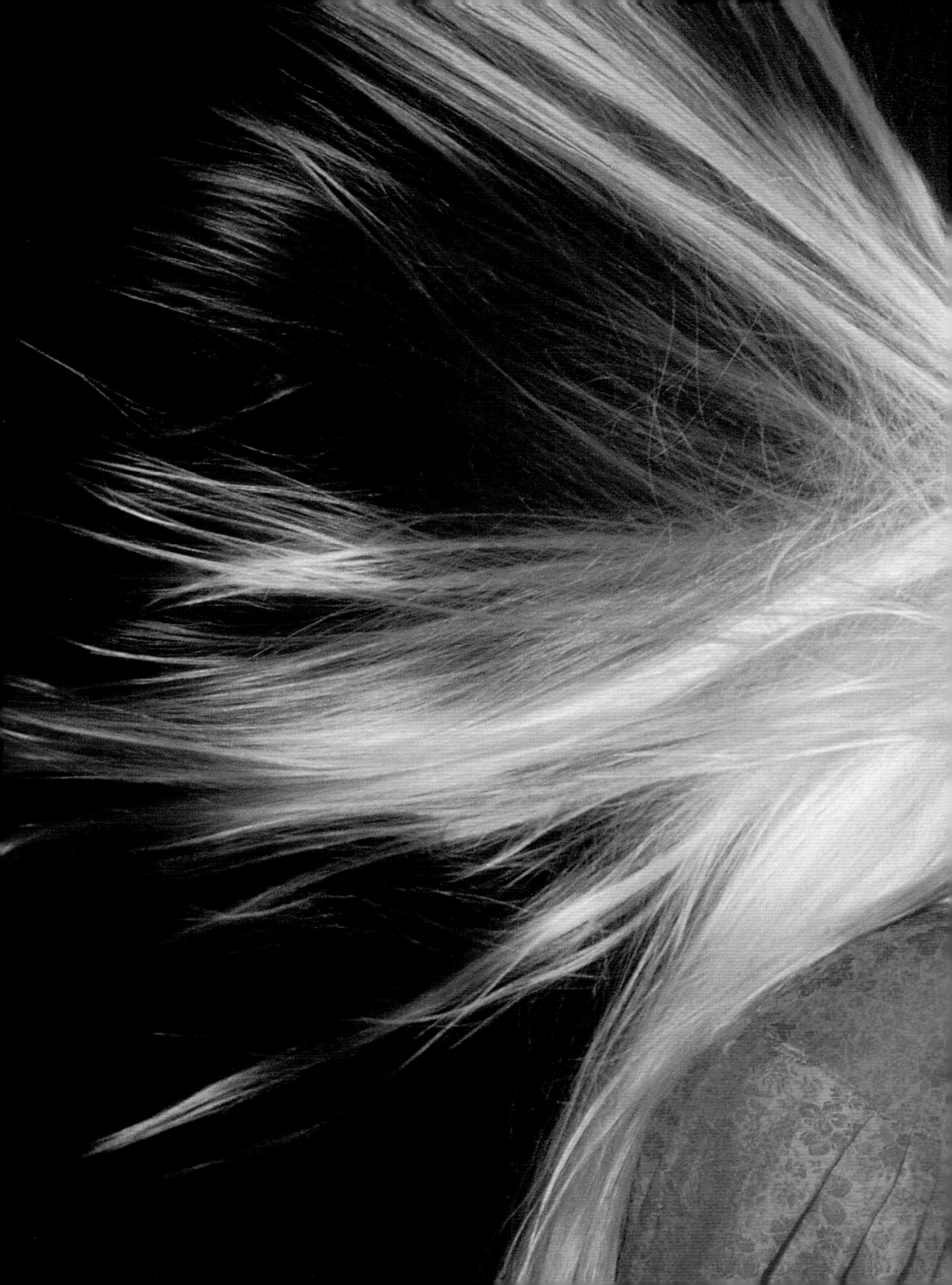

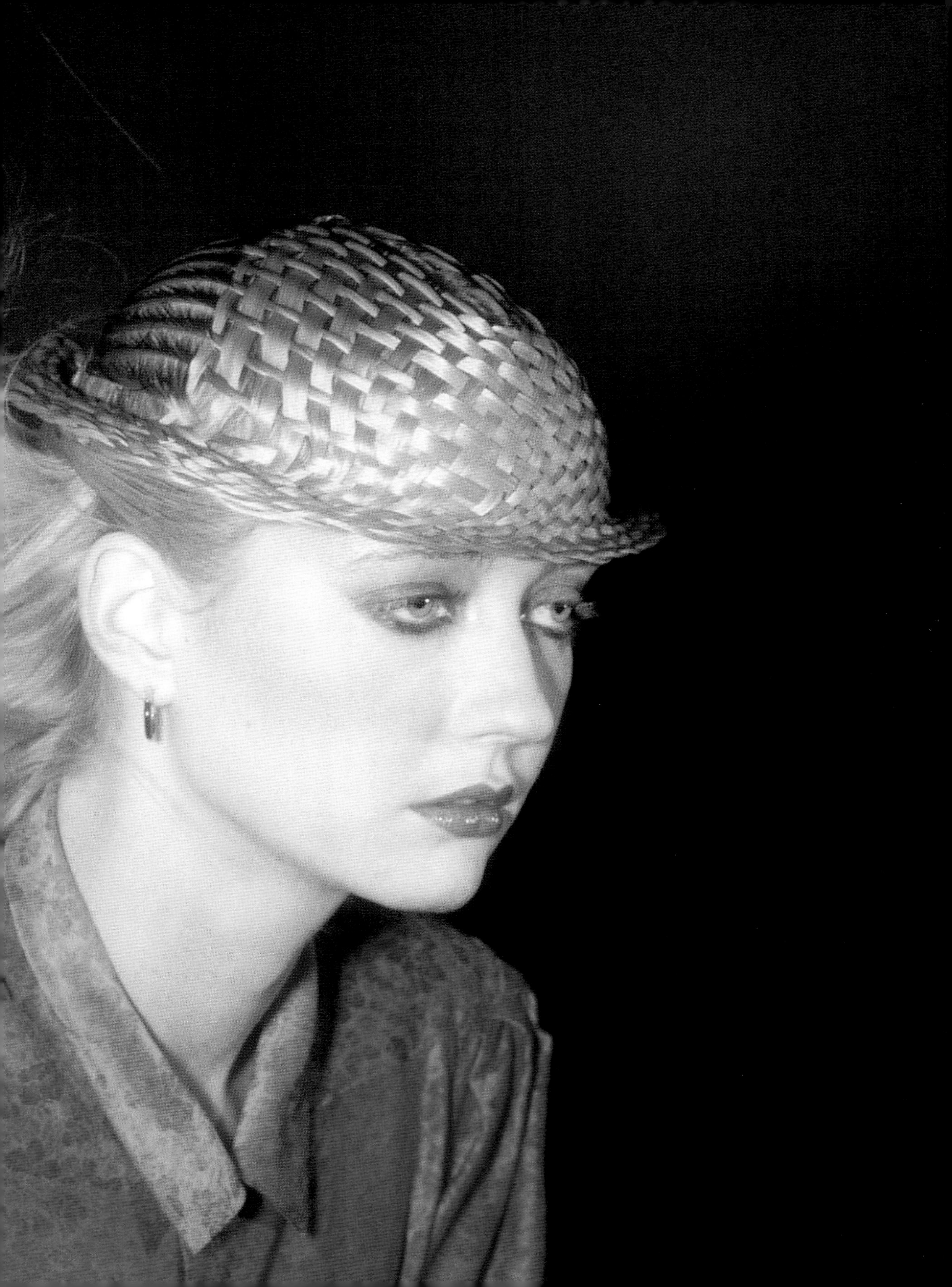

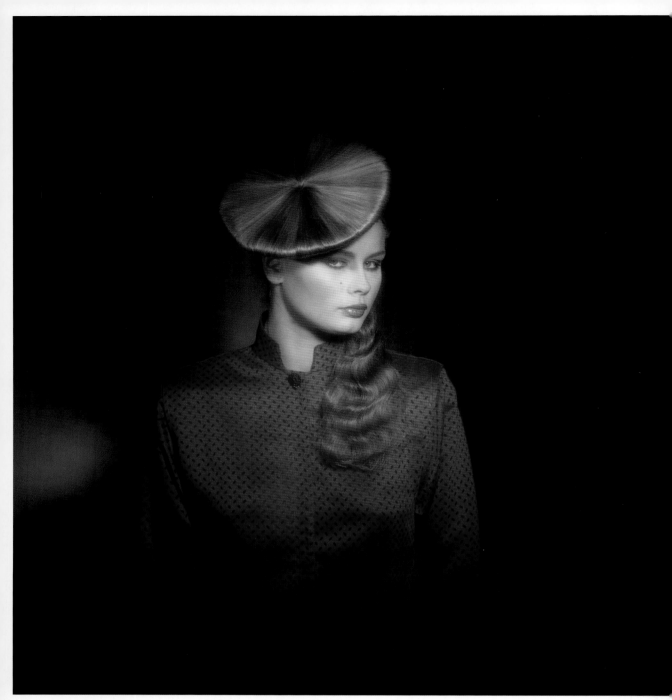

'Disc' hairstyle by Anthony
Mascolo for TONI&GUY, 1979

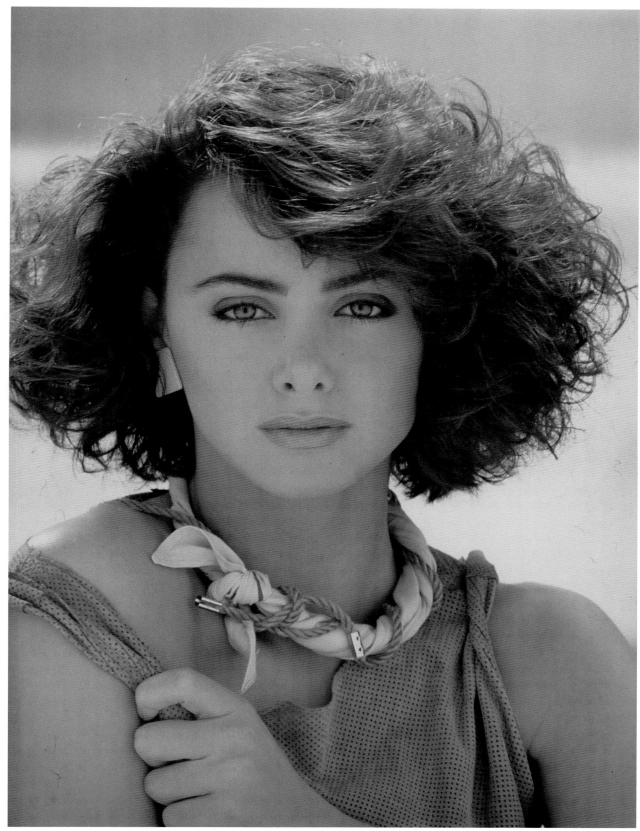

'The Scrunch' by Trevor Sorbie which utilised a revolutionary blow-drying technique, 1979

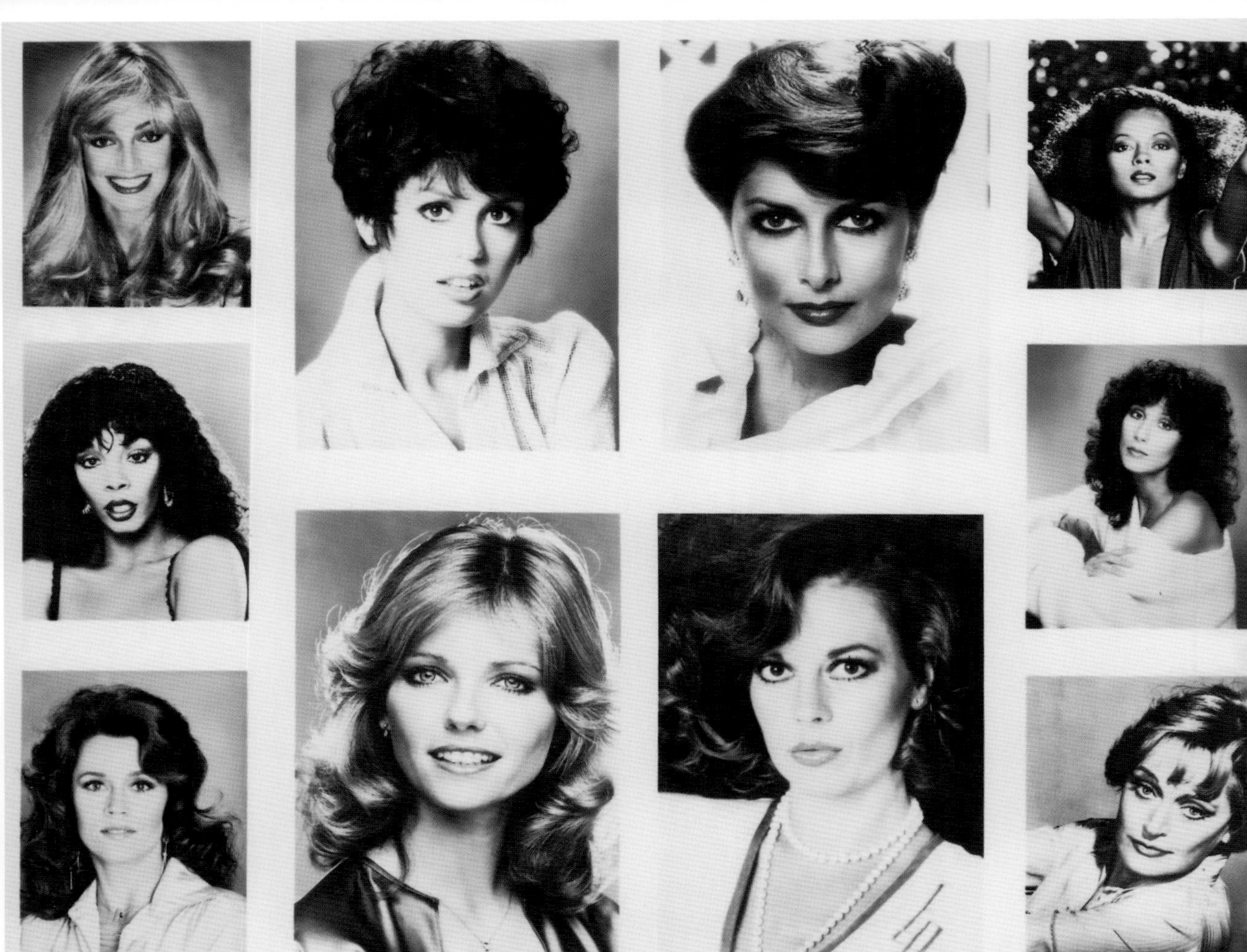

The Ten Best Coiffured Women of 1979, selected for the 23rd year by the Helene Curtis Guild of Professional Hairstylists, are: (clockwise, from upper left) actress/entertainer Susan Anton; singer Marie Osmond; model Cristina Ferrare Delorean; singer-actress Diana Ross; singer Cher; actress Alexis Smith; actress Natalie Wood; model/TV commentator Cheryl Tiegs; actress Jane Fonda; and singer Donna Summer.

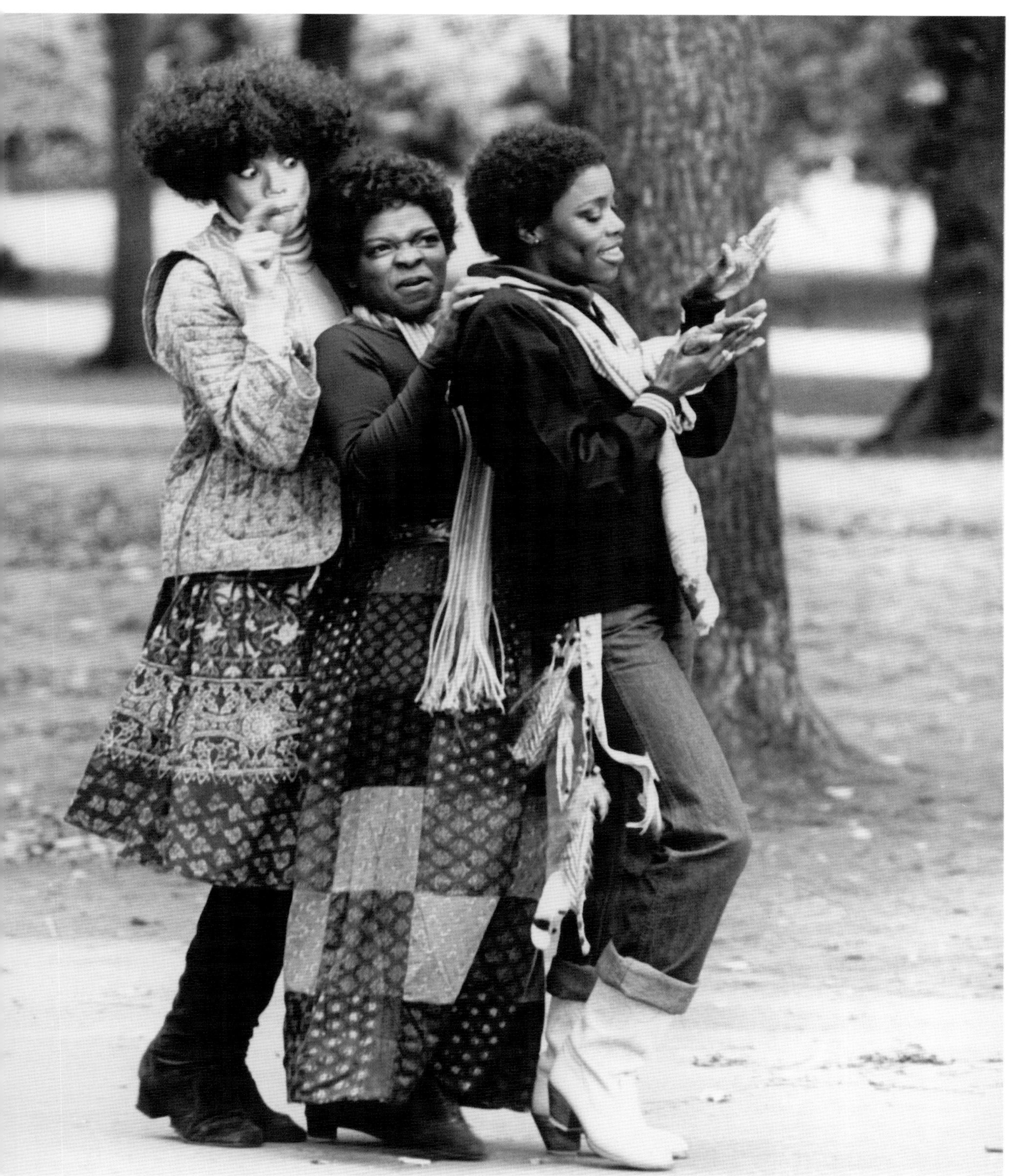

romotional photograph for the movie, 'Hair', showing
rudy Perkins, Nell Carter and Charlaine Woodard, 1979

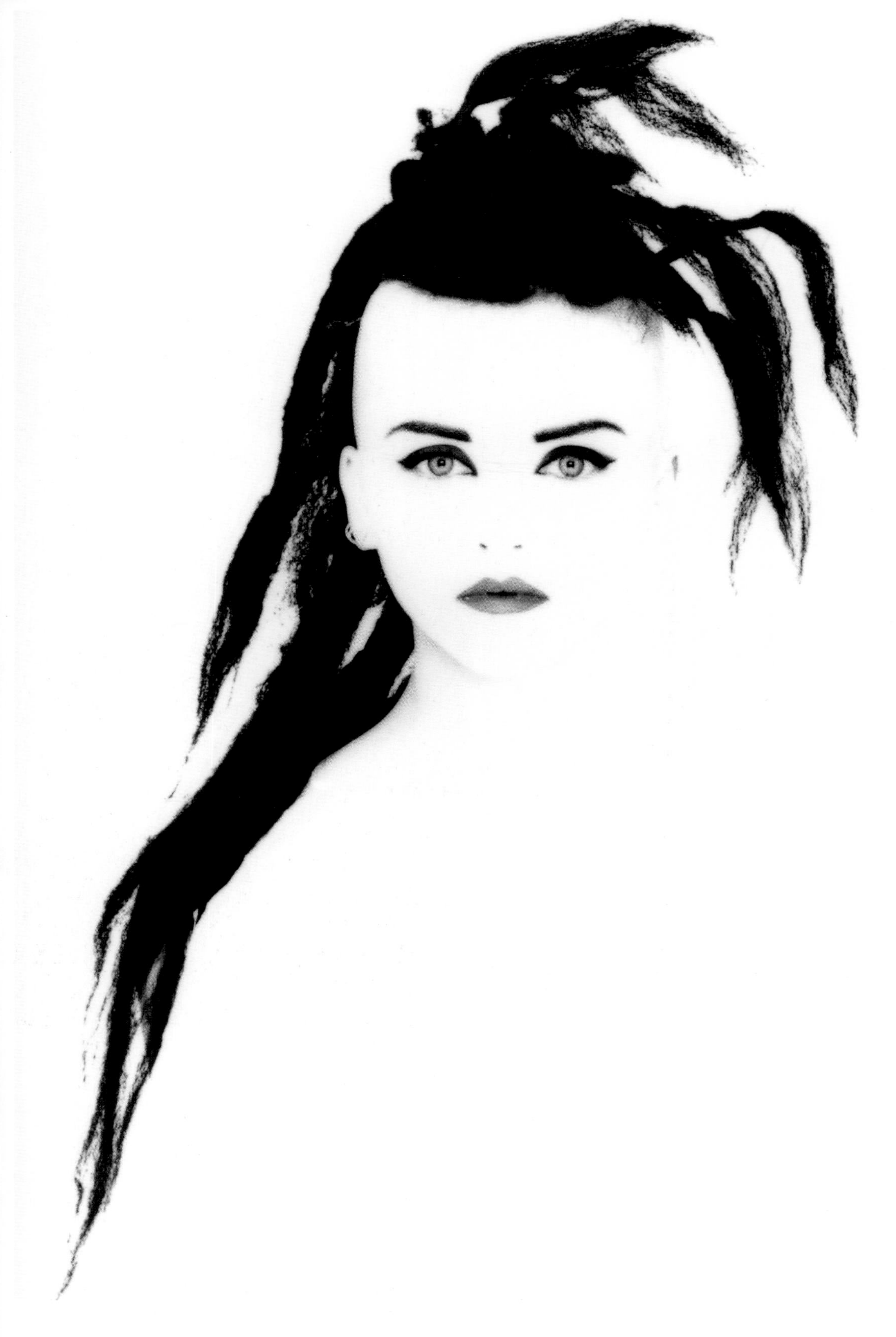

1980S

'oday, the Eighties is generally seen as a decade of hideous aux-pas fashions and it is only just entering into the vintage ollecting radar. Certainly it was a decade that saw some of he most unbelievably dreadful hairstyles, from ringlet perms hat looked wonderful on Italian teenagers (who were known n Italy as "chintz-girls") but looked absolutely appalling on nybody else, especially when the cork-screwing locks turned nto poodle-like frizz. Then there were the "big hair" dos hat were the coiffure equivalent of power dressing, the New omantic hairstyles with their eye-covering asymmetrical ringes or pirate-like spikes with headbands, and then, of ourse, the "Mullet" – perhaps the most ghastly hair fashion o ever make it onto anyone's head. So yes, the Eighties were esponsible for some memorably awful hairstyles, but at the ame time there were some really interesting things going on n the hair world during this period of intense social change. here were also a few highly talented practitioners who were ushing the boundaries, both technically and aesthetically. s *GQ* editor, Dylan Jones noted in his excellent *Haircults* book, In the style-obsessed eighties the world became a global atwalk. Narcissism plumbed new depths as haircuts reached ew heights. The eighties rapidly became the designer decade, here everyone had an alias, an ambition and an aerodynamic aircut to match."

A hairdresser whose work had a huge influence in the arly Eighties was Trevor Sorbie, who in 1979 invented "The crunch", a look that became hugely popular during the first ew years of the decade. As he recalled, "During this period, I vas a stylist at the John Frieda salon. His method of finishing t that time was finger-drying. It was a great technique but ook ages. One day I was extremely busy; I had three clients vaiting, and was under a great deal of pressure. My next client ad thick, red, porous, wavy hair and, of course, she wanted finger-dried. Because of the backlog of clients I asked her I could speed the process up by adding heat. I found that by aking a handful of hair, squeezing it in my hand and applying eat, then allowing the hair to cool, could create volume. I realised that I had inadvertently iscovered a new method of drying." This new method allowed airdressers to create mussed-up hair that had impressive olume and was radically different from anything that had one before.

Throughout the 1980s, Anthony Mascolo also continued to reate innovative trend-setting hairstyles that were notable or the way in which they always suited the wearer. As a firm eliever that the haircut should complement the personality f the wearer, Mascolo's hair-raising styles had a stylistic freshness that was completely at odds with the step-by-step formulaic approach of some other hairdressers. The extraordinary haircuts that were invented by Mascolo during this period, from the mane-like "Cavallo" hairstyle to the spiky "Diffusion" hairstyle, also reflected the growing significance of spectacular "hair shows" that were (and still are) such an essential vehicle for helping to promote hair products to other practitioners. Apart from his progressive work as a hairstylist, Anthony Mascolo is also a highly accomplished photographer and he was one of the first people to understand the importance of taking photographs under proper studio conditions in order to show hairstyles to their best effect. This understanding of professional presentation through photo shoots was key to the development of the Toni&Guy brand, as was Mascolo's infective enthusiasm for new seasonal concepts.

Another stylist who also significantly raised the bar for innovative hairdressing and hair-product retailing during the 1980s was Simon Forbes, who founded the legendary Antenna salon in London's Kensington Church Street in 1980. The same year, Forbes introduced his Monofibre extensions made from fine strands of acrylic that could either look like natural hair or come in shockingly bright colours. Using neither glue nor chemicals, the lightweight extensions were held in place with their own sealing system, which meant they were easy to wear. In 1980, Forbes also introduced "Bobtails" which were the first "white dreadlocks" intended for the Caucasian market. Reflecting the influence of Reggae on the music scene of the early 1980s, "Bob-Tails" were according to Forbes, "developed as a new way to wear one's hair to complement the clothes being worn [at the time]... They fitted in perfectly to the anti-fashion, hobo feeling. The success of them... inspired us to work with the concept of people buying 'hair off the shelf'... Now the taboo of not combing one's hair and washing it every other day has been thrown out the window. It has allowed us so much more freedom to create hairstyles along the lines of adding hair." In 1982, Forbes also invented "Ragtails" which were pieces of real or Monofibre hair that were combed and matted in large dreadlocks and then attached to the wearer's own hair to give a "white Rasta" look. Throughout the 1980s, Forbes continued to develop the technology behind extensions, including the introduction of "The Clamp" in 1984, and at the same time he experimented stylistically in order to create cutting-edge hairstyles that incorporated his Monofibre locks.

Another group of hairdressers that came to prominence during the 1980s were the colourists, most notably Nicky Clarke, Daniel Galvin and John Frieda, who were skilled at creating convincingly blonde tresses. Certainly the 1980s

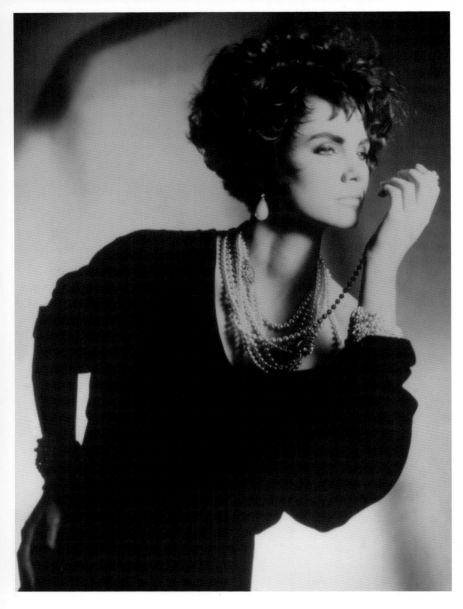

'Soft Top', by Elliot at Michaeljohn, 1980s

hairdressing mainstream was dominated by "streaked blonde" hairdos, often emulating those adopted by Princess Diana such as her much-copied layered pageboy hairstyle. There was, however, during the early 1980s a youthful revolt away from such seemingly conservative hairstyles and the blossoming of New Romanticism heralded in radical hairstyles with boys often looking like girls and girls looking like boys. The Blitz Kids of this new movement took the Punk spikes of the late Seventies and appropriated them into something far less rough-and-ready and infinitely more androgynously glamorous; a fitting hair response to a decadent age of economic boom that saw the increasing questioning of sexual taboos. We should perhaps remember, that like shoulder pads, the big hair of the Eighties also echoed the strengthening power of women in society and symbolised the newfound post-feminist confidence of the "have-it-all" superwoman... hair as a political gender statement.

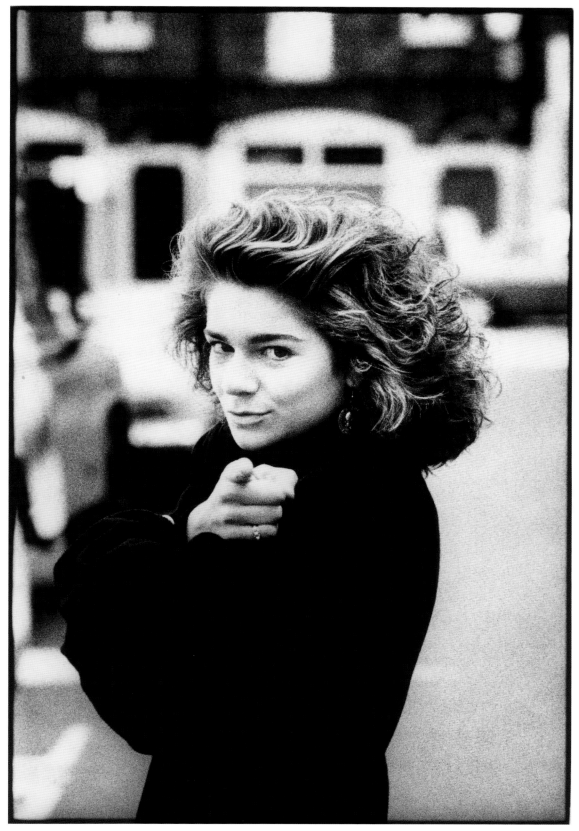

Hairstyle by Ted Reynell from Sissors hairdressers, Kings Road, London, 1980s

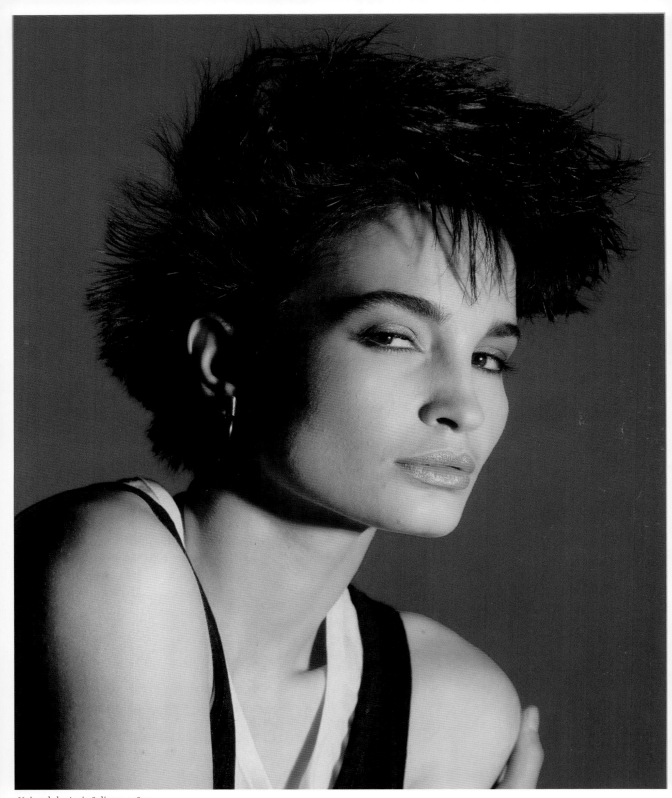

Hairstyle by Amir-Splinter, 1980s,
Wella Elite magazine

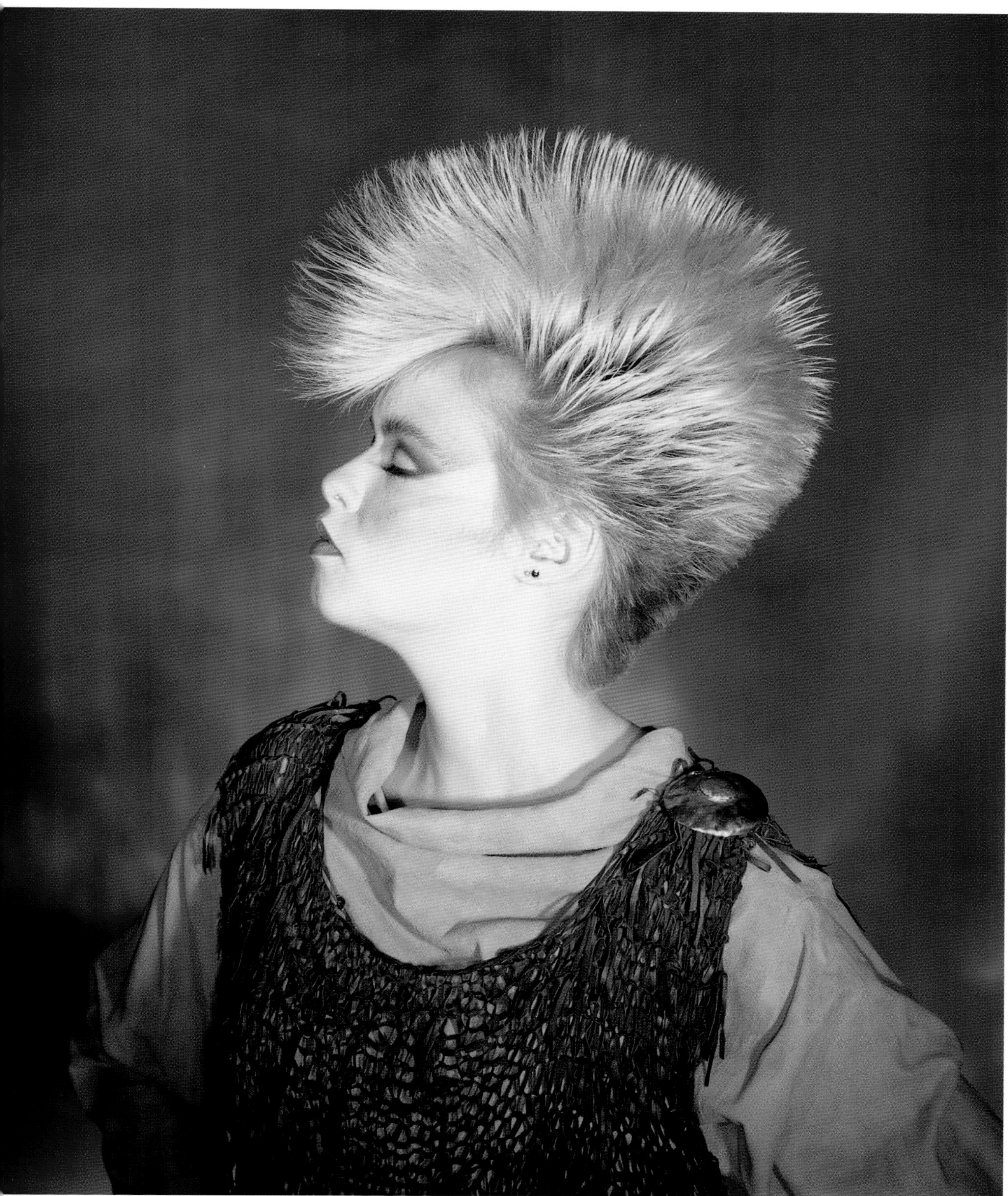

[Mo]hawk hairstyle by Anthony [M]ascolo for TONI&GUY, 1982

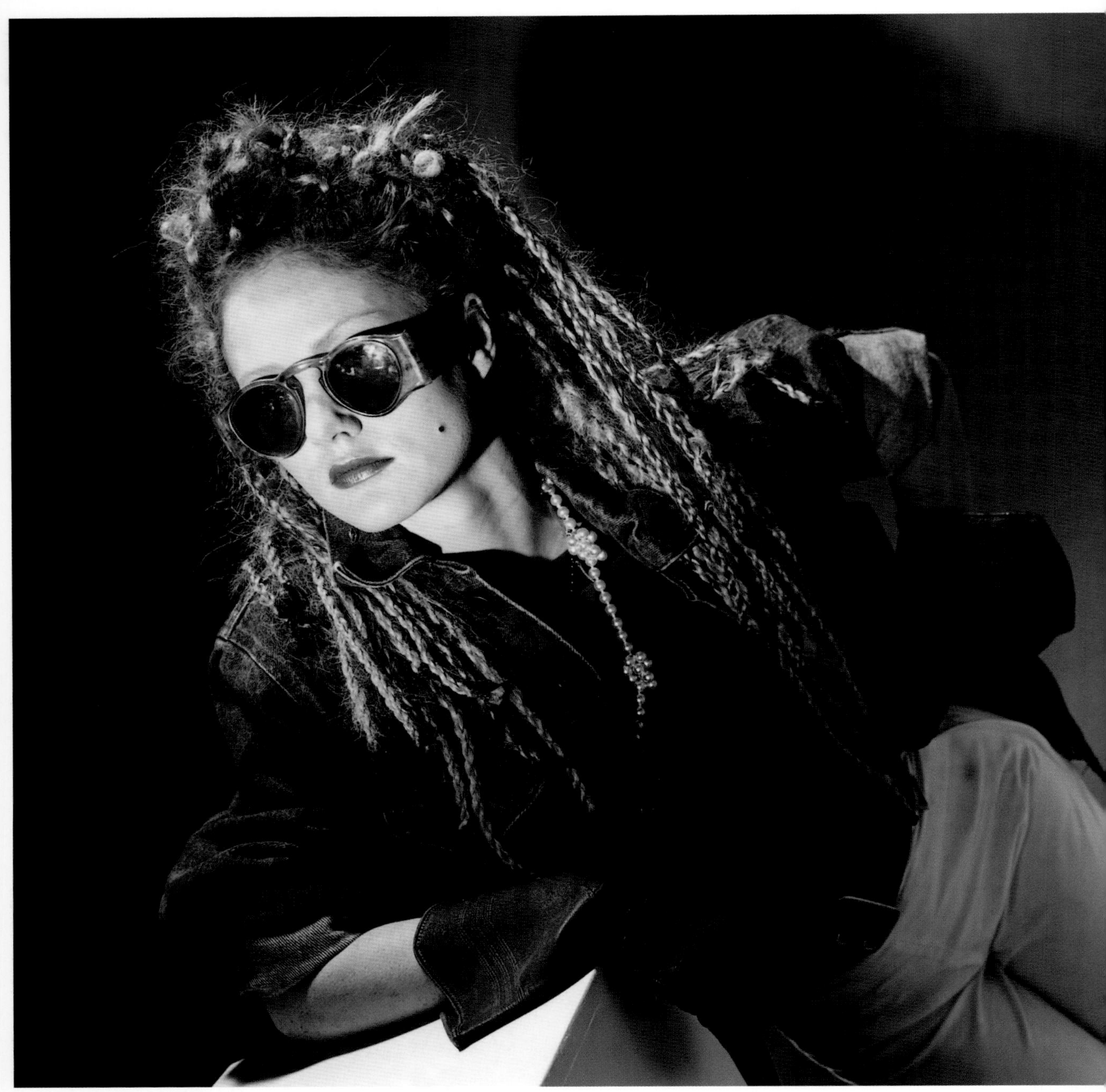

'Braids' hairstyle by Simon Forbes
for Antenna, 1980

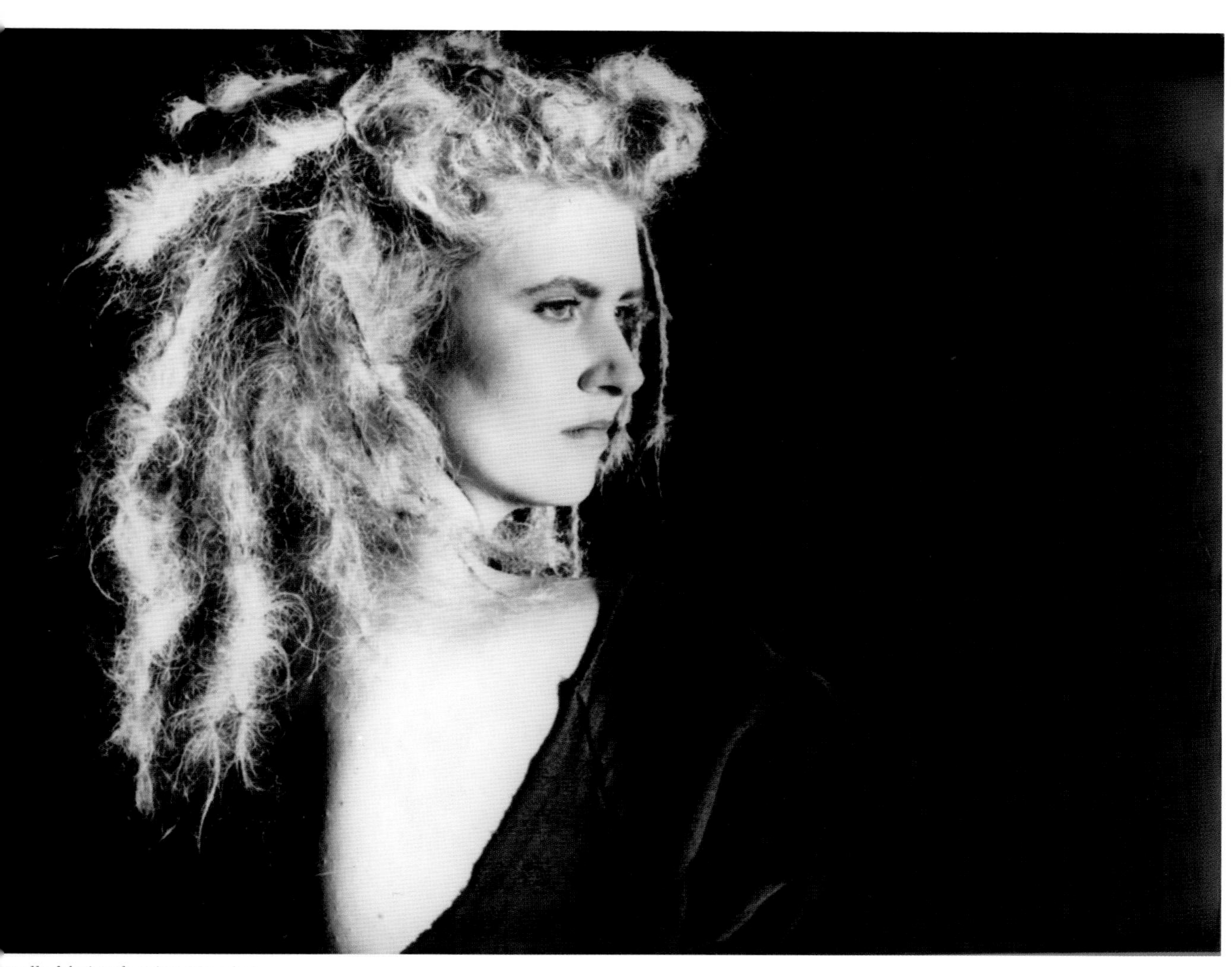

readlock hairstyle using extensions
y Simon Forbes of Antenna, 1980

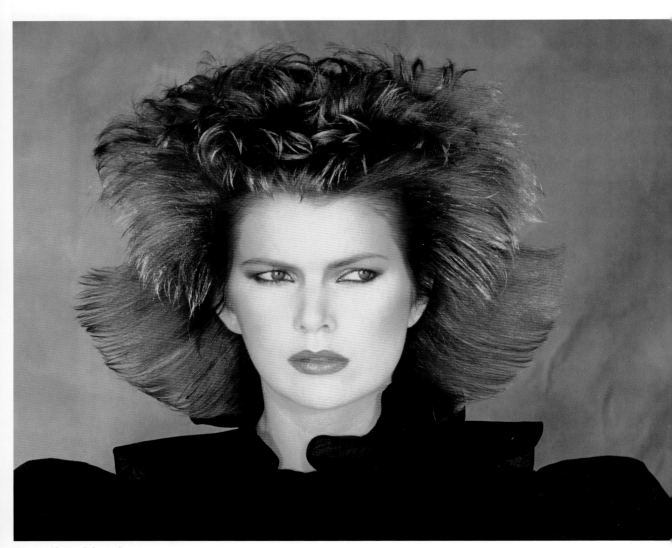

'Fantasy' hairstyle by Anthony Mascolo for TONI&GUY, 1982

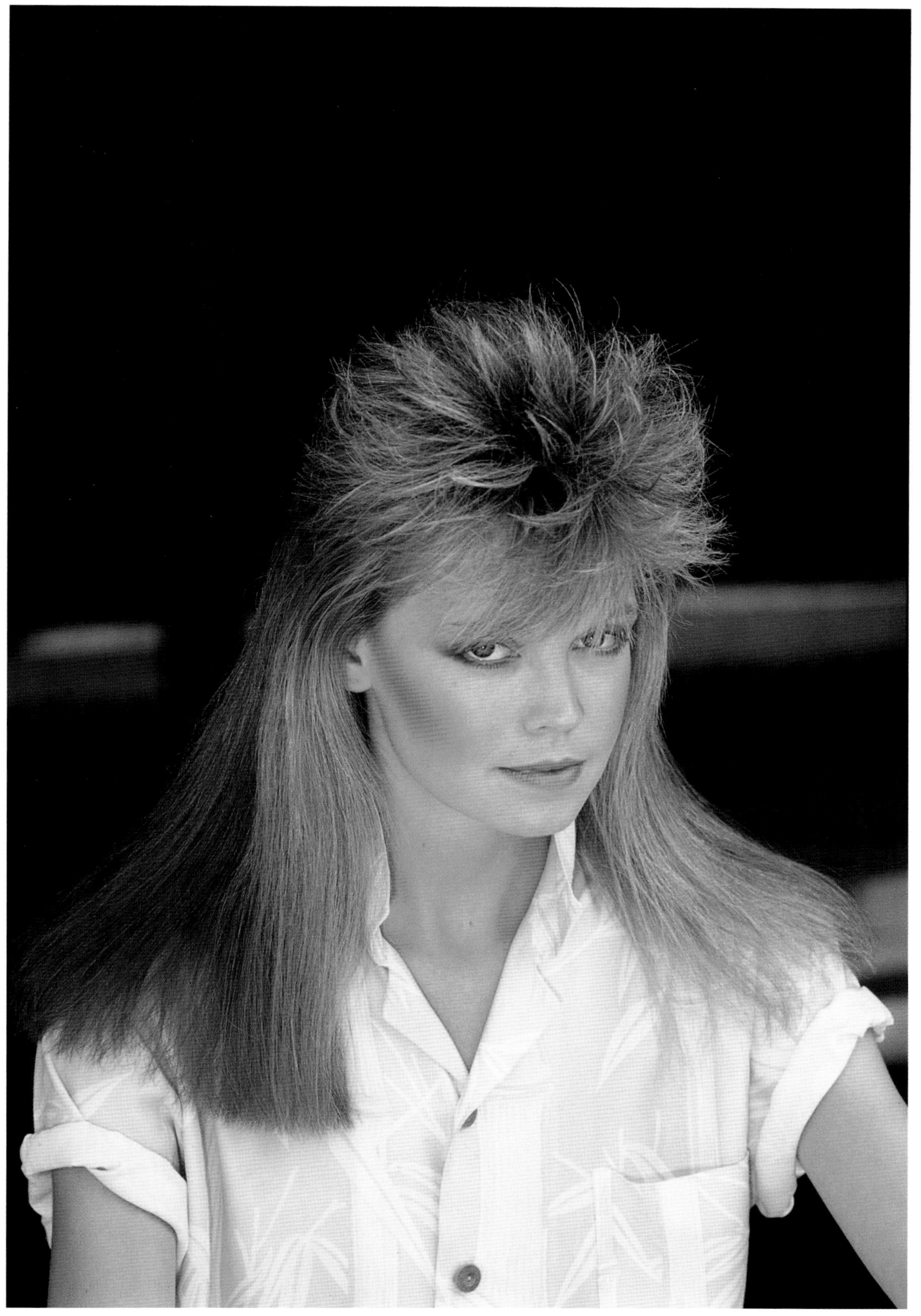

'California' hairstyle by Anthony Mascolo for TONI&GUY, 1982

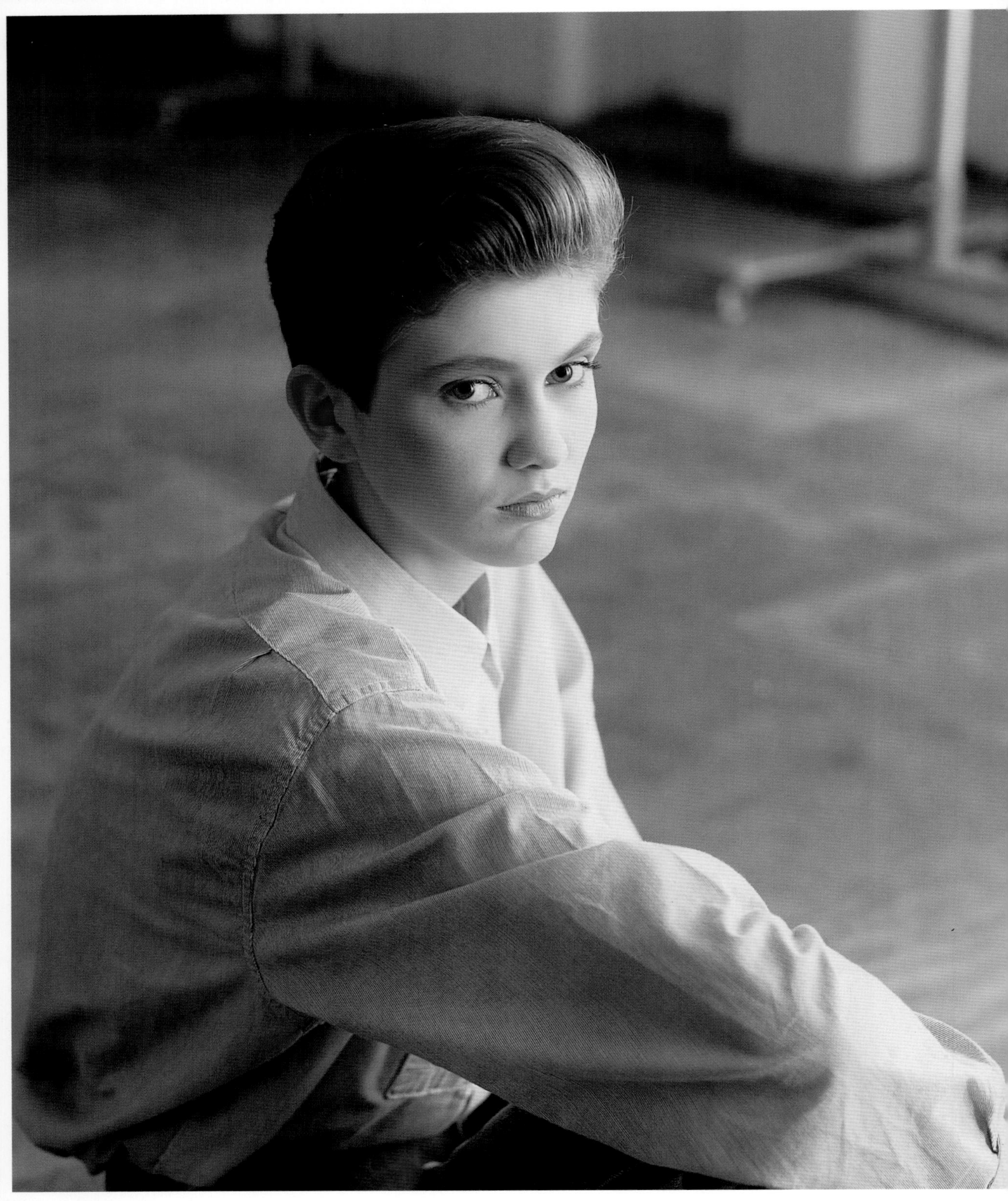

Hairstyle by Keith Wainwright
of Smile, c.1982

Hairstyle by Keith Wainwright
f Smile, c. 1982

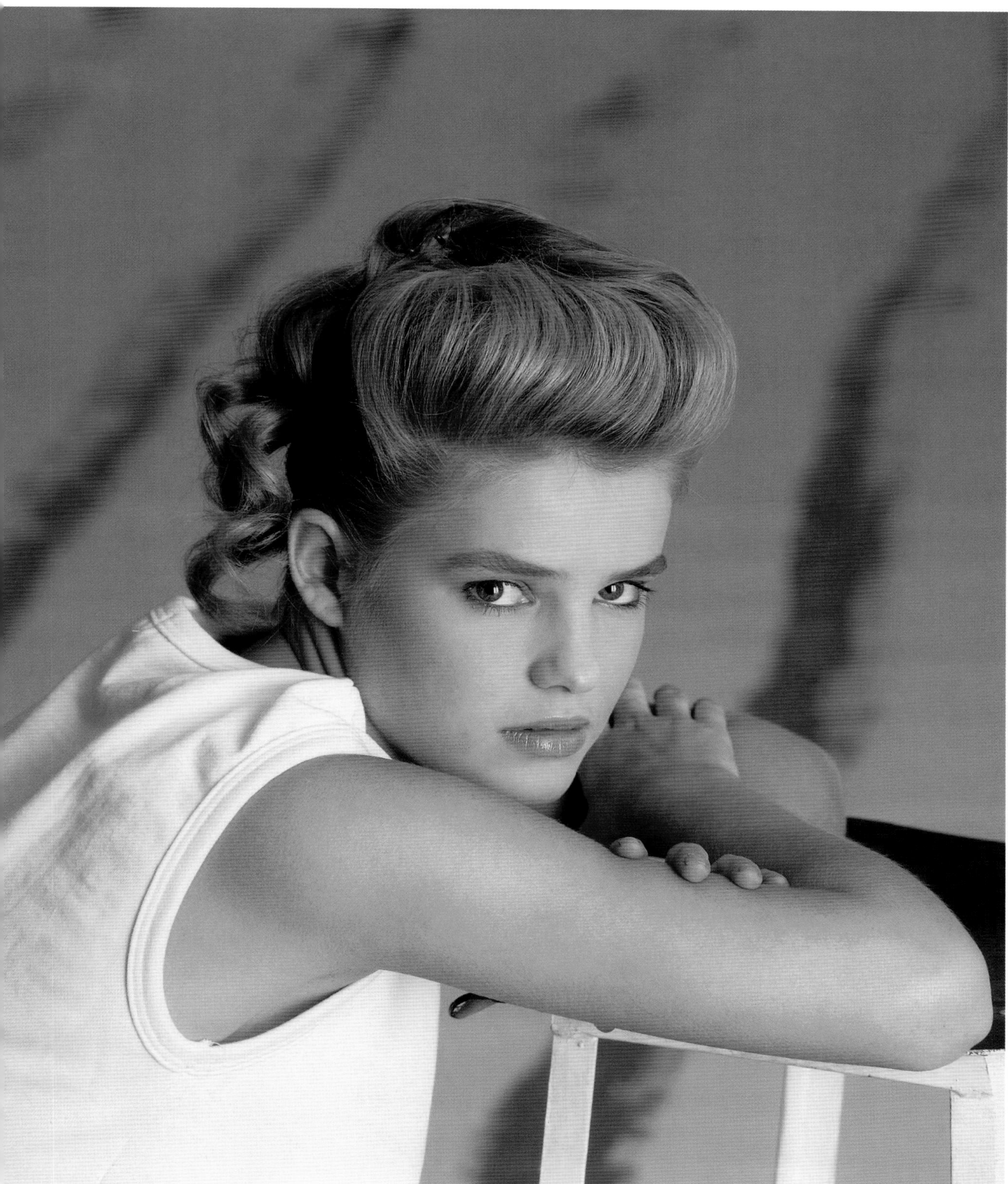

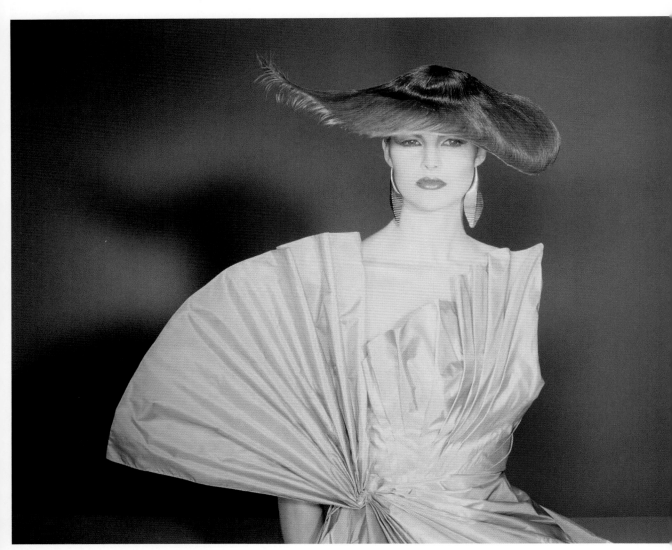

Hairstyle by Anthony Mascolo
for TONI&GUY, 1981

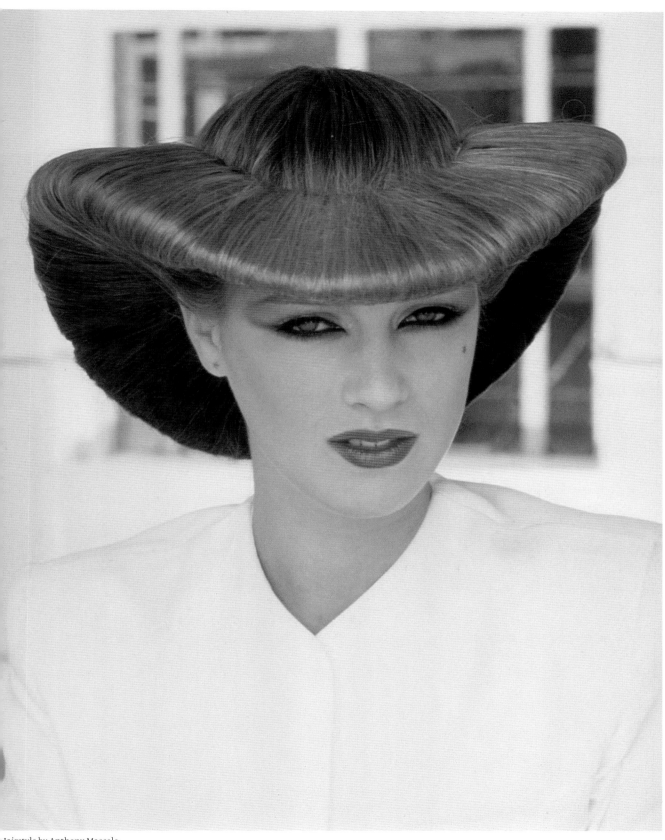

Hairstyle by Anthony Mascolo
for TONI&GUY, 1984

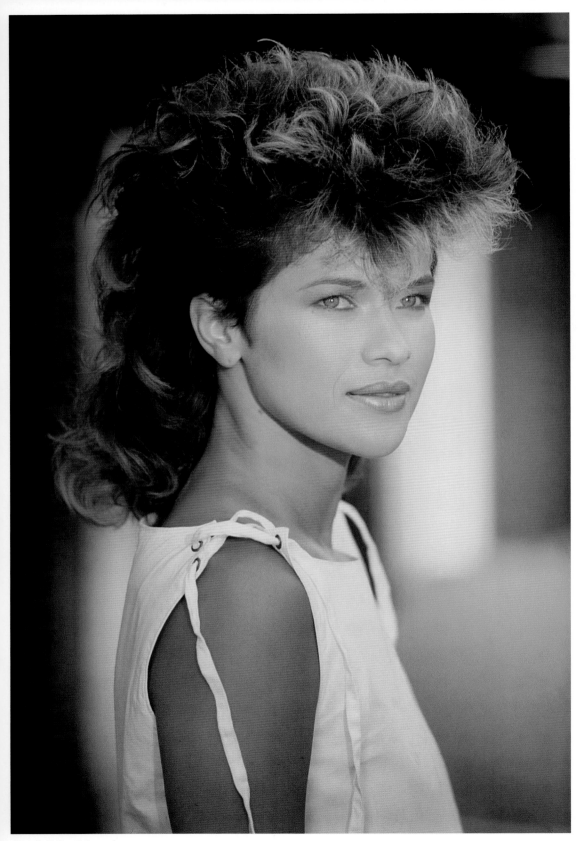

'Cavallo' hairstyle by Anthony Mascolo for TONI&GUY, 1984

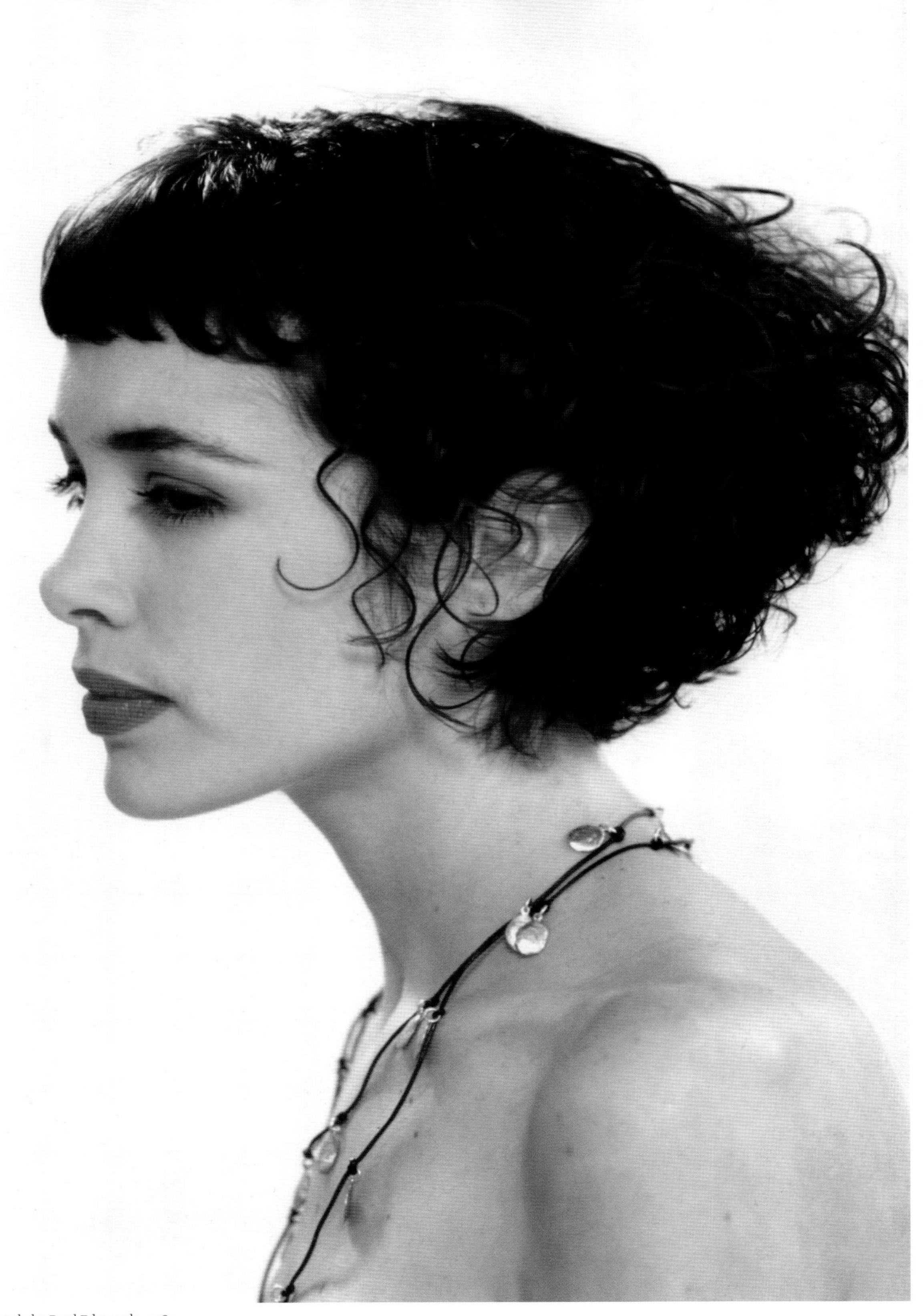

Hairstyle by Paul Edmonds, 1984

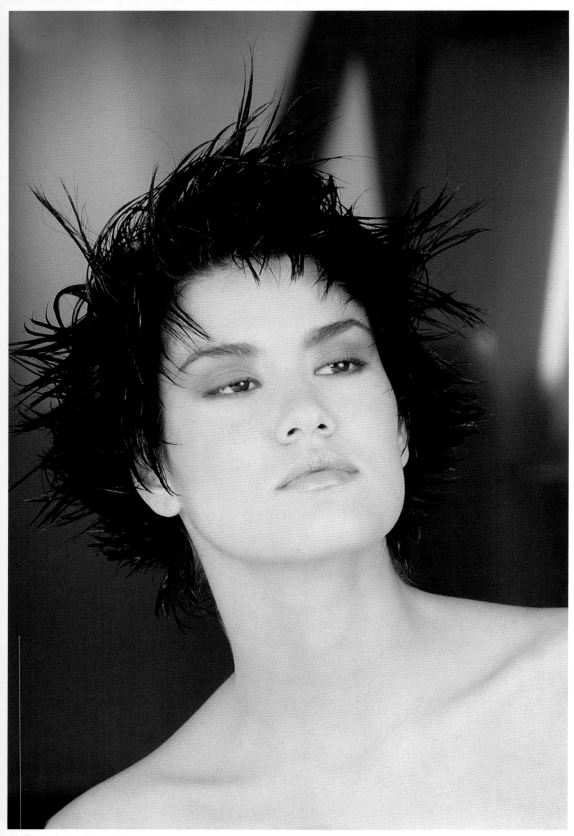

'Diffusion' hairstyle by Anthony Mascolo for TONI&GUY, 1985

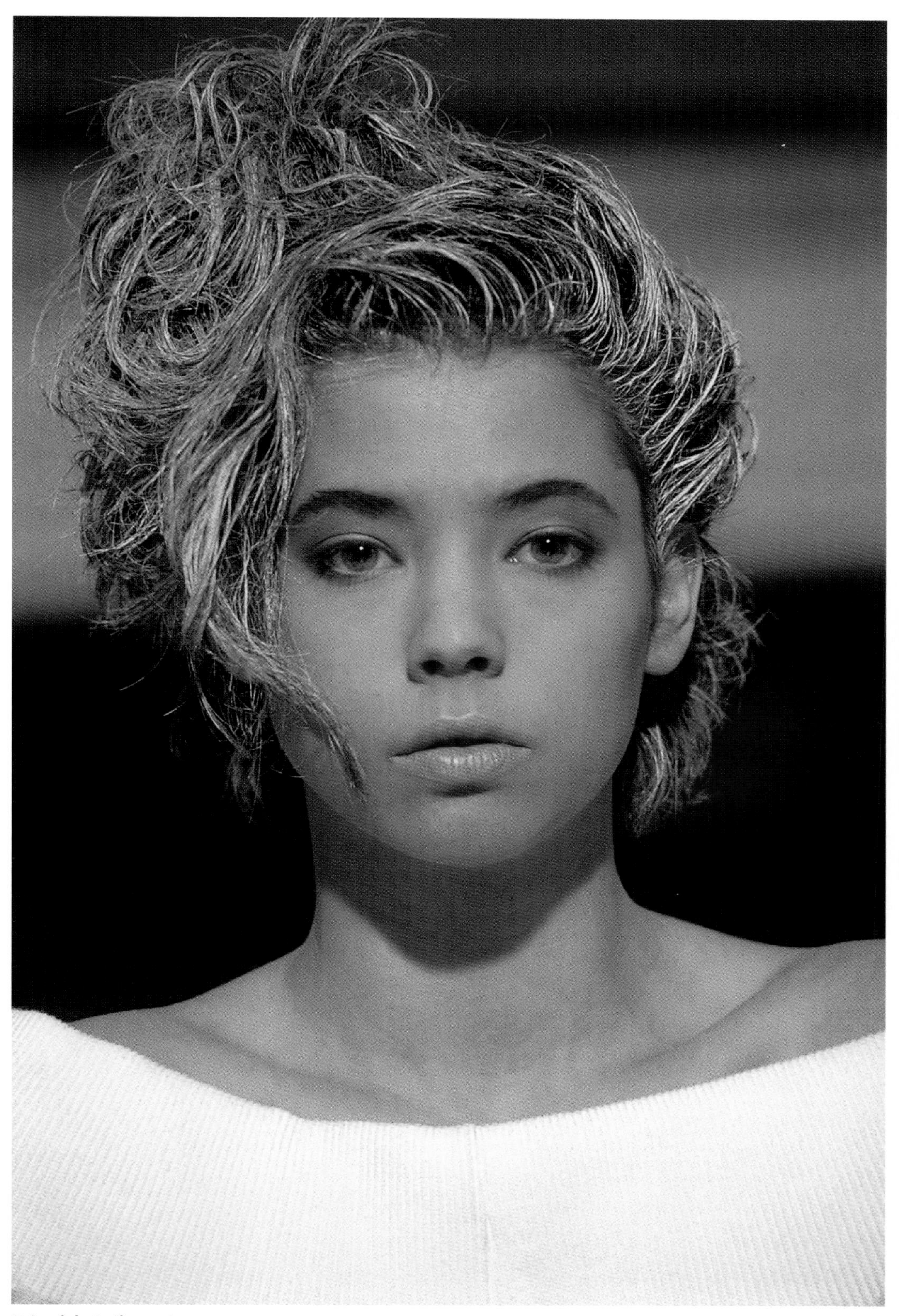

Hairstyle by Smile, c. 1985

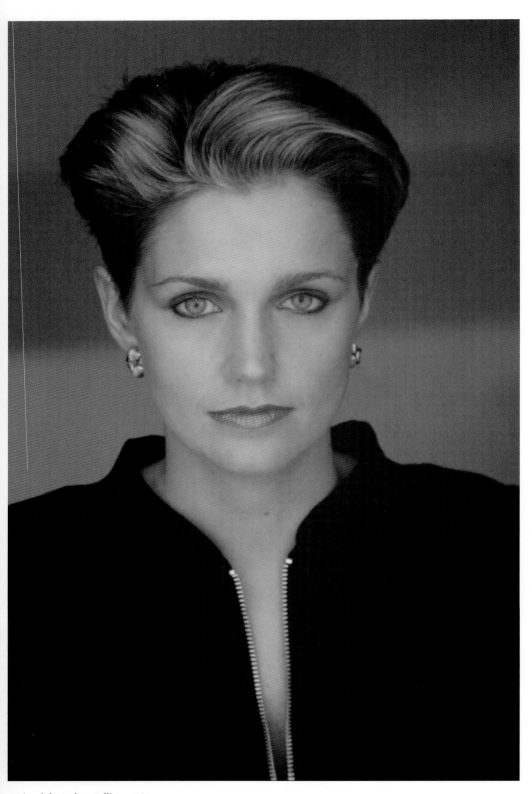

Hairstyle by Andrew Collinge, 1985,
photographed by Craig Johnston

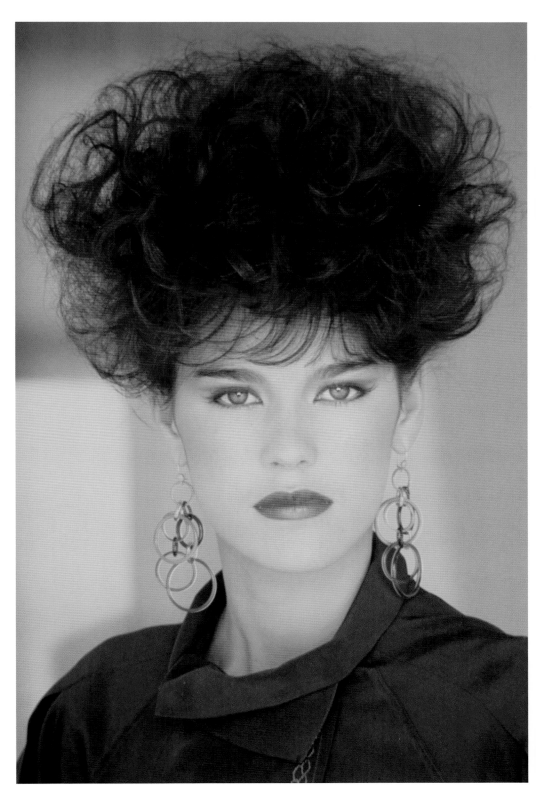

Hairstyle by Andrew Collinge, 1987

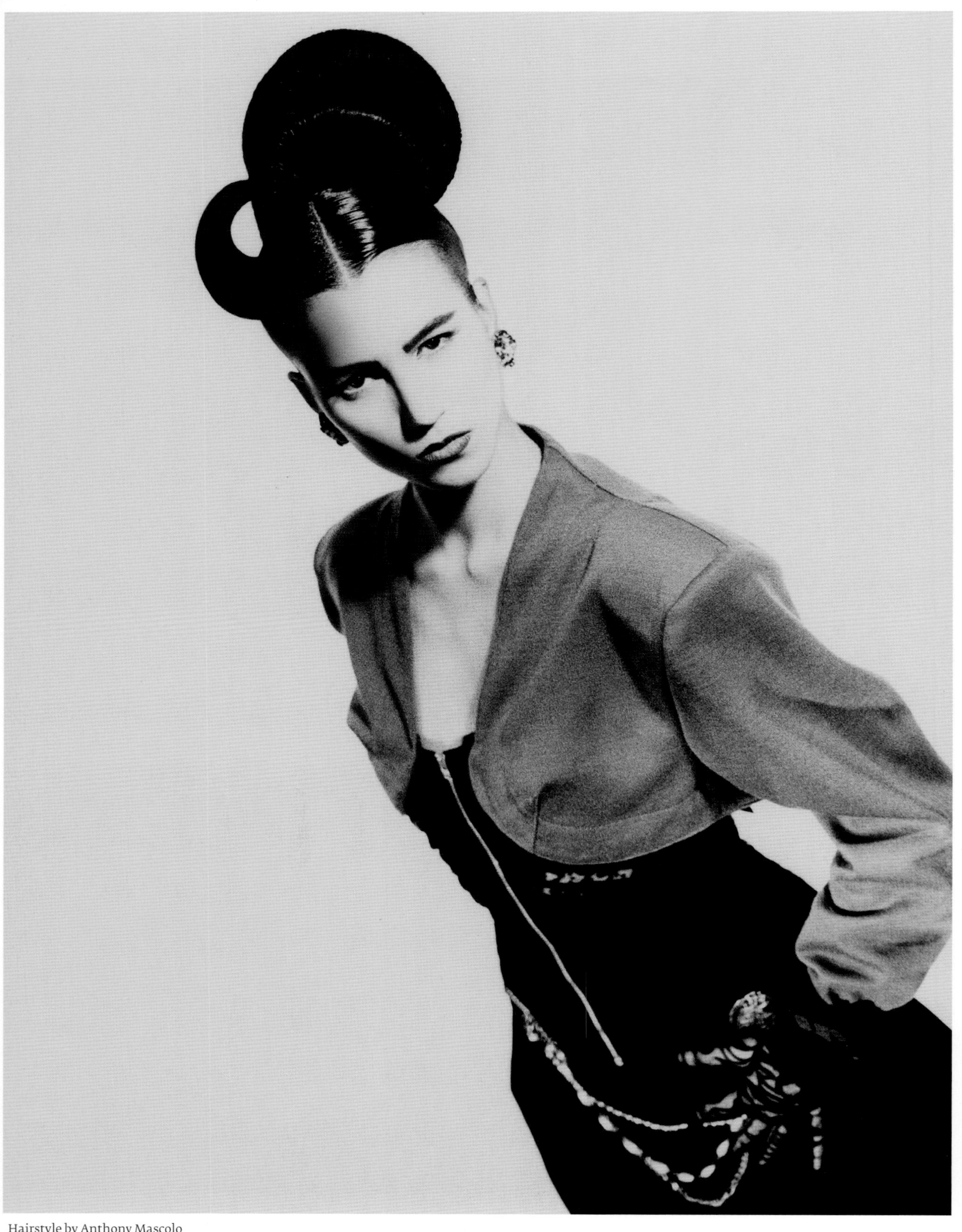

Hairstyle by Anthony Mascolo
for TONI&GUY, 1987

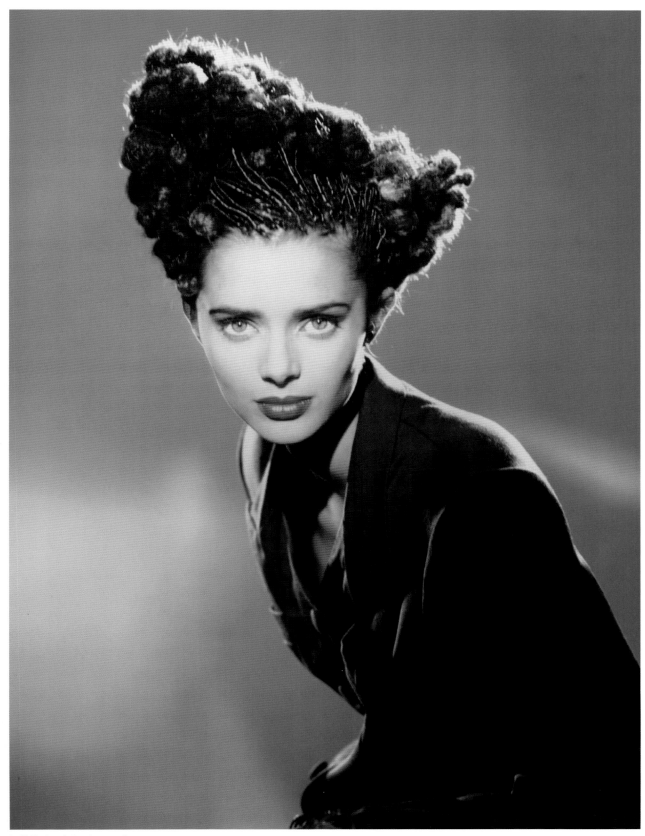

'Balls' hairstyle by Simon Forbes
for Antenna, 1986

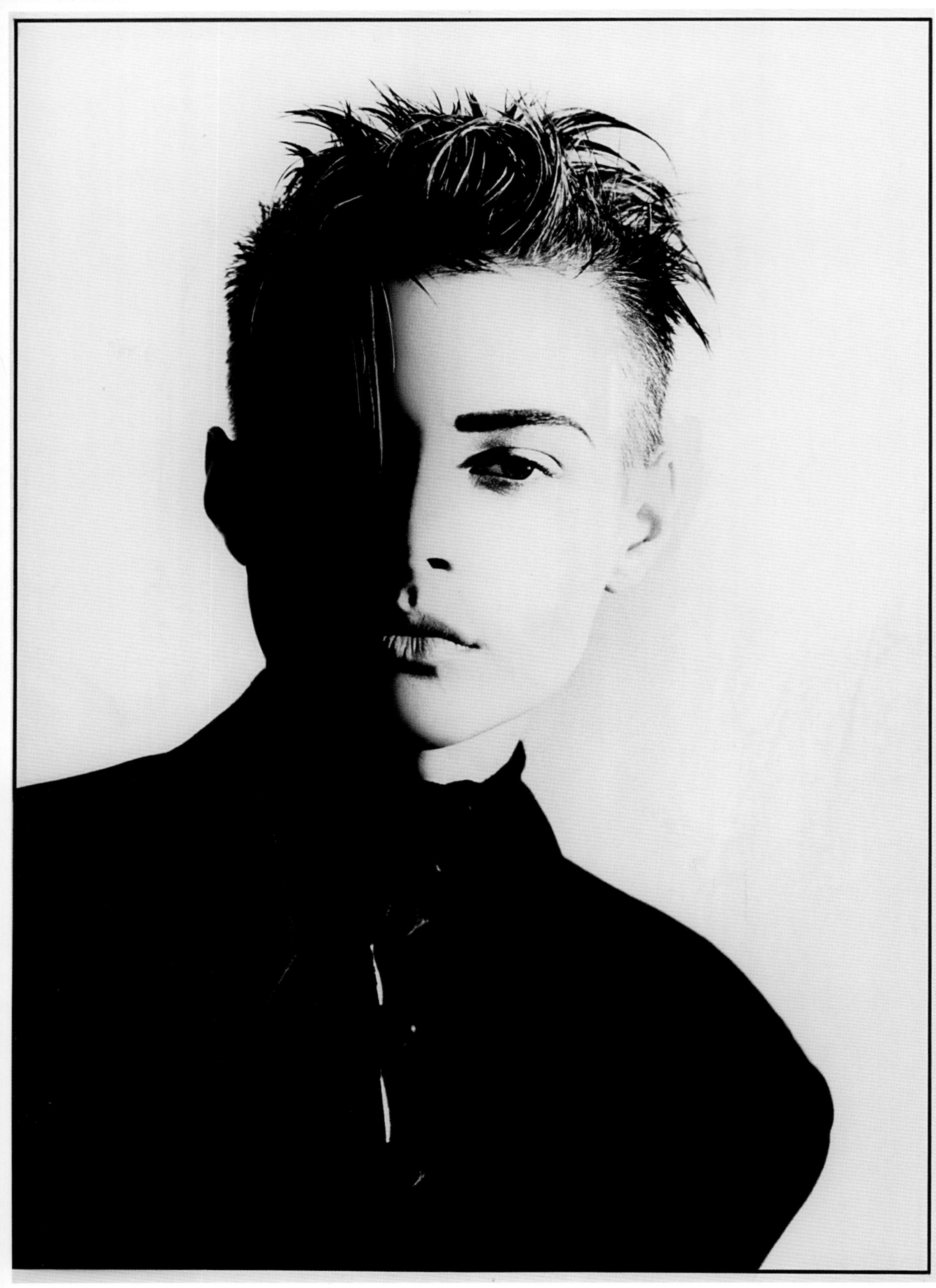

'Silhouette' hairstyle by Anthony Mascolo for TONI&GUY, 1987

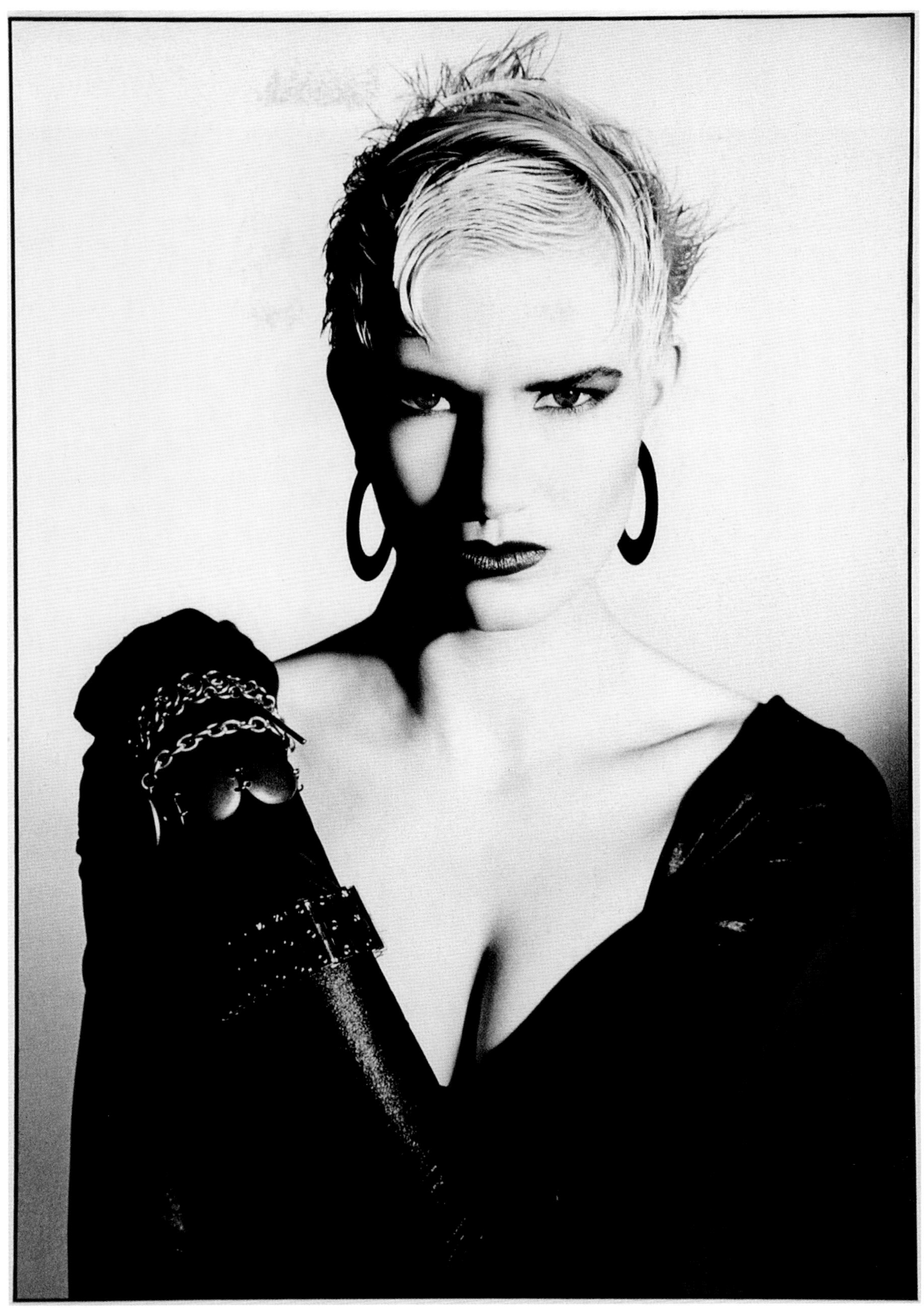

'Graphic' hairstyle by Anthony Mascolo for TONI&GUY, 1988

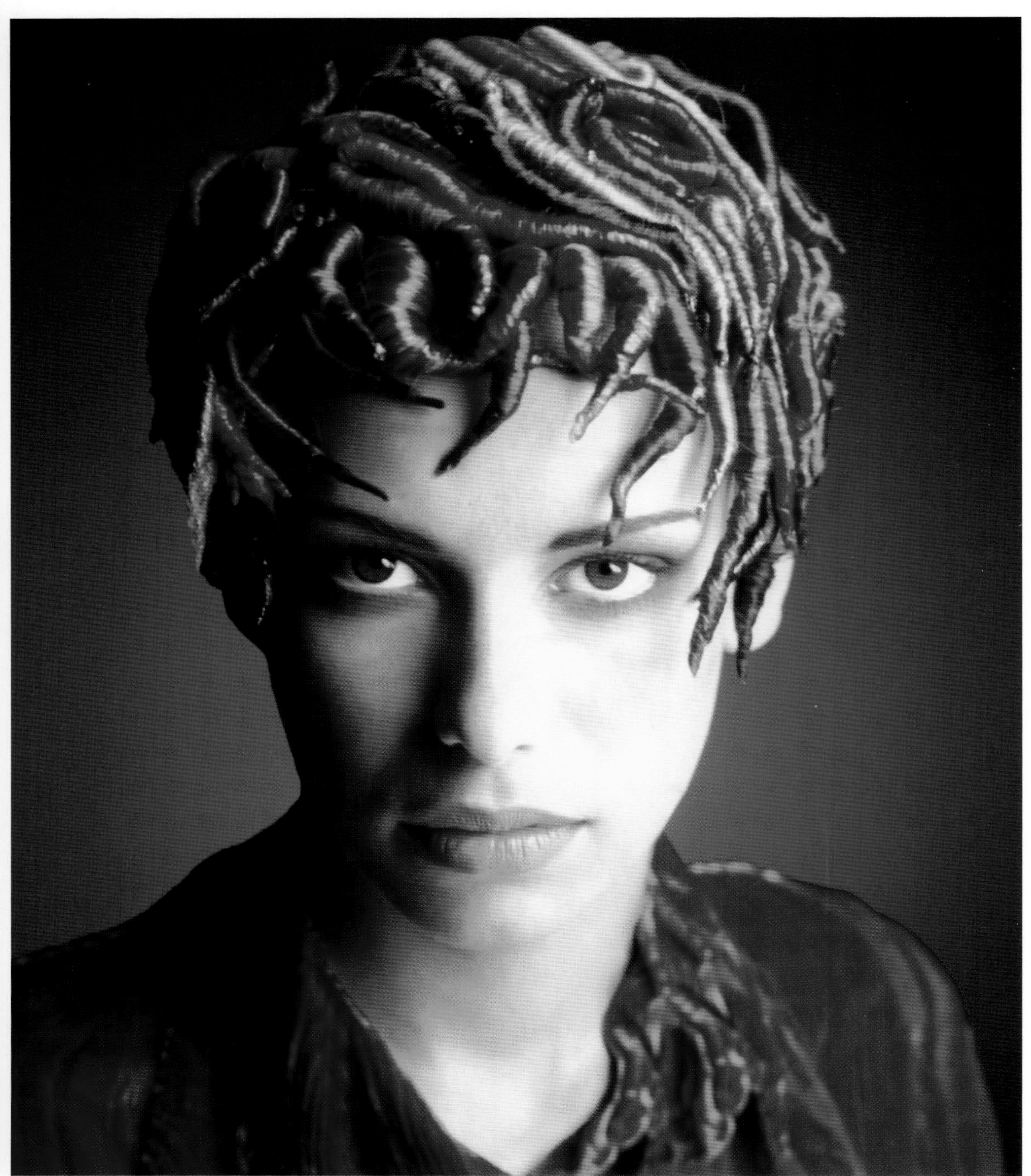

'Chilli Pepper' hairstyle by Simon Forbes for Antenna, c.1987

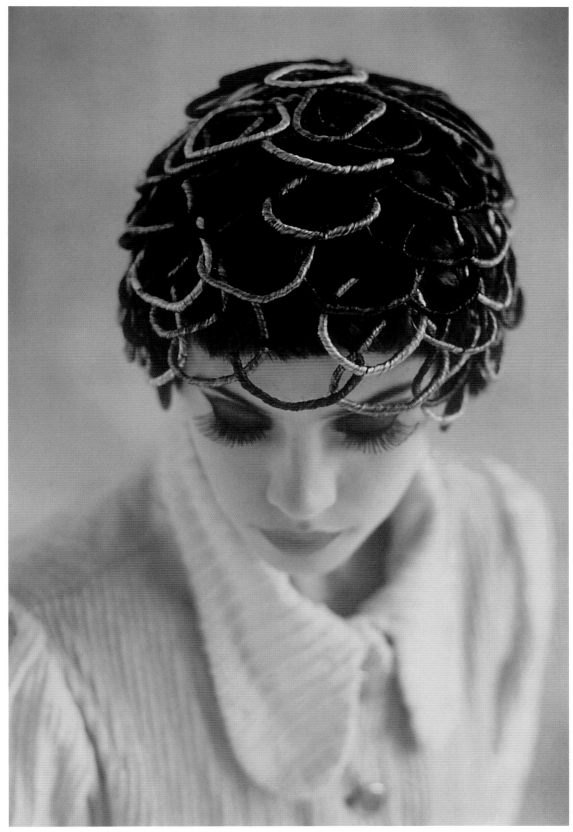

'The Loop' hairstyle by Simon Forbes for Antenna, 1988

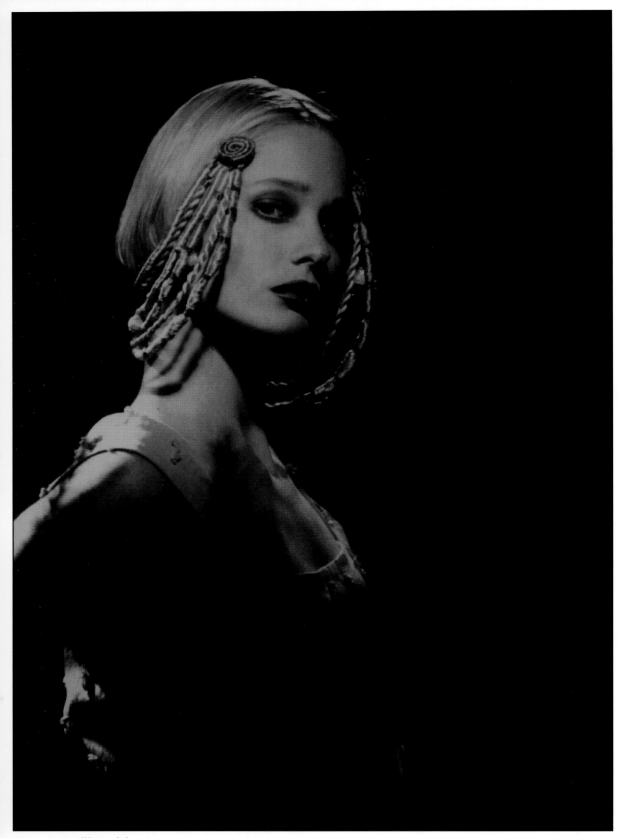

'Decorative Braid' hairstyle by
Simon Forbes for Antenna, 1988

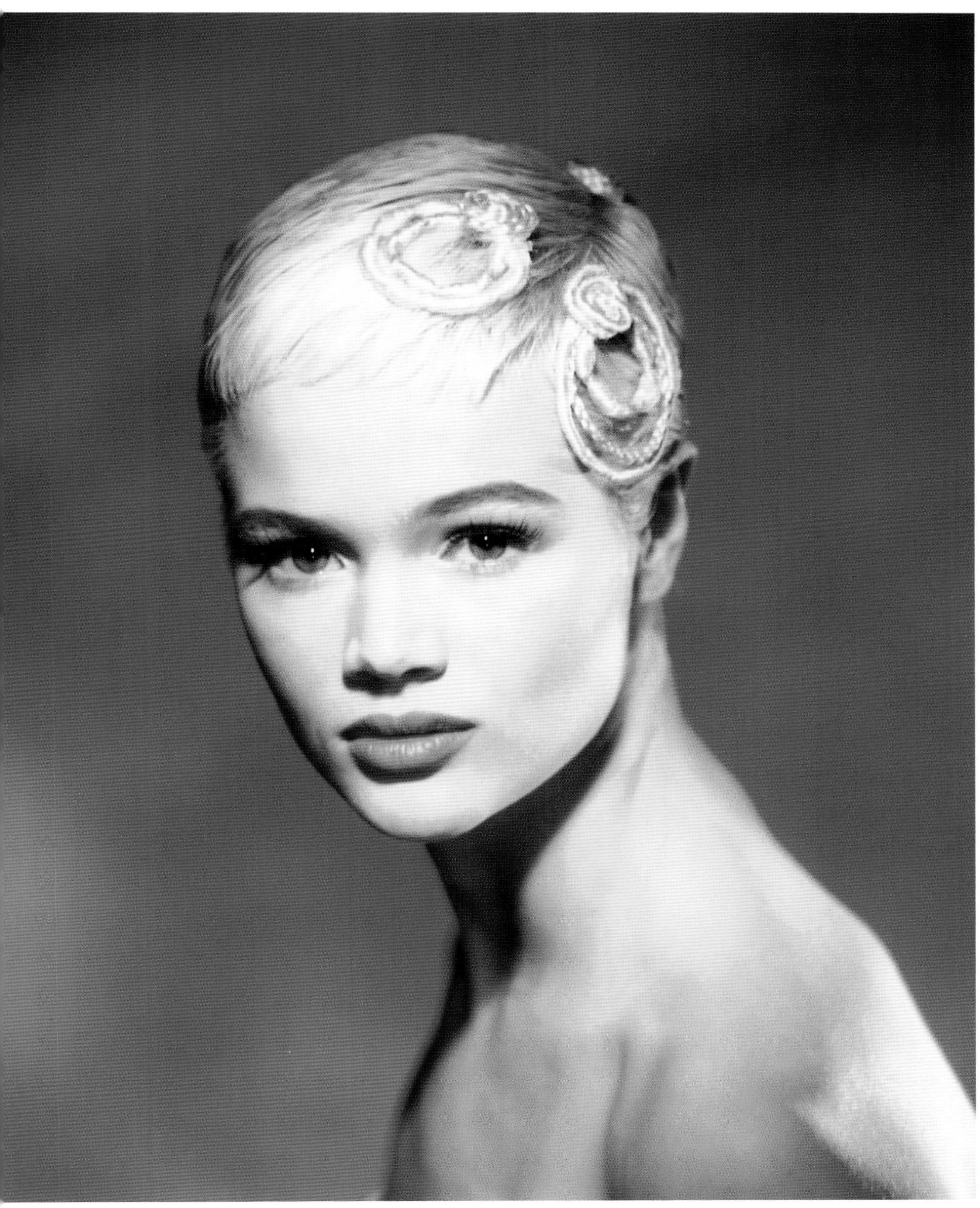

Decorative Braid' hairstyle by
Simon Forbes for Antenna, 1988

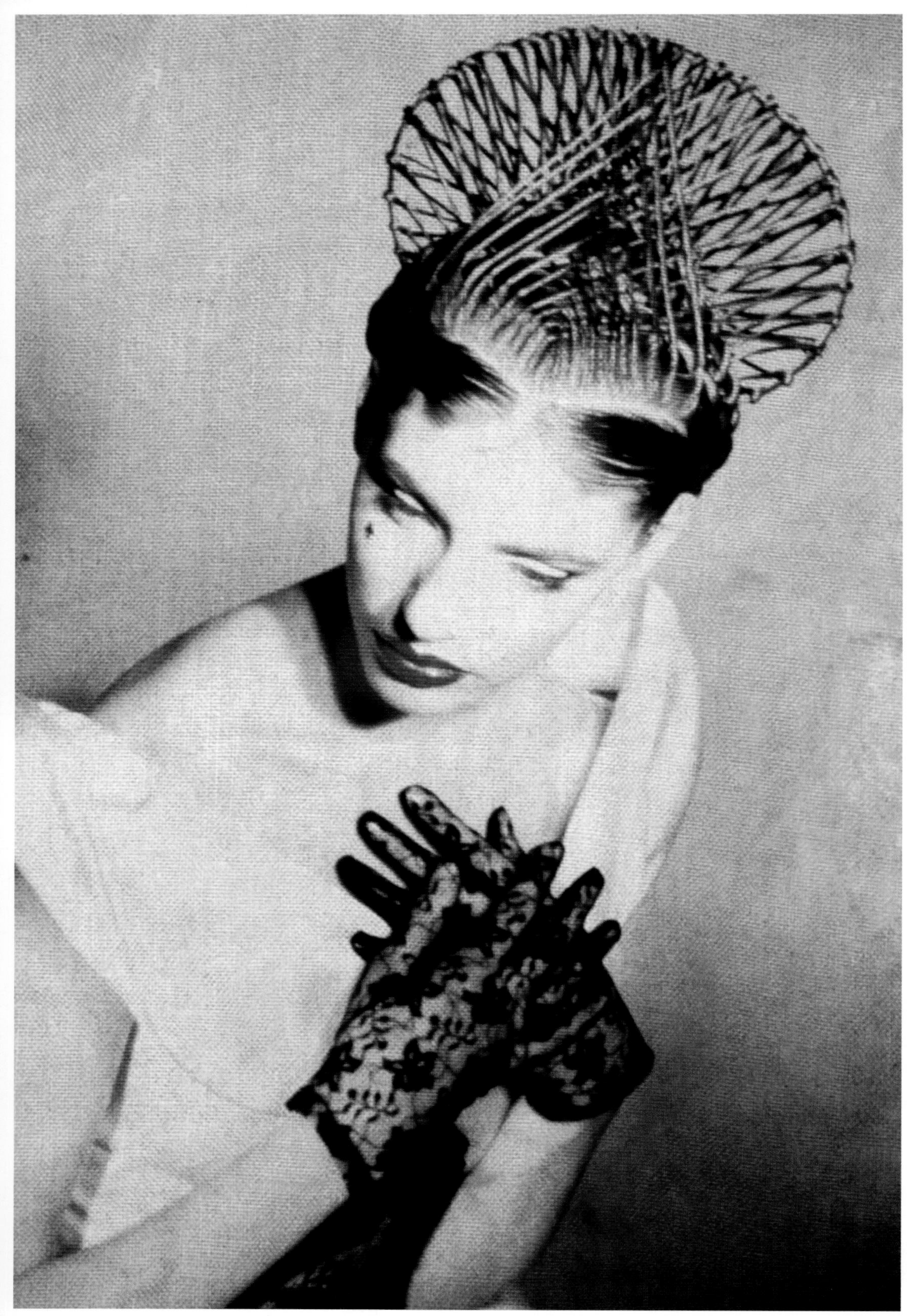

'Canvas' hairstyle by Anthony Mascolo for TONI&GUY, 1988

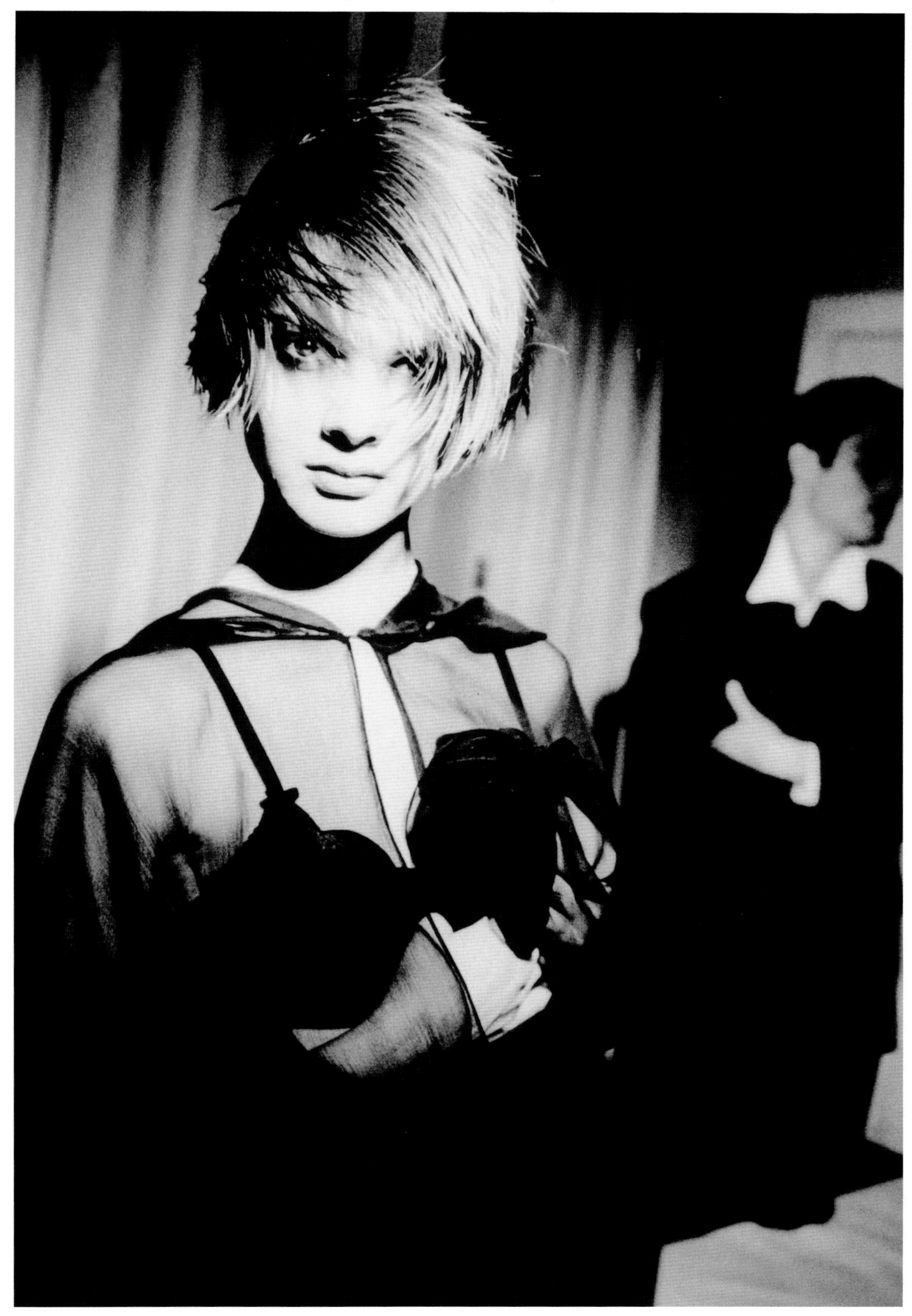

'Reportage' hairstyle by Anthony Mascolo for TONI&GUY, 1989

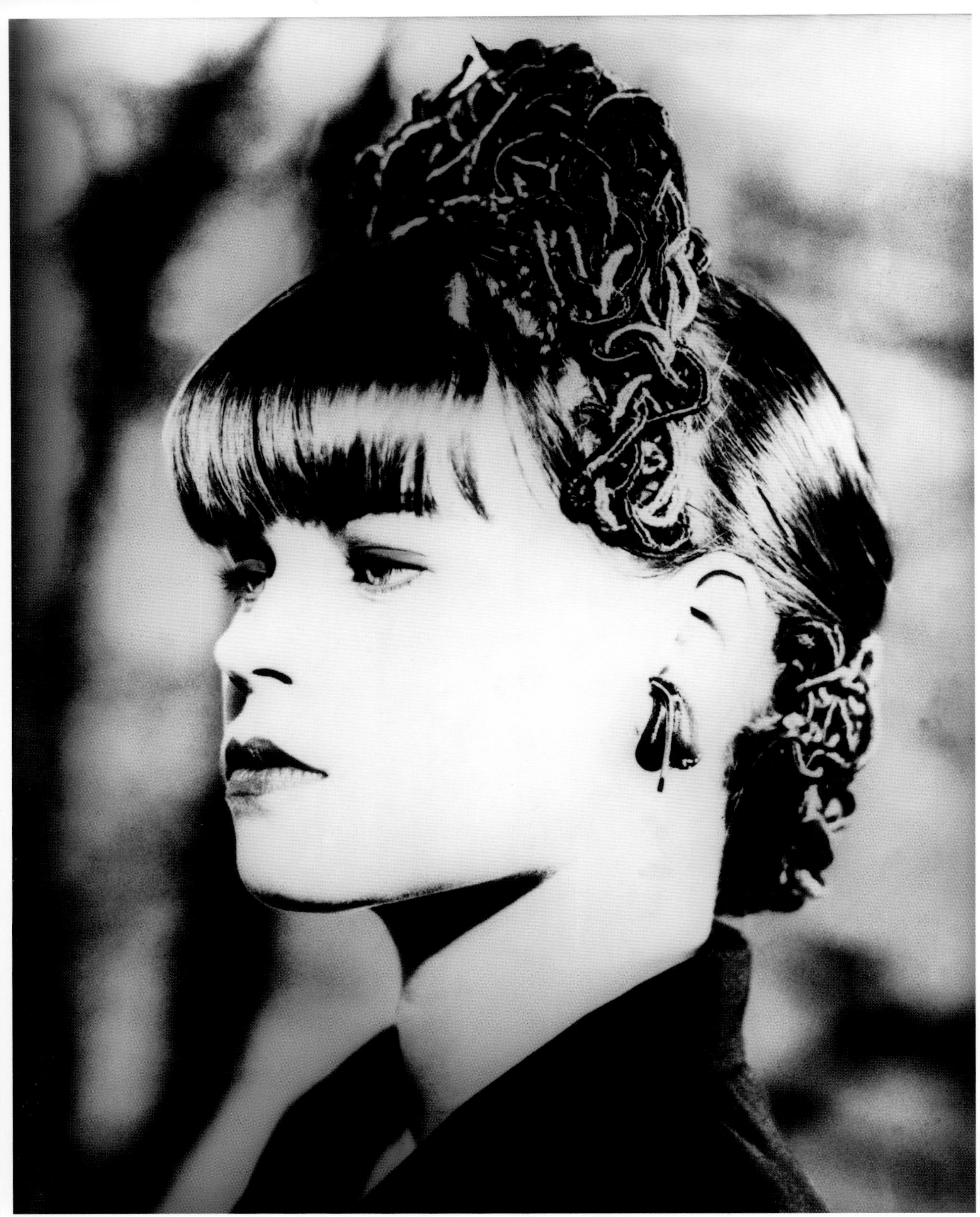

'Chignon' hairstyle by Simon Forbes for Antenna, 1989

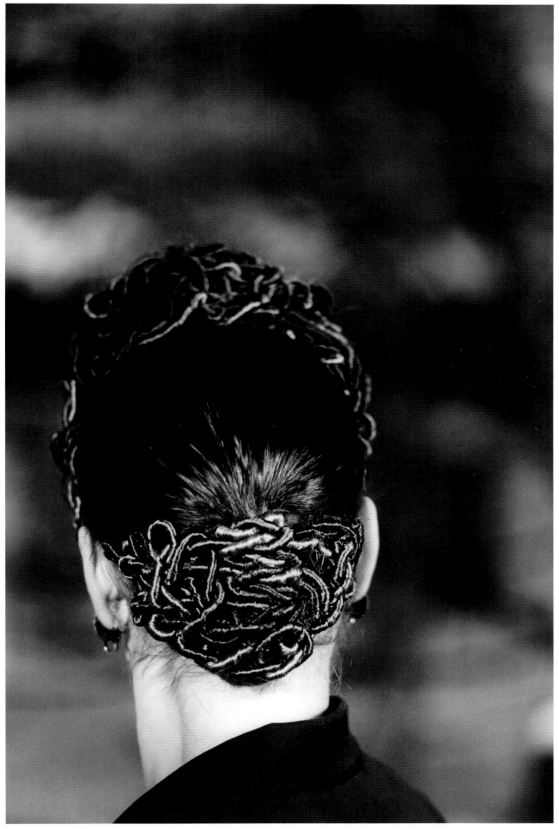

'Chignon' hairstyle by Simon Forbes for Antenna, 1989

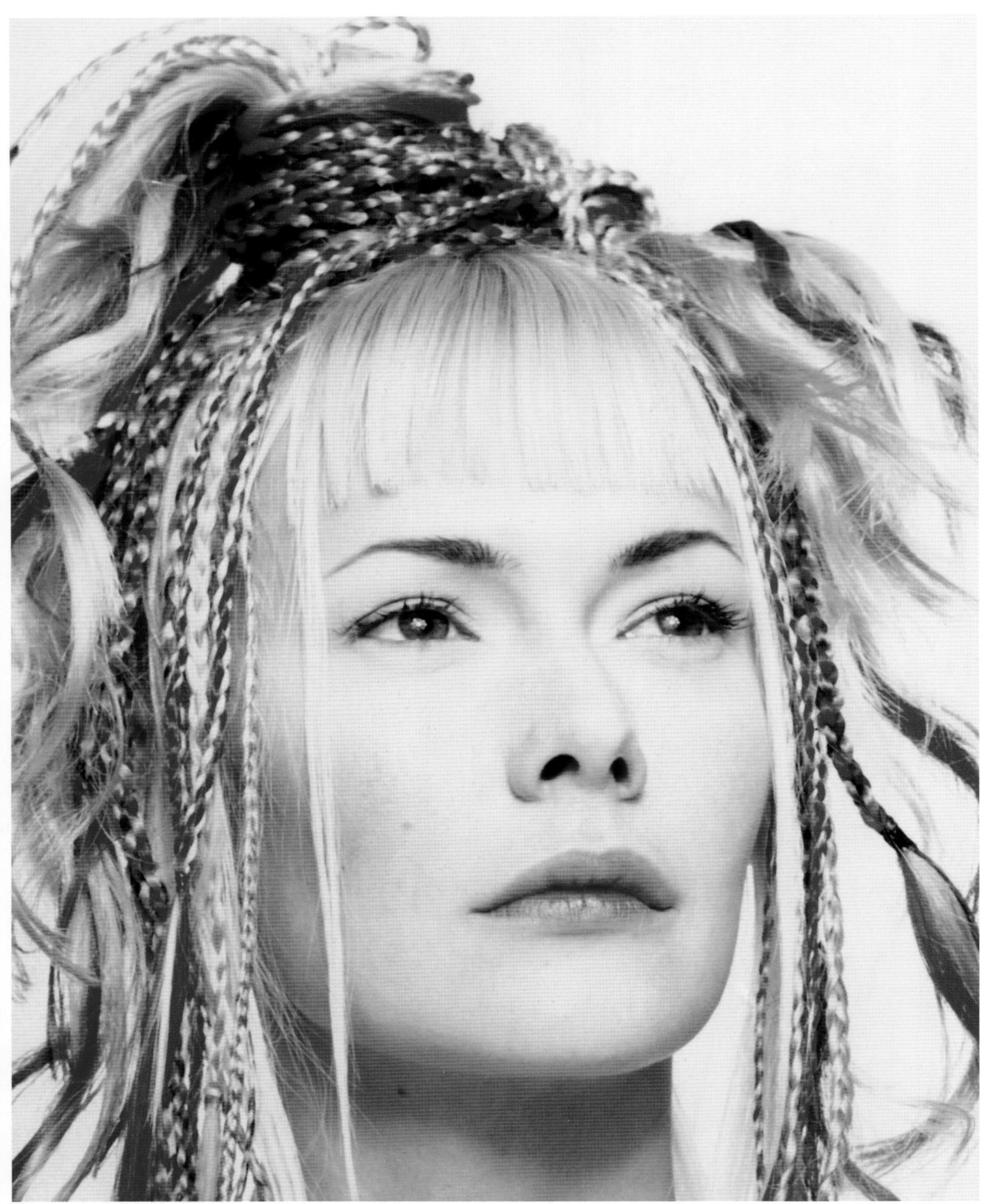

'Cult Colour' hairstyle by Simon Forbes for Antenna, 1989

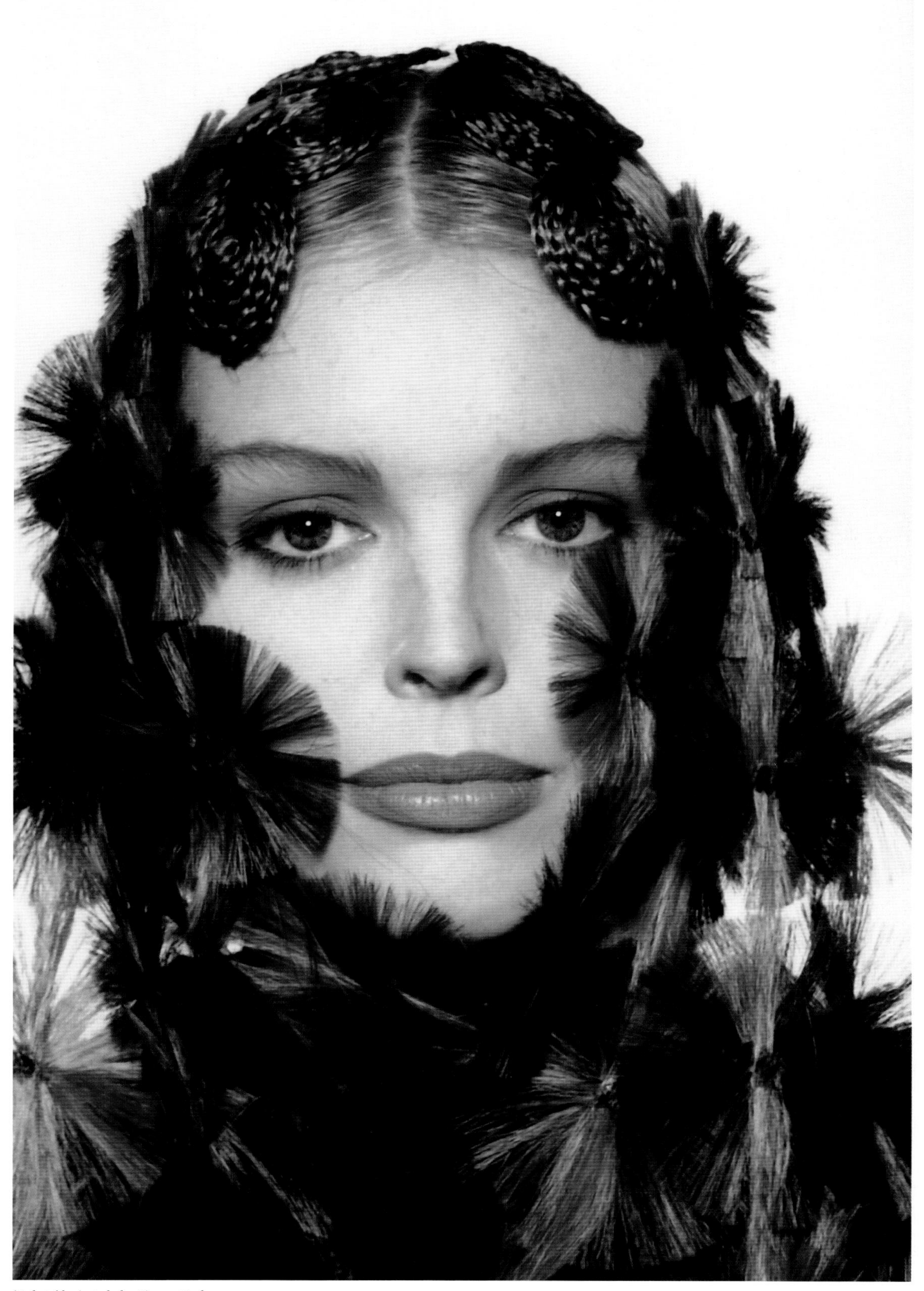

'Splatz' hairstyle by Simon Forbes
for Antenna, 1989

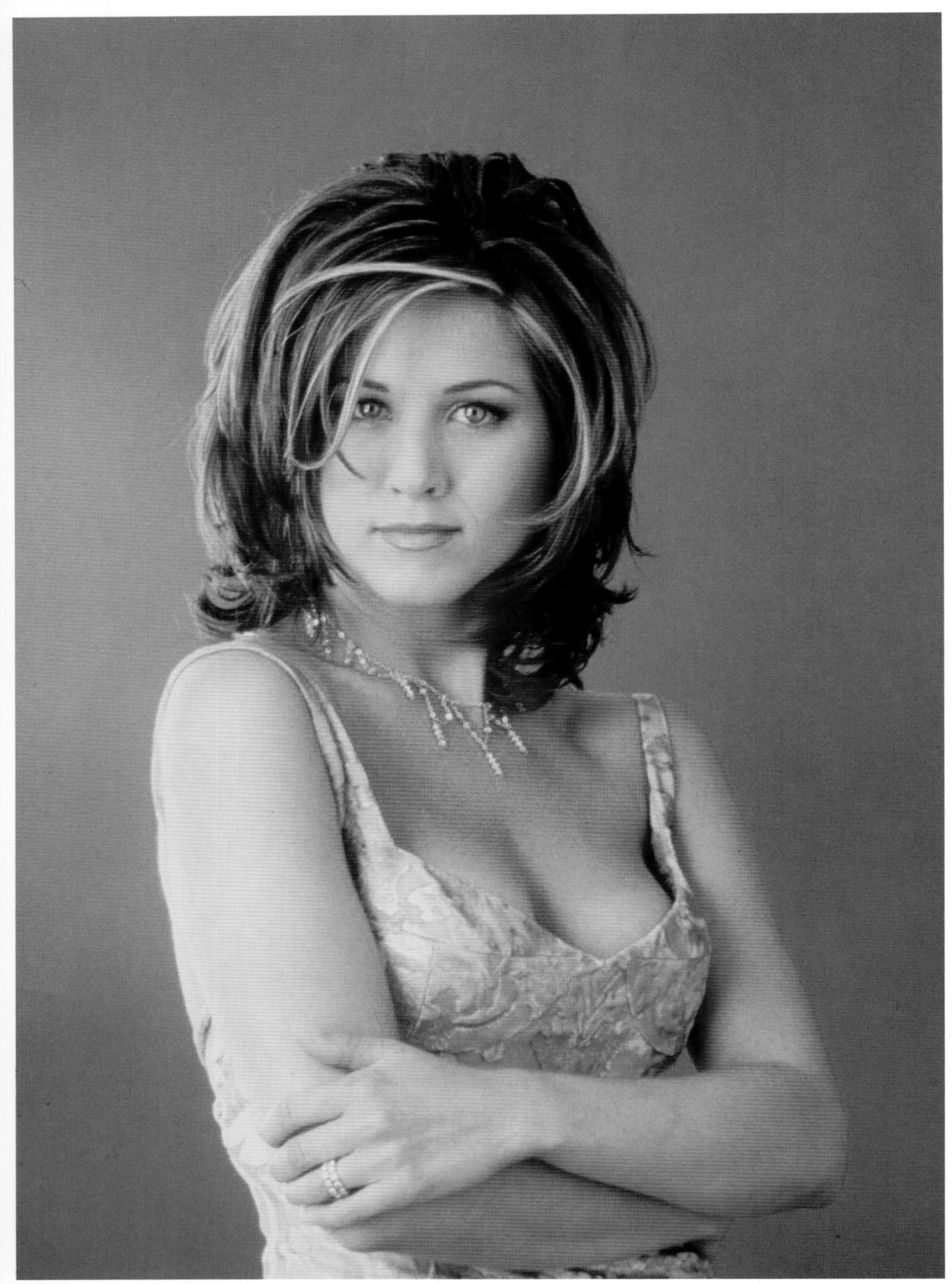

'The Rachel', created by Chris MacMillan for *Friends* actress, Jennifer Aniston, was the most requested cut of the decade, 1996

1990S

The Nineties saw the complete and utter rejection of the overtly styled hairdos of the previous decade. Instead, a more natural look was desired, and in the early Nineties women began growing out their previous haircuts – as they did this, new feathered, layered and shaggy styles became fashionable. At this stage there seemed more emphasis on trimming than cutting, and also easy-to-wear/easy-to-maintain styles became increasingly popular. There was also an obsession with the actual quality of the hair and numerous flower-based and cocoa-butter based products came onto the market in order to provide, so they claimed, an extra-healthy shine. The emphasis was also on natural-looking hair colour rather than the bright and often artificial look of the Eighties era.

During the mid-to-late Nineties, "Up-Do Princess" styles were very fashionable, especially for bridal hairstyles, however, the most popular hairstyle of the decade by far, was the "Rachel" named after Jennifer Aniston's character in the long-running sitcom, "Friends". Shoulder-length and straight, the honey-coloured "Rachel", created by Chris McMillan, was the antithesis of the Eighties power-do and reflected a new kind of knowing sexy femininity. By the late 1990s there was a marked resurgence in the use of hair straighteners and as a result the predominant look was super-straight long hair. The Nineties also saw the increasing use of hair extensions to either lengthen hair instantly or thicken it so that it appeared to have more luxurious volume.

Significantly the 90s saw the advent of new digital media, which enabled hair fashions to spread rapidly from one country to another, so you were just as likely to see the same haircut in New York as you were in Stockholm or Paris. New media, most notably the Internet, also helped to increase the pace of globalisation, and this in turn helped turn hair into a really big business. This led to increased specialisation within the industry, with hairdressers falling into four distinct camps: the salon stylist, the session stylist, the competition/show stylist and the celebrity stylist. During this decade numerous celebrity hairstylists launched or licensed their own hair product ranges and made a fortune, and increasingly their hairstyles became a means to shift ever more lucrative product. Hair shows also became progressively more lavish and were an important vehicle for prominent stylists to promote the use of their "product" to other members of the industry. Overall, the Nineties were marked by a greater degree of professionalism within the industry as a whole, and high-maintenance straightened hair became the defining look of this "good hair" obsessed decade.

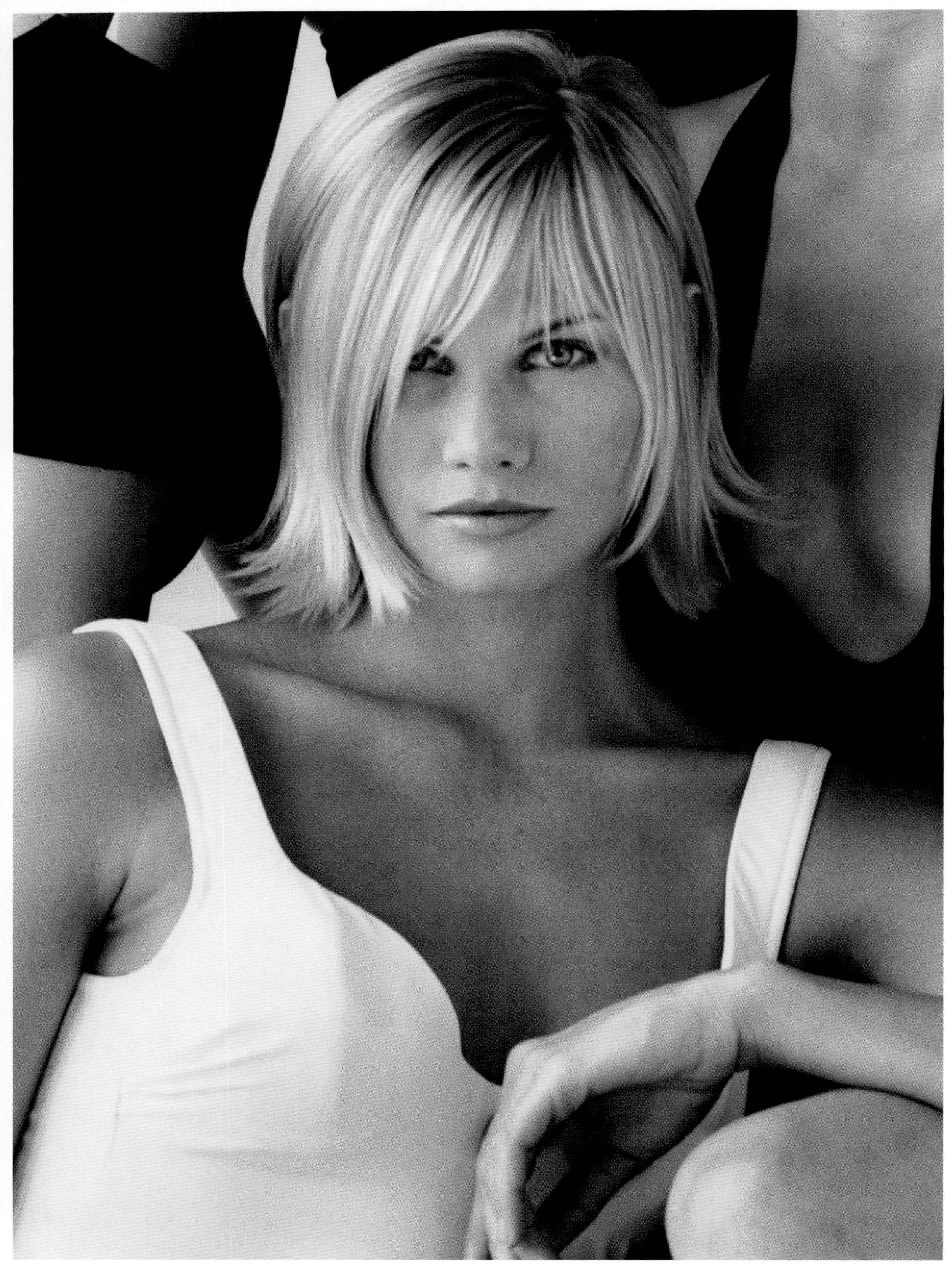

'Transient' hairstyle by Anthony Mascolo for TONI&GUY, 1992

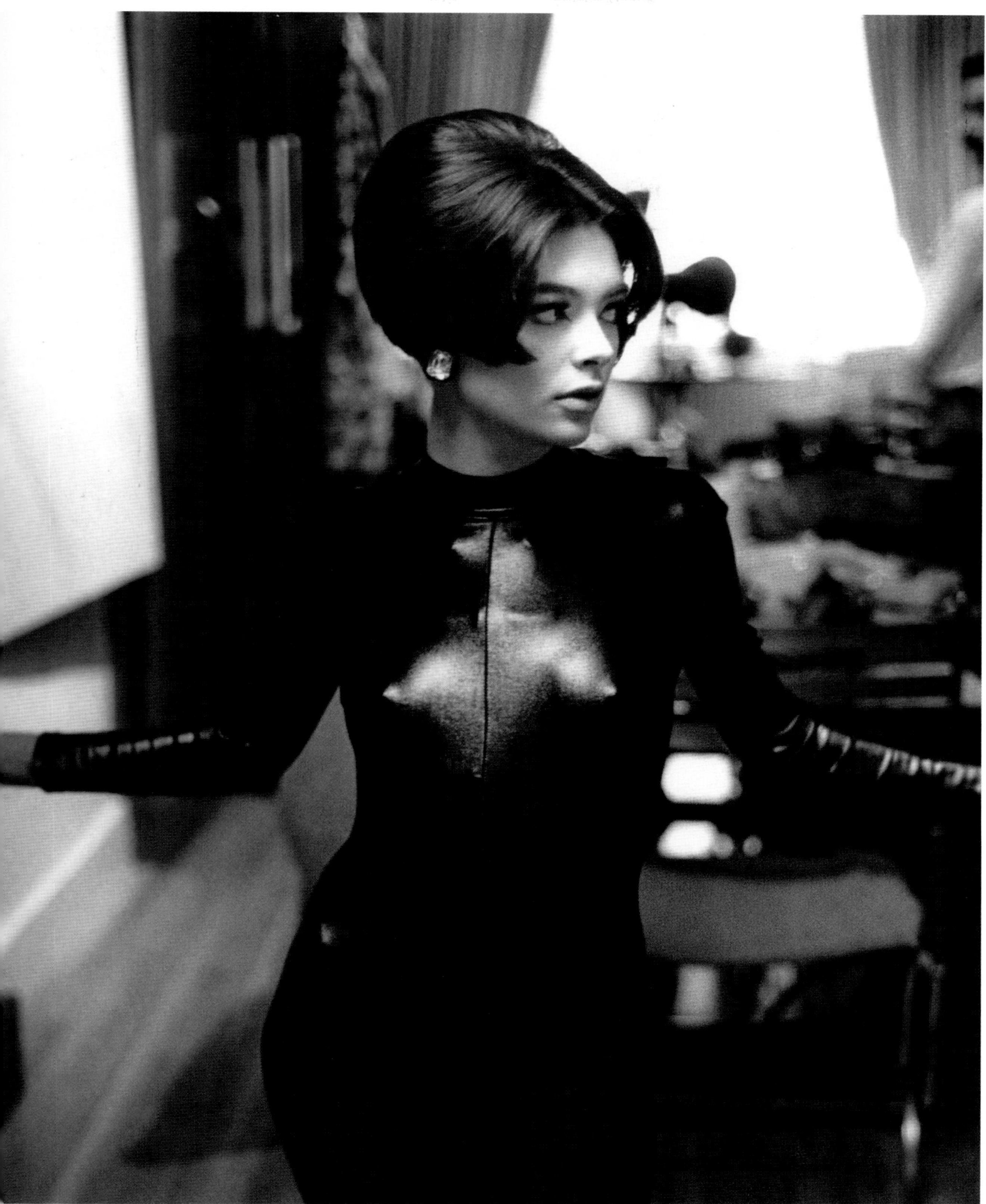

bbed hairstyle by Paul
monds, 1992

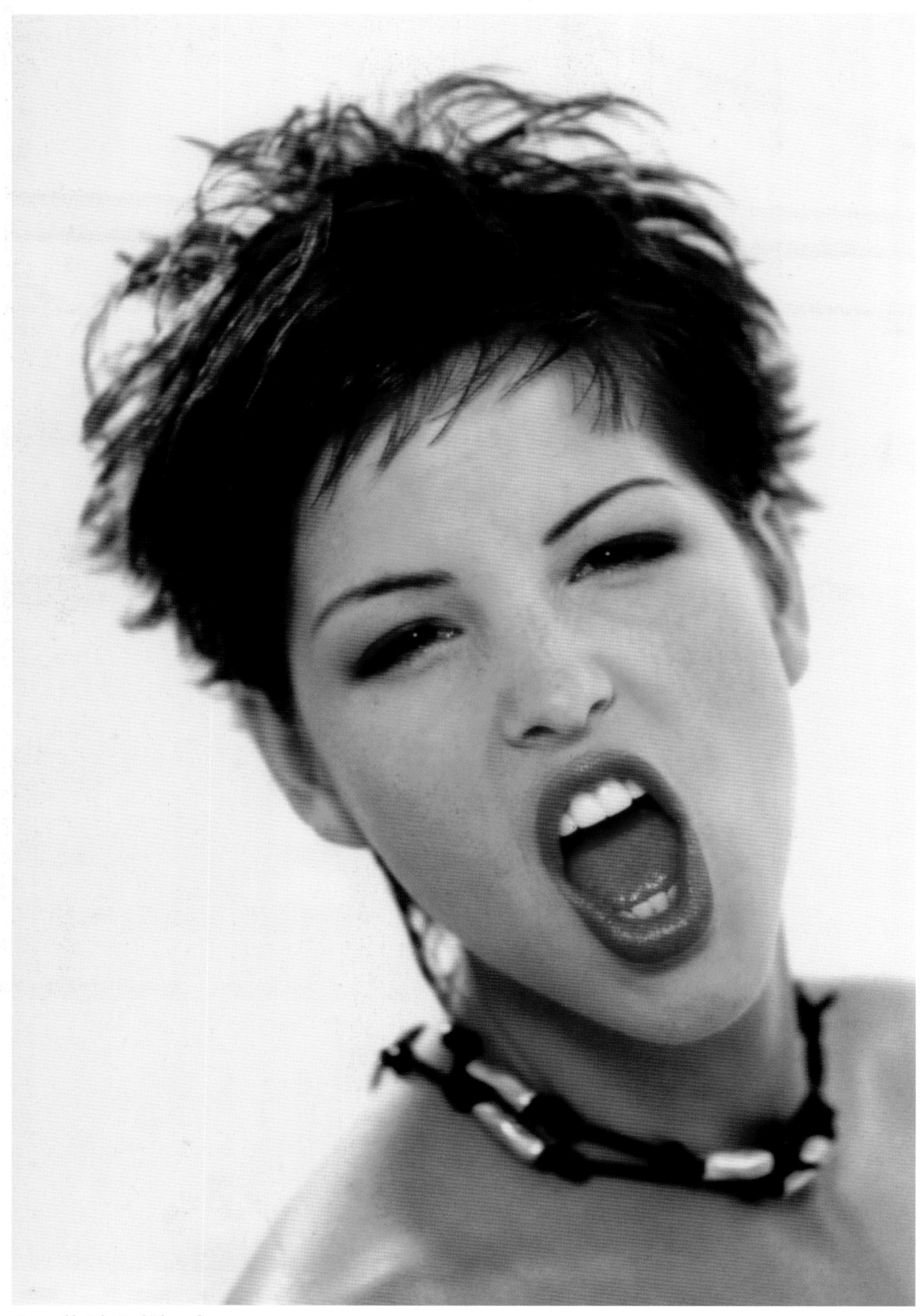

Cropped hair by Paul Edmonds, 1993

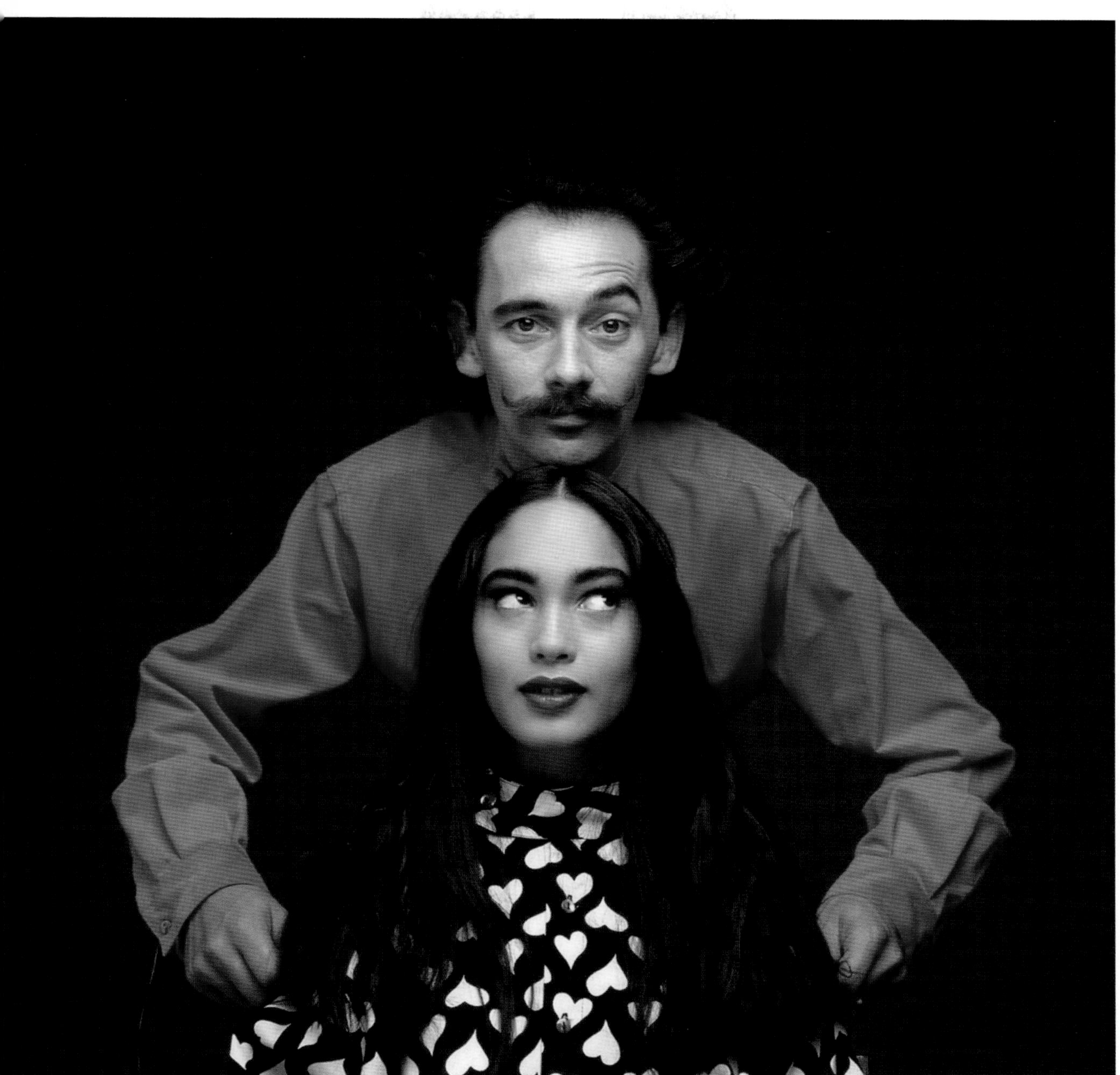

Hairstylist, Paul Edmonds, styling hair, early 1990s

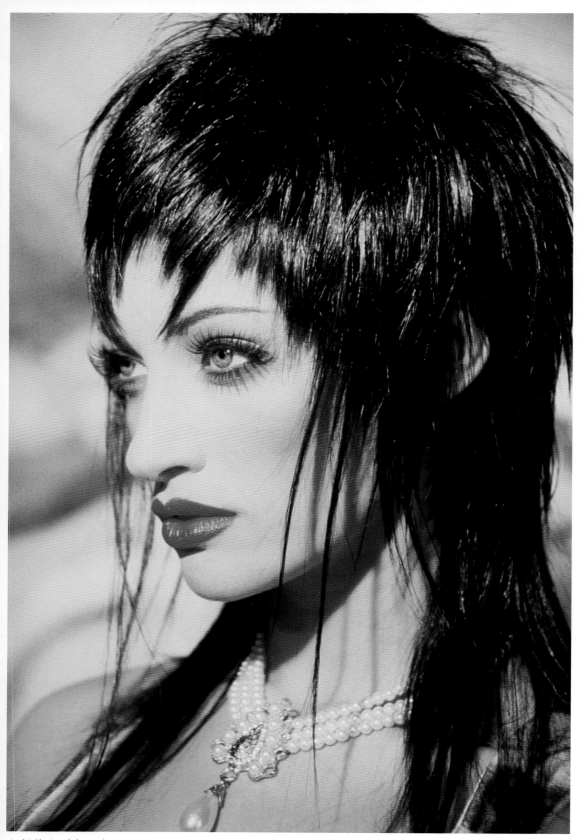

'Celtic' hairstyle by Anthony Mascolo for TONI&GUY, 1994

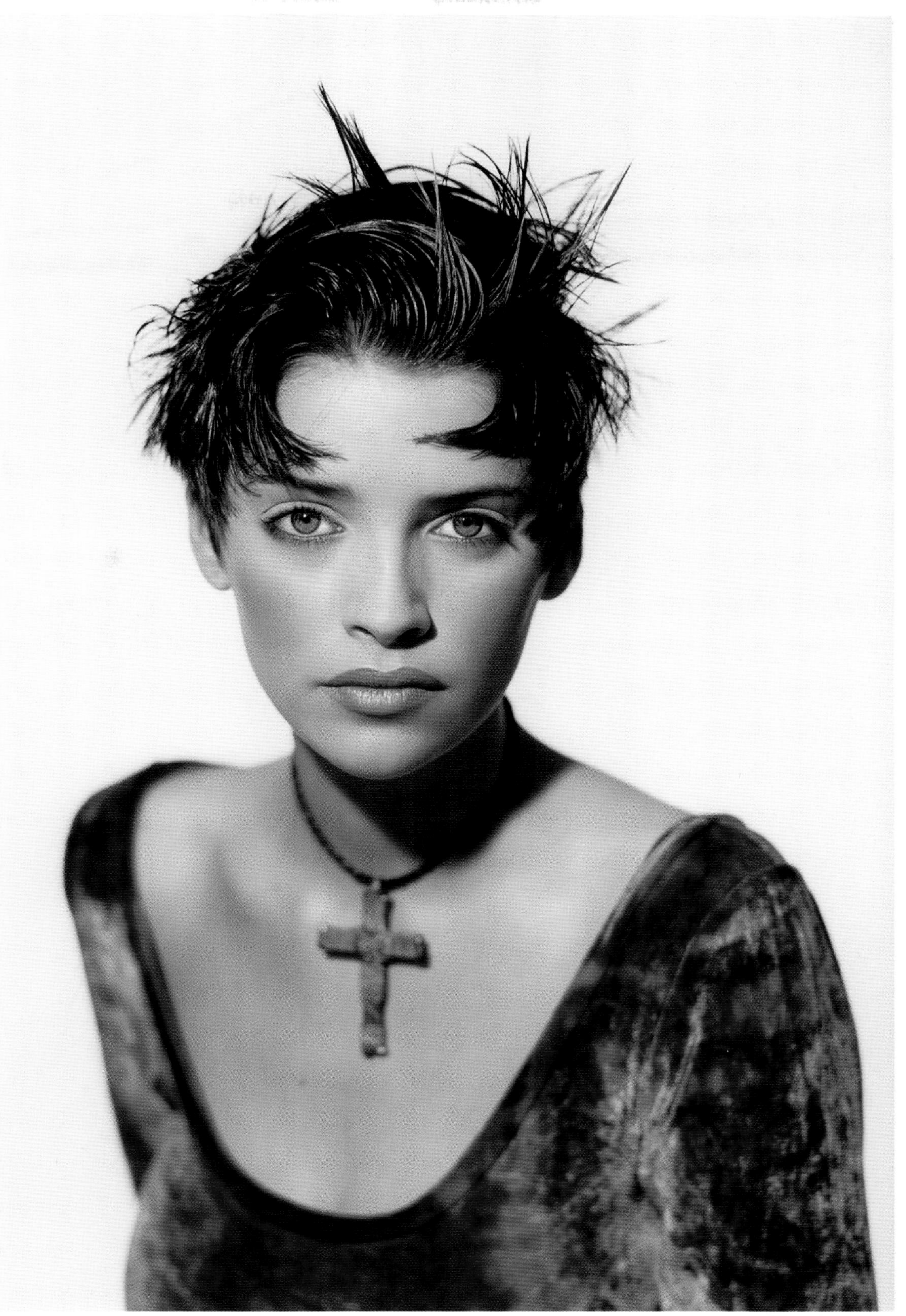

'Clarity' hairstyle by Anthony Mascolo for TONI&GUY, 1994

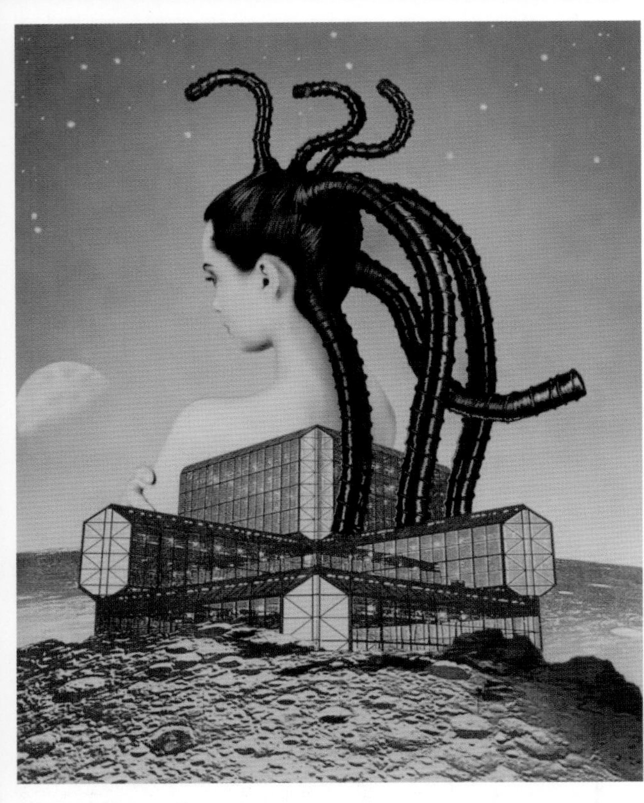

Hairstyles by Michael Barnes, the first Architecture Collection for the Alternative Hair Show, 1994

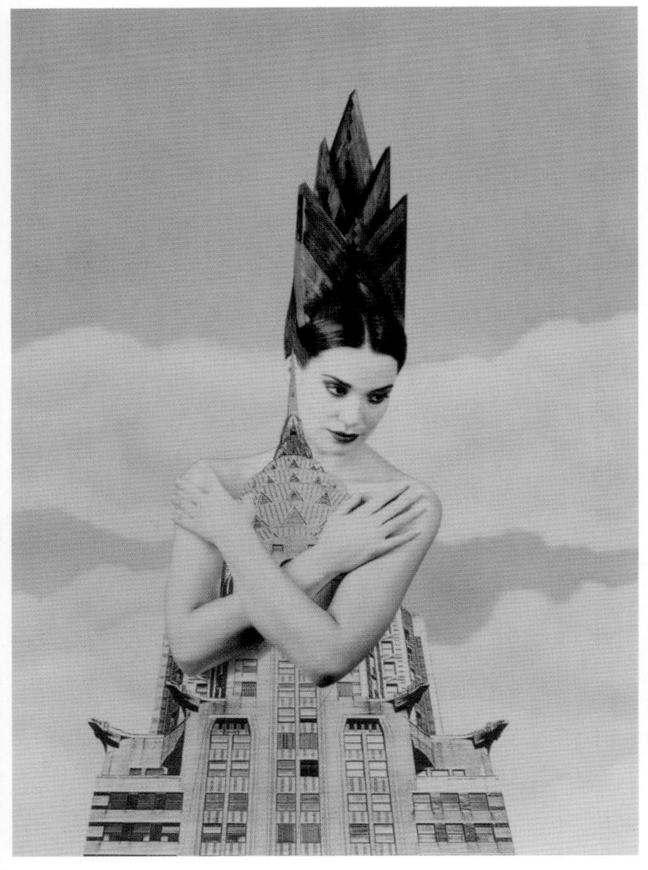

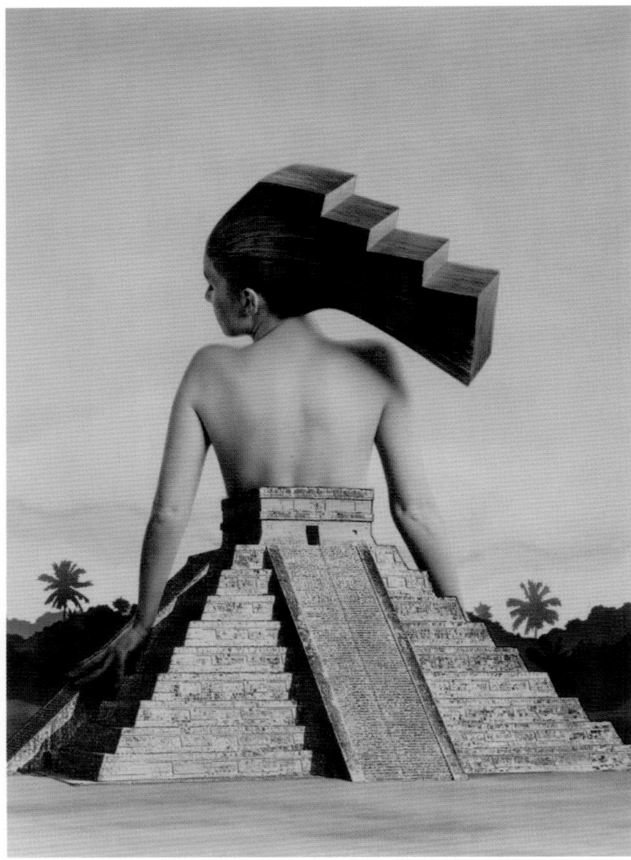

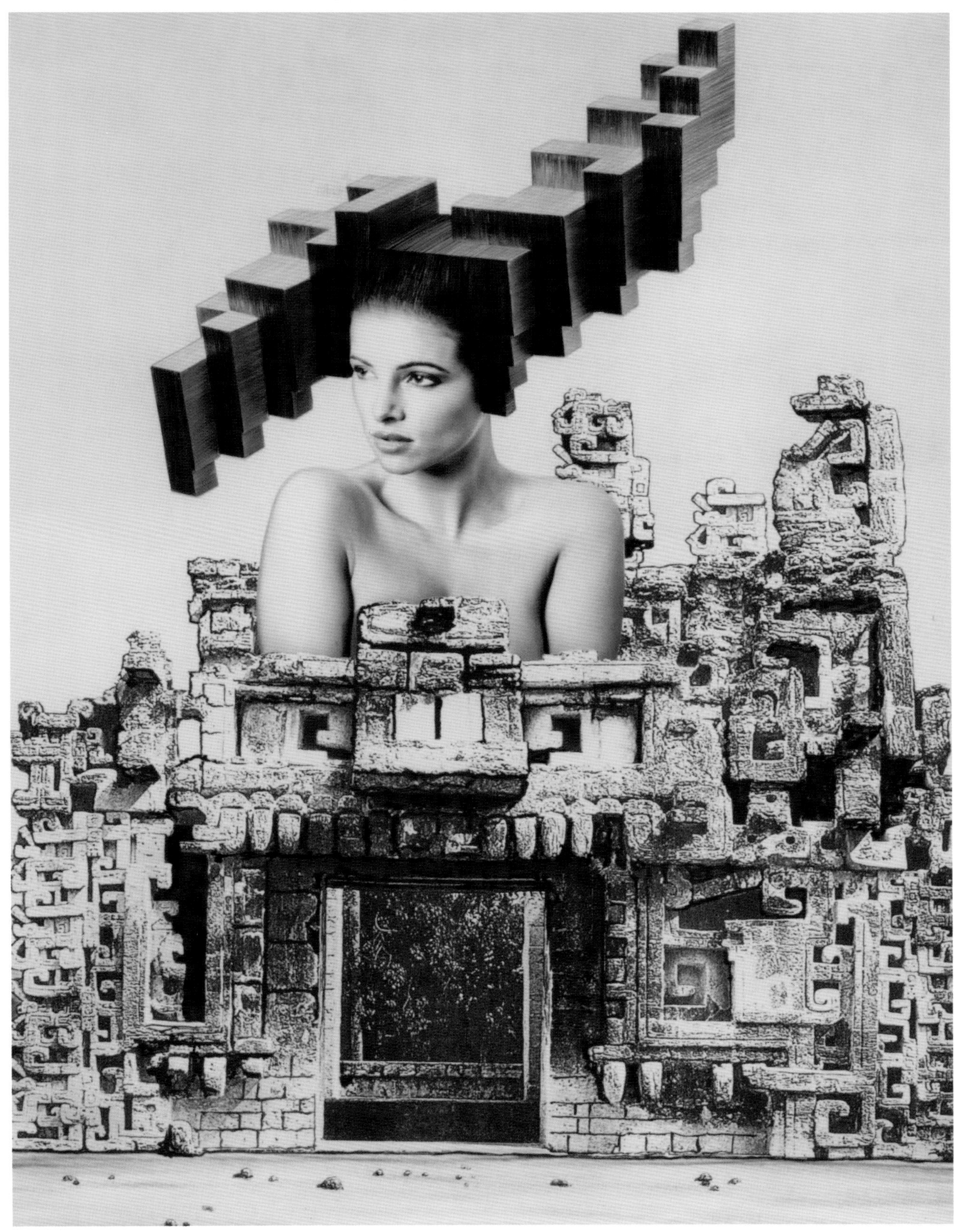

'Aztec' by Michael Barnes, the first Architecture Collection for the Alternative Hair Show, 1994

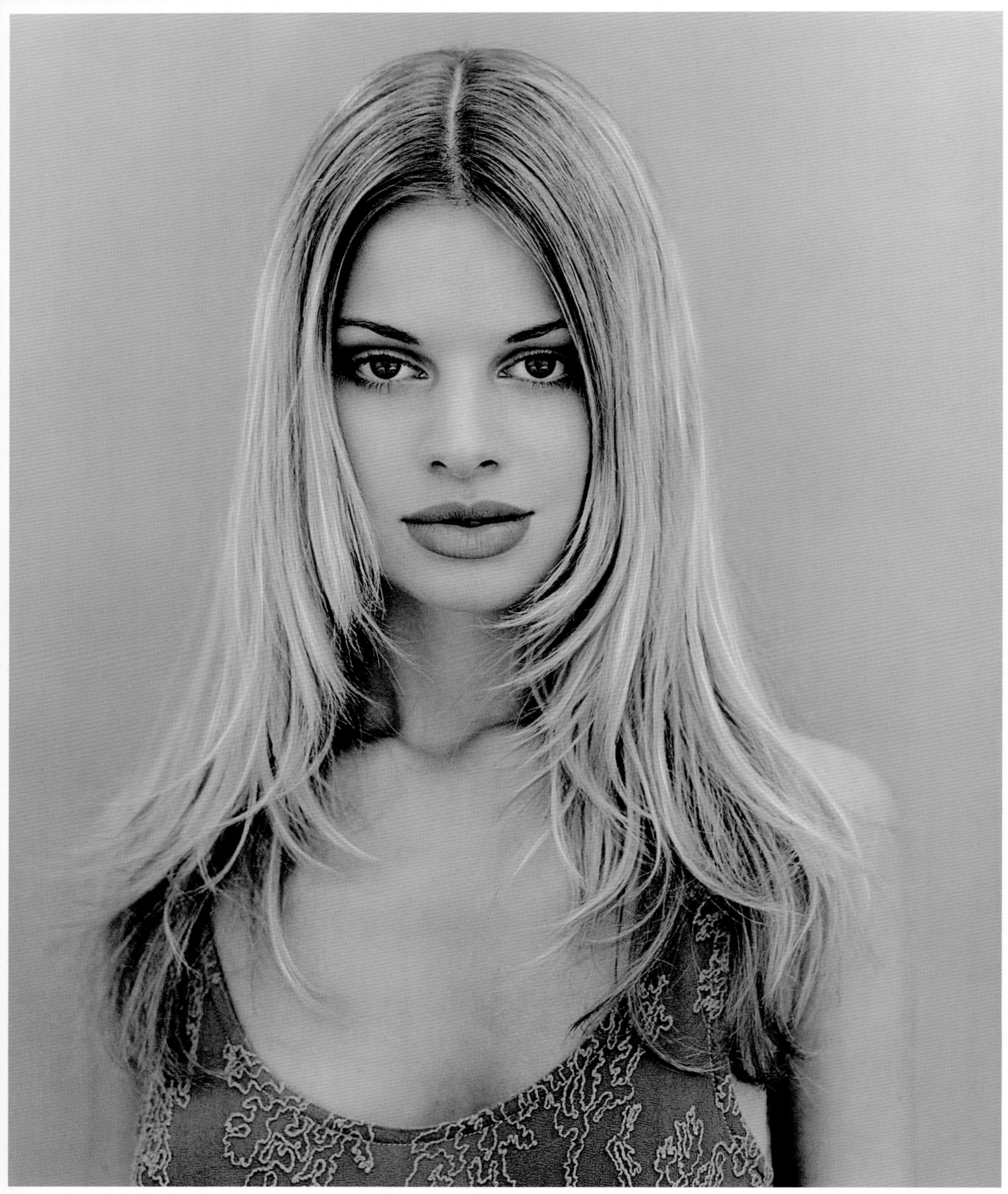

Hairstyle by Anthony Mascolo for
TONI&GUY, 1995

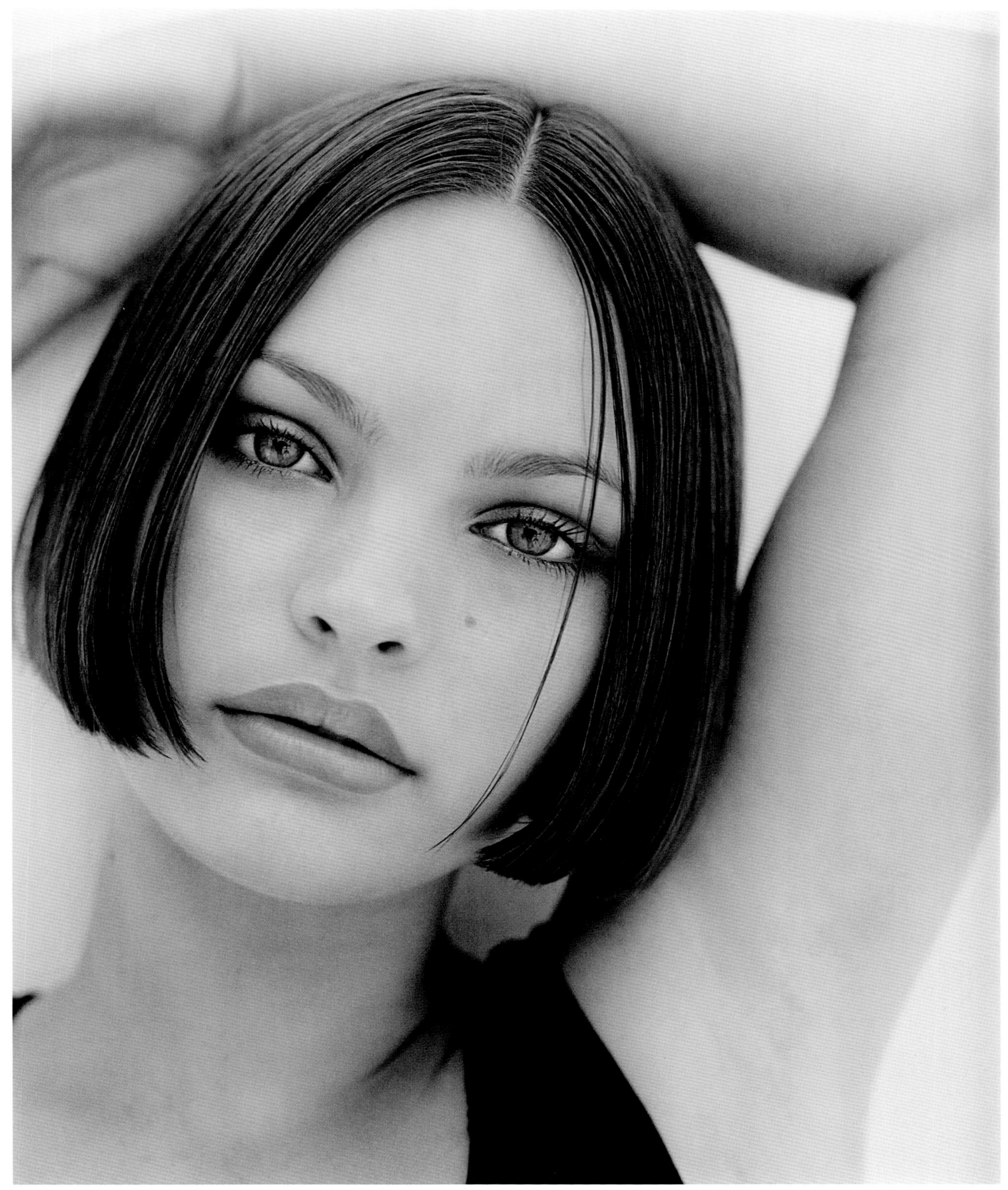

Hairstyle by Anthony Mascolo for TONI&GUY, 1995

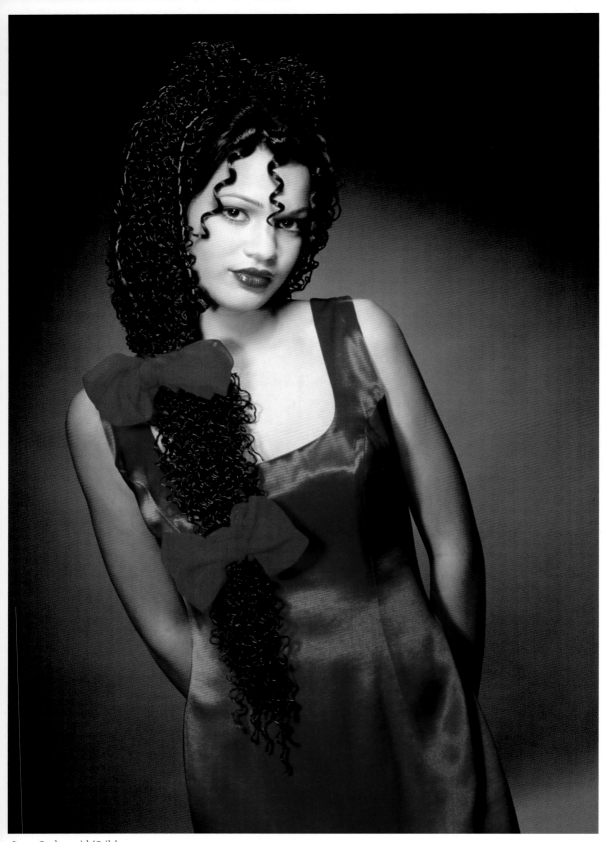

Stacey Gardner with 'Coils'
hairstyle by Rona O'Connor, 1995

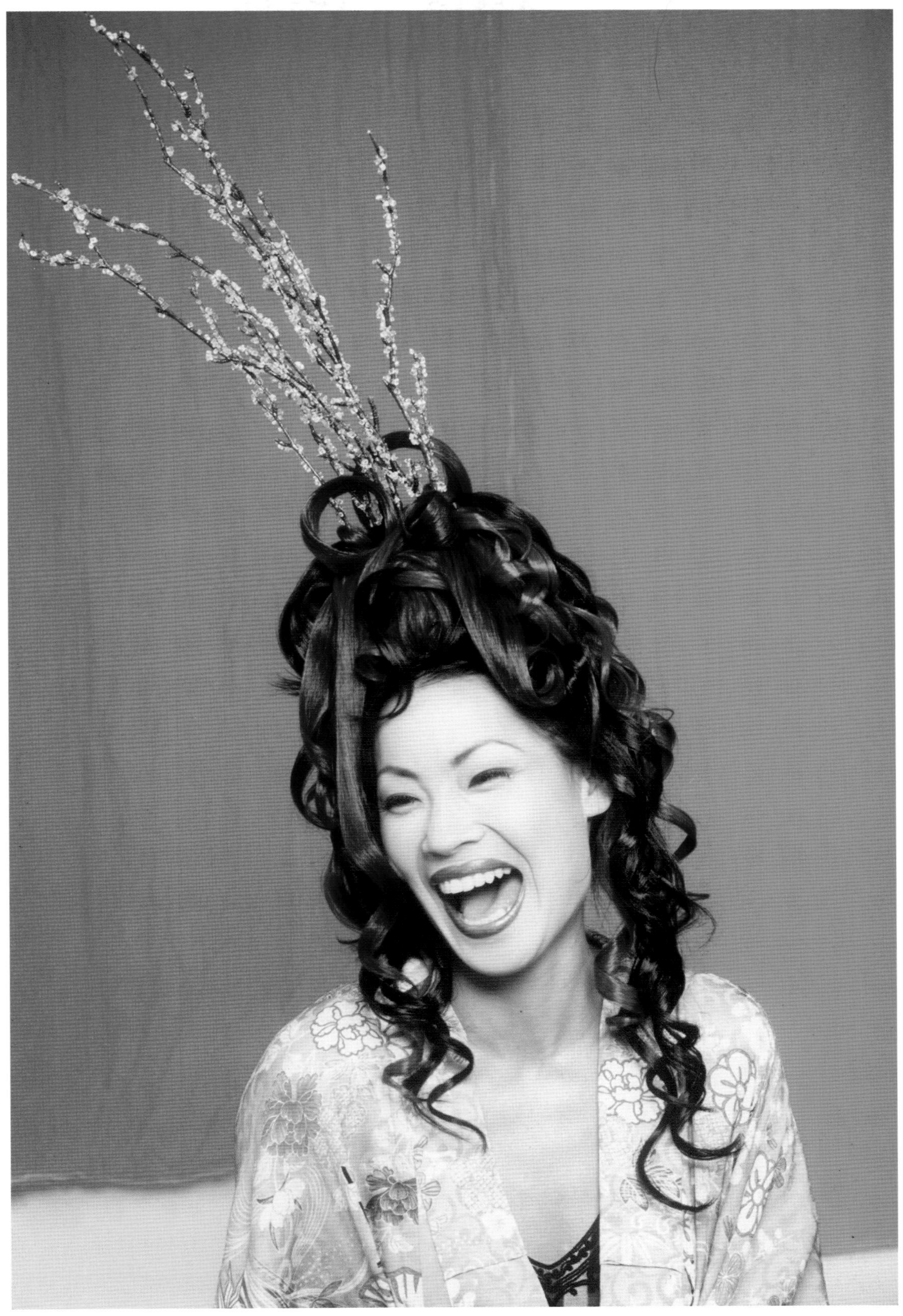

Lucy Liu with hairstyle by Rona O'Connor, Luke O'Connor, and Julie Watson, 1996

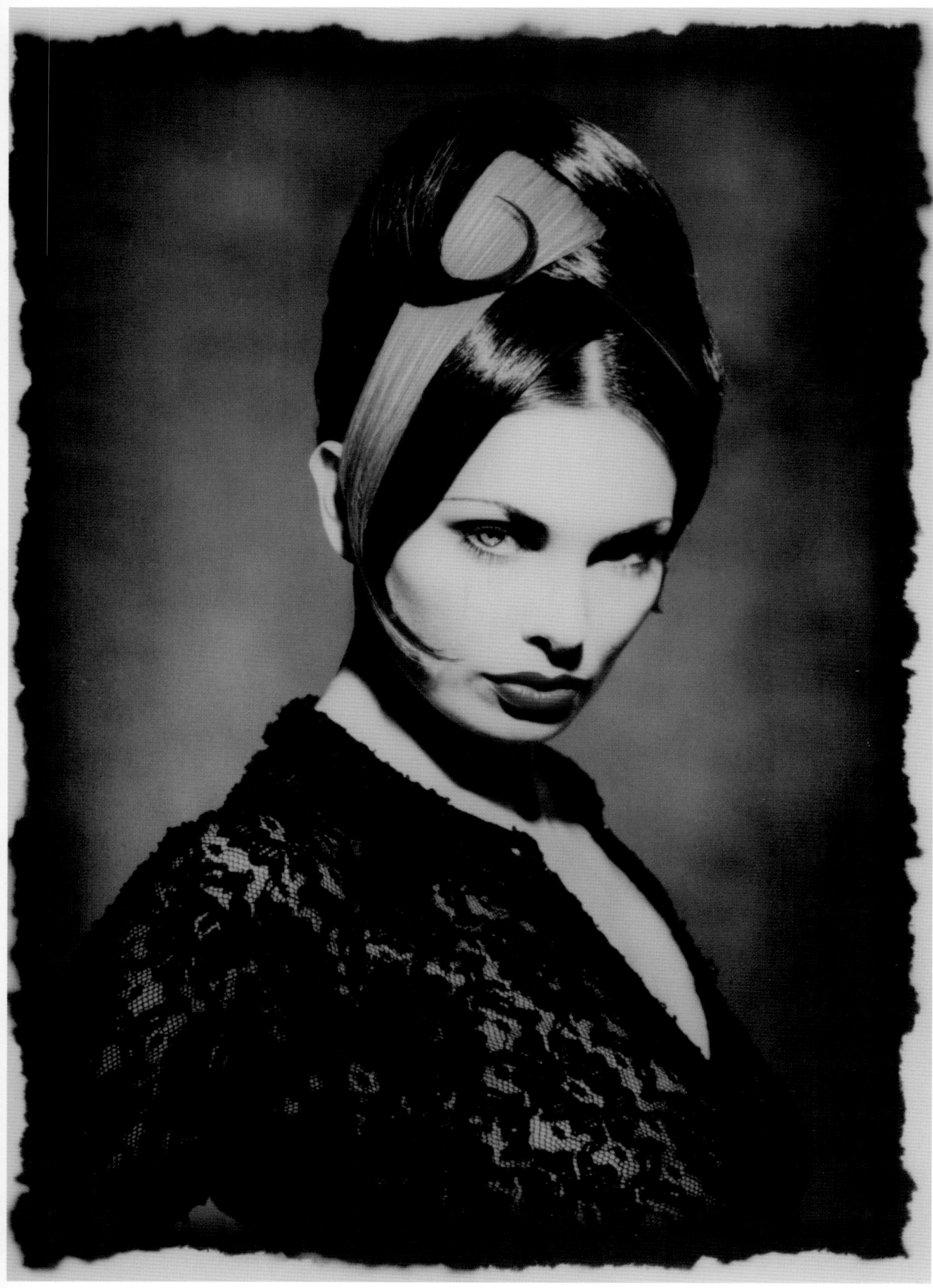

Hairstyles from Painted Ladies
Collection, Michael Barnes, 1995

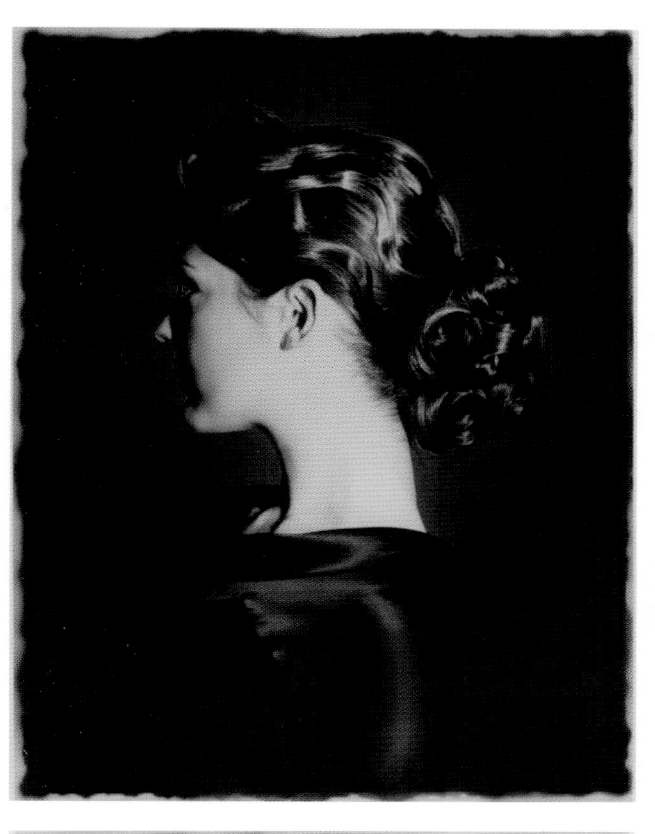

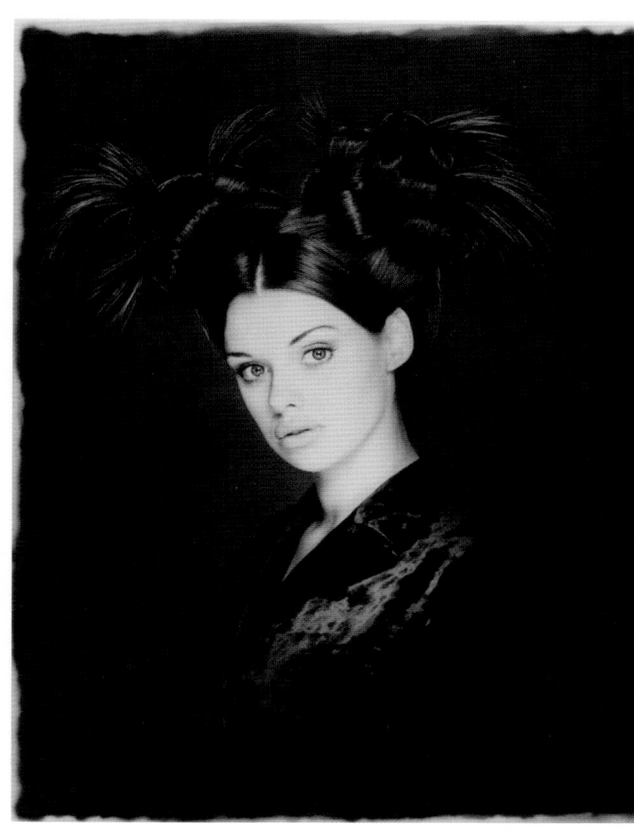

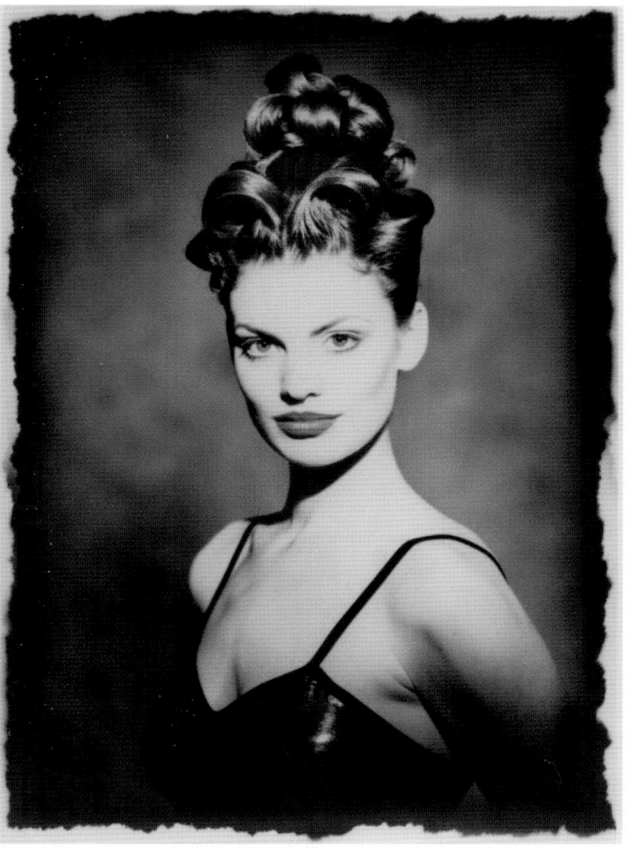

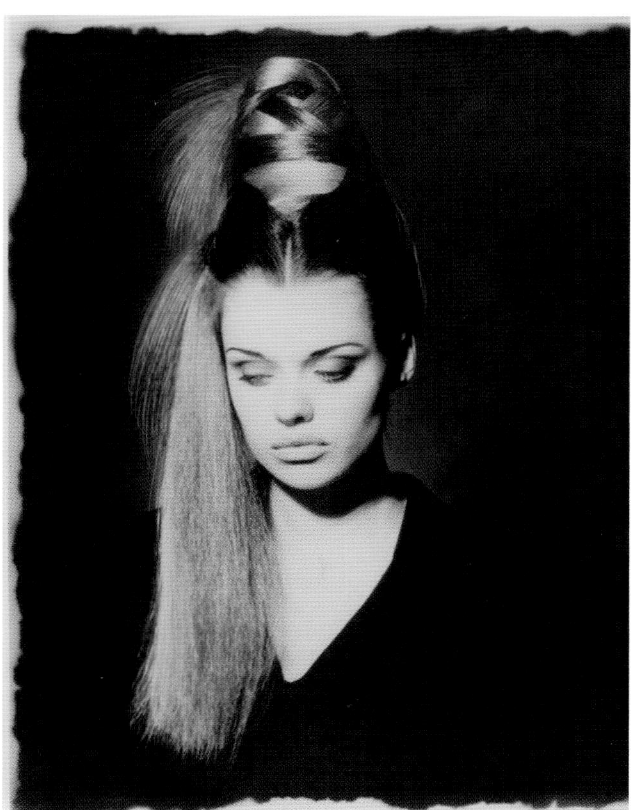

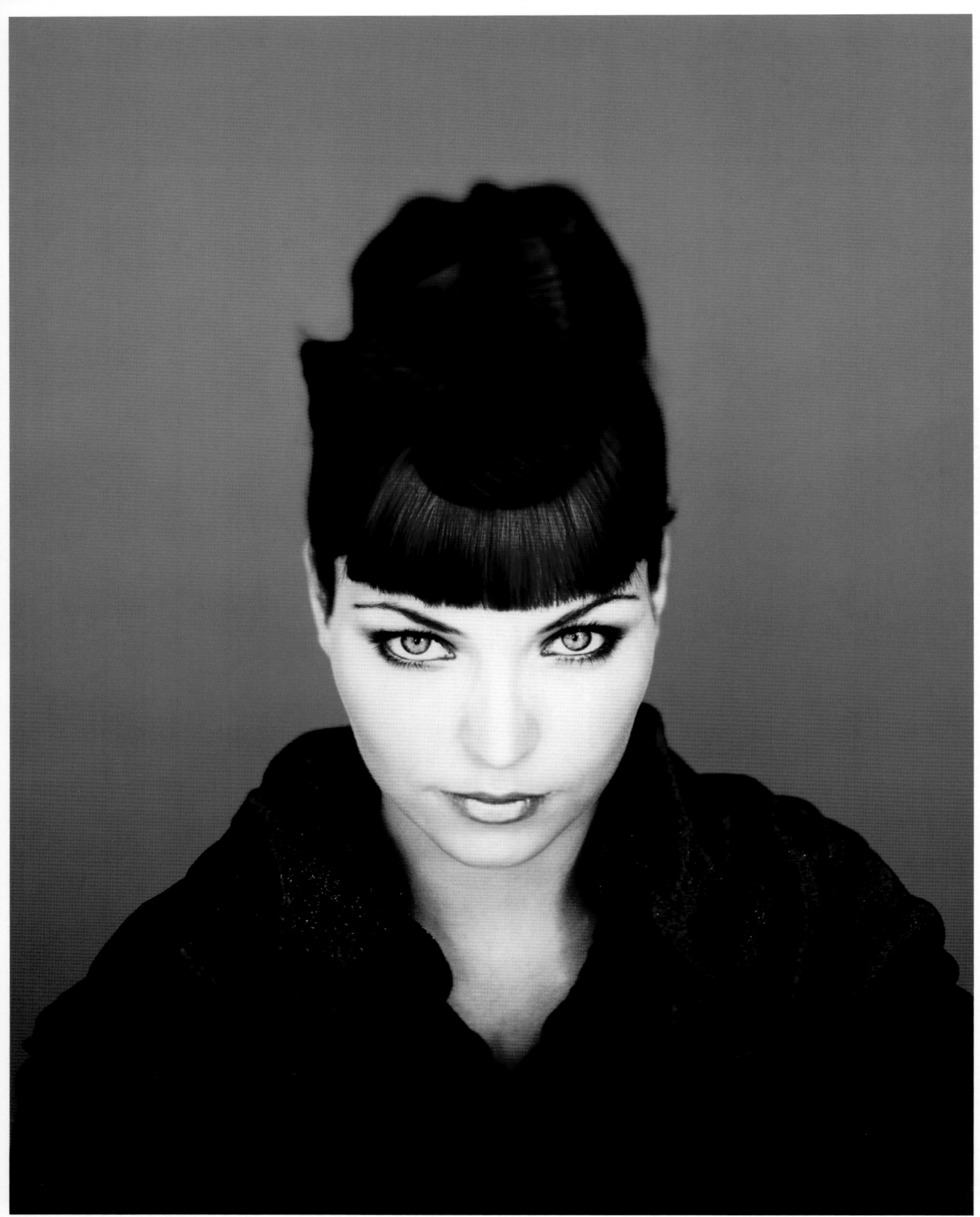

Hairstyle by Paul Edmonds, 1997

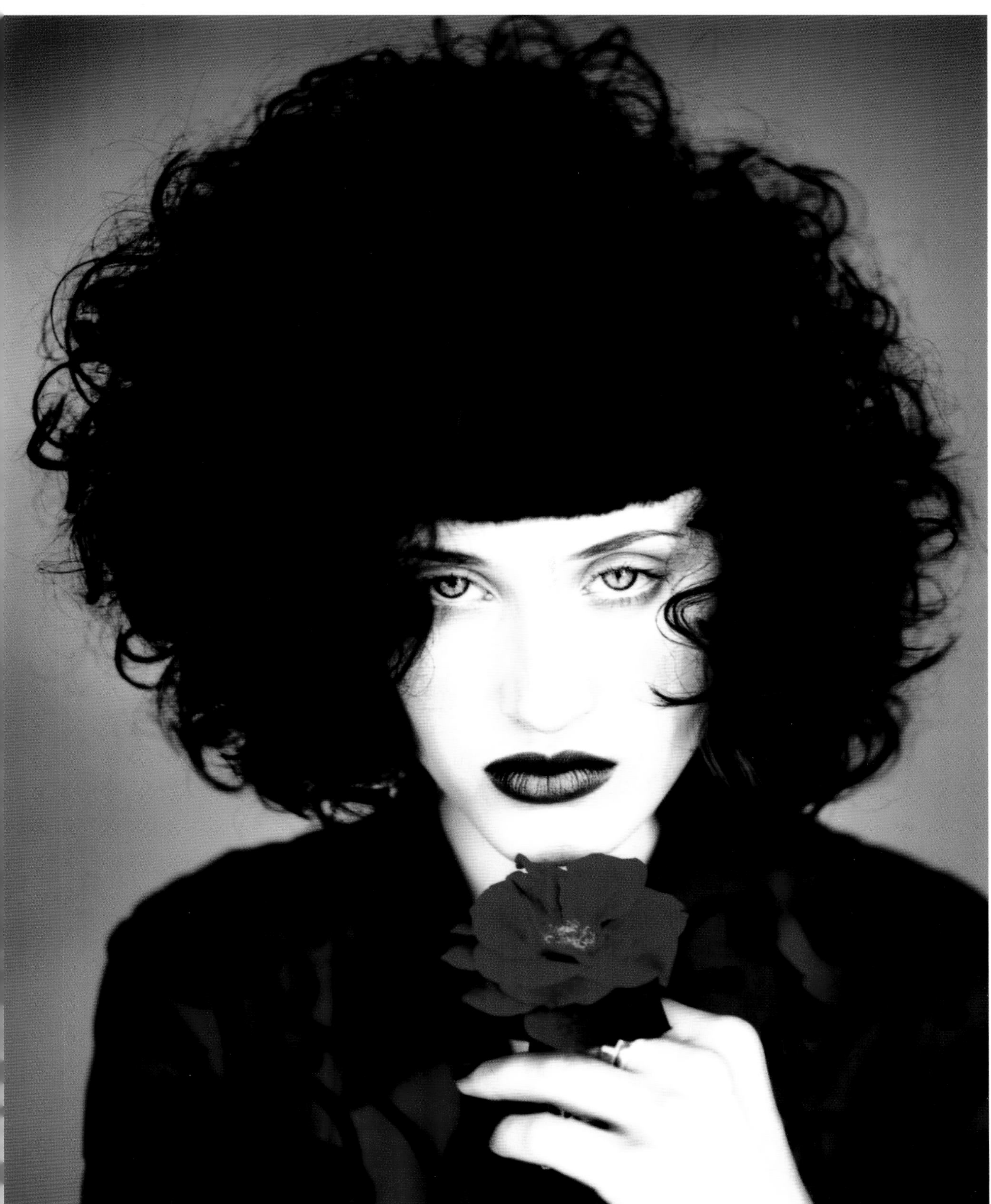

Hairstyle by Paul Edmonds, 1997

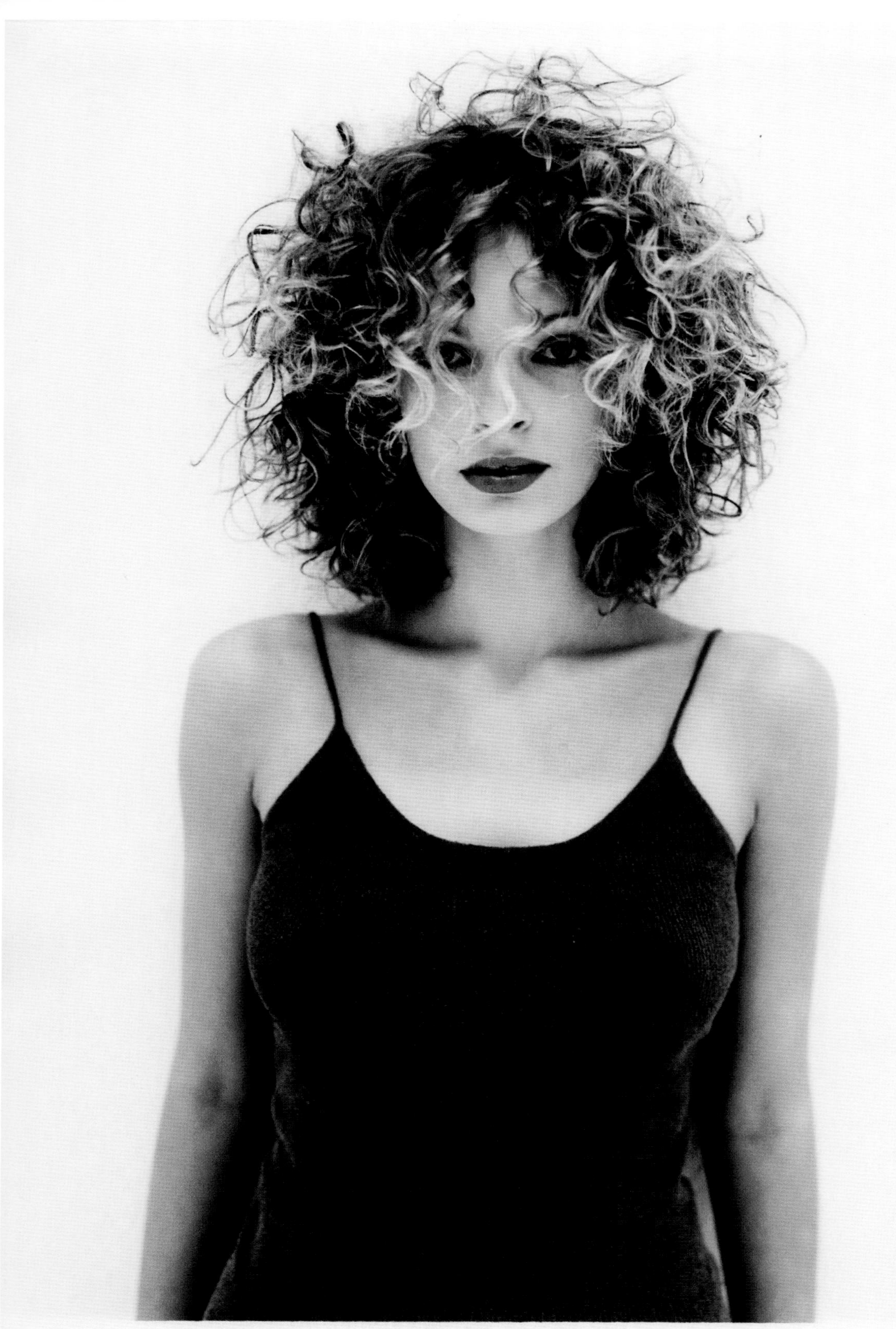

‘Raw’ hairstyle by Anthony
Mascolo for TONI&GUY, 1997

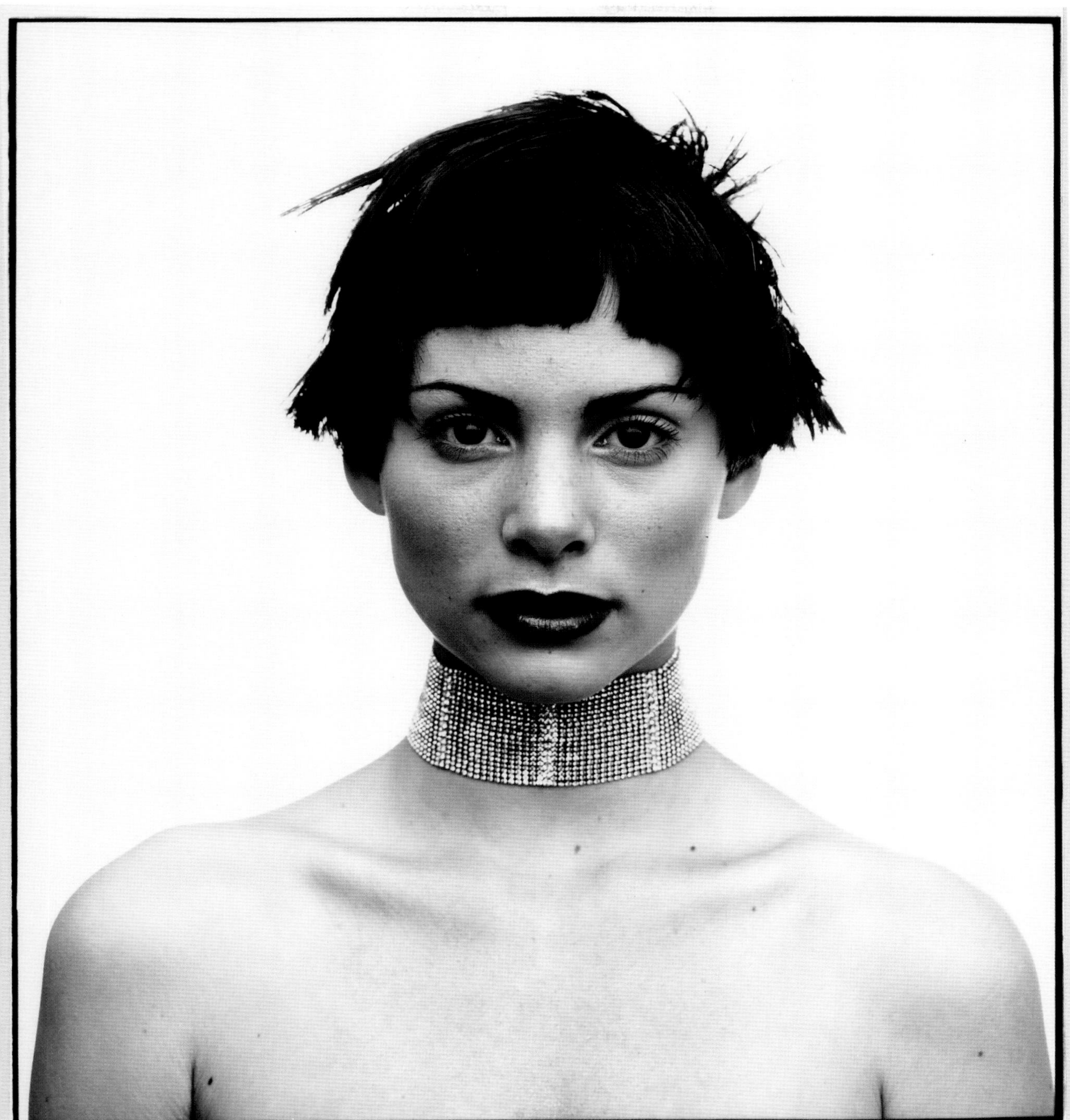

Nation' hairstyle by Anthony
Mascolo for TONI&GUY, 1997

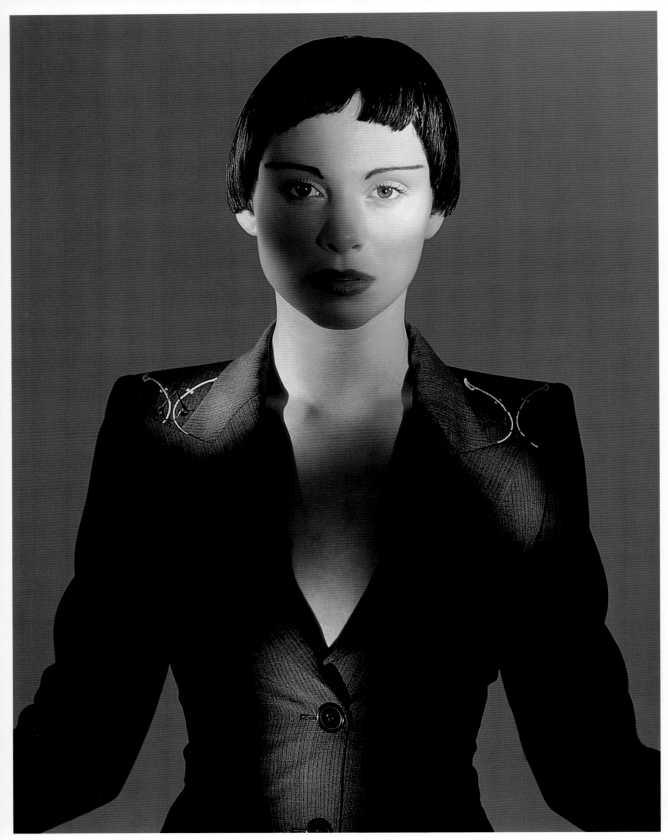

'On the Edge' hairstyle by Anthony Mascolo for TONI&GUY, 1998

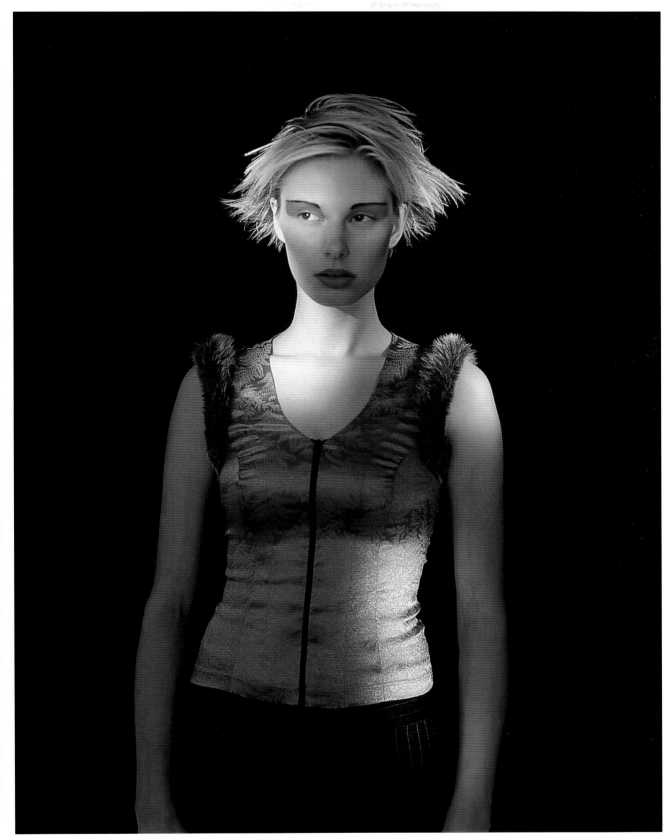

'On the Edge' hairstyle by Anthony Mascolo for TONI&GUY, 1998

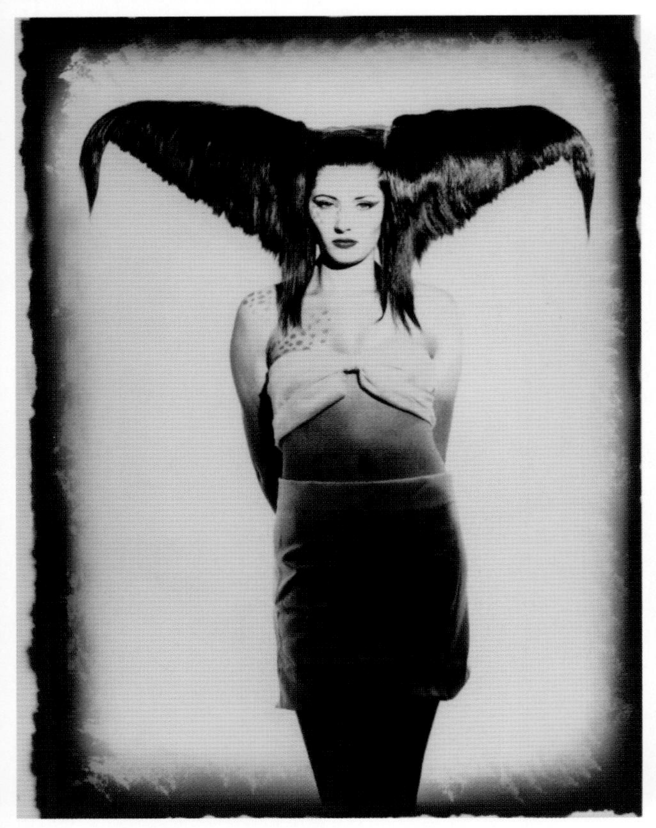
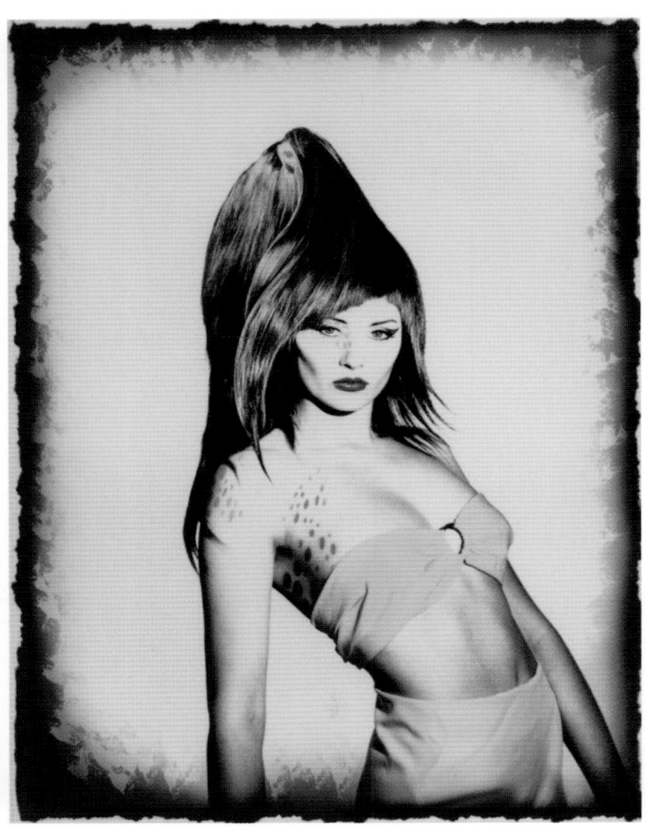
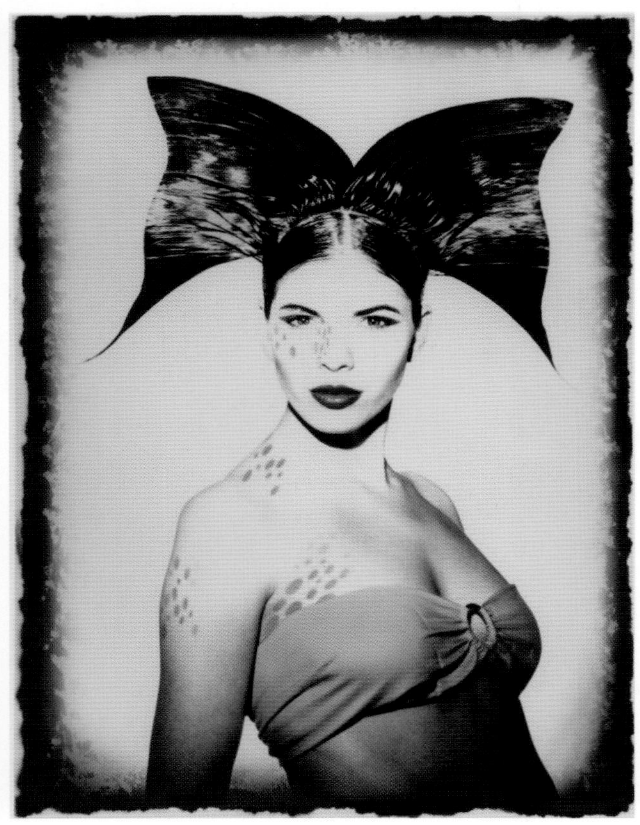
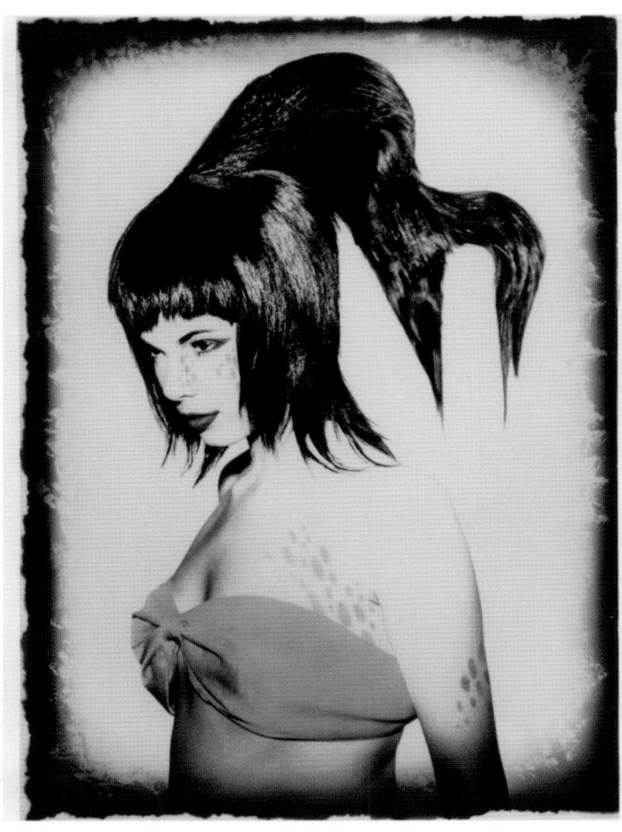

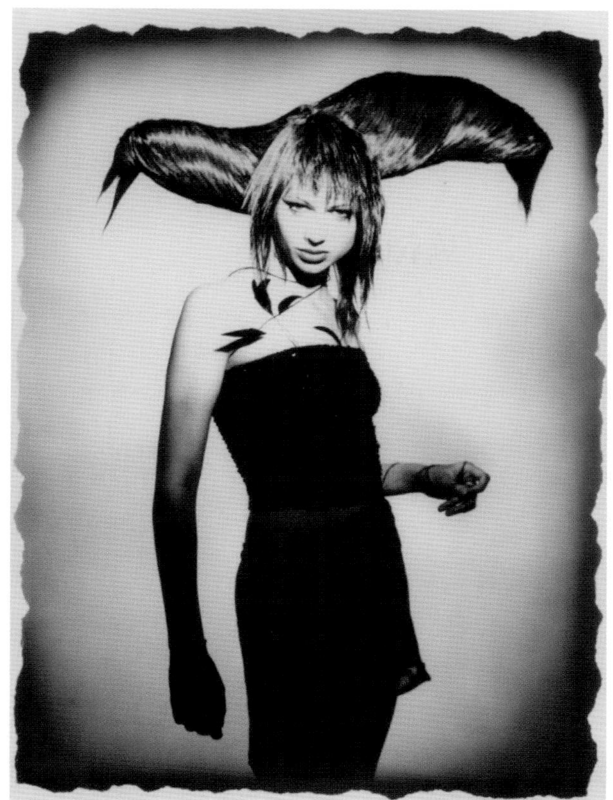

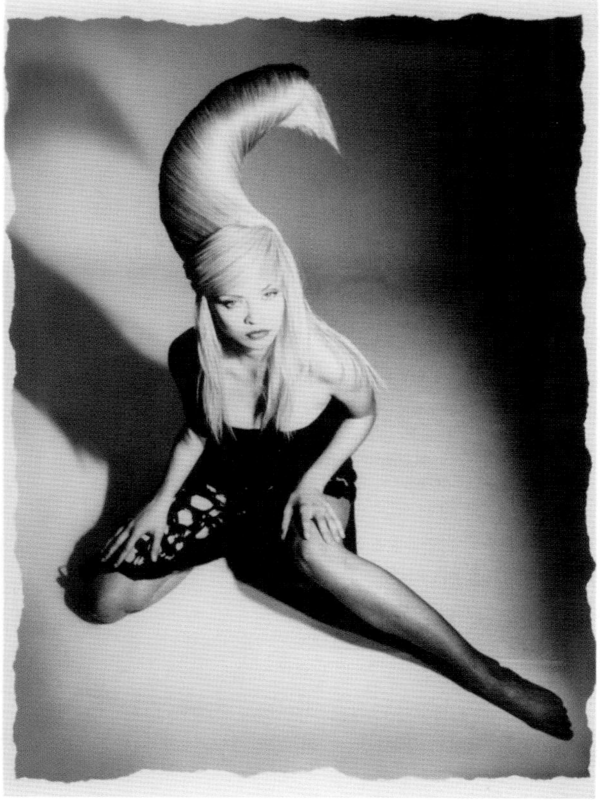

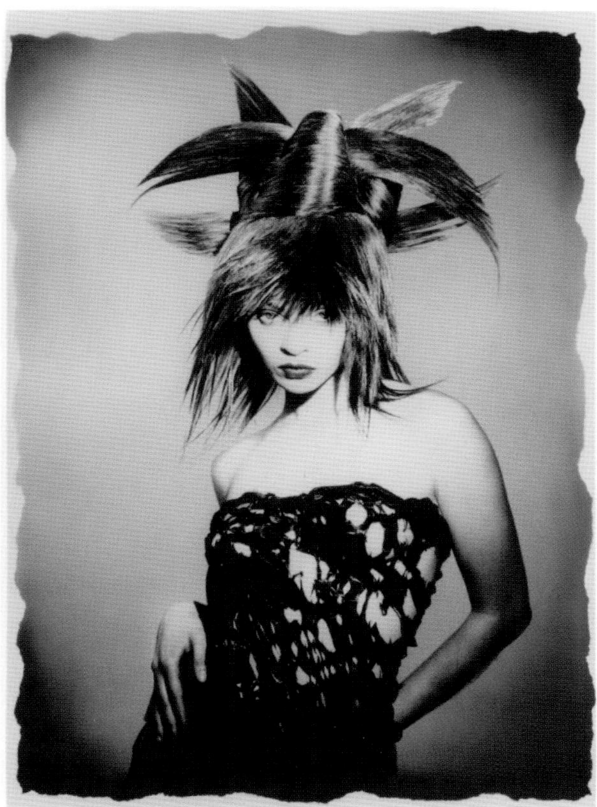

Hairstyles from the
Animal Nitrate Collection
by Michael Barnes, 1998

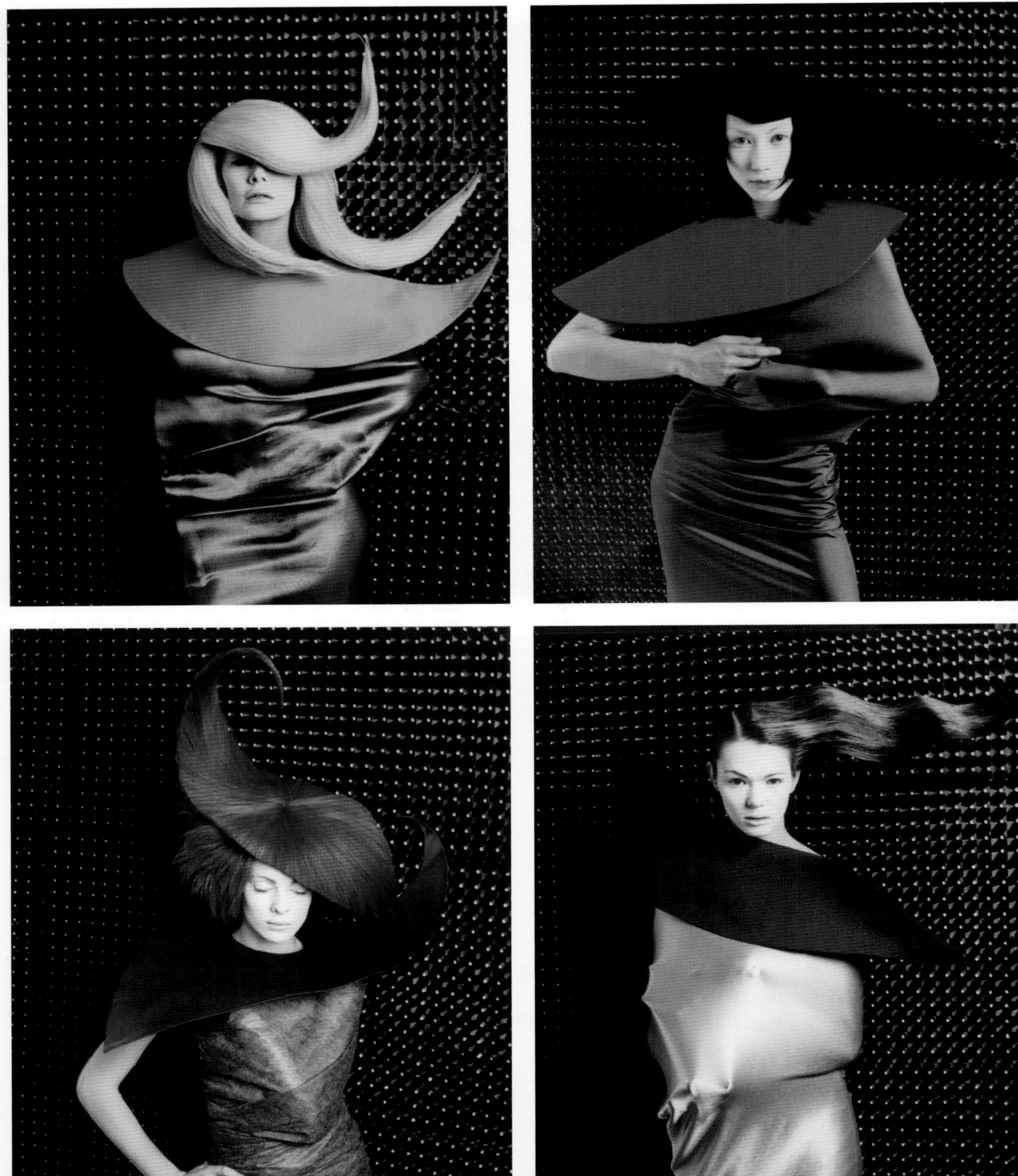

Hairstyles from the Wrapped Collection
by Michael Barnes, 1999

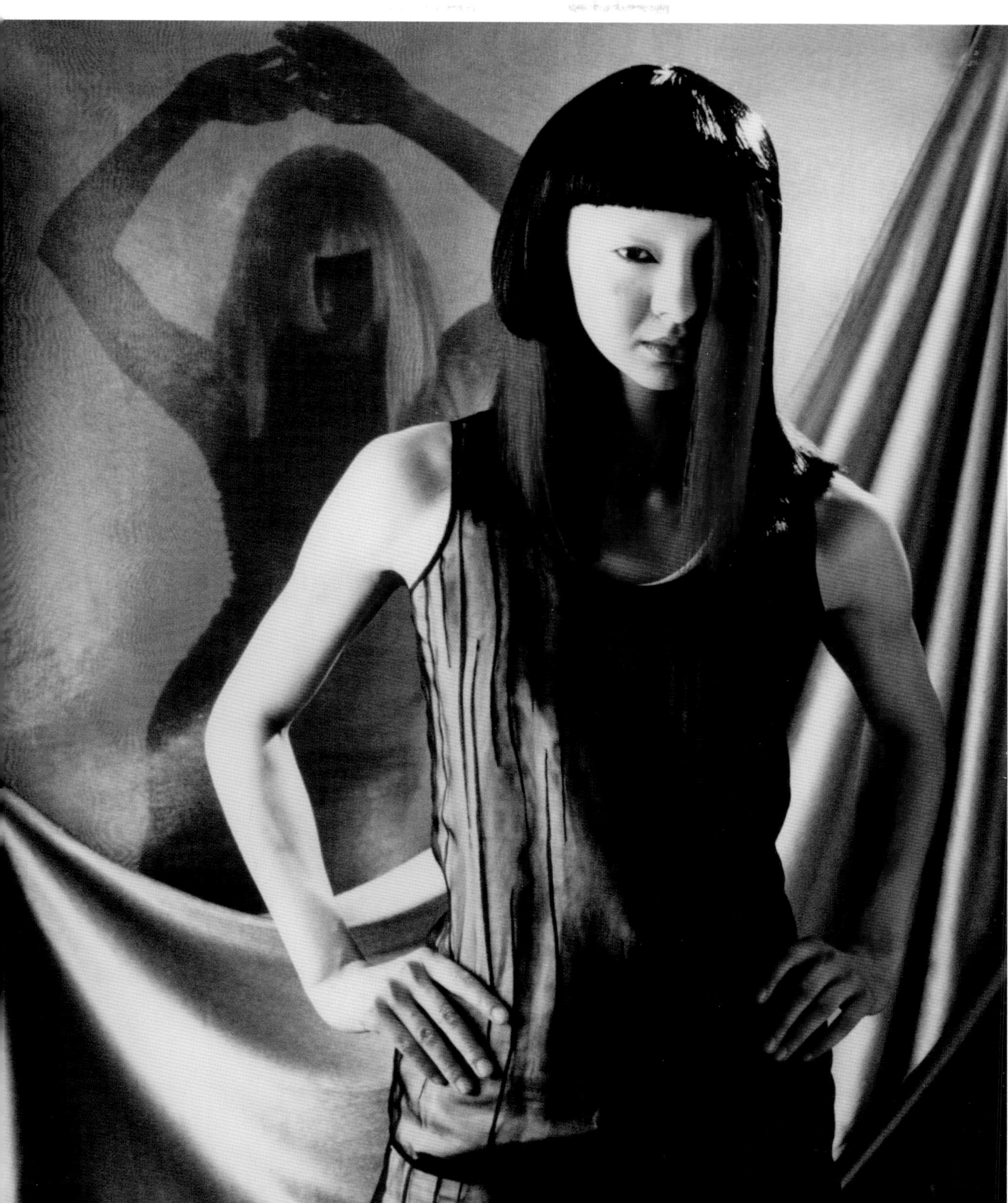

Hairstyle from the Shadow Collection by Michael Barnes, 1999

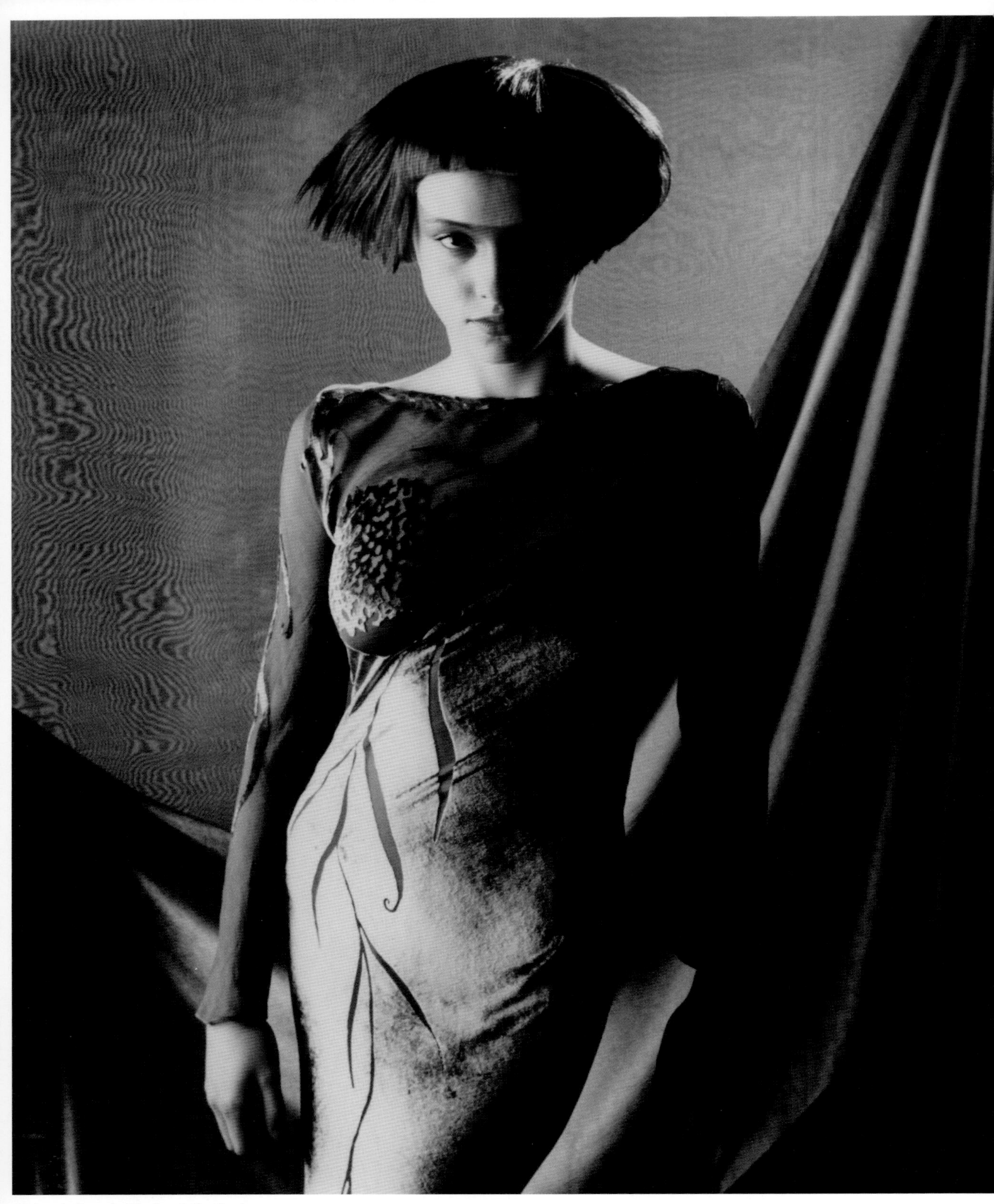

Hairstyle from the Shadow Collection by
Michael Barnes, 1999

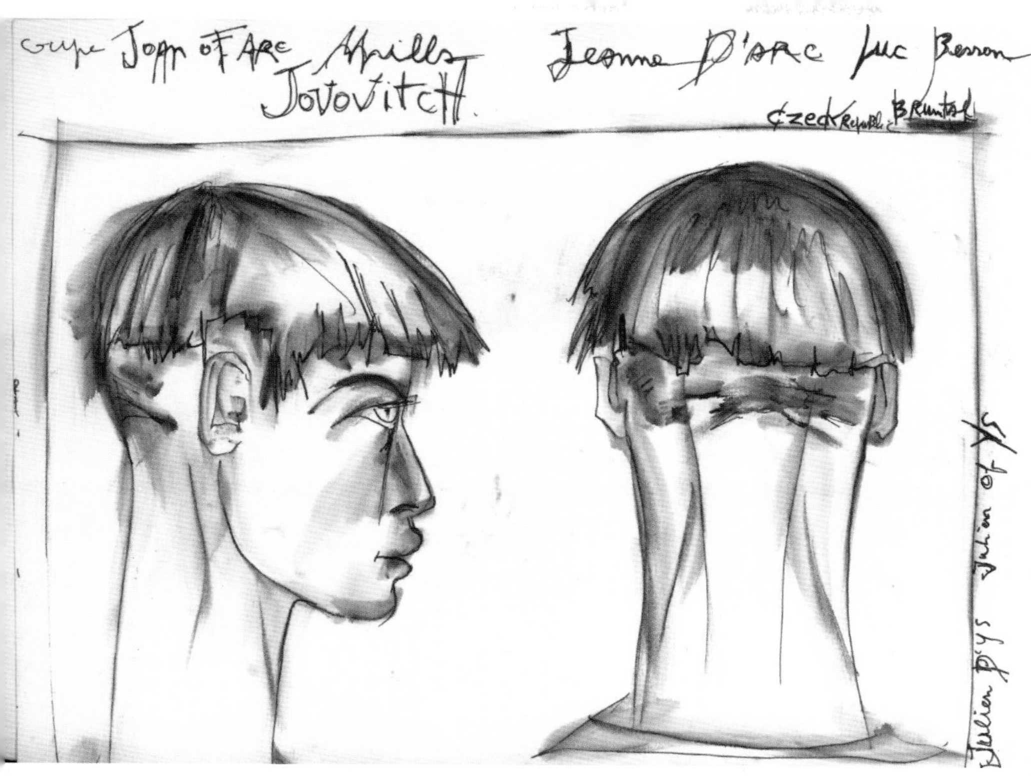

Preparatory sketch for Milla Jovovich's hairstyle for the Luc Besson film, *Joan of Arc: The Messenger*, by Julien d'Ys, 1999

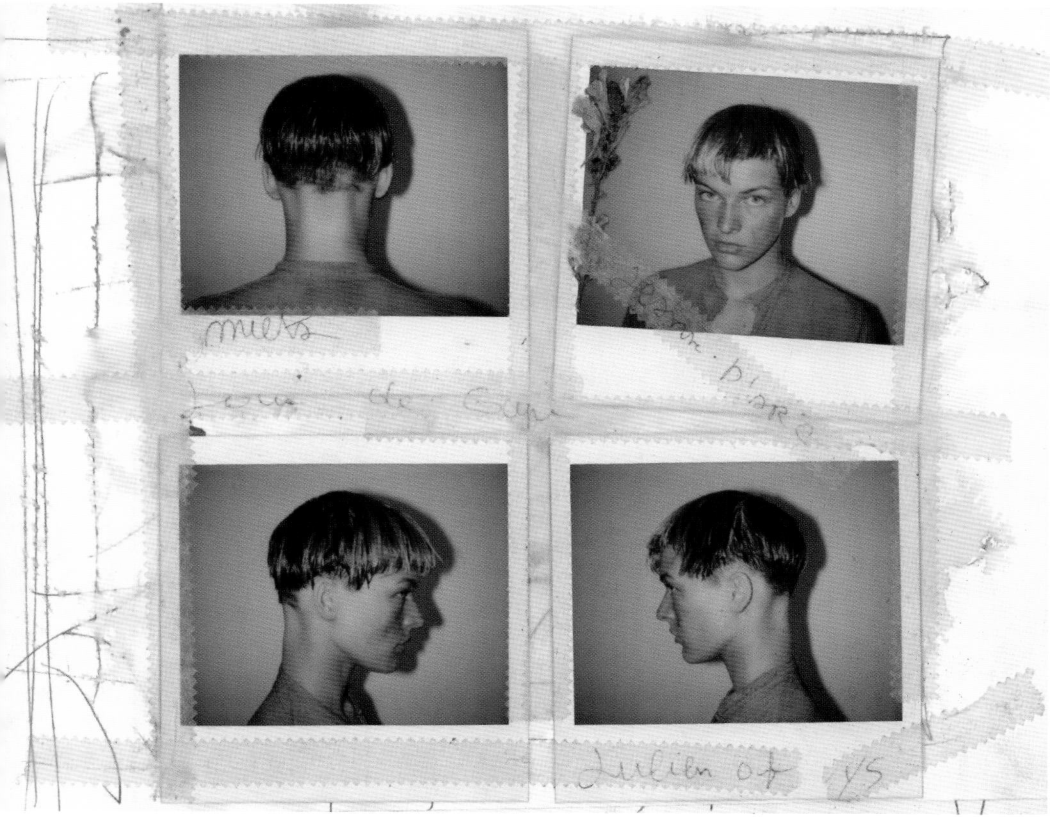

Milla Jovovich with hairstyle for the Luc Besson film, *Joan of Arc: The Messenger*, by Julien d'Ys, 1999

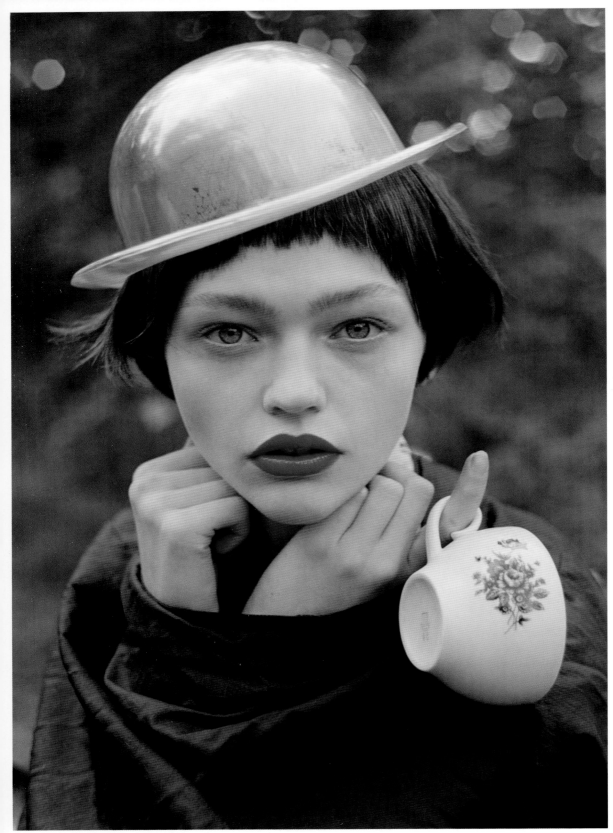

Sasha Pivovarova with hair by Gianni Scumaci, 2006,
photographed by Tim Walker for British Vogue

2000S

'he "Noughties" have witnessed a new experimental onfidence within hairstyling, while as a discipline it ıas become much more closely linked to fashion, art and nusic. This in turn has led to the increasing importance of ıairstylists within the fashion image-making industry. For xample, Gianni Scumaci has worked closely with the fashion hotographer Tim Walker, while Anthony Mascolo has worked vith various fashion designers including Vivienne Westwood nd Christopher Kane. The 21st century has also seen a marked tylistic divergence between the high-street haircut and the rogressive coiffures created for fashion shoots or hair shows.

During the early 2000s, mainstream hairstyles were redominantly long and straight. GHD's hair straighteners vere a veritable revelation when they were first launched in 001 and made the sleek tamed-mane look achievable for most ıair types. By 2005, GHD was selling so many of its ceramic traighteners that it was ranked Britain's fastest growing ompany by *The Sunday Times Fast Track*. Unlike the shoulder-ength hair of the 1990s, in the 2000s there was a fashion for ery long hair that was poker-straight. This ever-so-straight tyle contrasted strongly with the extraordinary fashion-led ıairstyles created for ad campaigns and hair shows during the arly 2000s. For example, the ground-breaking themed photo hoots Anthony Mascolo art directed during this period are like tories which capture, as he put it, "a fashion feel". They were ıot about promoting a specific hairstyle; in fact Mascolo freely cknowledges his hair designs and imagery are inspired by utting-edge street style, modestly describing them as a look t "what young people are doing". Often the hairstyles created or such campaigns and shows were and still are eccentric antasies that function in much the same way "haute couture" loes in the fashion world, ultimately filtering down to the ıigh street in a somewhat diluted form.

During the early 2000s, the "Emo" haircut comprising a long ringe brushed over one side of the forehead to cover part of he face became a global youth culture phenomenon that was ultimately a rejection of the overly straightened "perfect" hair of the mainstream. Another haircut known as the "Fanni" created by Gianni Scumaci in 2000 (named after the Swedish model, Fanni Bostrom) also became hugely influential and spawned many imitations. Certainly during the late 2000s and early 2010s there has been a move away from the long straight look, and shorter and chunkier styles with more texture have become fashionable. At the time of writing, the luminous long blonde tresses that seem to be the preserve of footballers' wives are, however, still popular among a certain class of celebrity and are often embellished with real hair extensions – a case of rich women buying poorer women's hair just as they did in Ancient Rome or 18th century France. There does, however, seem to be a move away from blonde locks among the younger generation, with blonde highlights being seen as slightly old-fashioned; instead, various hues of red have become the must-have hair colouring of today. Certainly, we seem to be in the midst of a definable "hair moment", and this publication is part of this ongoing reappraisal of the hairstylist's craft – an art form that has had it highs and lows, its extravagant follies and its stylistic disasters. As a design discipline that has had its virtuoso maestros and its eccentric geniuses, hairstyling is a cultural phenomenon that has at its heart a creative and vibrant energy, which has shaped and defined women over the centuries. Inherently linked to status and power throughout the ages, and a significant cultural marker of civilization, ultimately, the story of hair mirrors the story of women. And let us not forget that above all hair has been central to our concept of alluring female beauty, as Alexander Pope noted:

> "Fair tresses man's imperial race ensnare,
> And beauty draws us with a single hair."
>
> ("The Rape of the Lock", 1712)

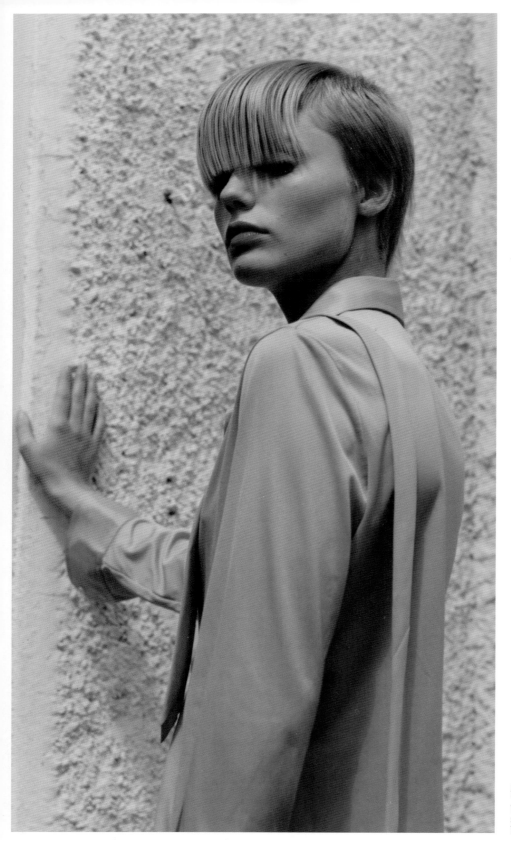

Model Fanni Bostrum with 'The Fanni' undercut hairstyle, by Gianni Scumaci for Vidal Sassoon, 2000, photographed by Tomoko Nagakawa

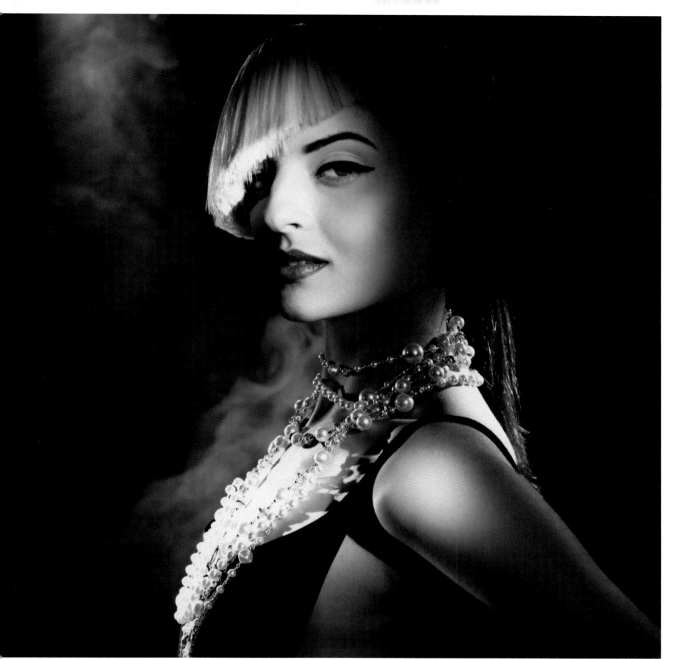

Hairstyle by Anthony Mascolo (International Creative Director of TIGI), for TIGI, 2000s

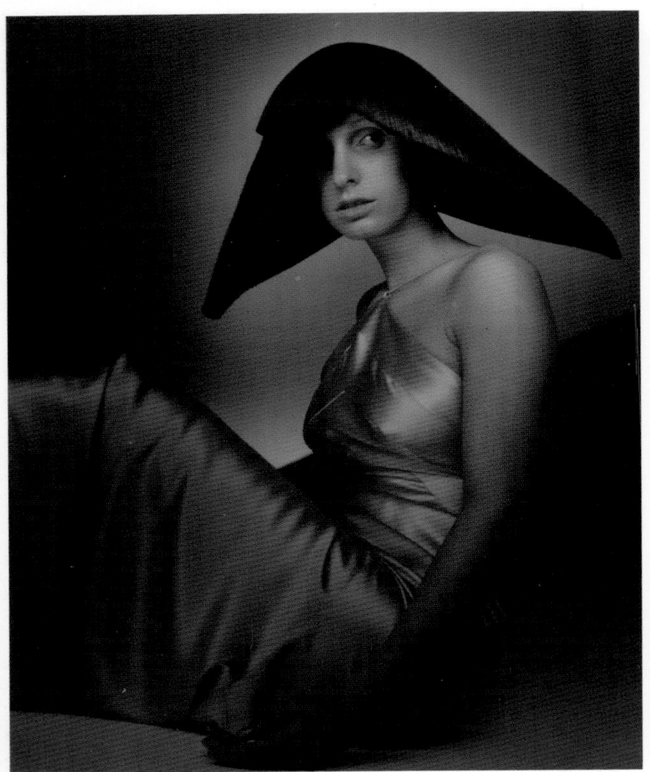

'Black Purple' by Michael Barnes, White Geisha Collection, 2000

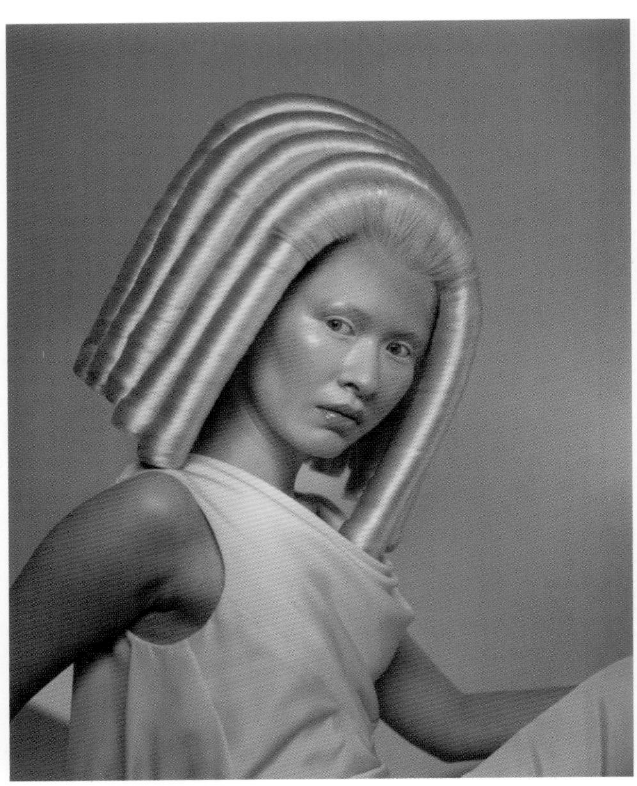

'Connie' by Michael Barnes, White Geisha Collection, 2000

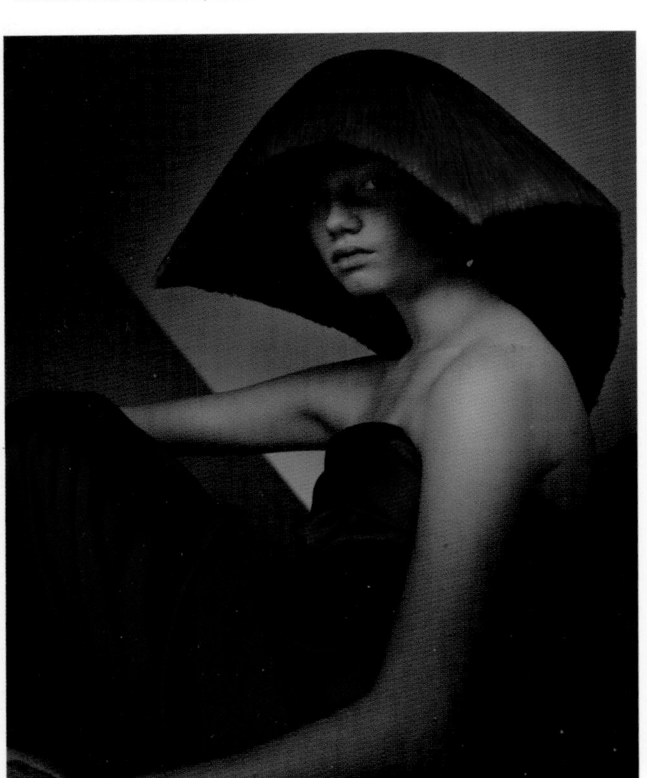

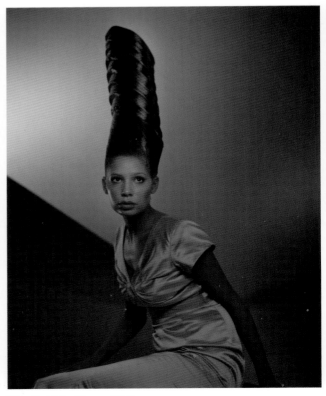

'Samurai' by Michael Barnes, White Geisha Collection, 2000

'Slices' by Michael Barnes, White Geisha Collection, 2000

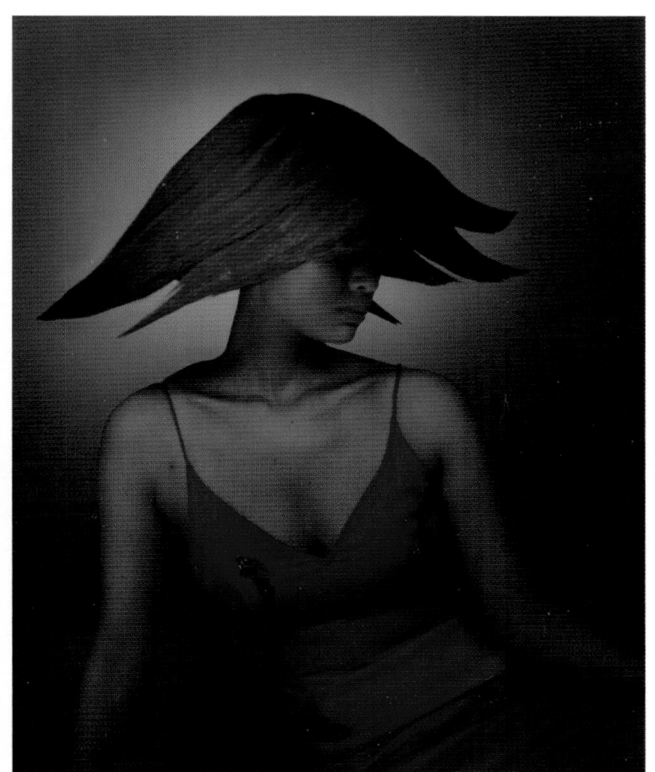

'Maki' by Michael Barnes, White Geisha Collection, 2000

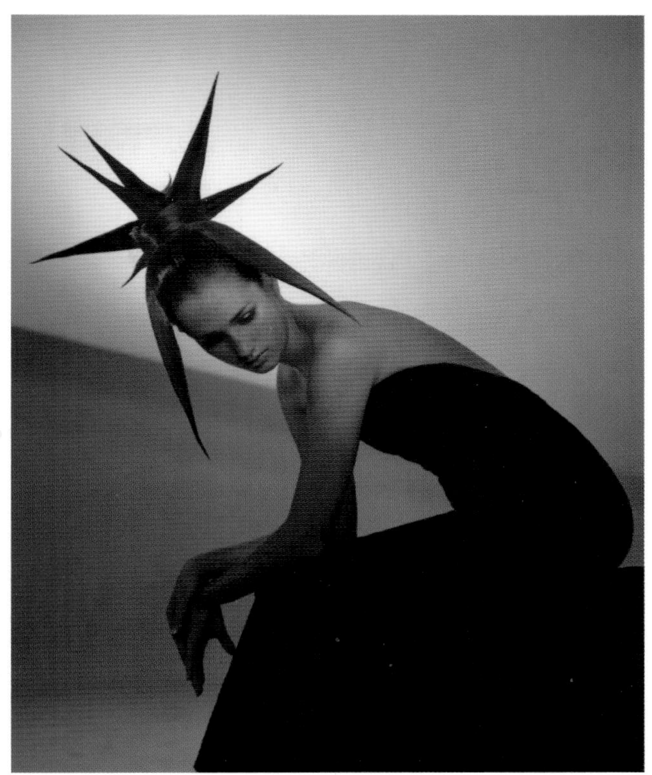

'Manga' by Michael Barnes, White Geisha Collection, 2000

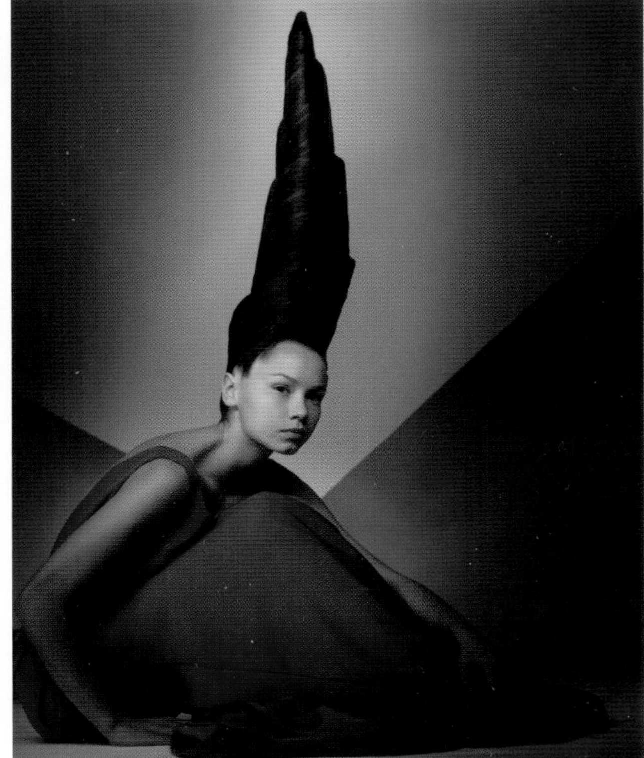

'Tornado' by Michael Barnes, White Geisha Collection, 2000

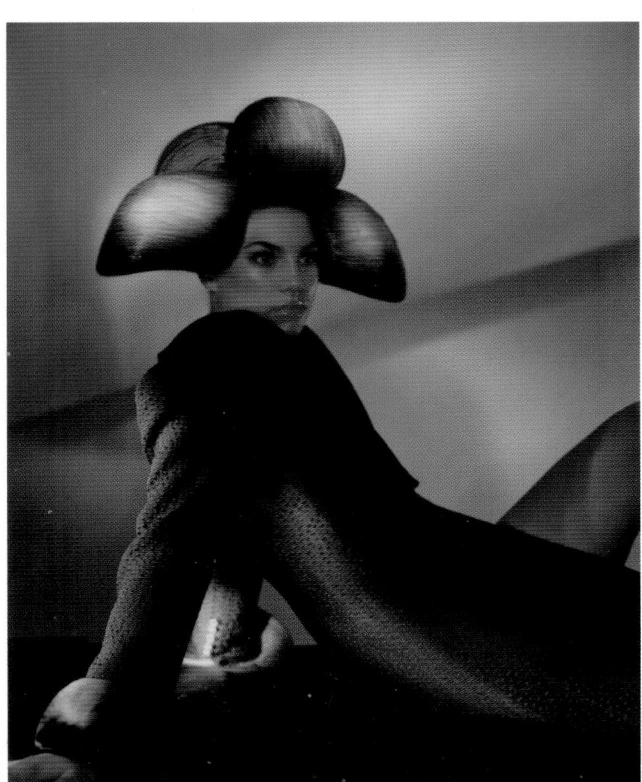

'White Geisha' by Michael Barnes, White Geisha Collection, 2000

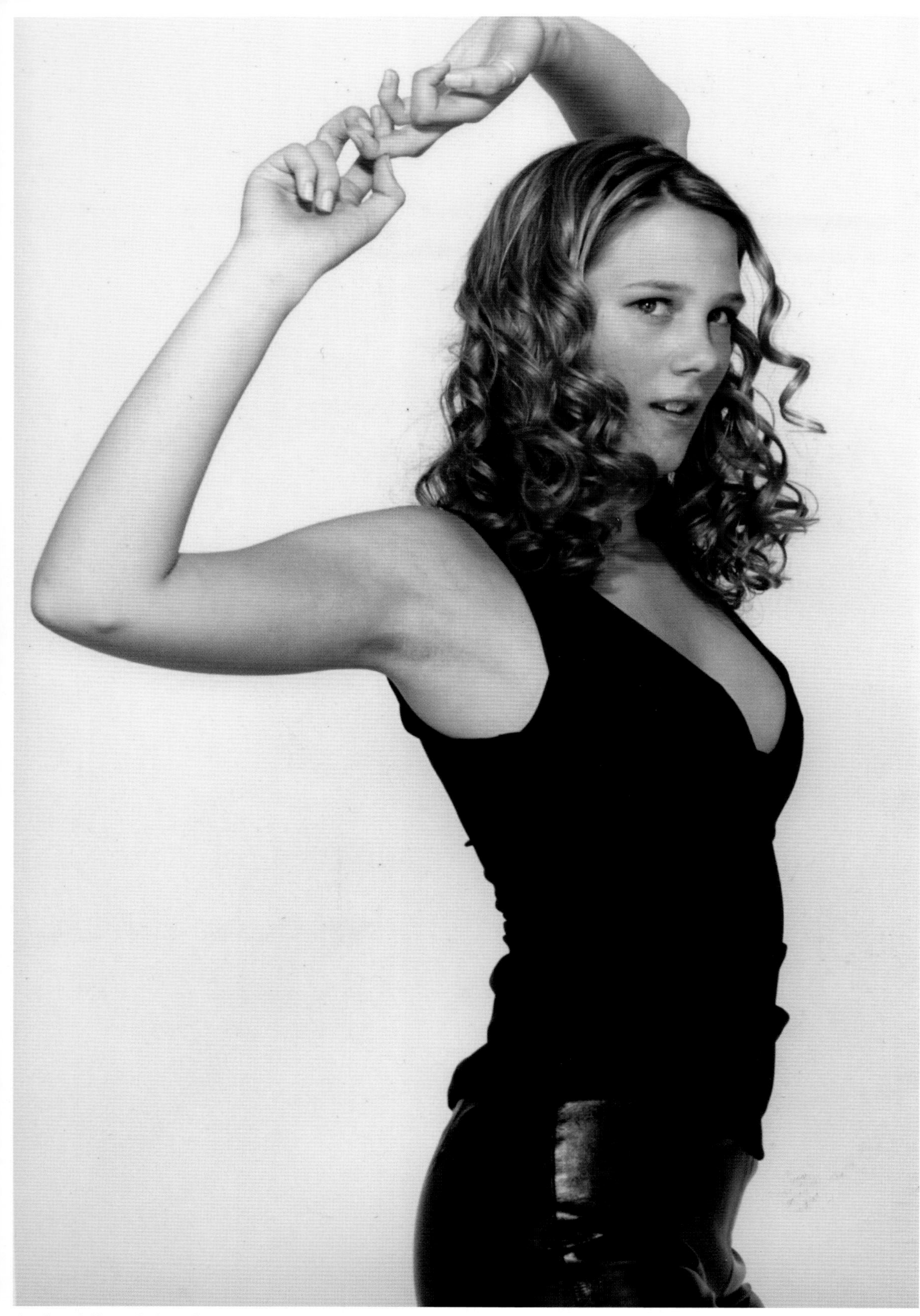

'Curly Style' by Paul Edmonds, 2000

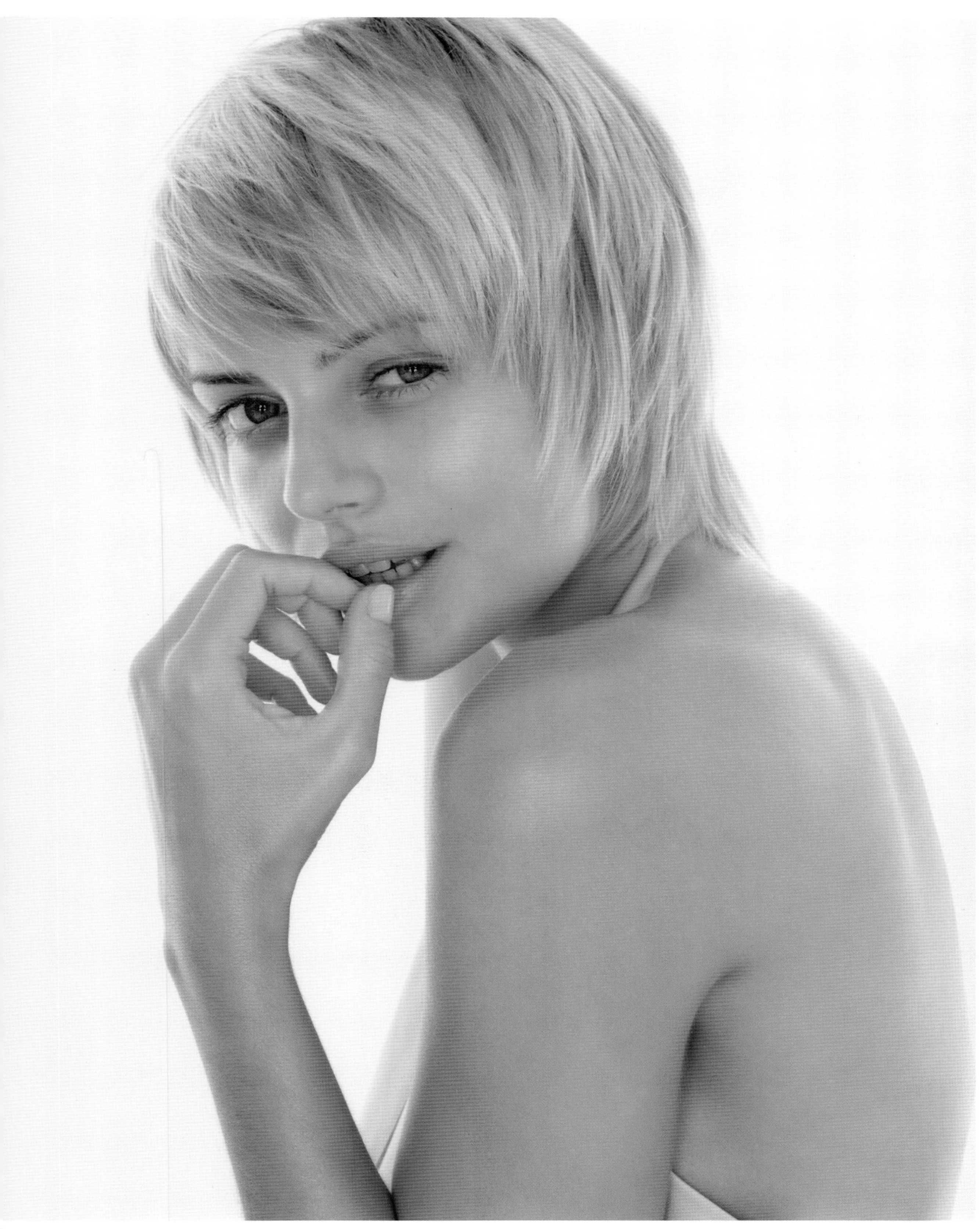

'Sand' hairstyle from the award-winning Blondes Collection, Lisa Shepherd, 2004

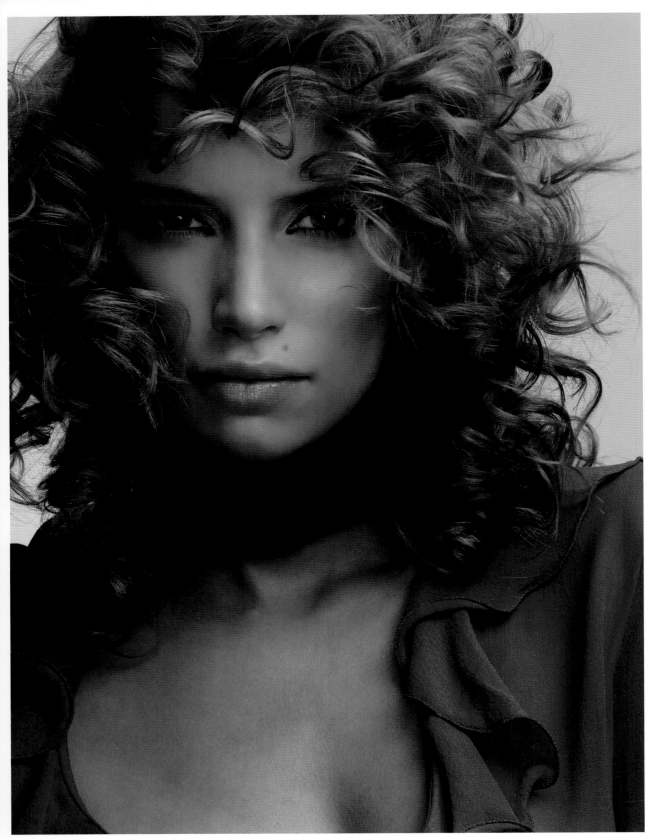

British Hairdresser of the Year award-winning hairstyle from the Touchable Collection, Lisa Shepherd, 2005

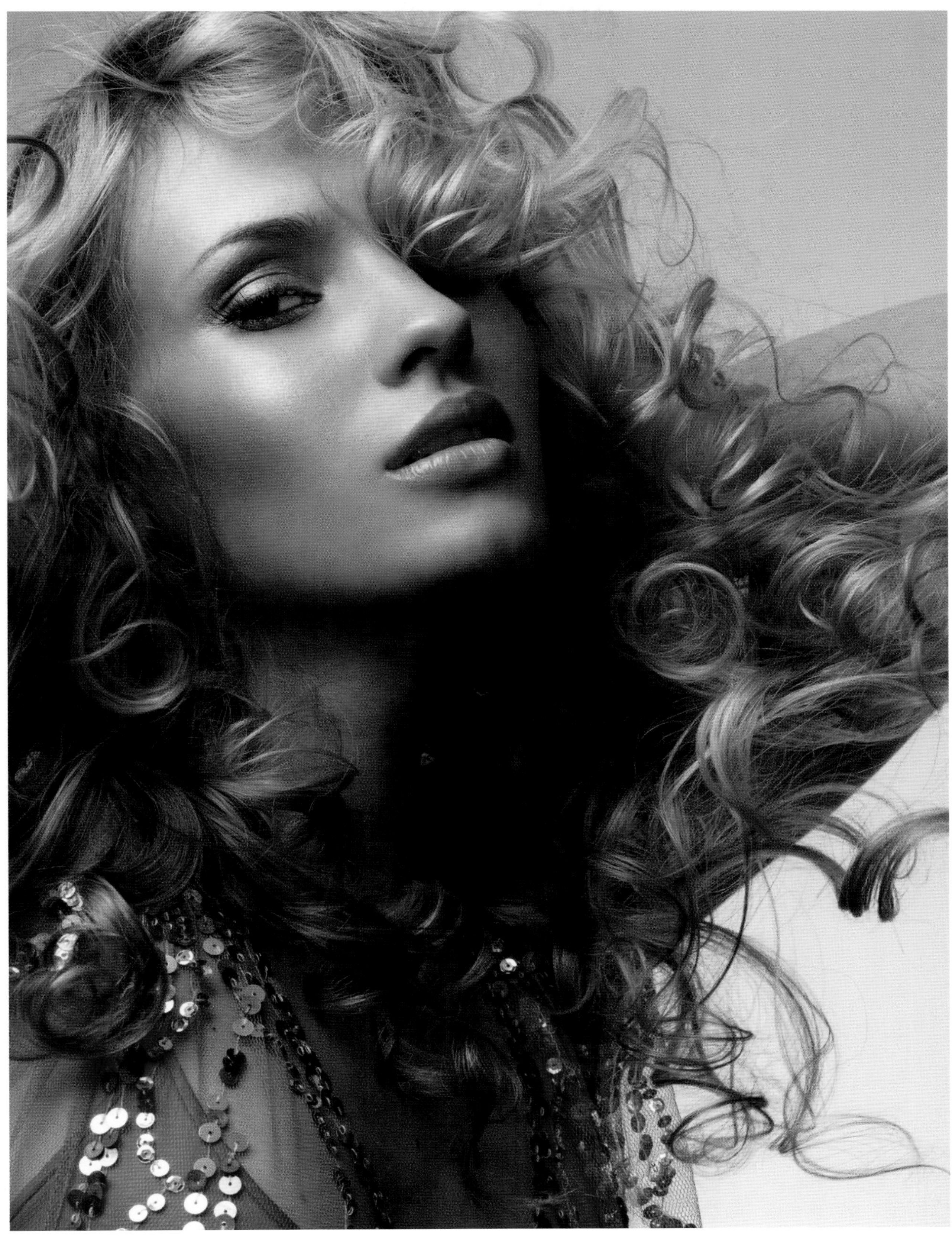

British Hairdresser of the Year award-winning hairstyle
from the Touchable Collection, Lisa Shepherd, 2005

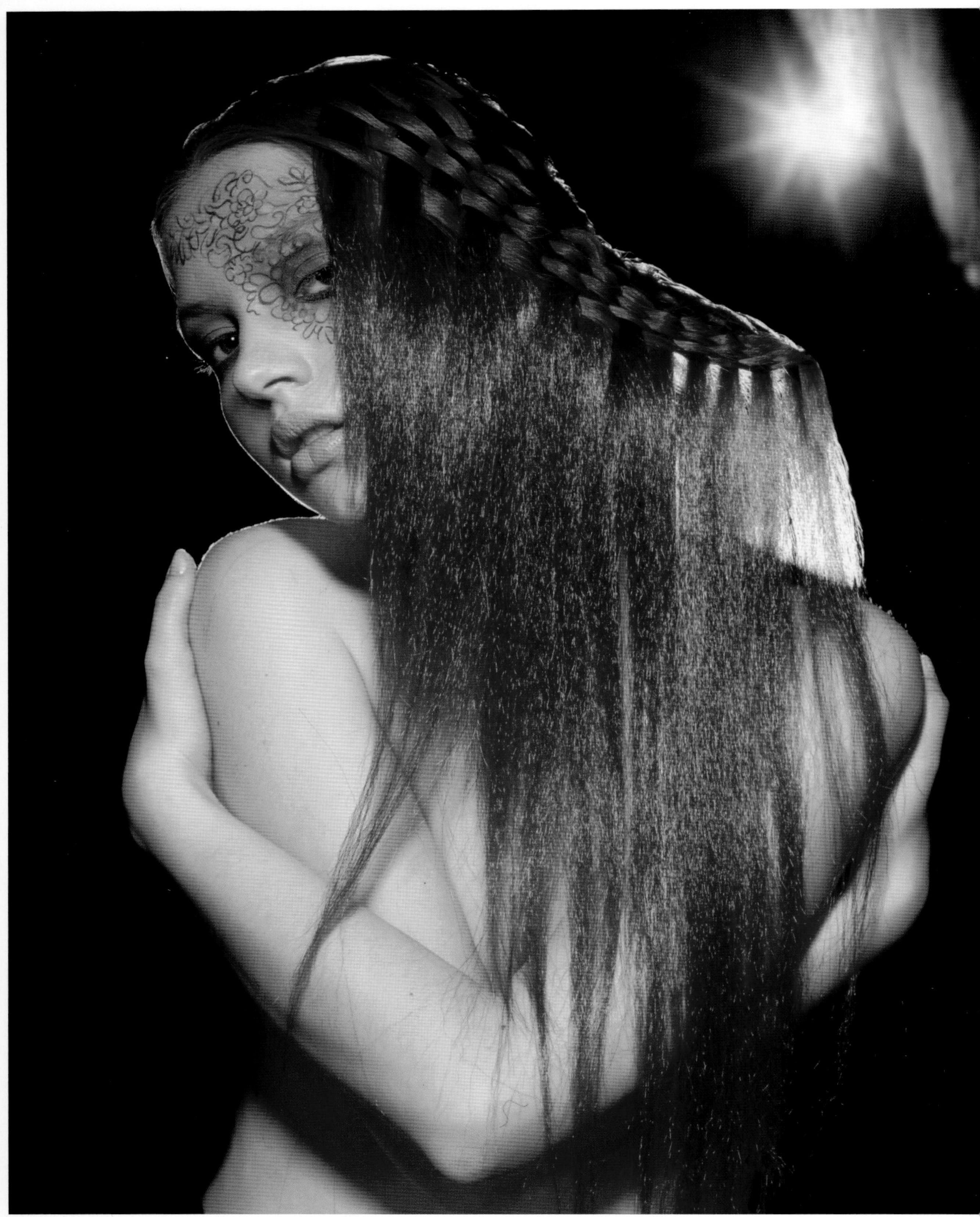

'Crimson' woven hairstyle from the Bohemian Ladies Collection by Michael Barnes, 2005

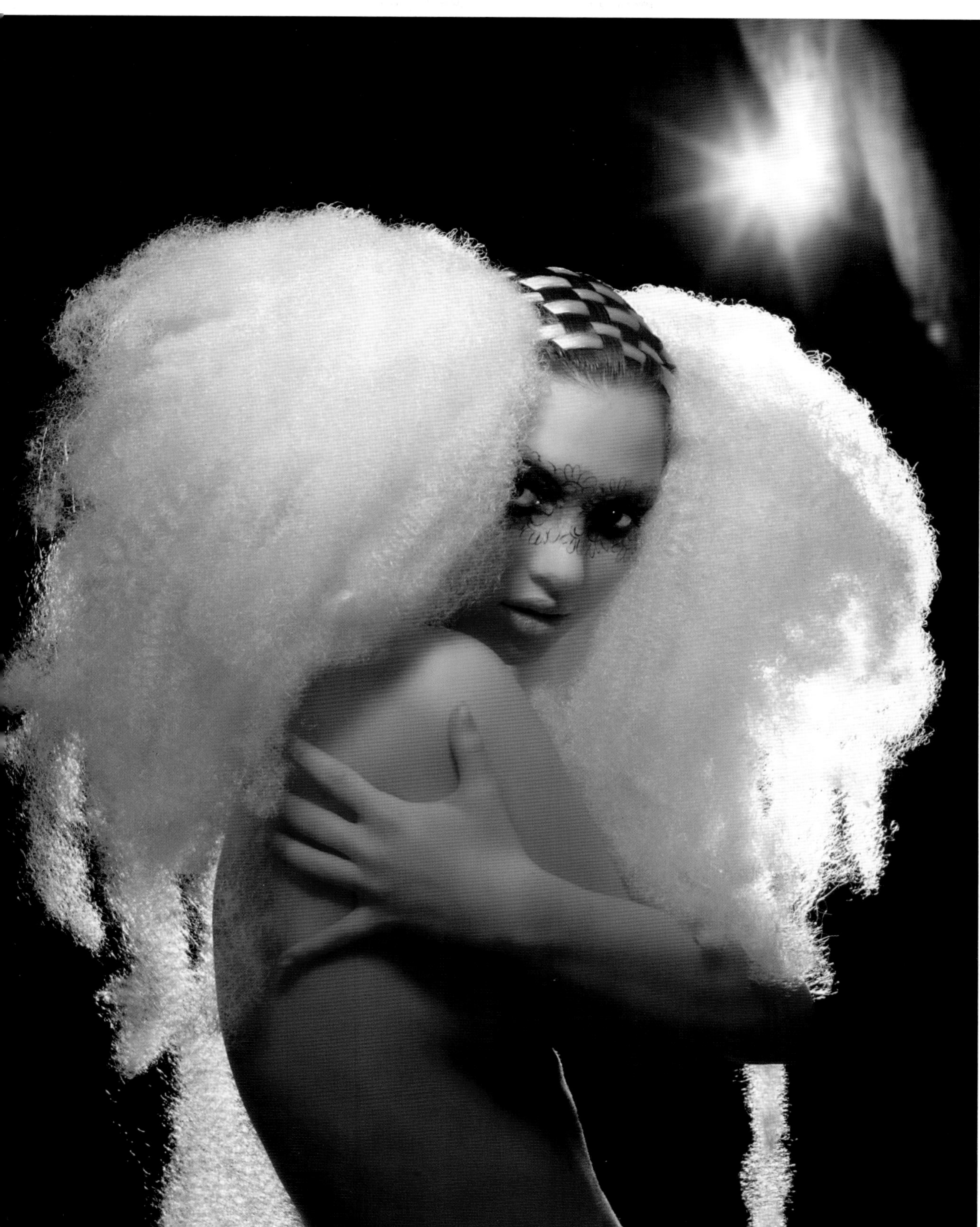

:andyfloss' snow-white dreadlocks from the
ohemian Ladies Collection by Michael Barnes, 2005

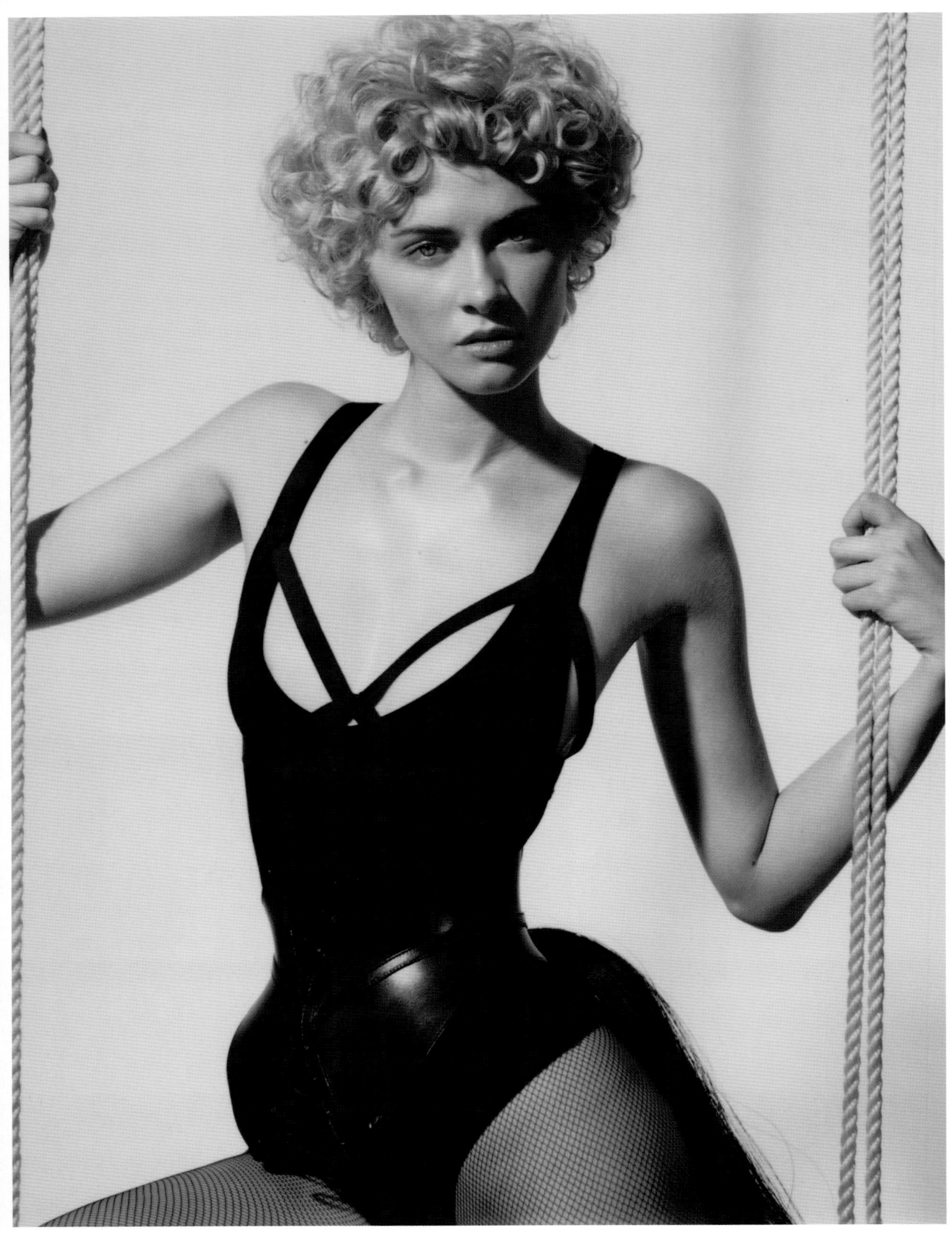

'Blonde on Swing' hairstyle by
Antoinette Beenders, 2006

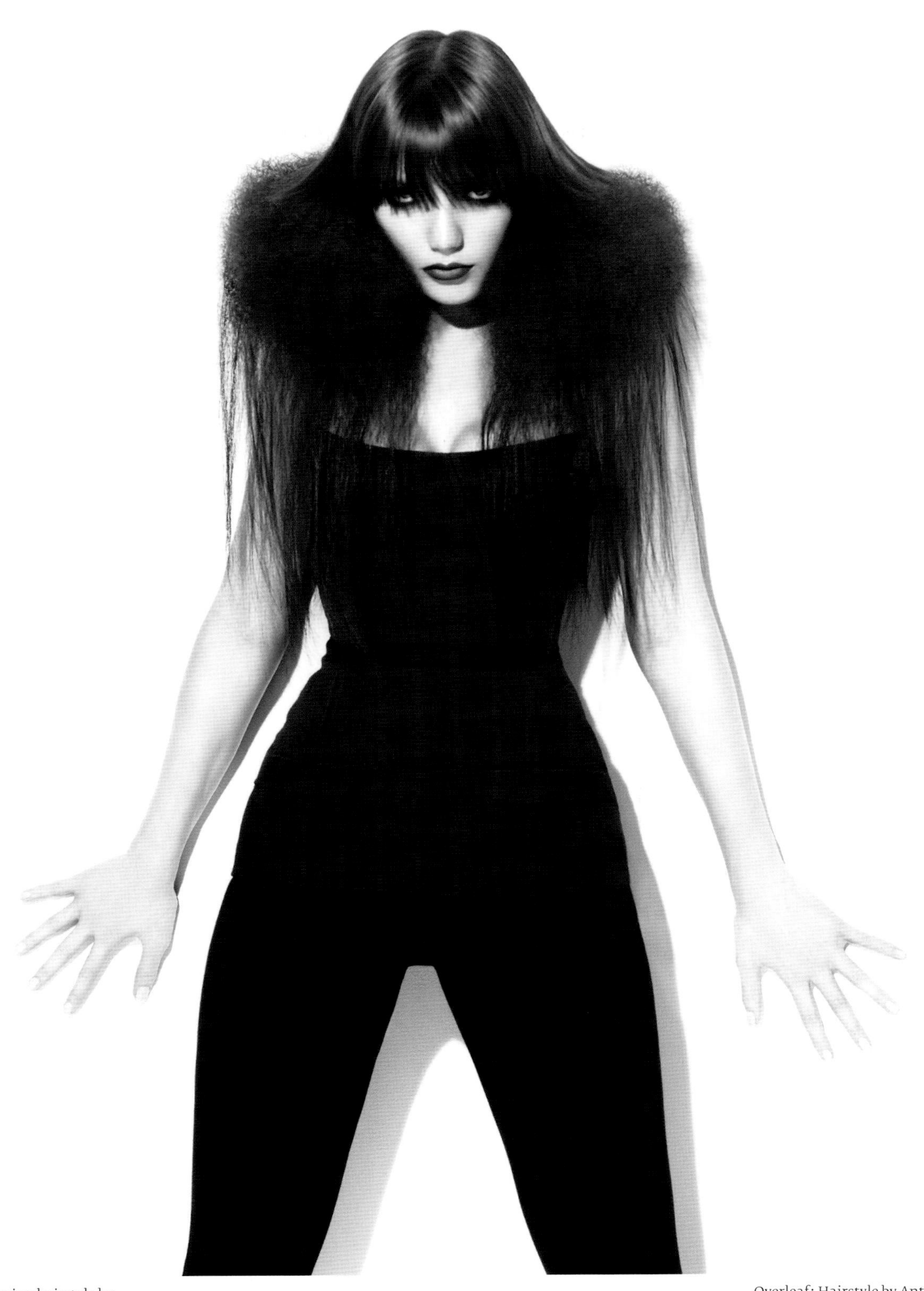

Award winning hairstyle by Antoinette Beenders, 2005

Overleaf: Hairstyle by Anthony Mascolo (International Creative Director of TIGI), for TIGI, 2006

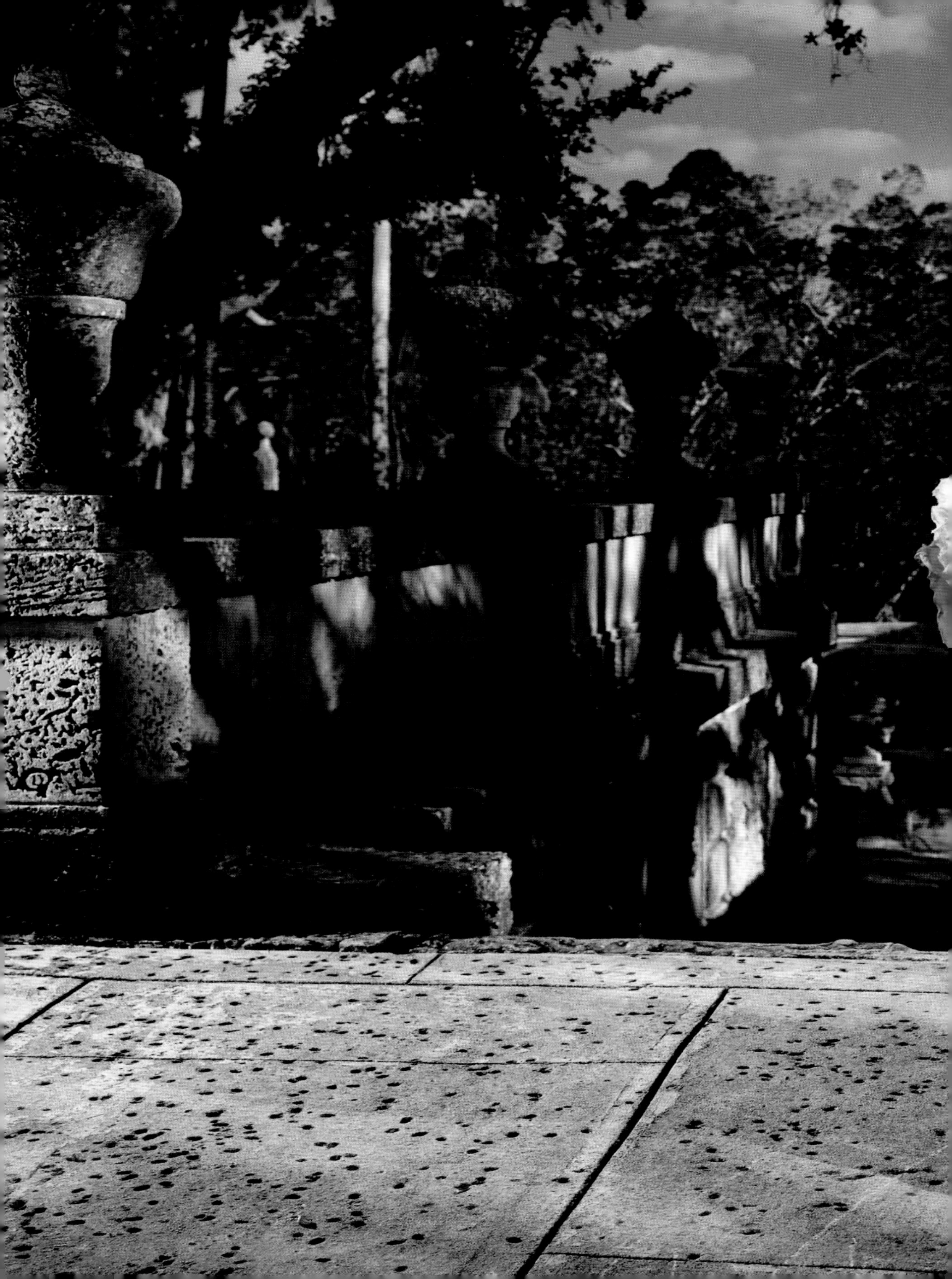

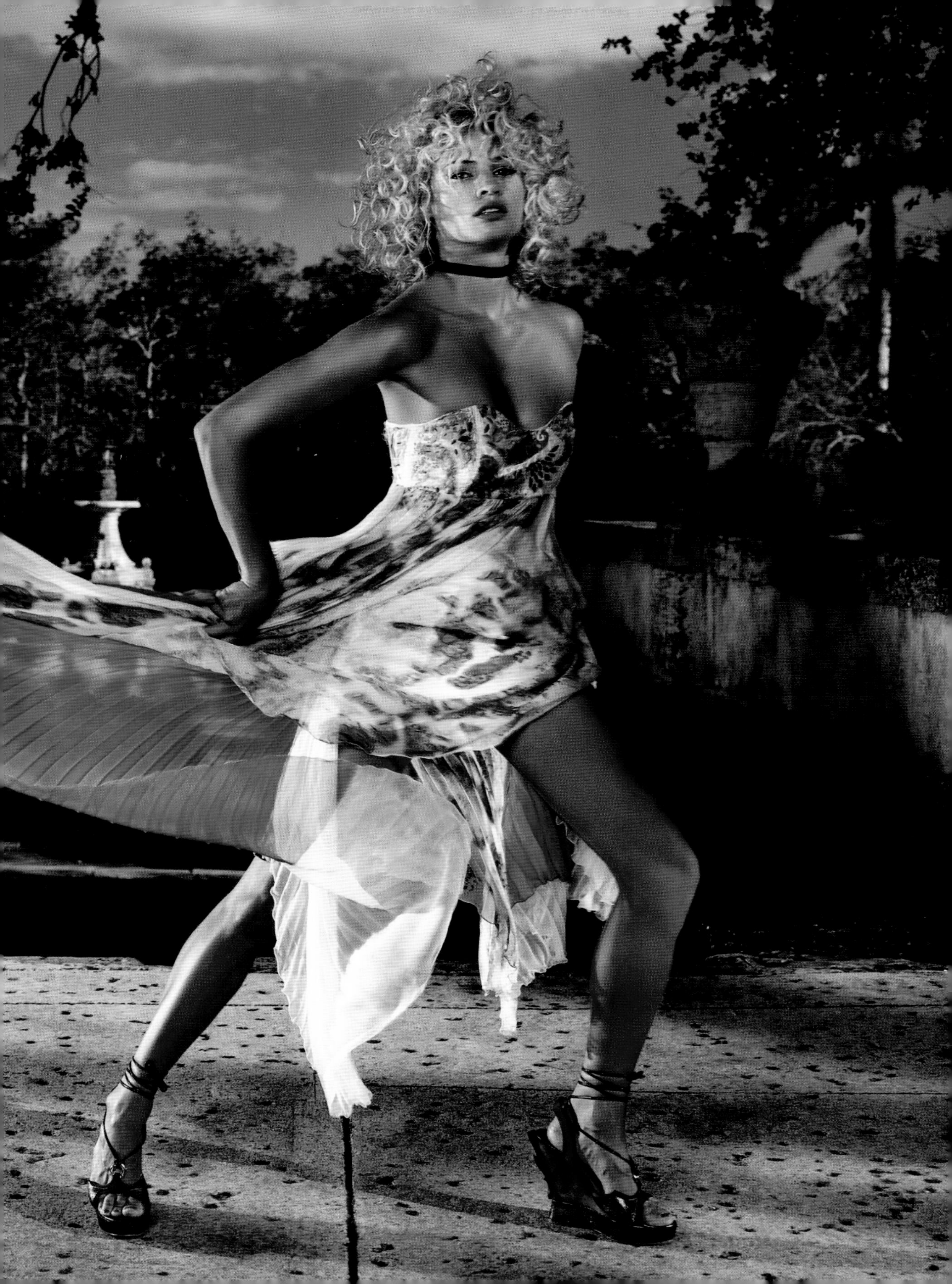

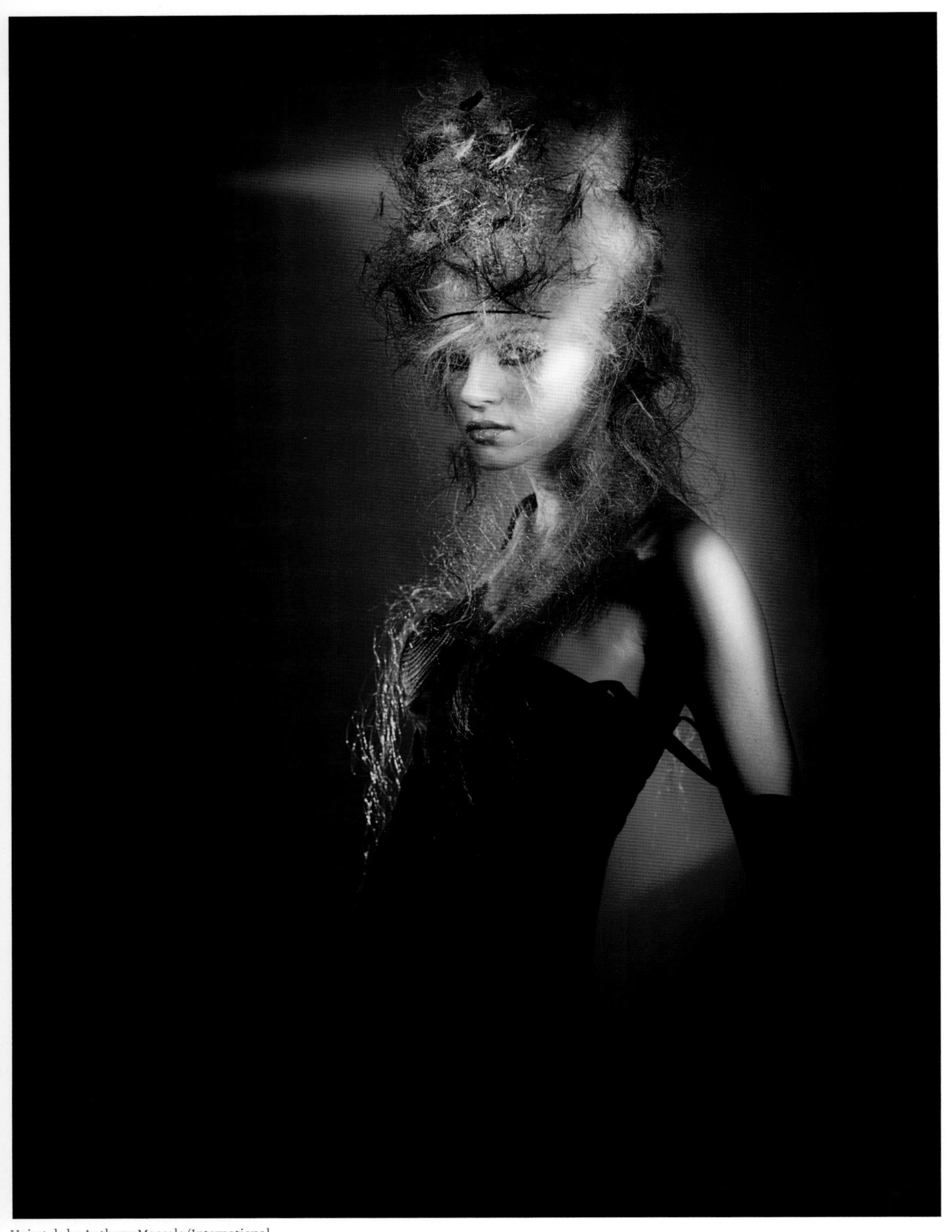

Hairstyle by Anthony Mascolo (International Creative Director of TIGI), for TIGI, 2006

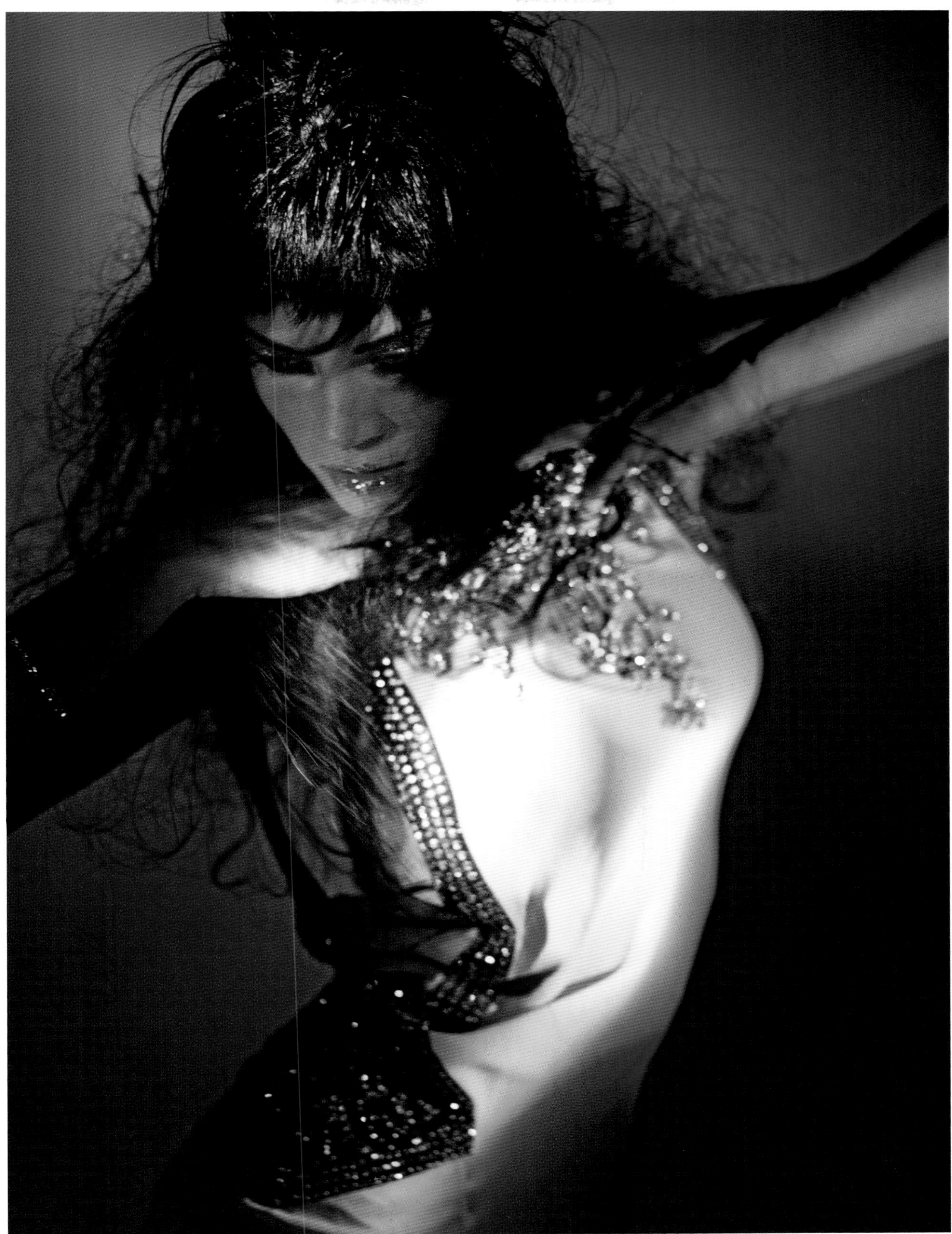

Hairstyle by Anthony Mascolo (International Creative Director of TIGI), for TIGI, 2006

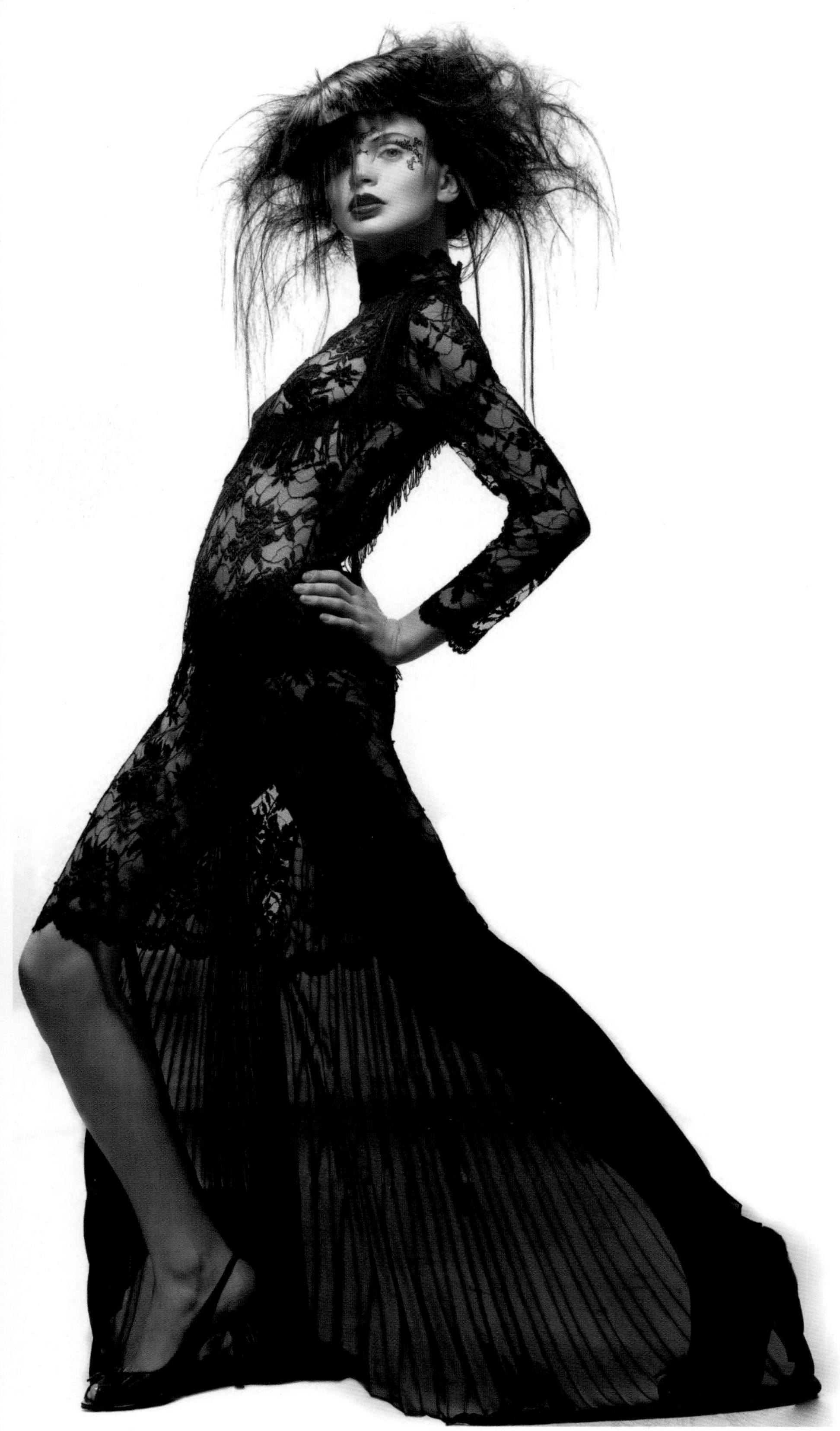

'Raven' hairstyle by Anthony Mascolo (International Creative Director of TIGI) for TIGI, 2006

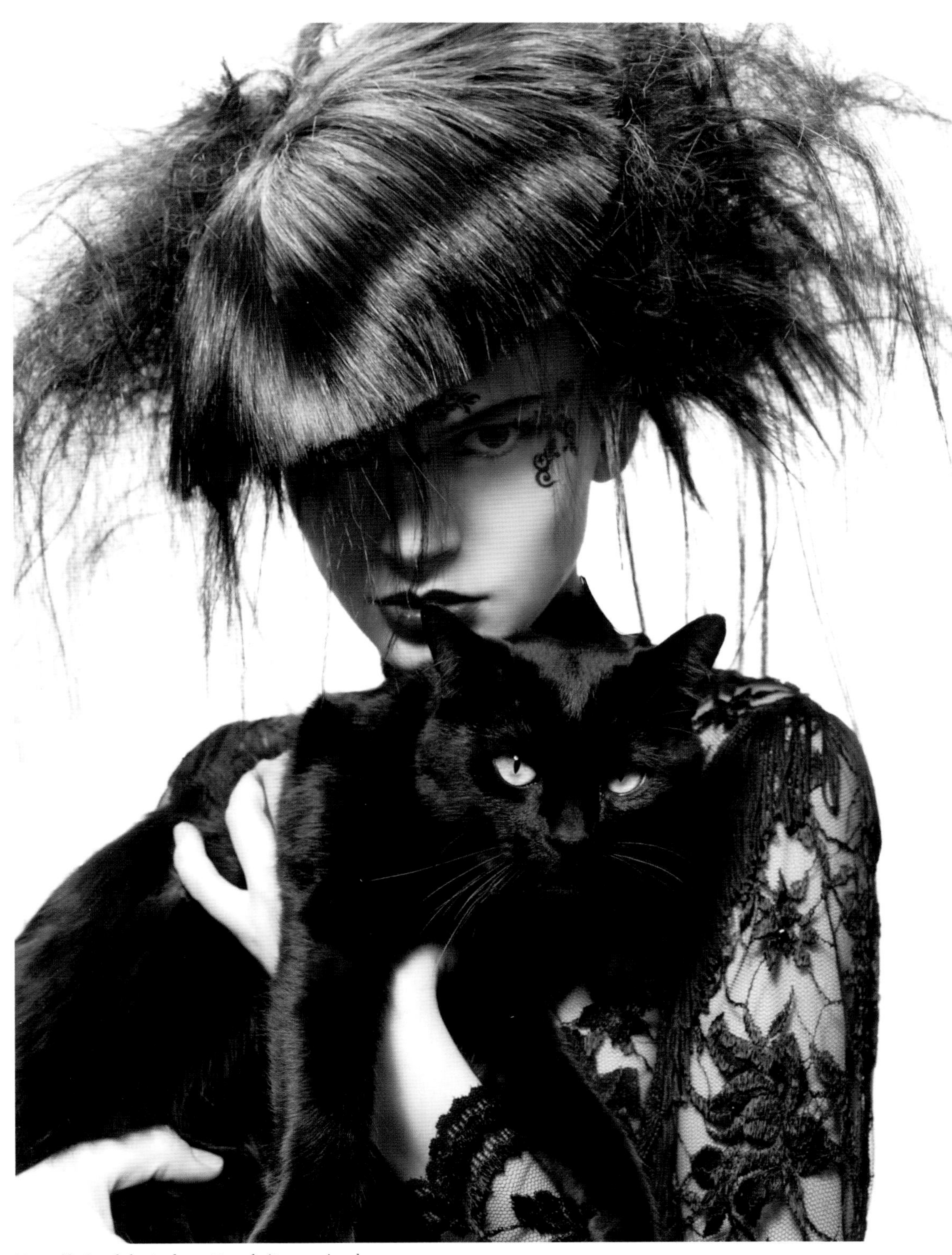

'Raven' hairstyle by Anthony Mascolo (International Creative Director of TIGI) for TIGI, 2006

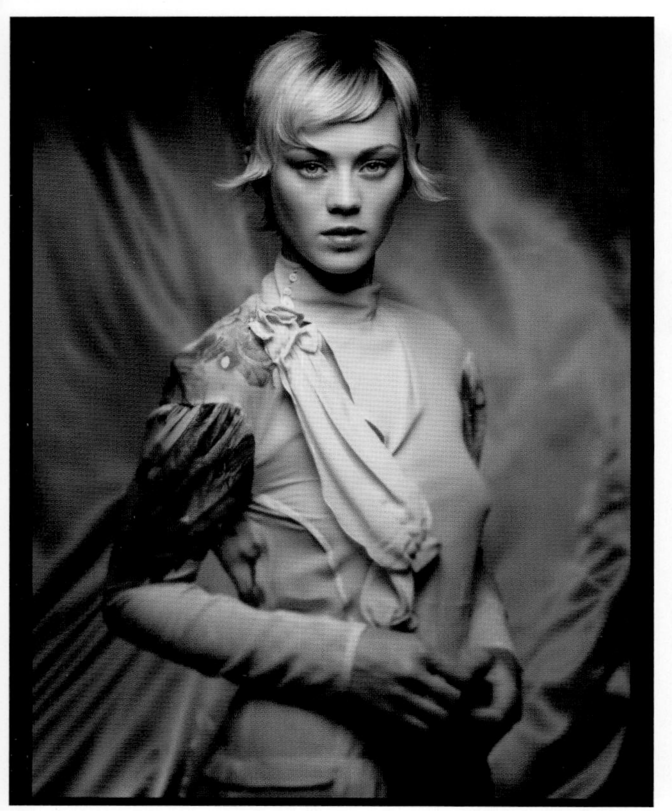
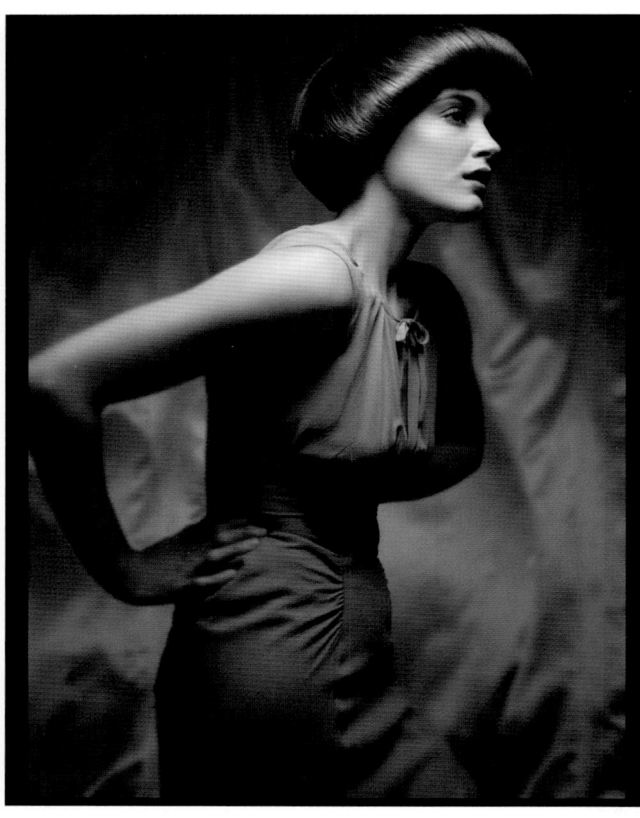
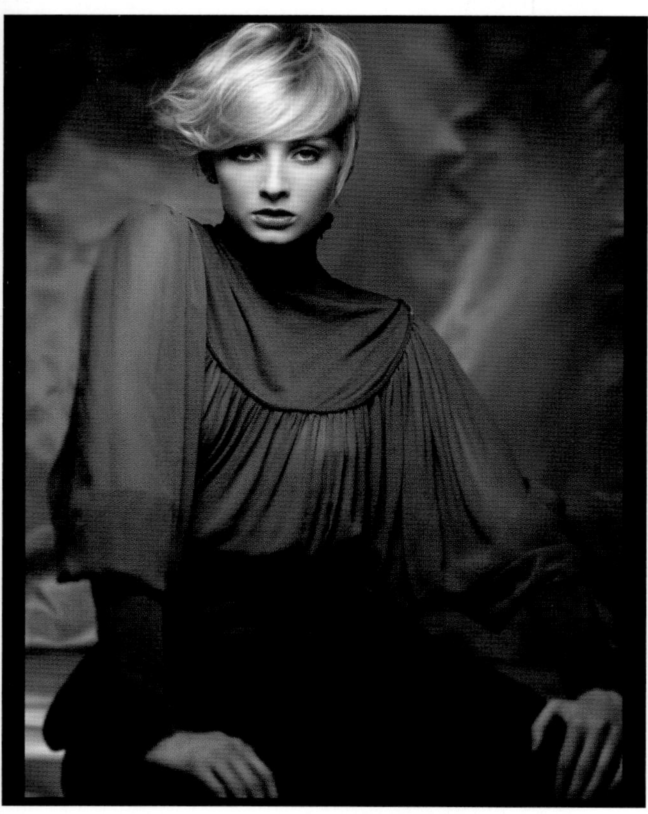
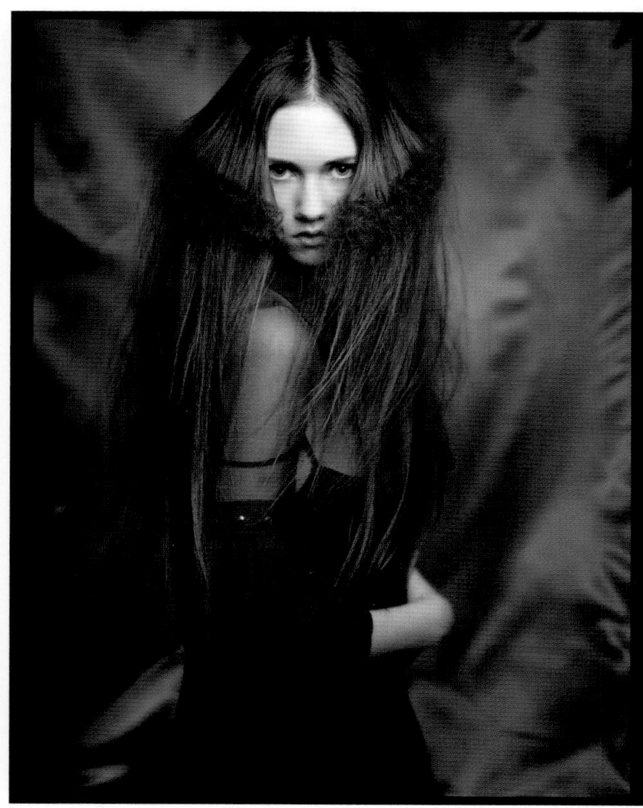

Hairstyles from the London Hairdresser of the Year Award winning Satine Collection by Sally and Jamie Brooks at Brooks&Brooks, London, 2006

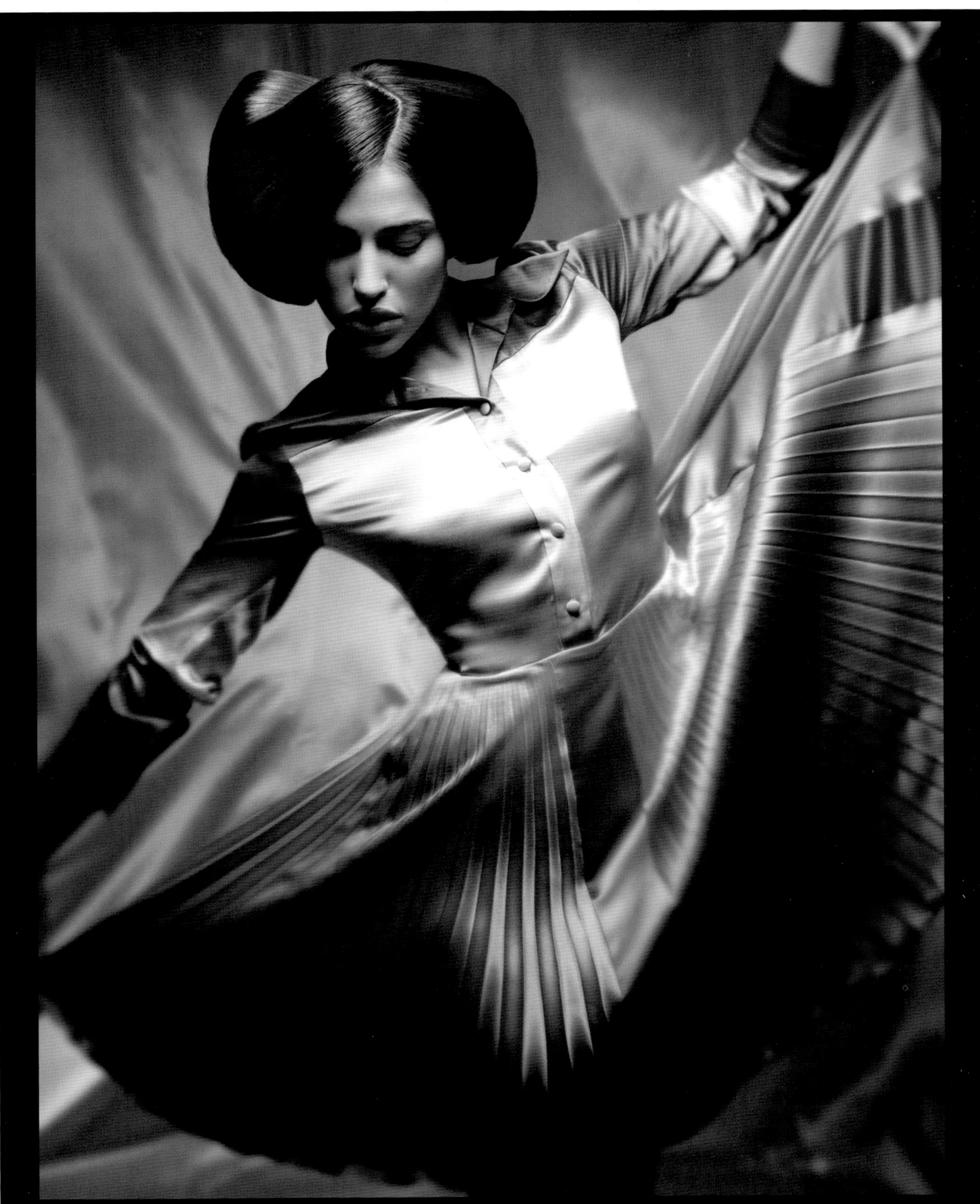

Hairstyle from the London Hairdresser of the Year Award winning Satine Collection by Sally and Jamie Brooks at Brooks&Brooks, London, 2006

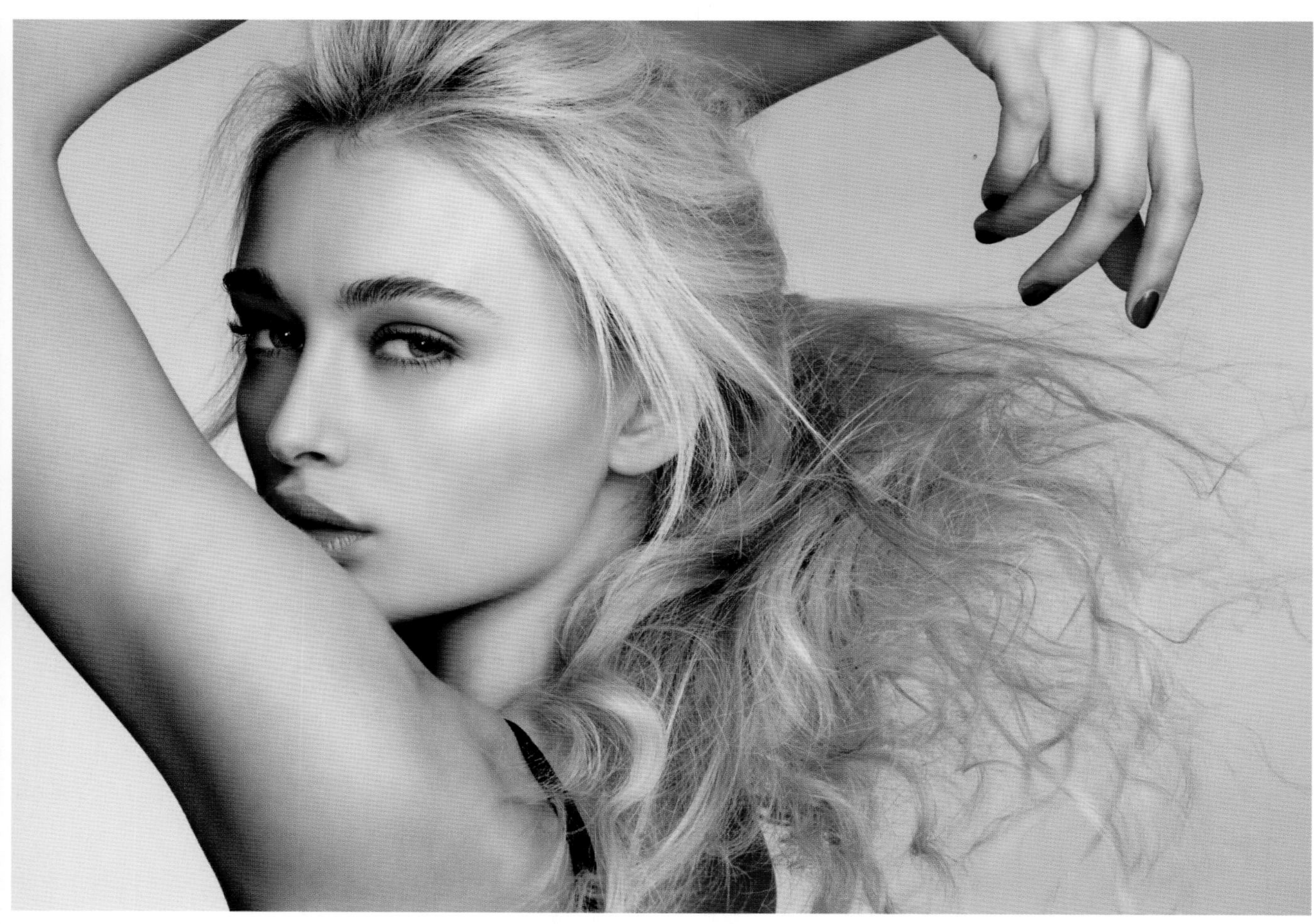

'Messy Pony' from the Allure Collection by Lisa Shepherd, 2006

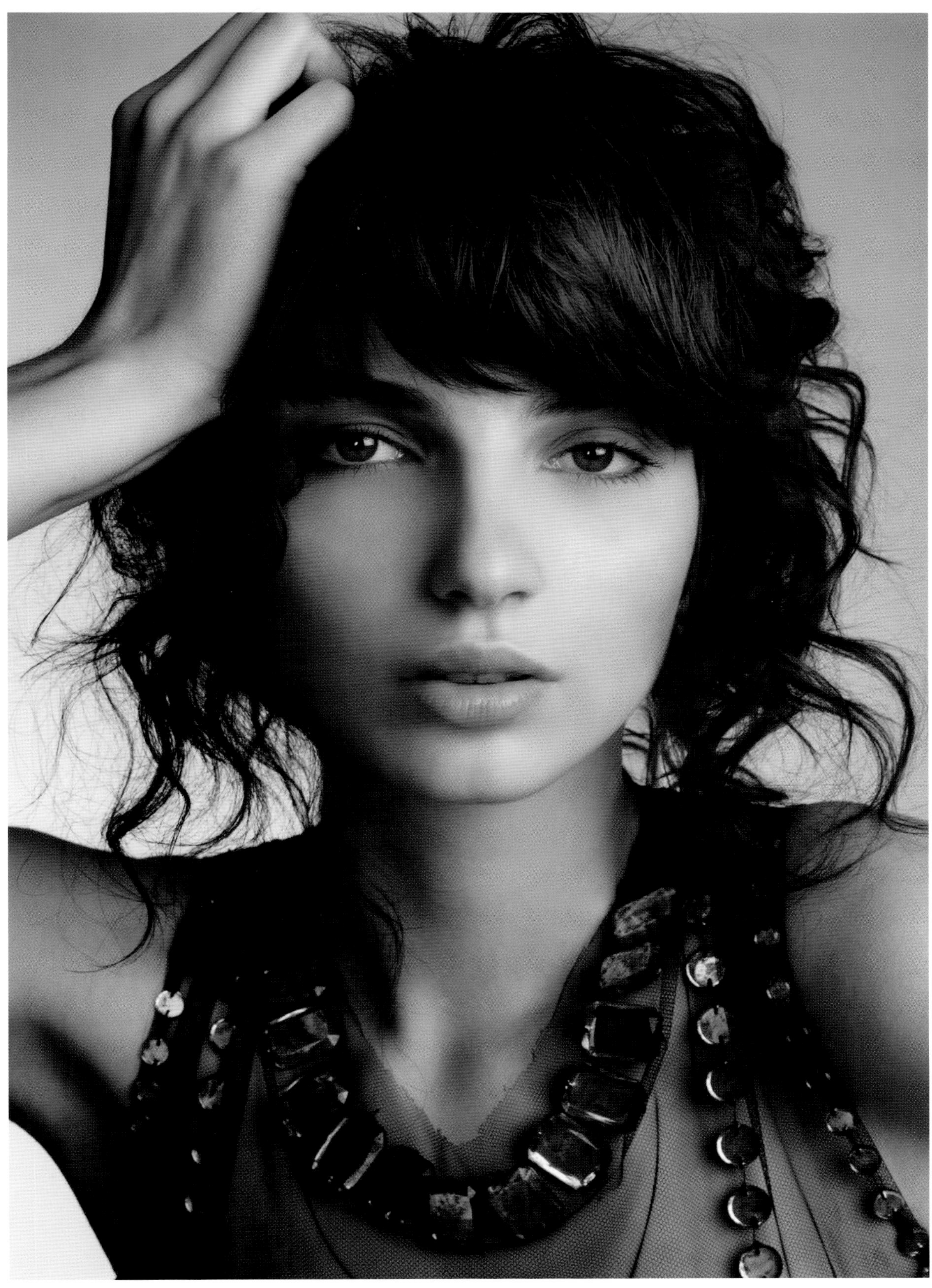

'Blue Girl' from the Allure Collection
by Lisa Shepherd, 2006

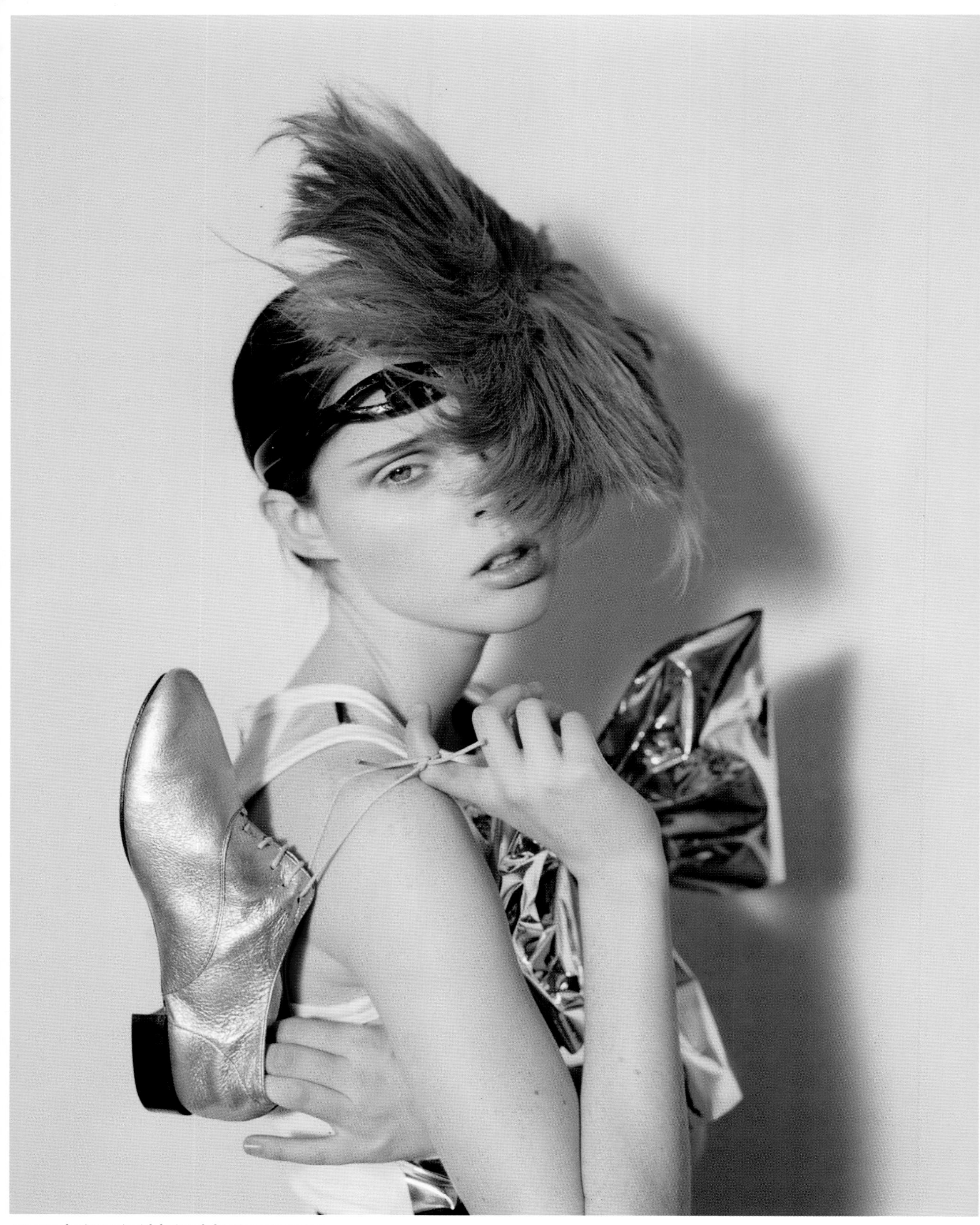

Coco Rocha (Storm) with hairstyle by Gianni Scumaci, photographed by Tim Walker, 2006

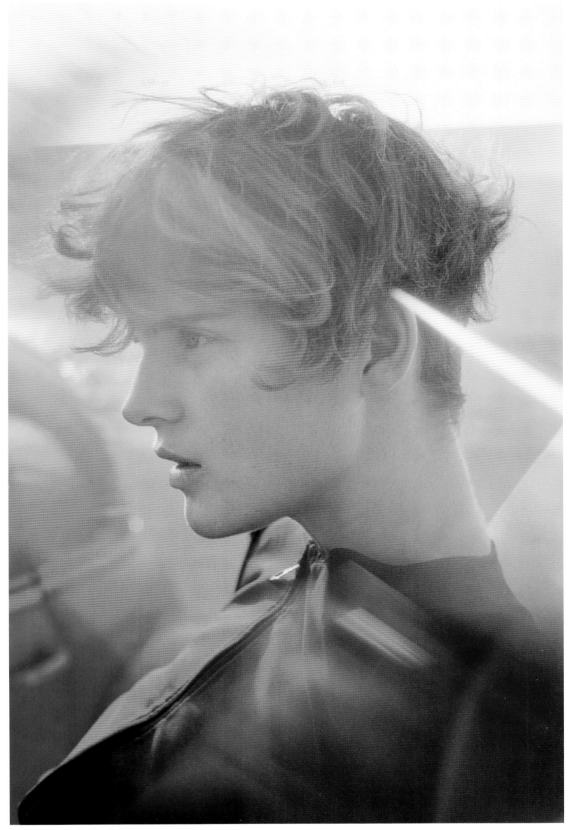

Stella Tennant (Select) with hairstyle by Gianni Scumaci, photographed by Tim Walker, 2007

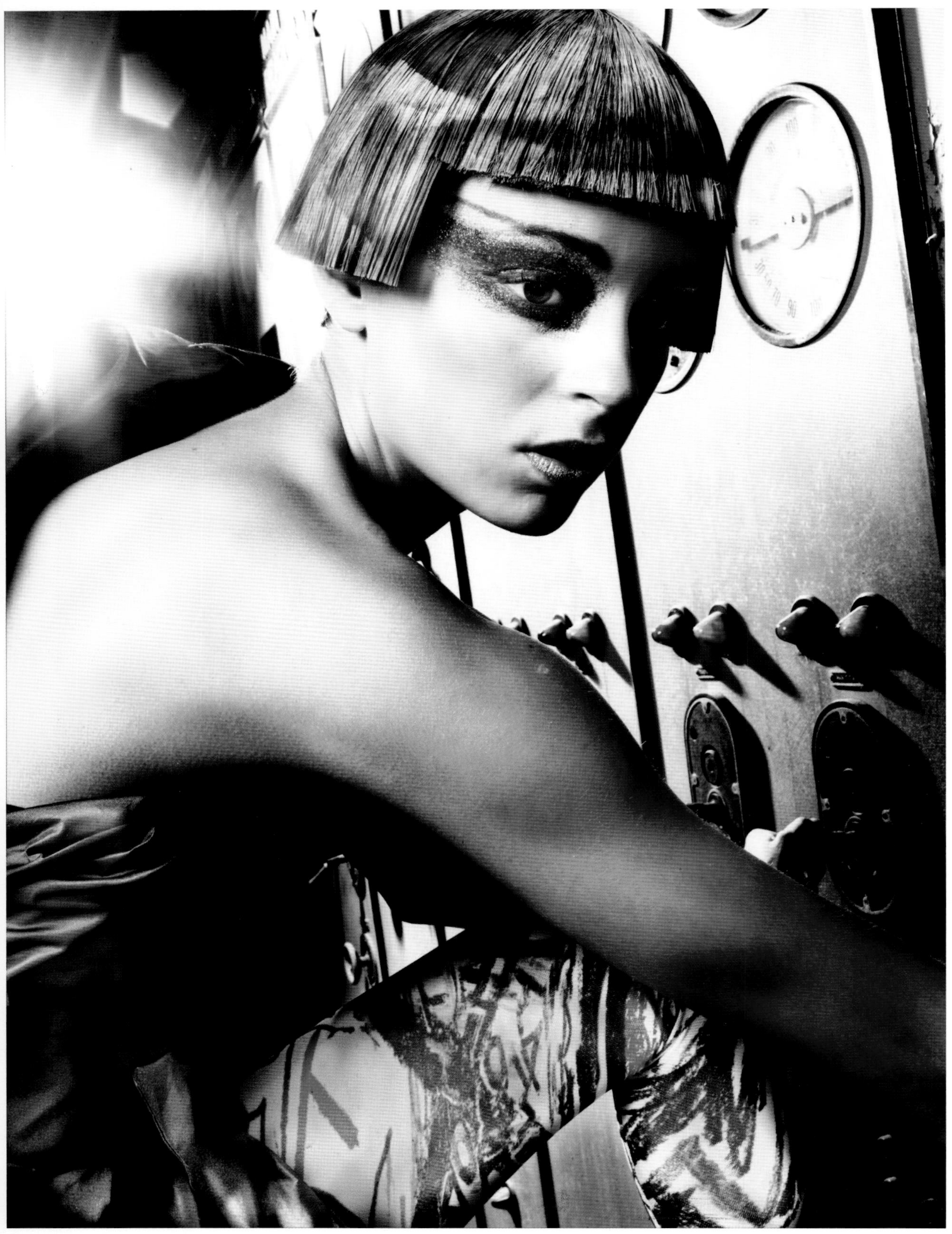

Hairstyle from *Alta Moda*, collaborative project between TIGI and Vivienne Westwood, hairstyle by Anthony Mascolo (International Creative Director of TIGI), for TIGI, 2007

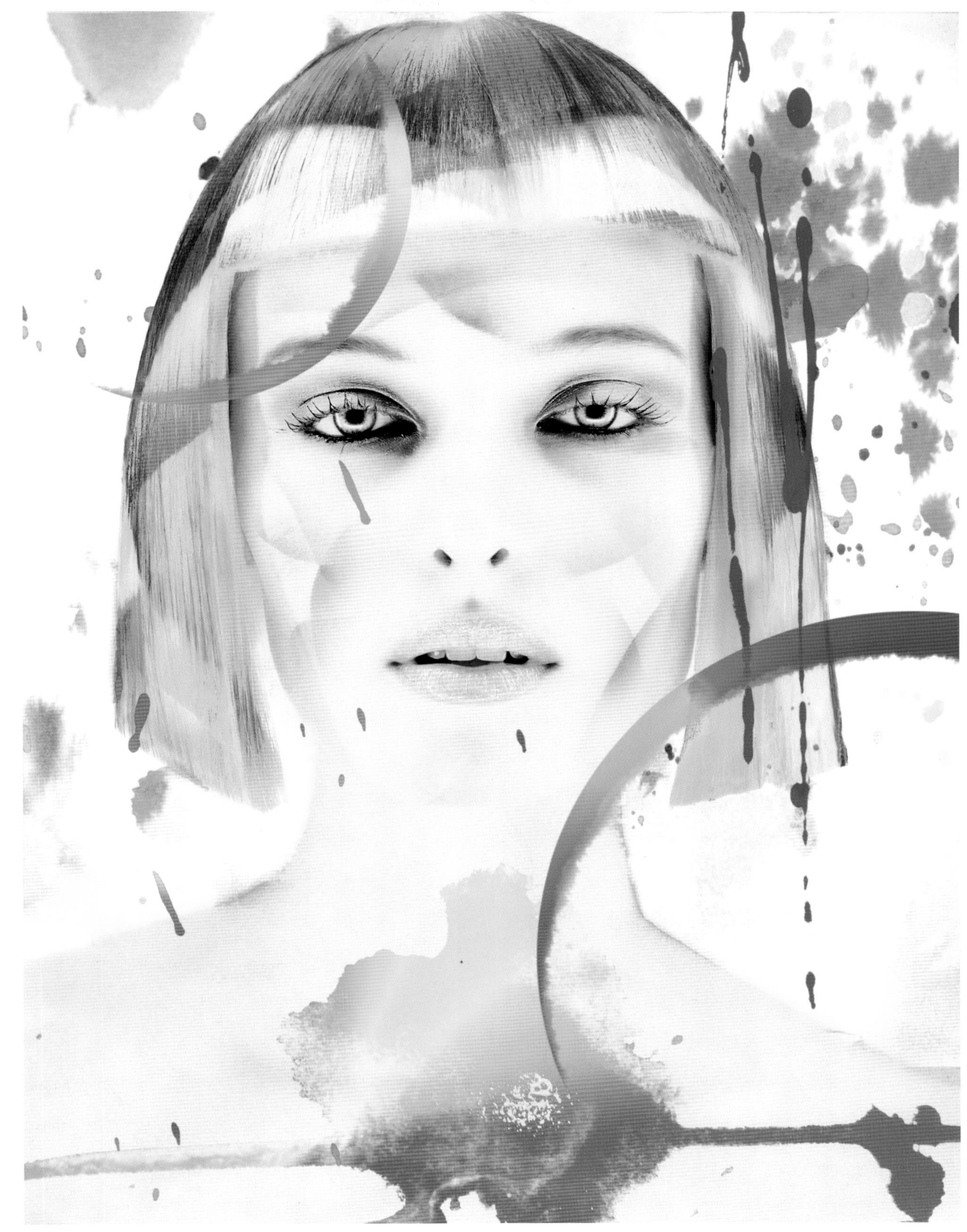

Hairstyle from *Alta Moda*, collaborative project between TIGI and Vivienne Westwood, hairstyle by Anthony Mascolo (International Creative Director of TIGI), for TIGI, 2008

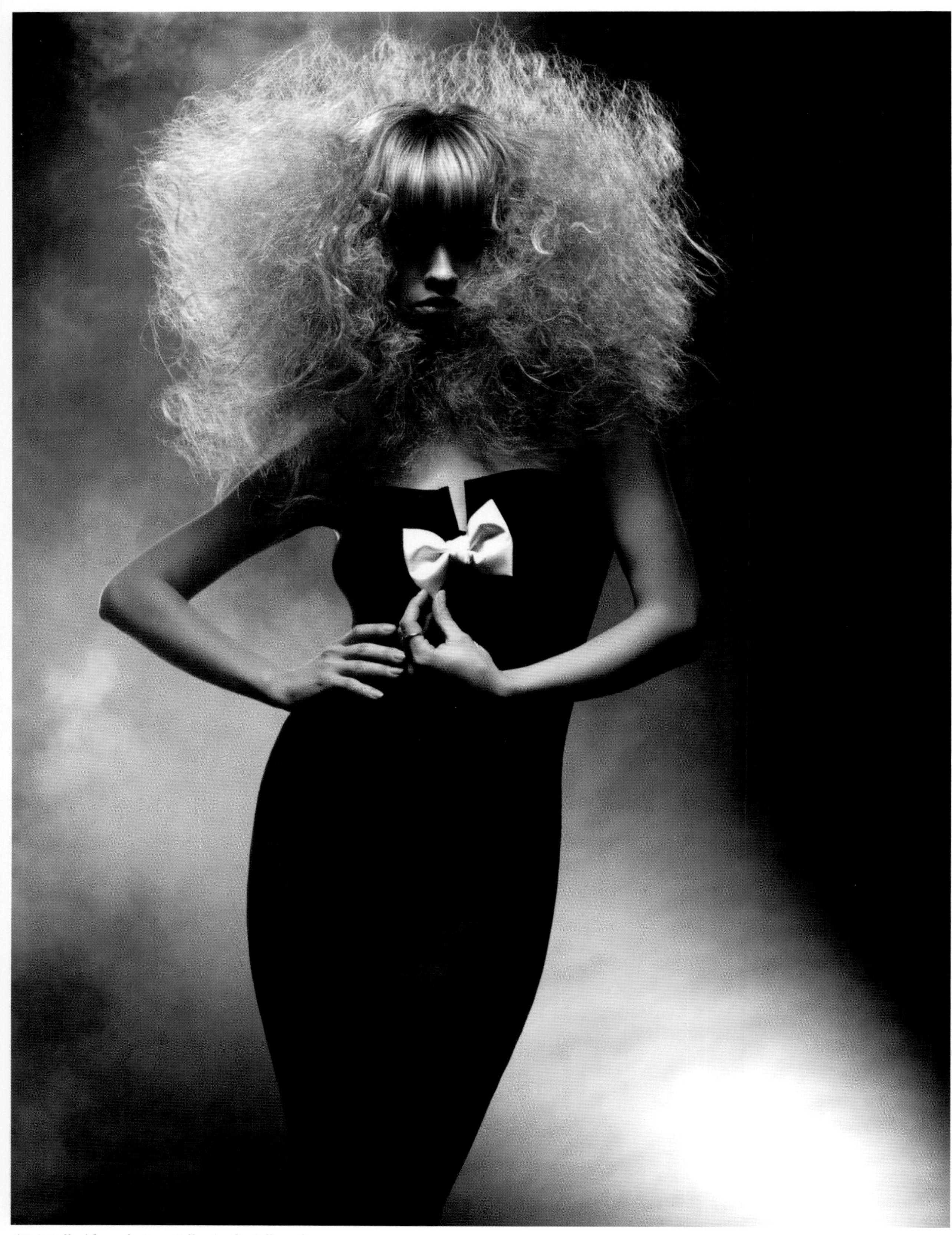

'Hair Collar' from the Lace Collection by Sally and Jamie Brooks at Brooks&Brooks, London, 2007

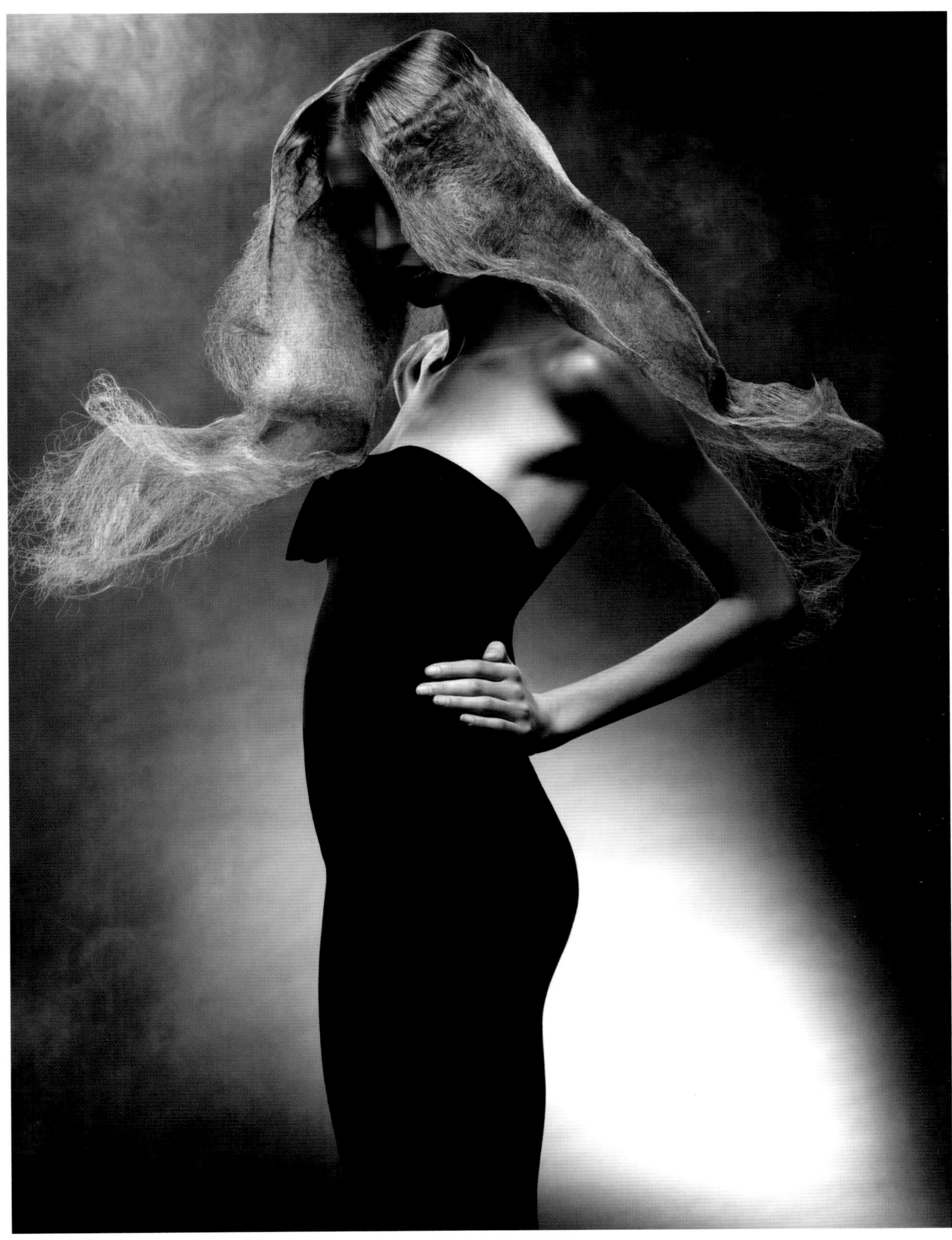

'Lace Sheet' from the Lace Collection by Sally and Jamie Brooks at Brooks&Brooks, London, 2007

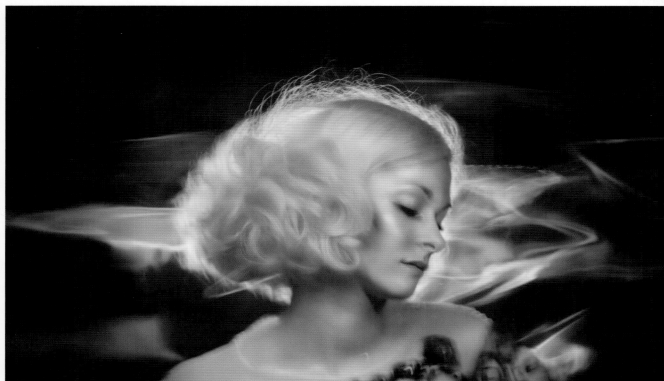

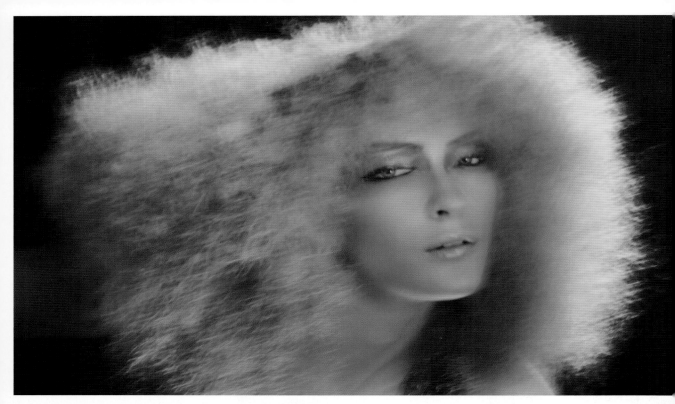

'Disco Diva' from the Aura Collection
by Antoinette Beenders, 2007

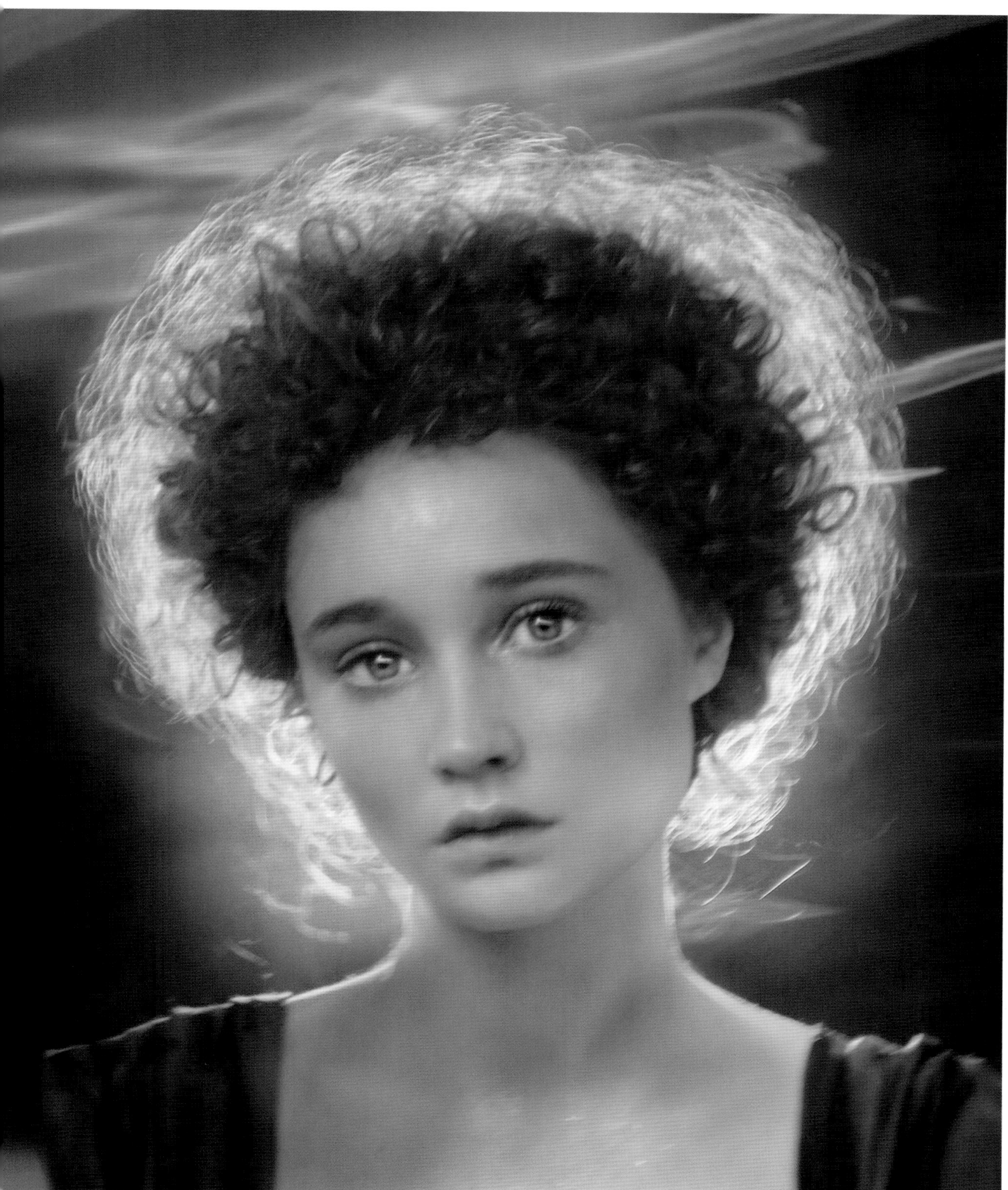

ngel Face' from the Aura Collection
Antoinette Beenders, 2007

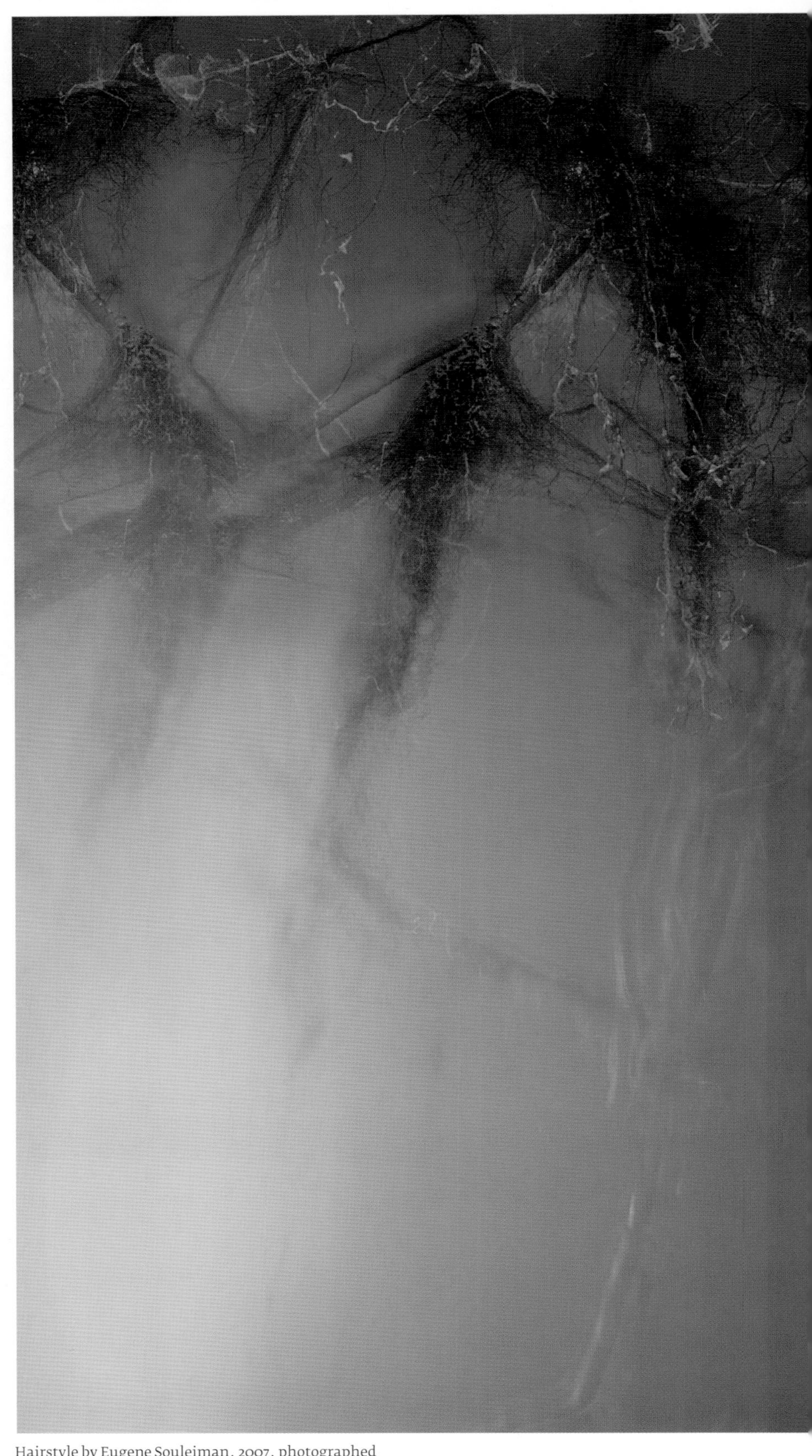

Hairstyle by Eugene Souleiman, 2007, photographed
by Warren du Preez and Nick Thornton Jones

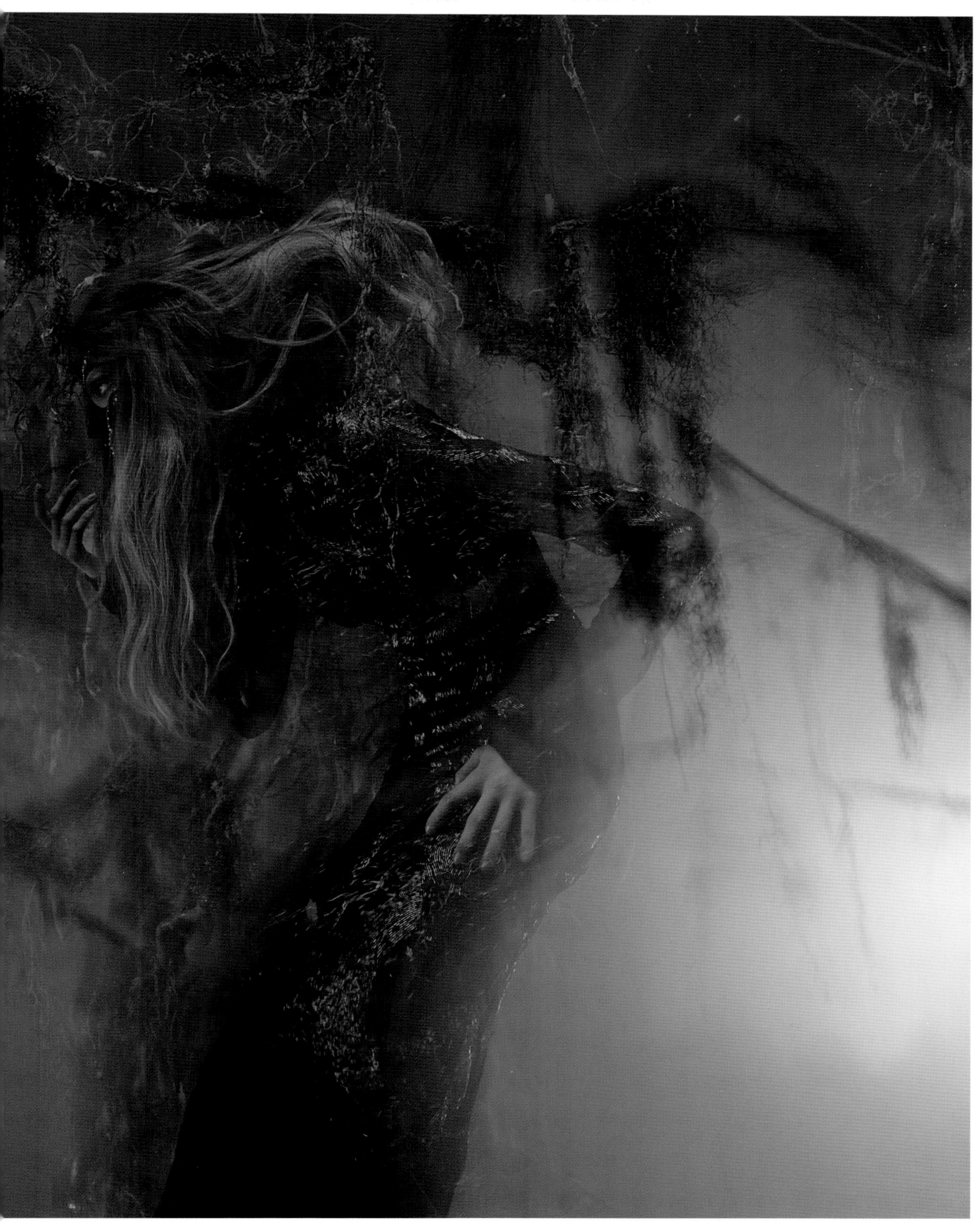

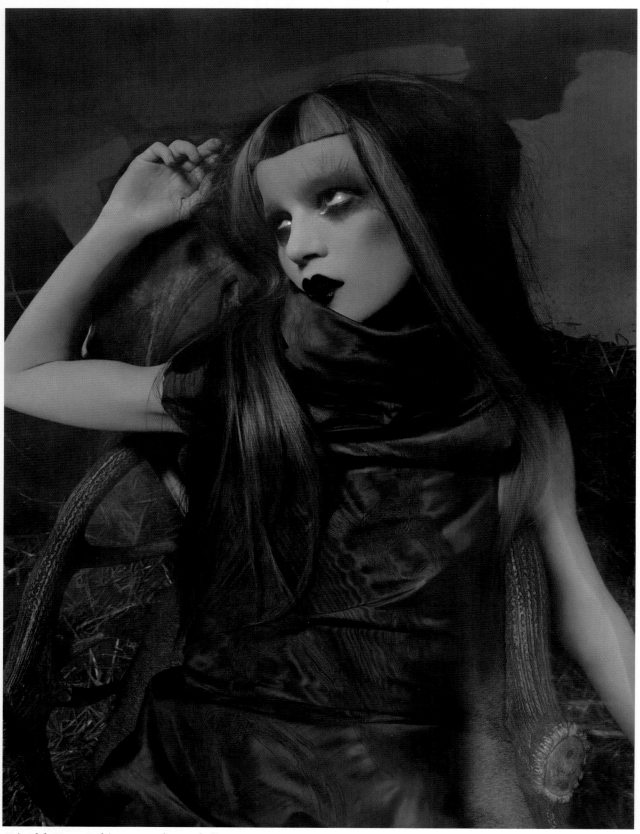

Hairstyle by Eugene Souleiman, 2007, photographed by Warren du Preez and Nick Thornton Jones

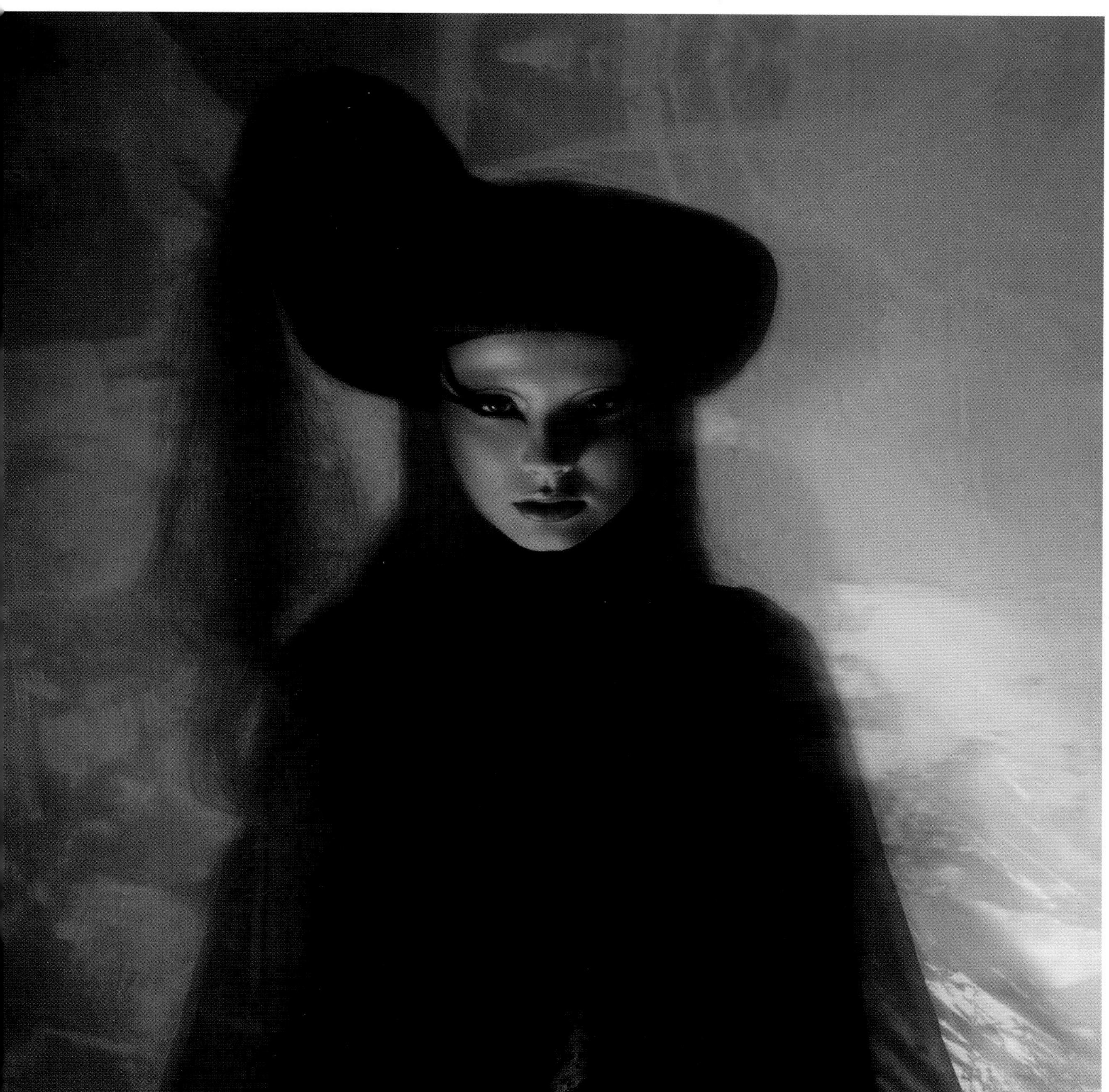

Hairstyle by Eugene Souleiman, 2007, photographed by Warren du Preez and Nick Thornton Jones

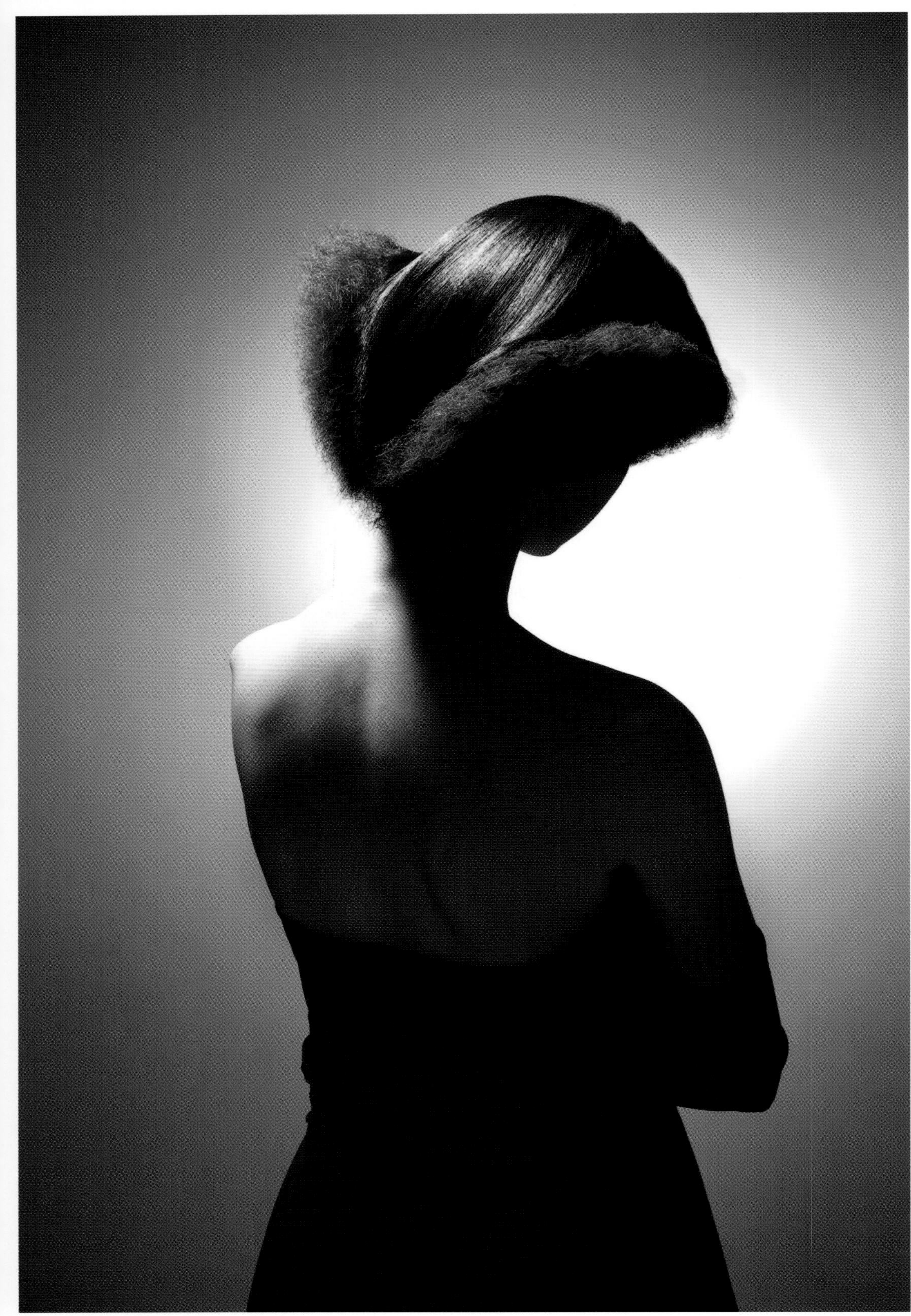

Hairstyle by Andrew Collinge, 2008,
photographed by John Swannell

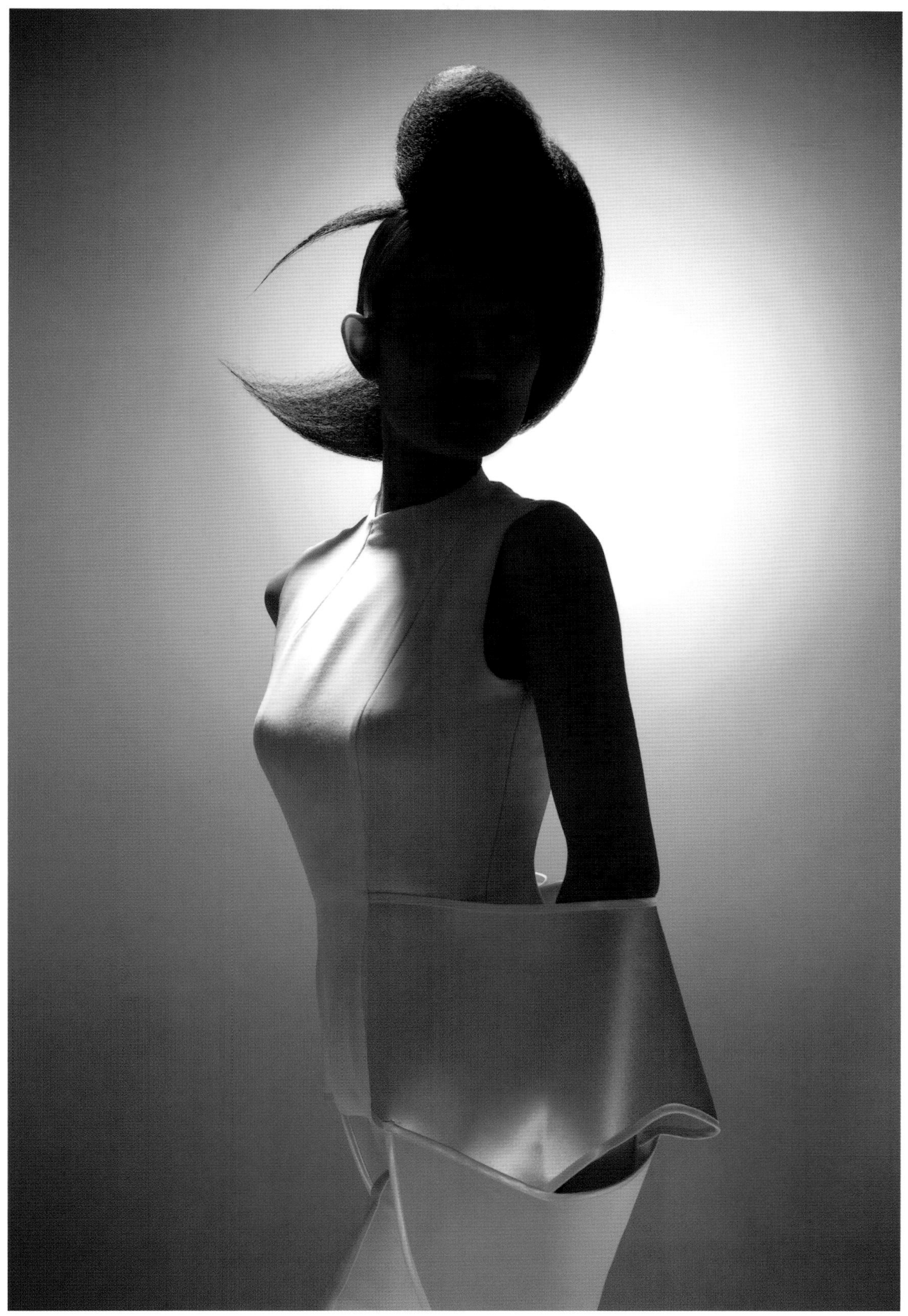

Hairstyle by Andrew Collinge, 2008, photographed by John Swannell

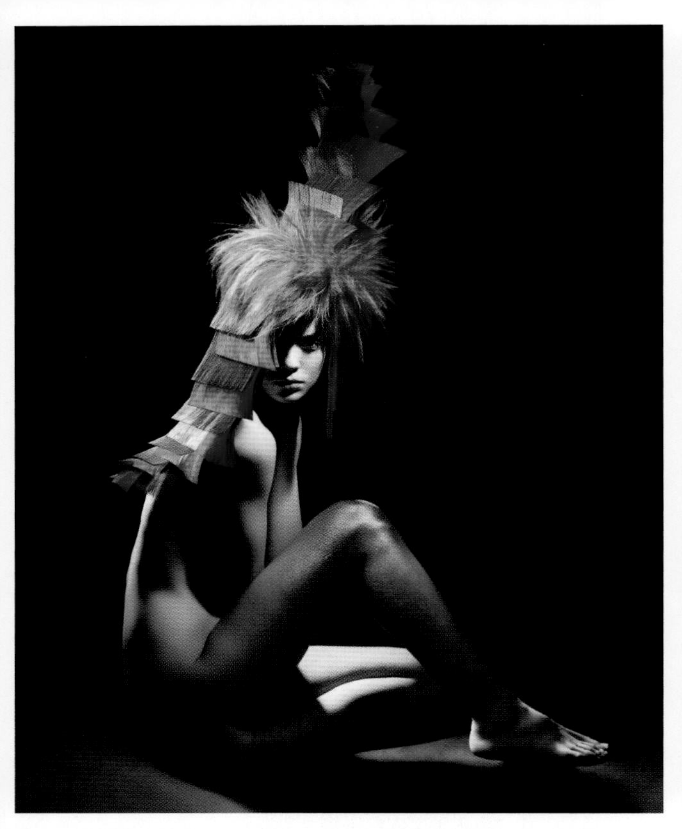

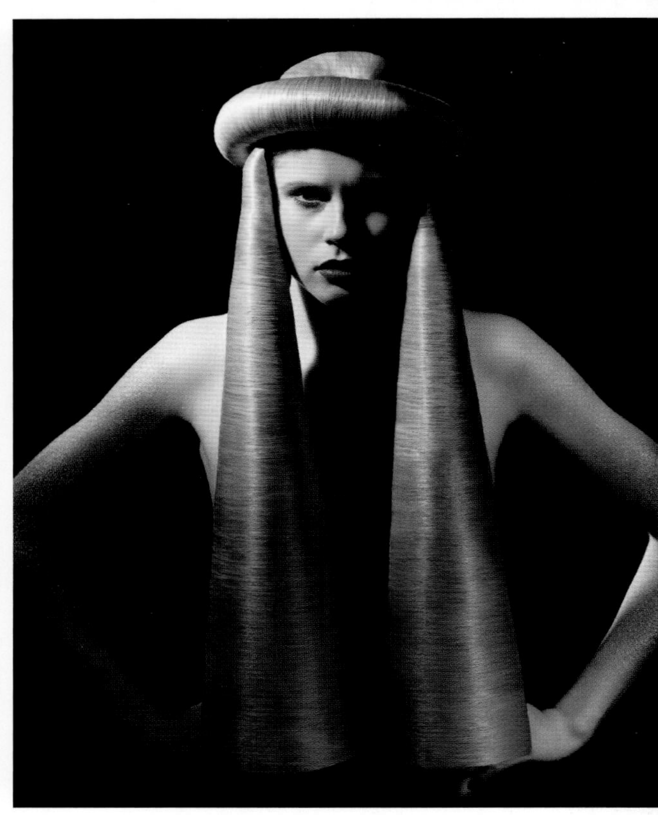

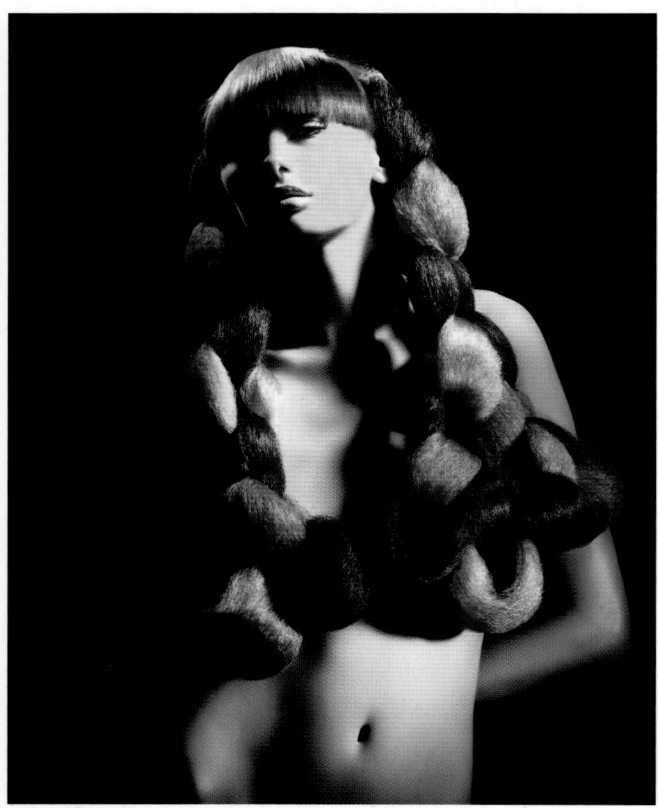

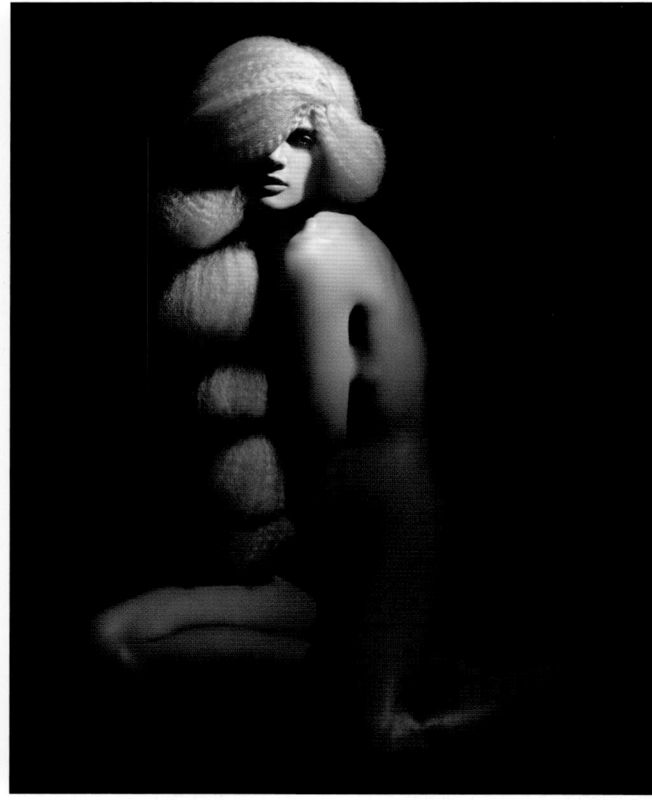

Hairstyle from the Midsummer Night's Dream Collection by Michael Barnes for Goldwell, 2008

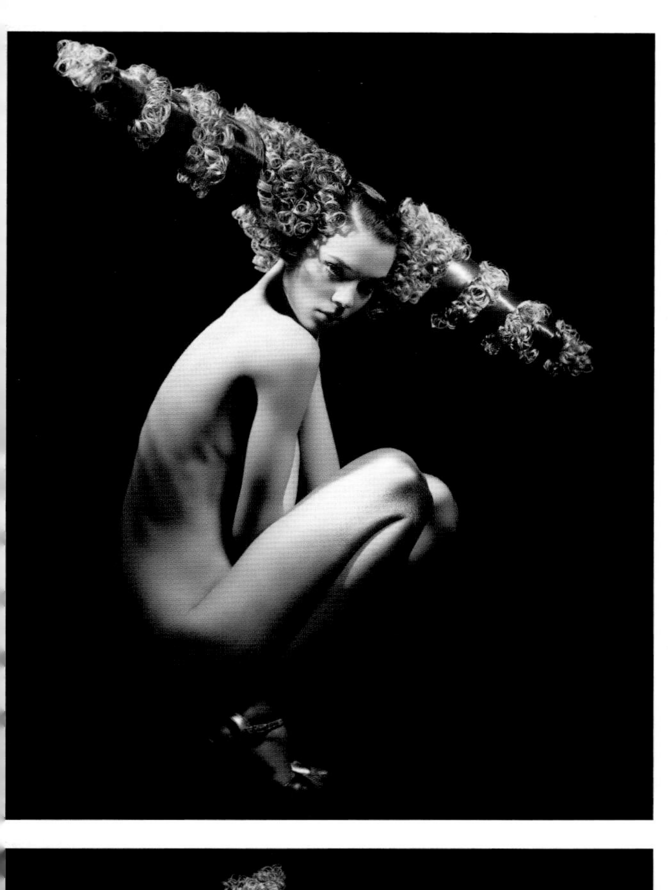

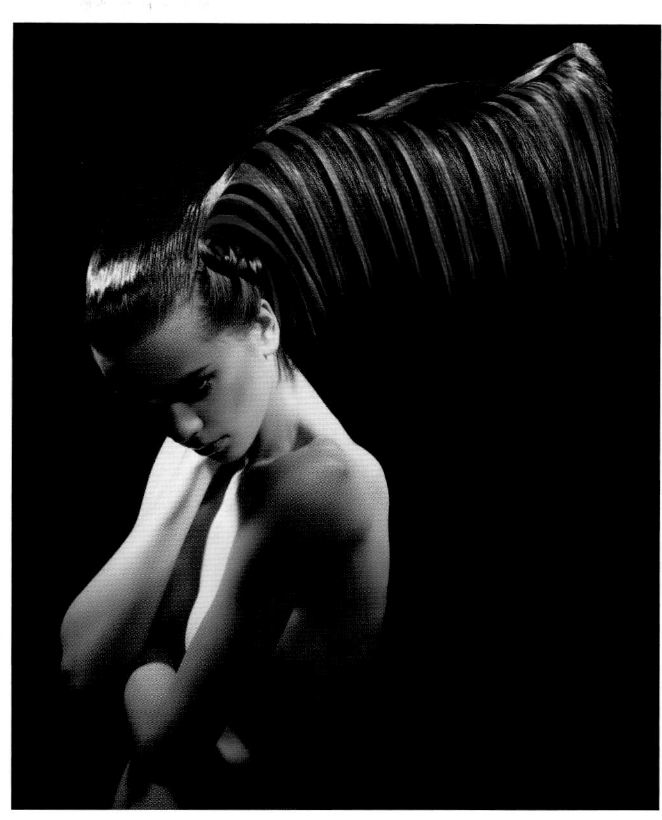

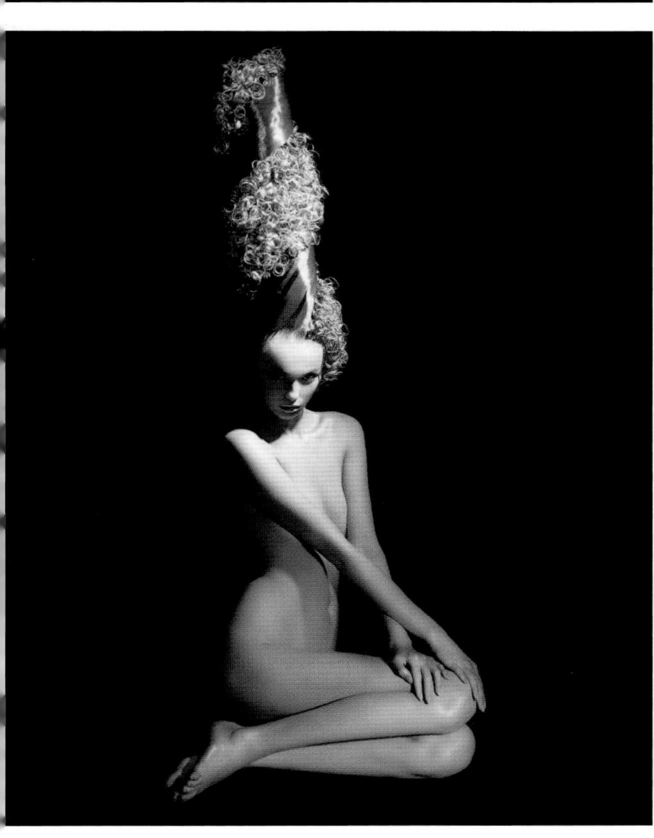

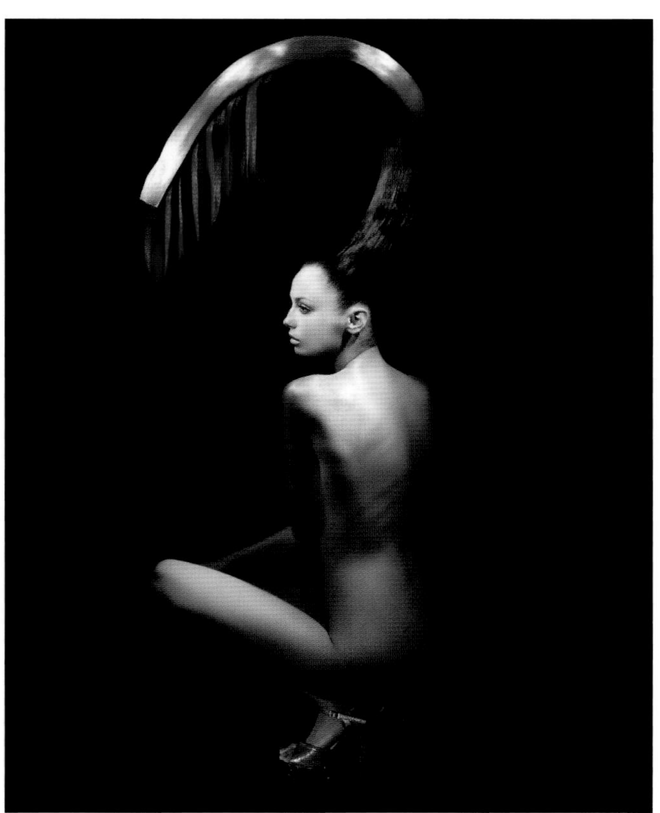

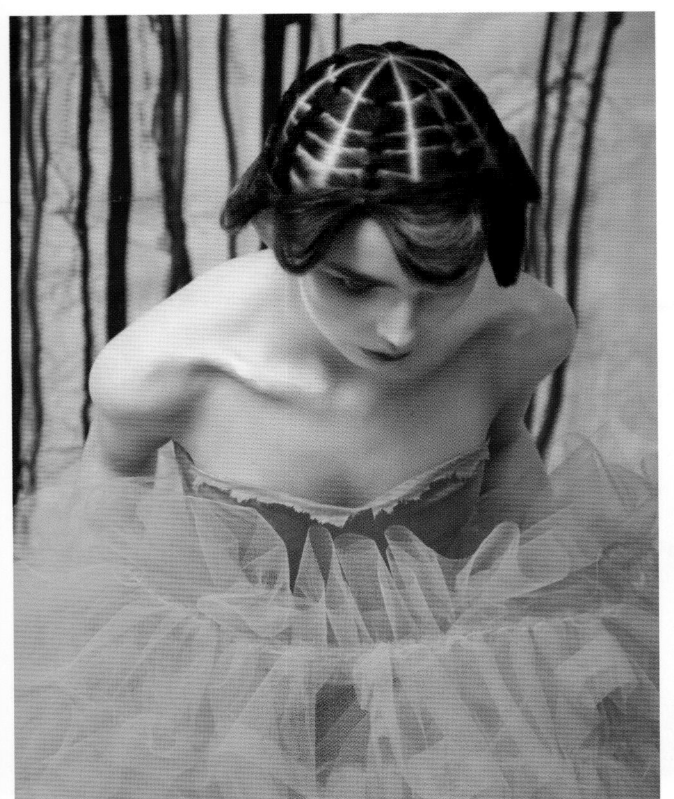

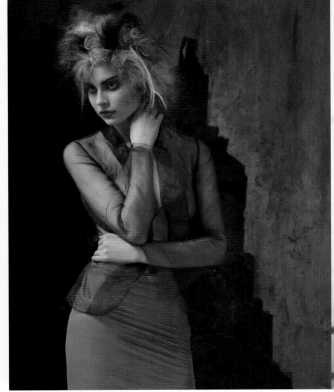
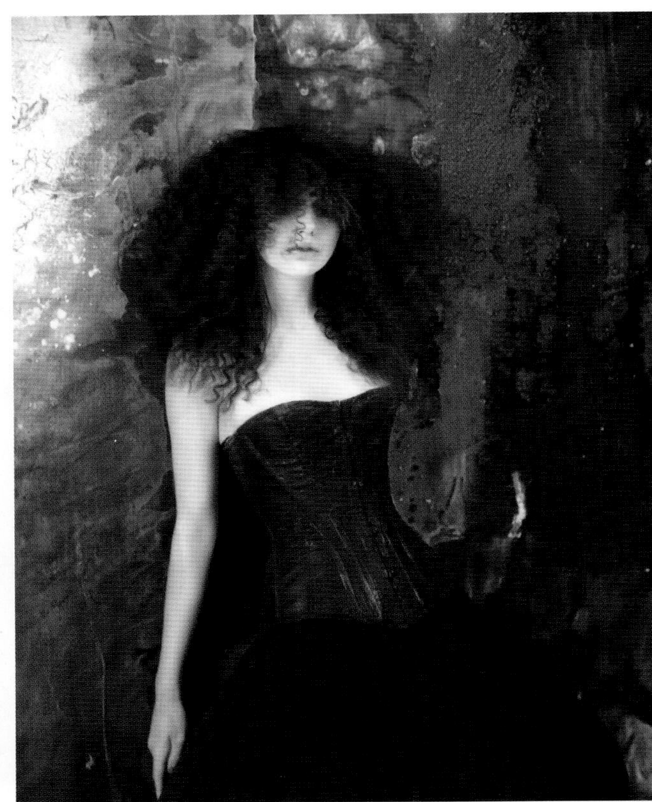
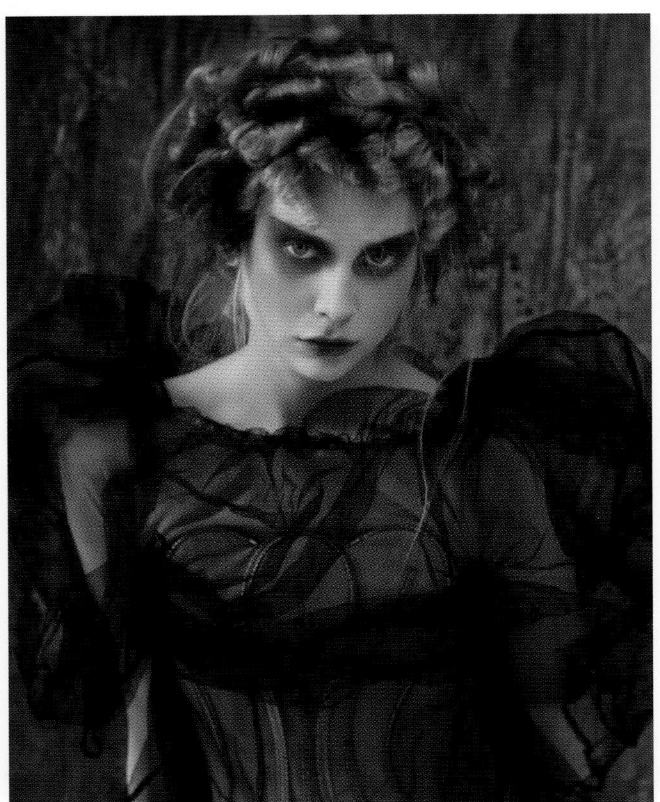

'Avant garde' hairstyles by Louis Byrne, 2000s

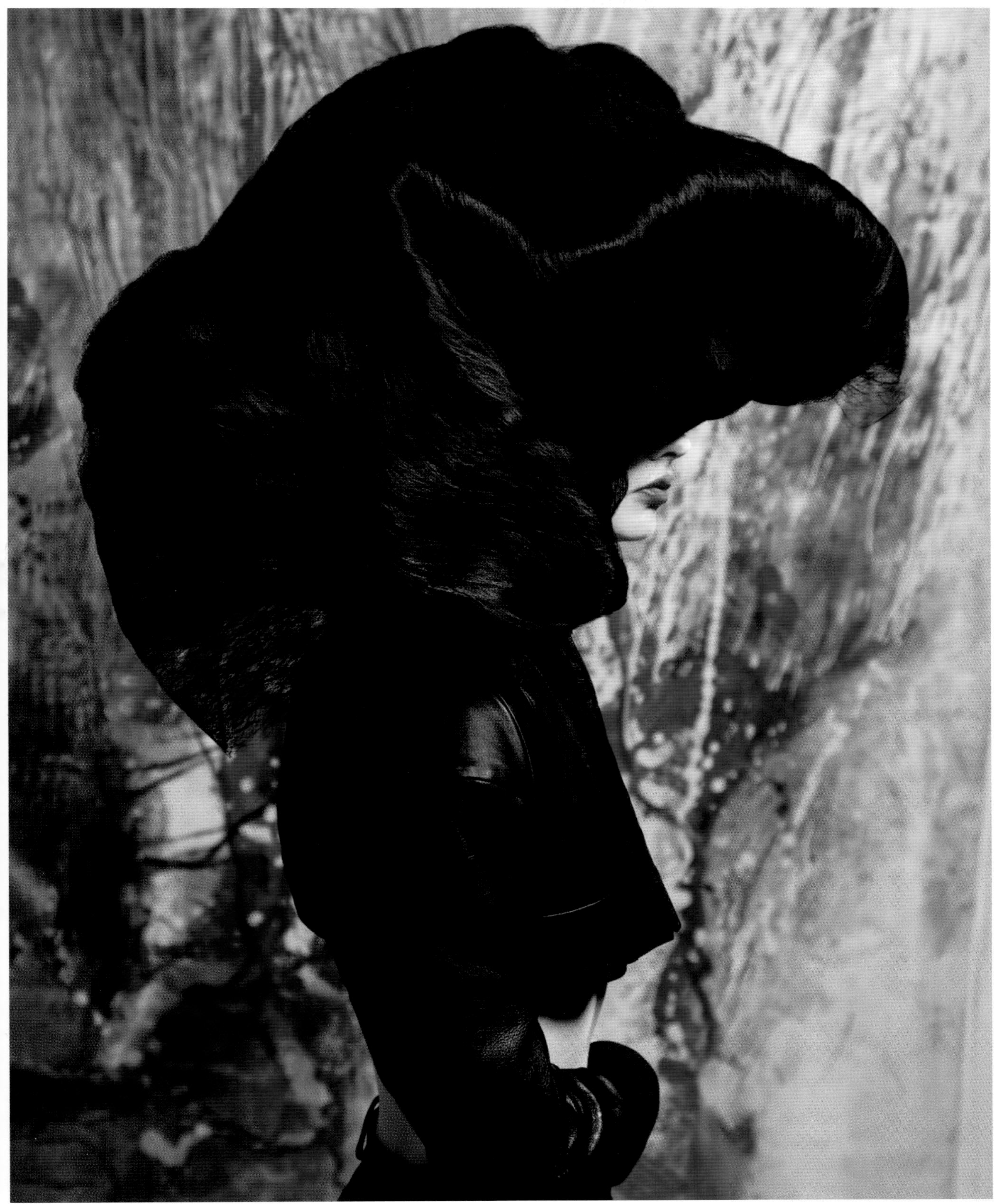

'Avant garde' hairstyle by Louis Byrne, 2000s

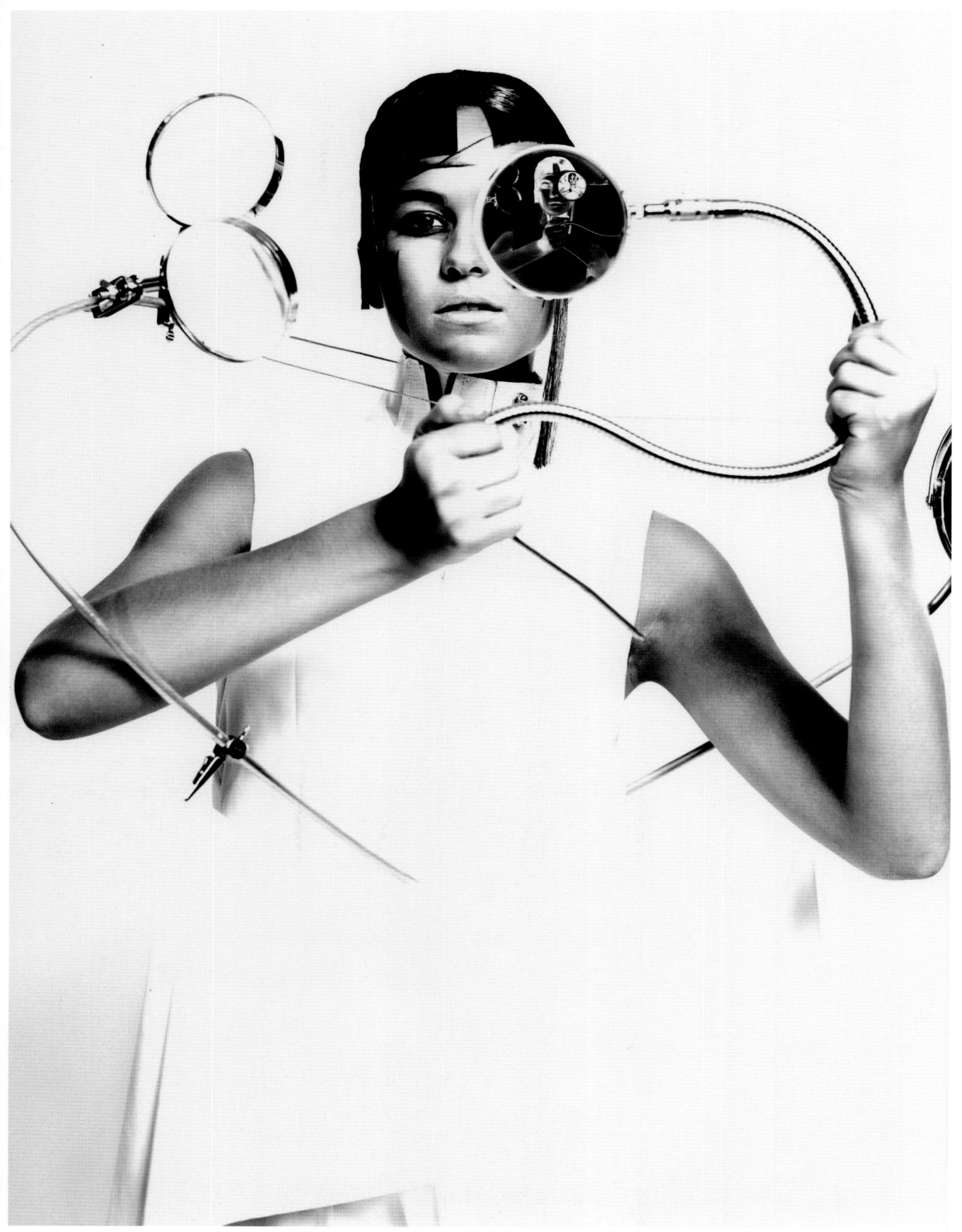

Hairstyle by Anthony Mascolo (International Creative Director of TIGI), for TIGI, 2008

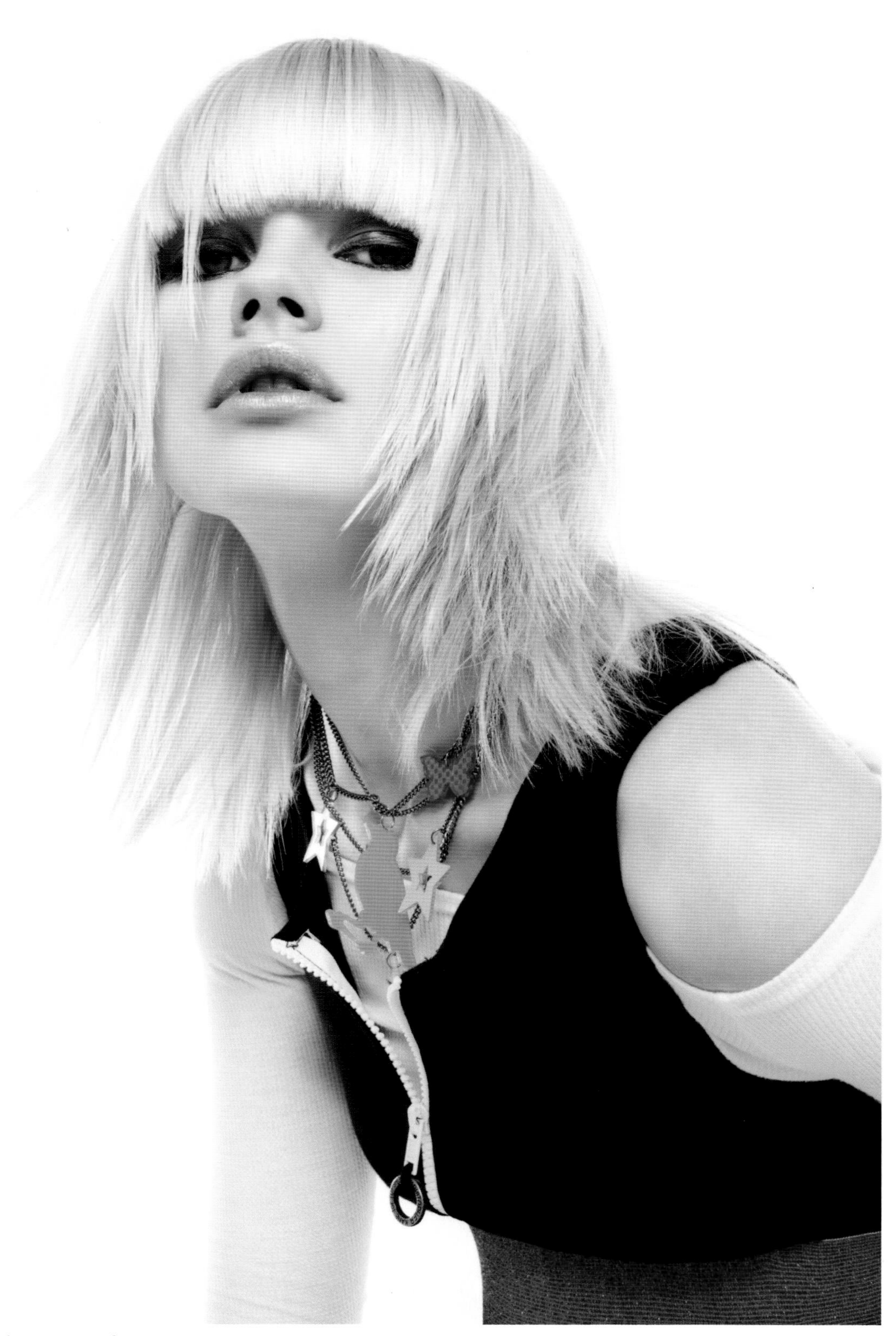

Hairstyle by Anthony Mascolo (International Creative Director of TIGI), for TIGI, 2007

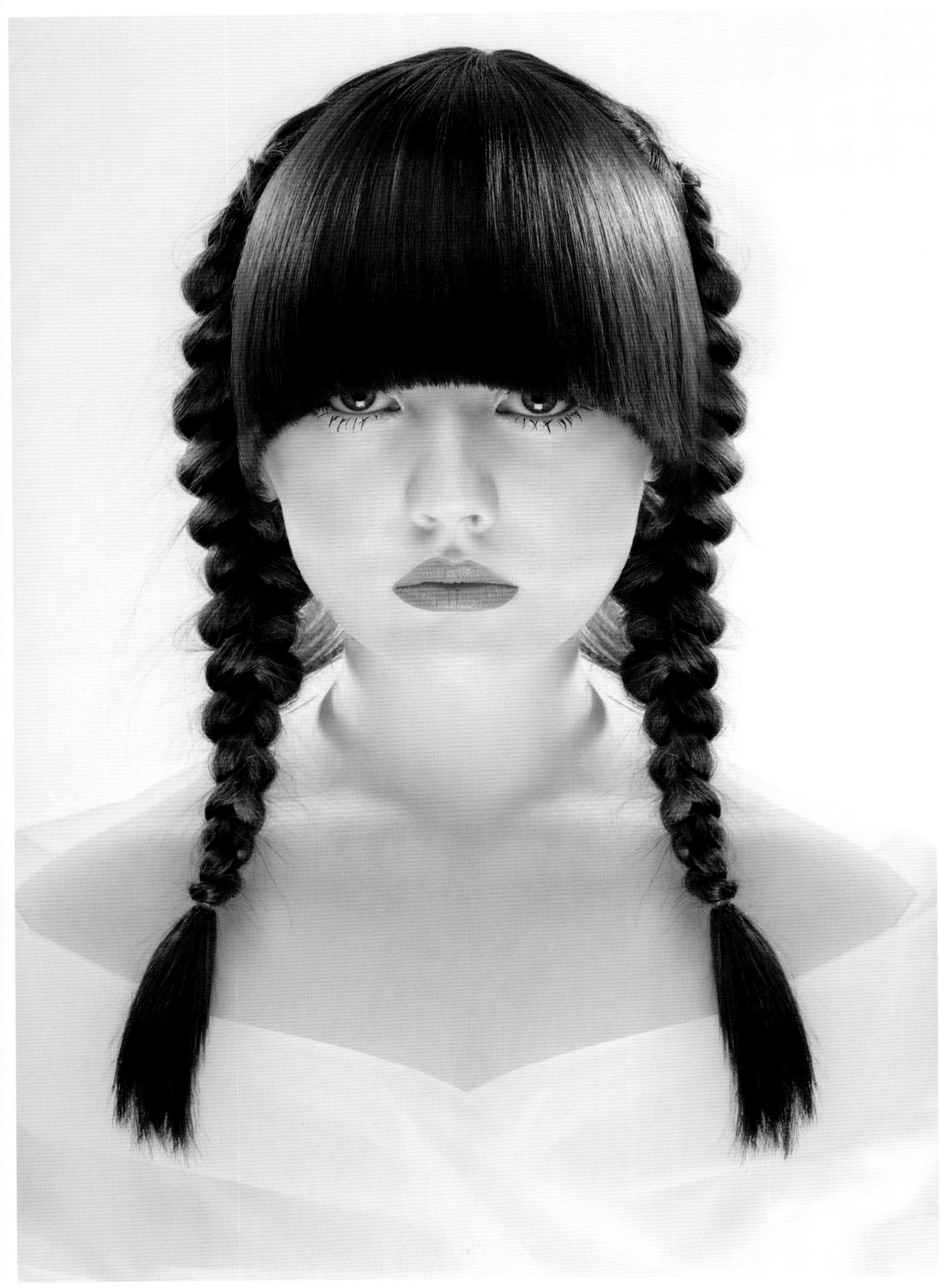

Hairstyle from Pure Collection by
Michael Barnes for Goldwell, 2008

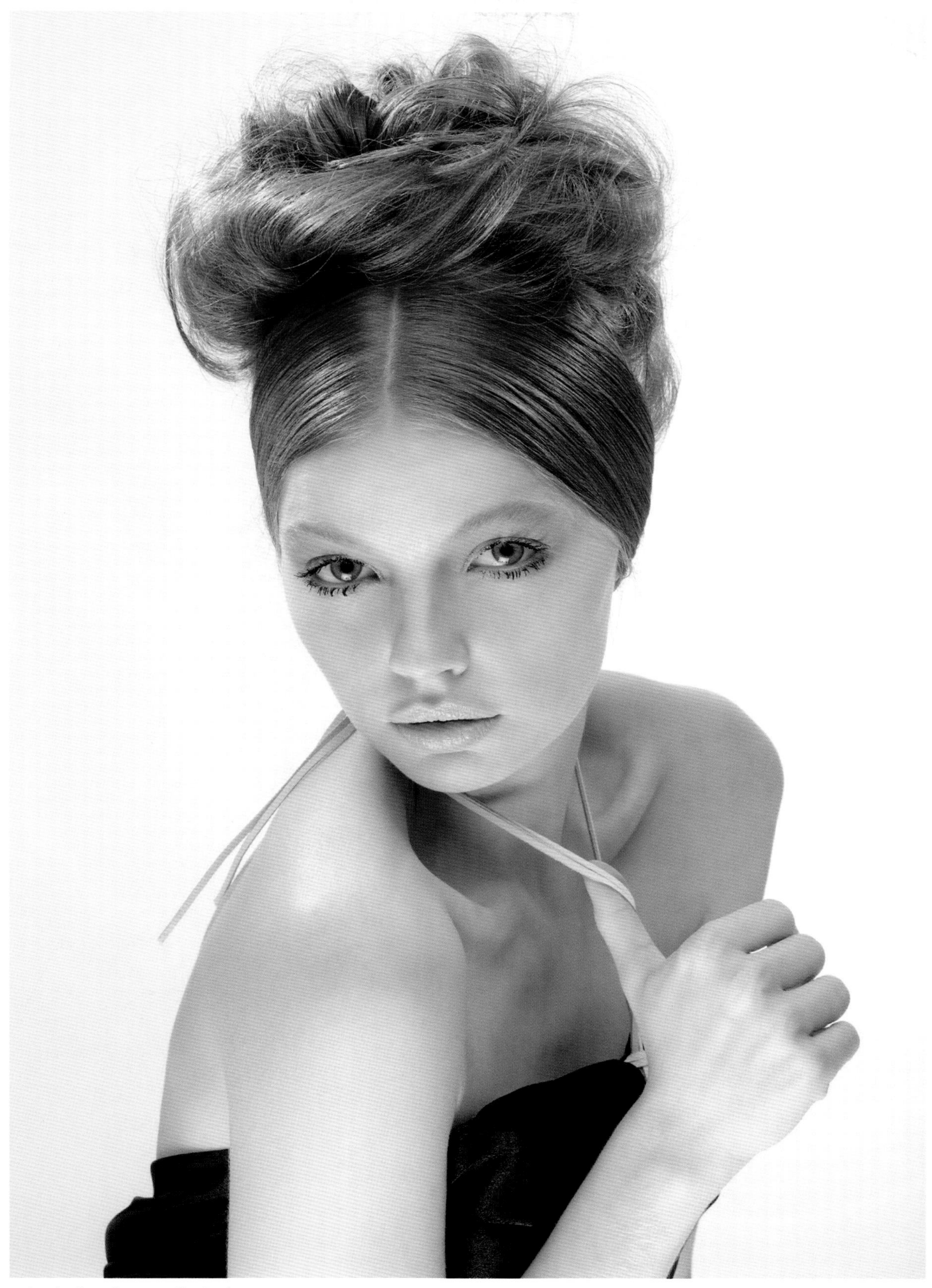

Hairstyles from the Pure Collection by
Michael Barnes for Goldwell, 2008

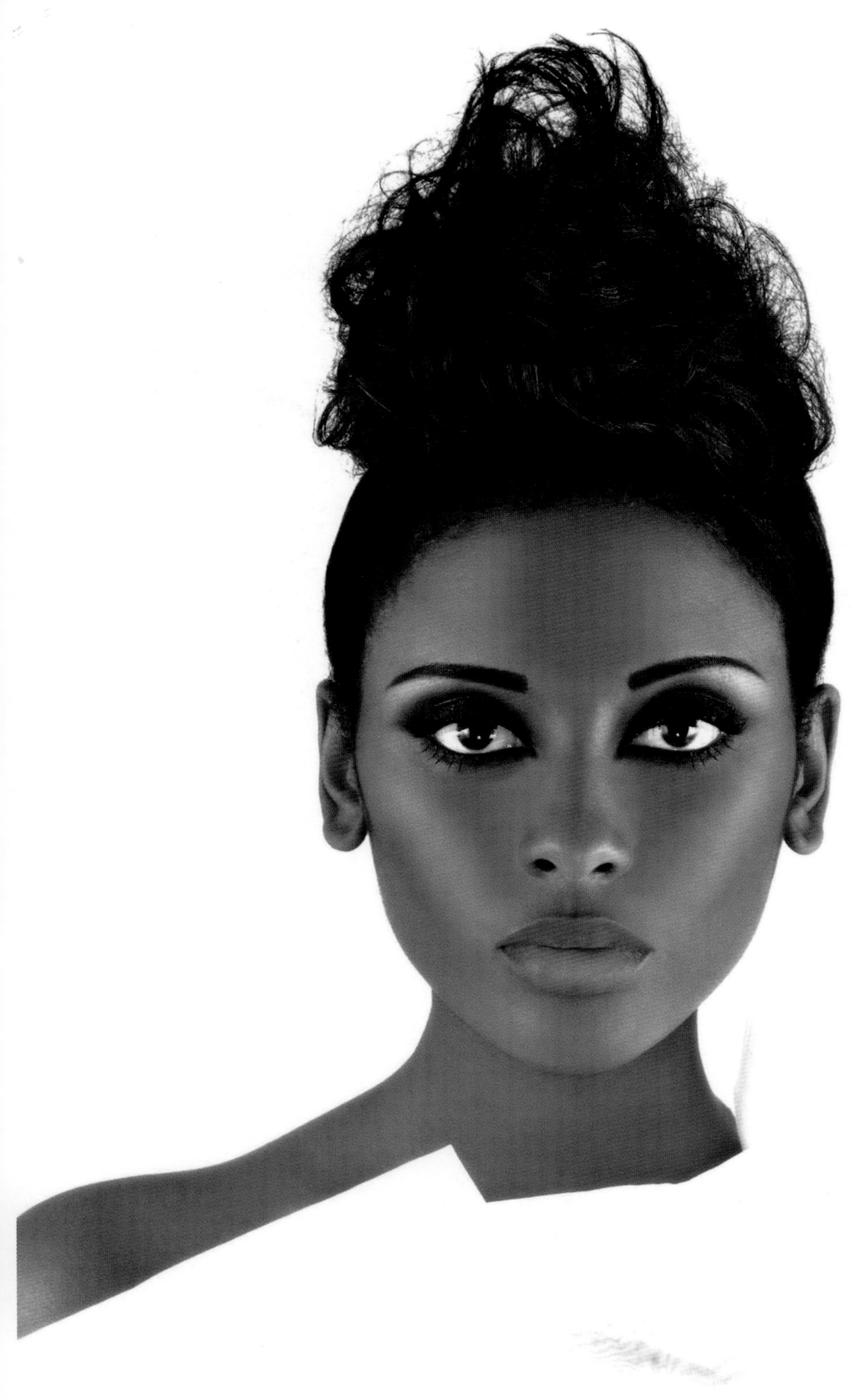

Hairstyle from the Afro Collection by Michelle Thompson (Francesco Group), 2008

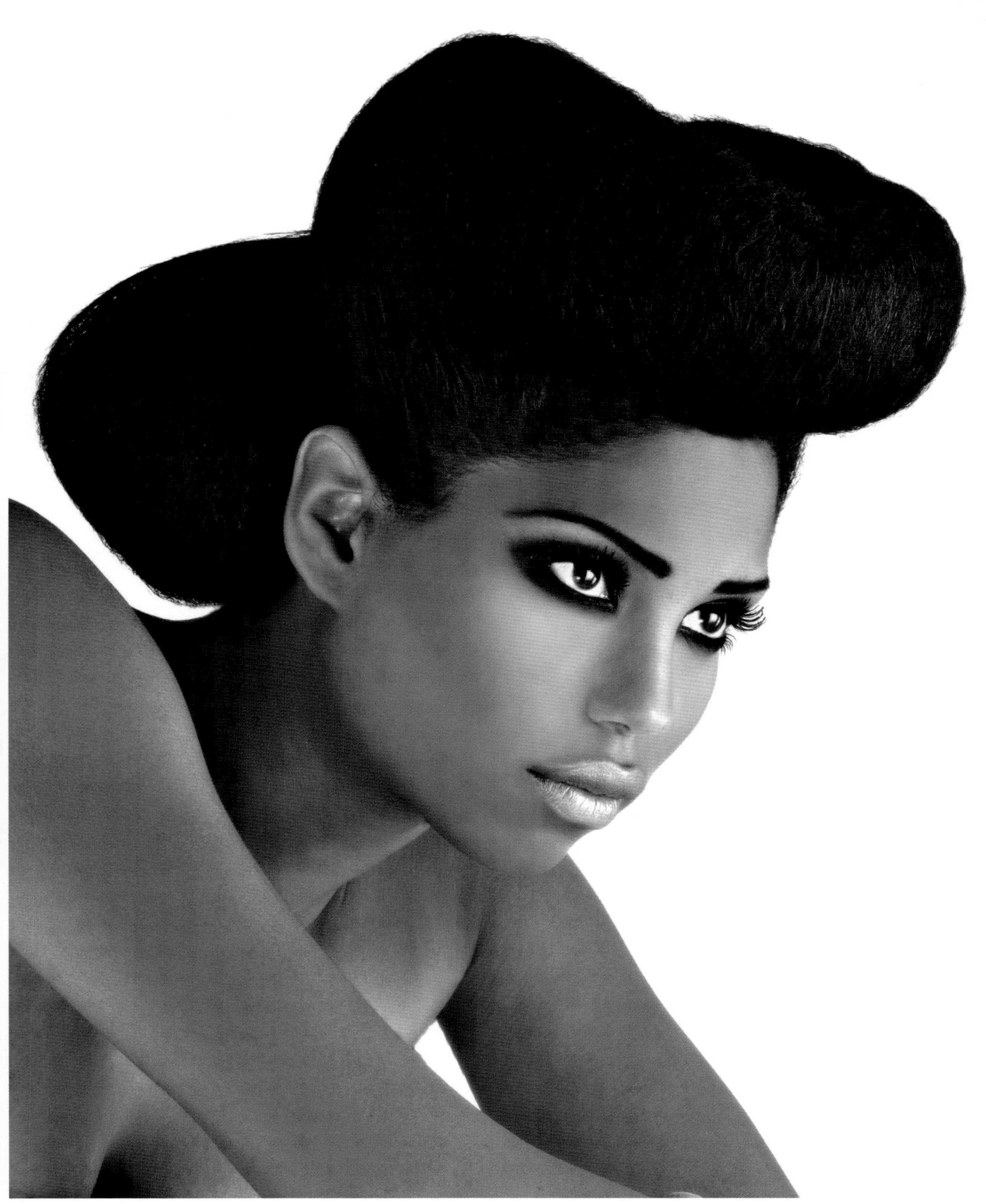

Hairstyle from the Afro Collection by Michelle Thompson (Francesco Group), 2008

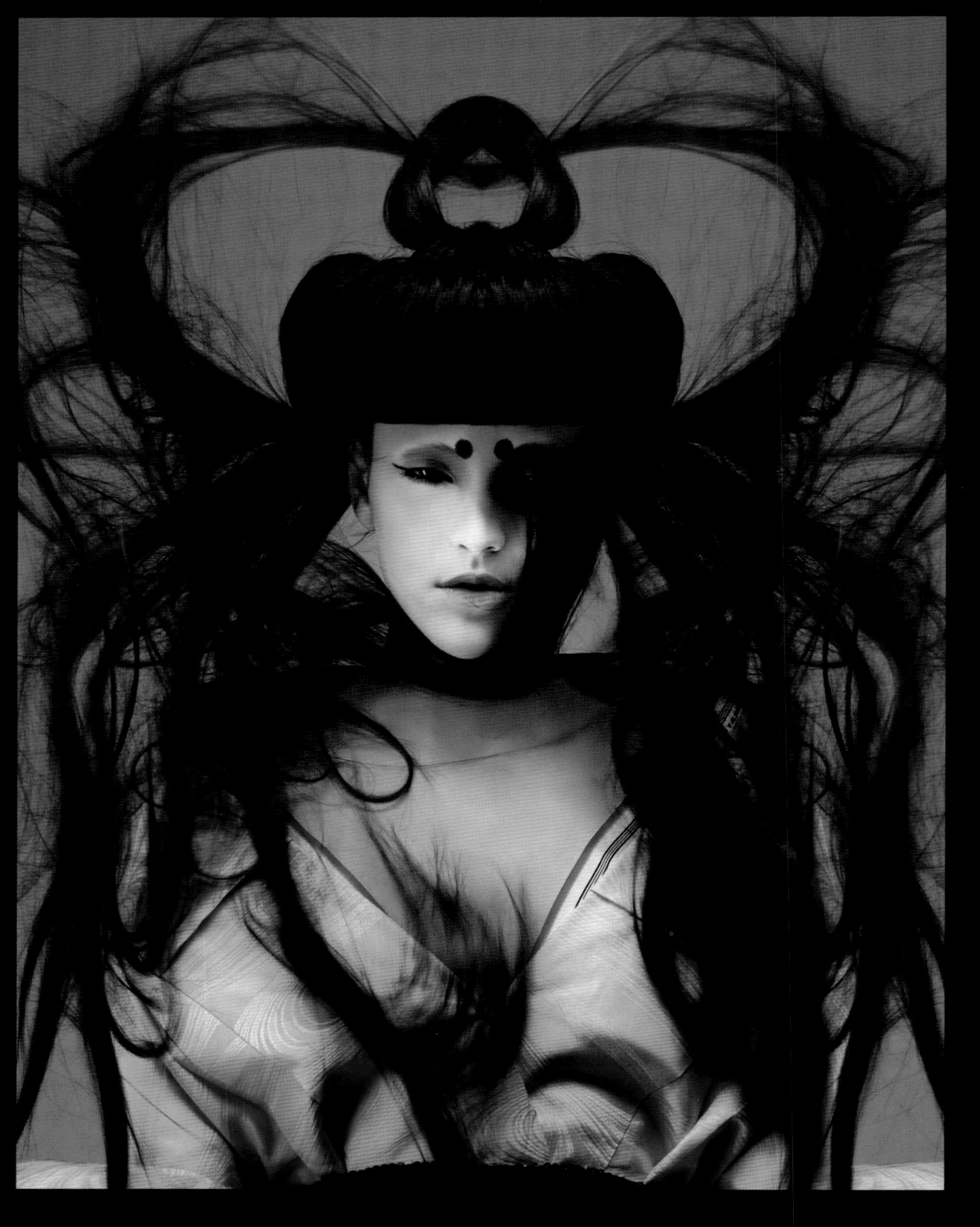

Hairstyle from the Tanabata
Collection by Michael Barnes, 2008

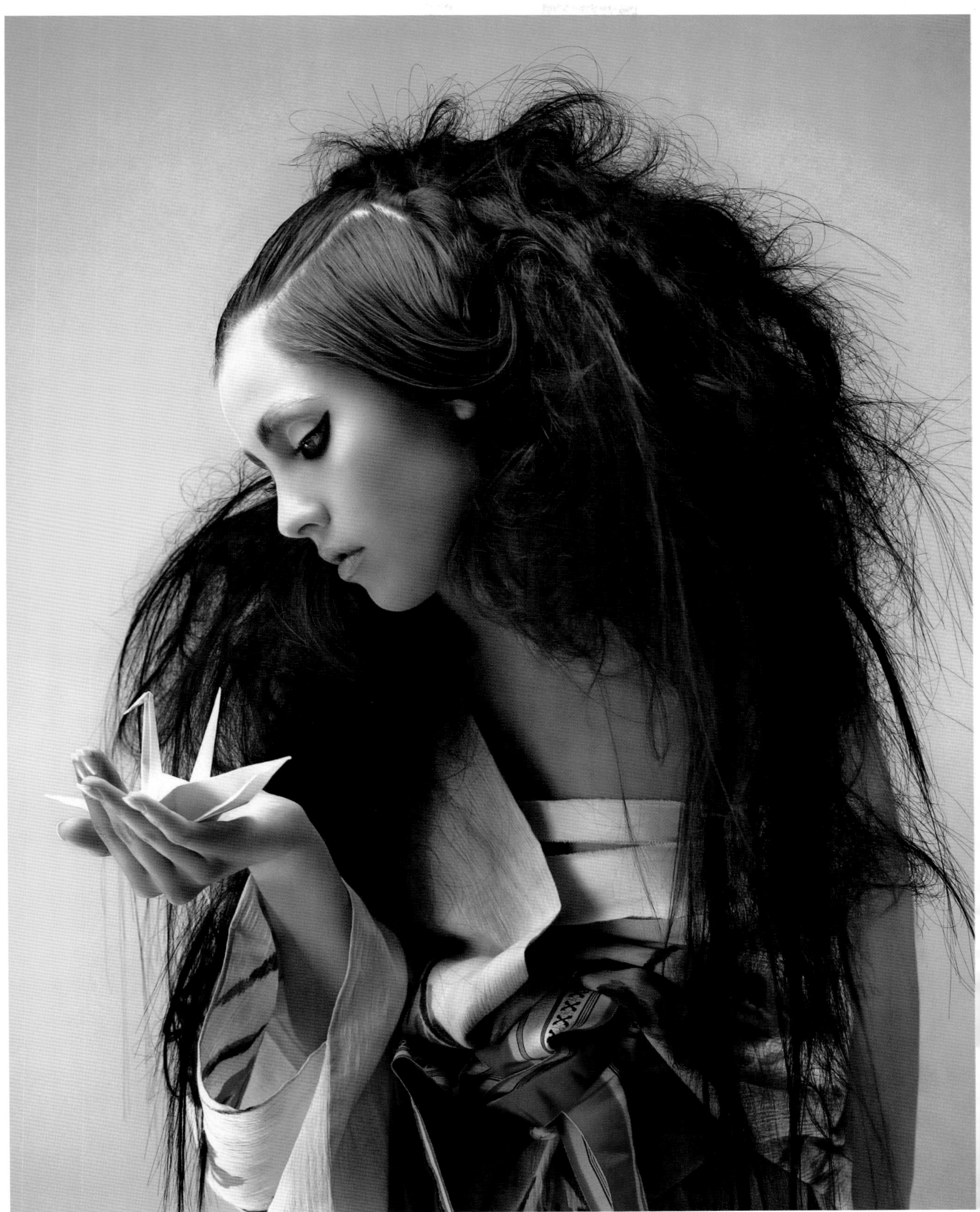

Hairstyle from the Tanabata
Collection by Michael Barnes, 2008

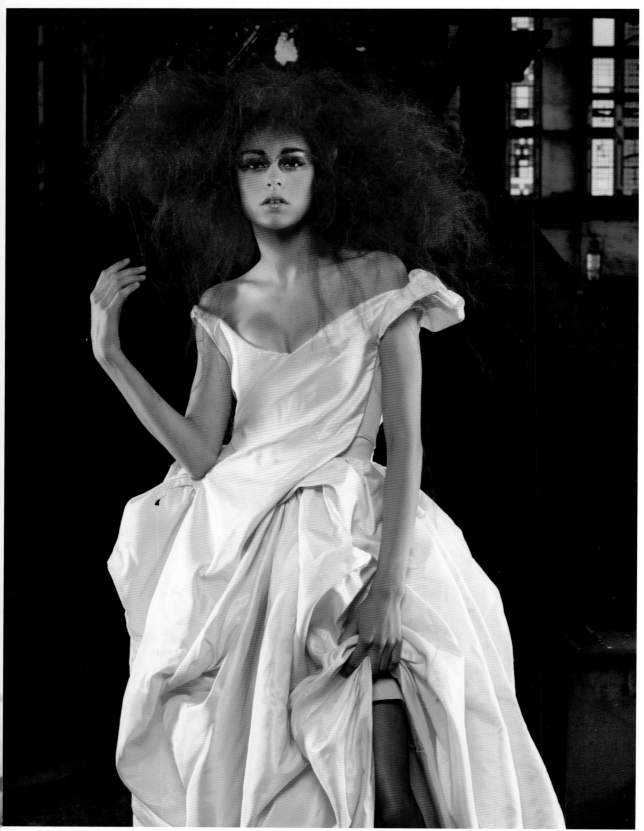

Hairstyle by Anthony Mascolo (International Creative Director of TIGI), for TIGI, 2009

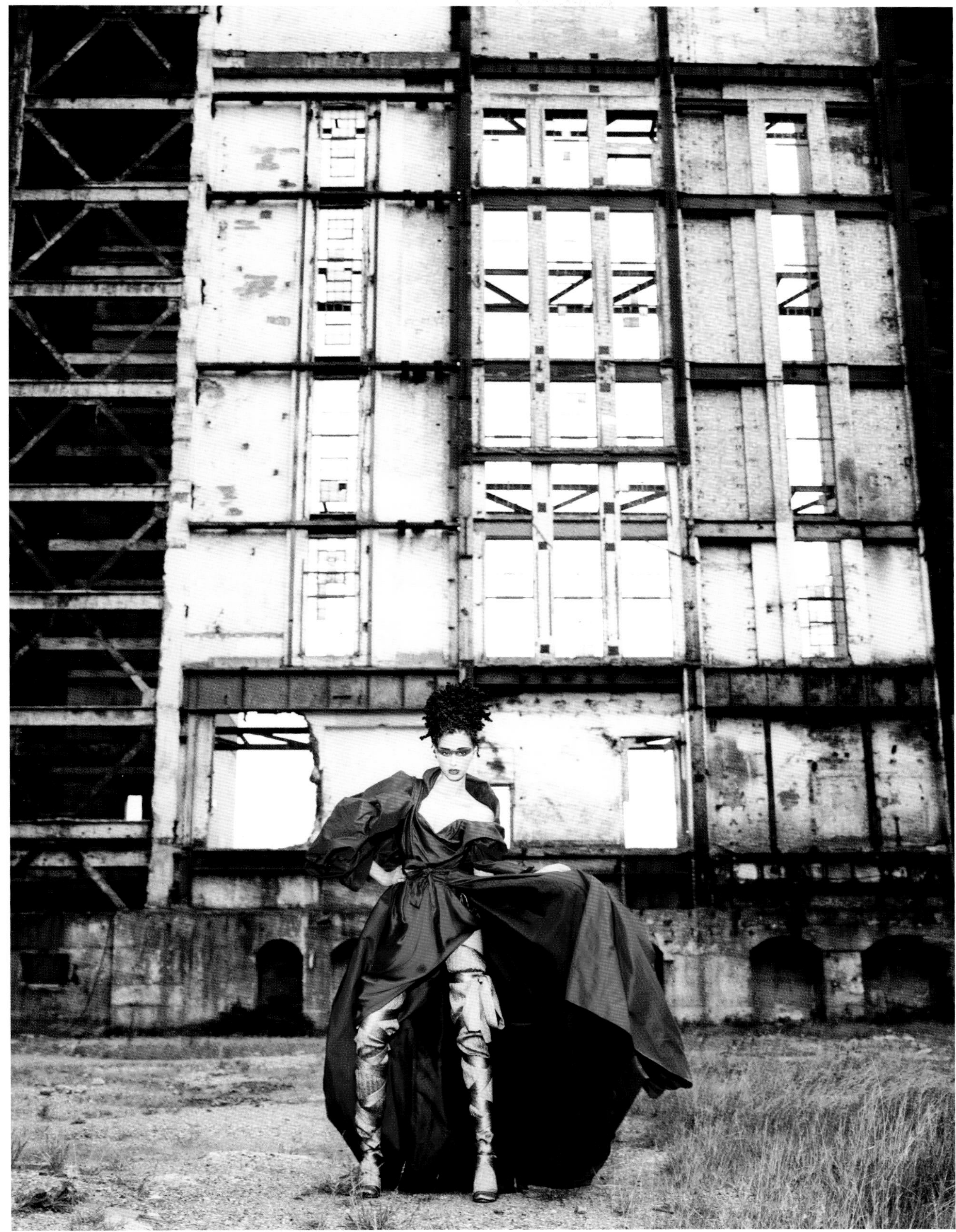

Hairstyle by Anthony Mascolo (International Creative Director of TIGI), for TIGI, 2009

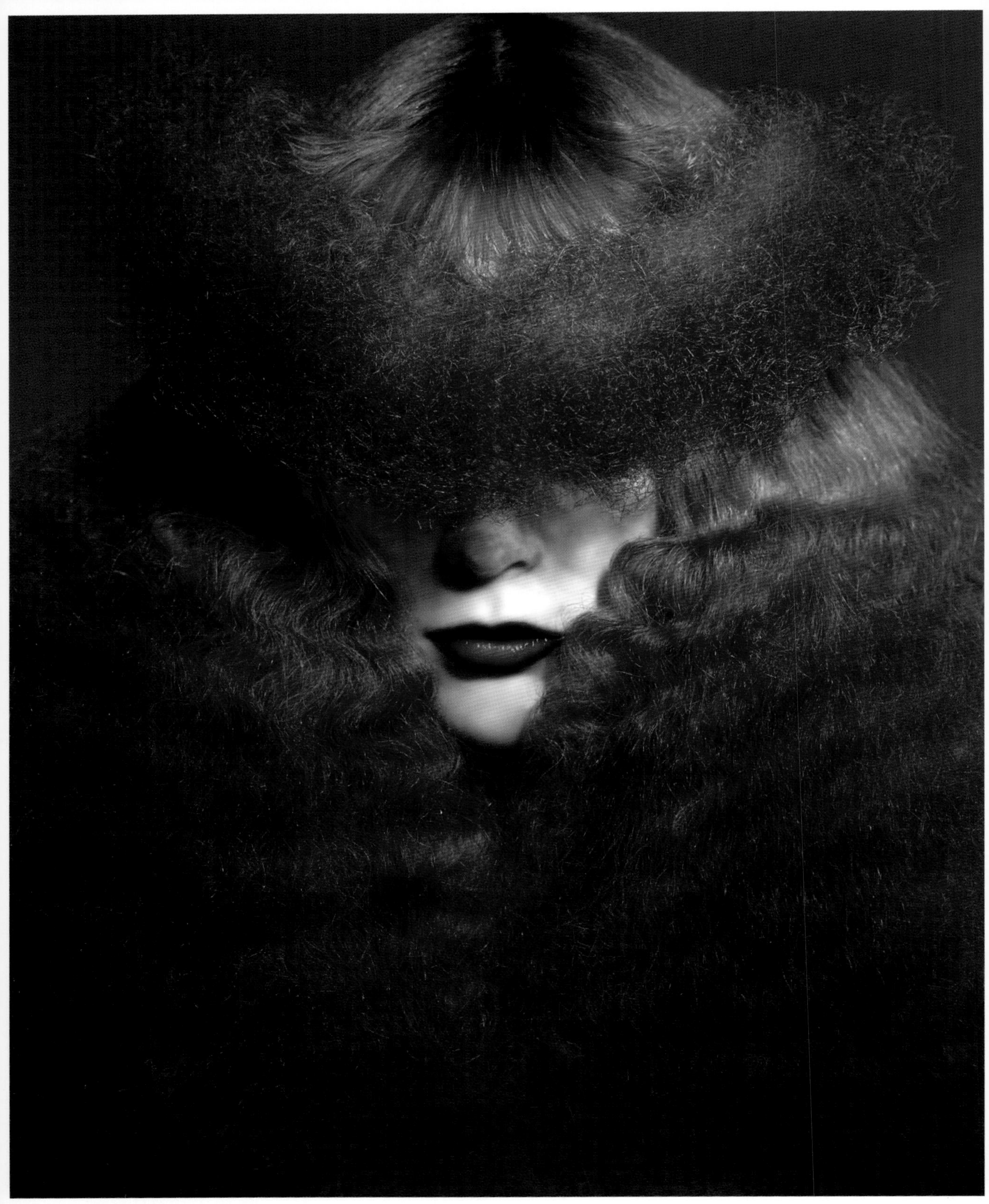

'Naomi' hairstyle by Louis Byrne, 2000s

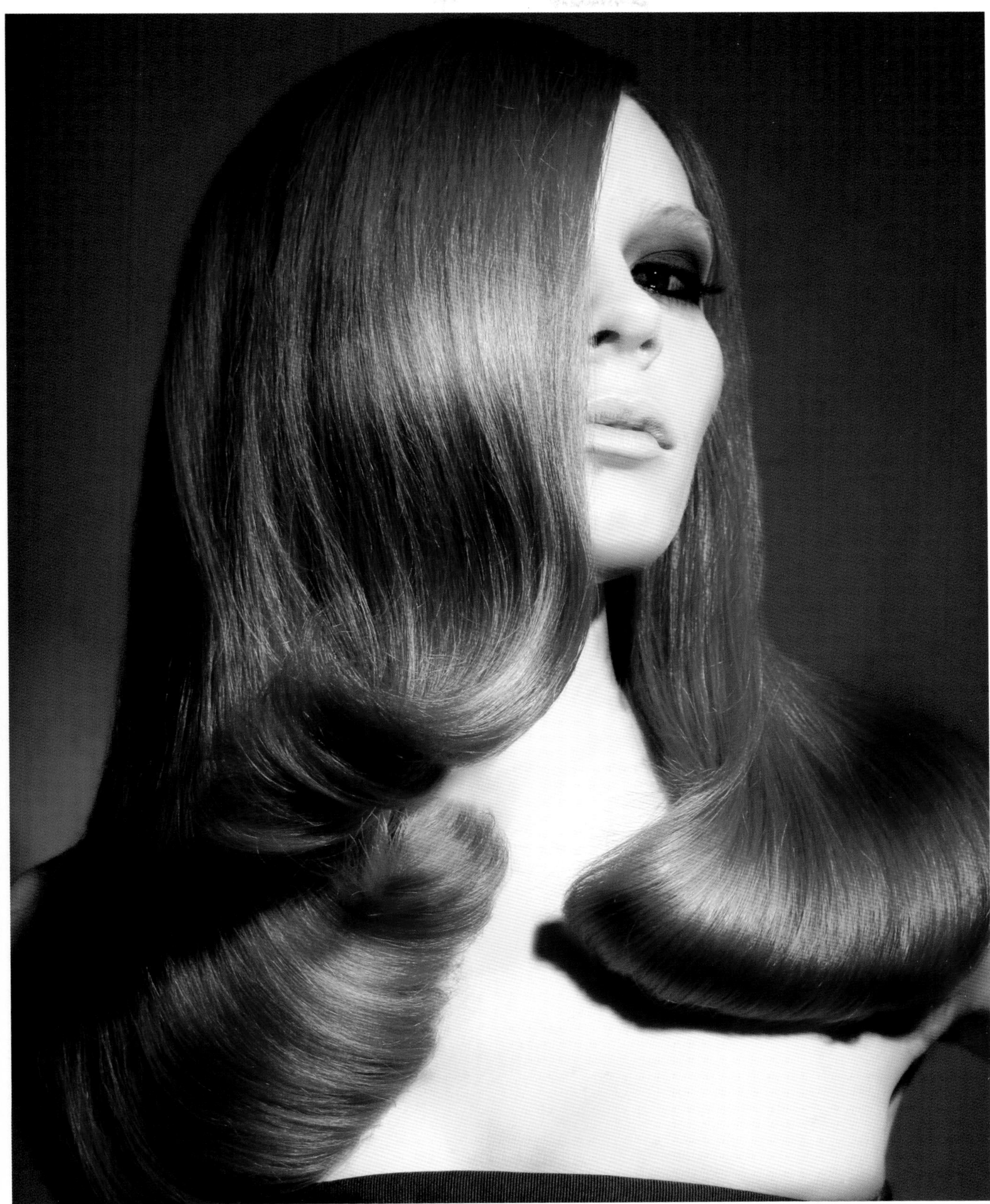

Hairstyle by Louis Byrne, 2000s

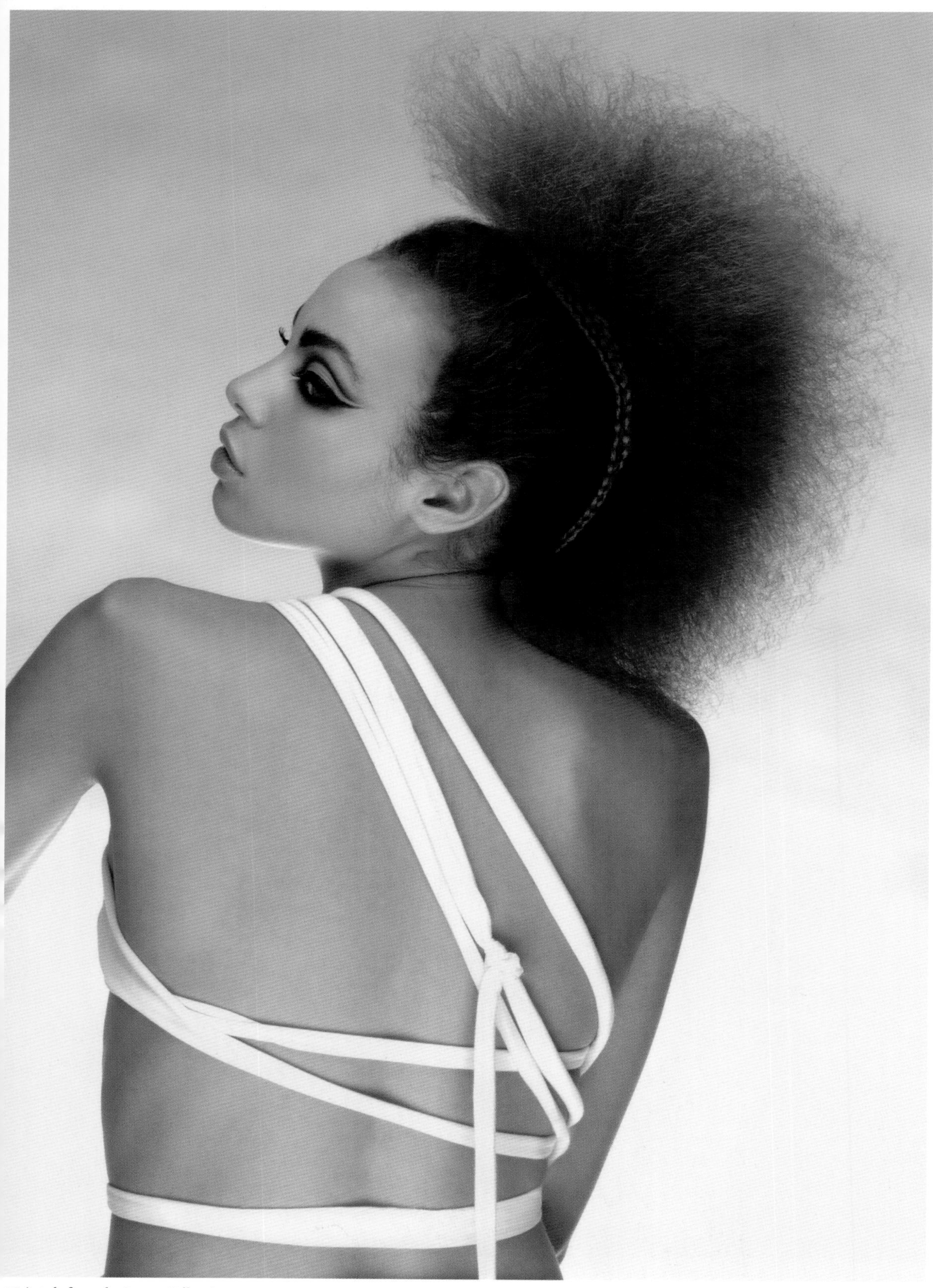

Hairstyle from the Serene Collection
by Michael Barnes, 2009

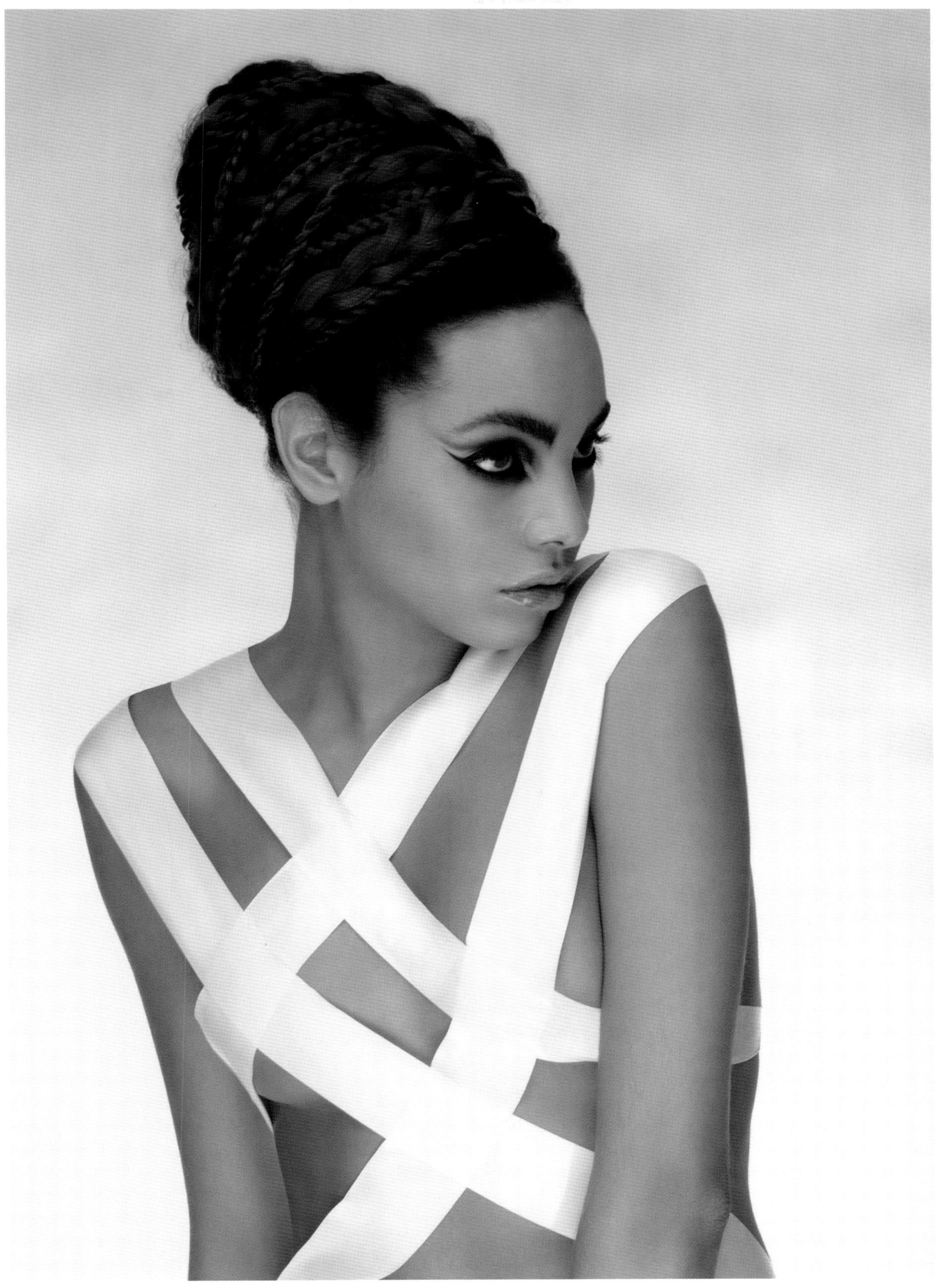

Hairstyle from the Serene Collection
by Michael Barnes, 2009

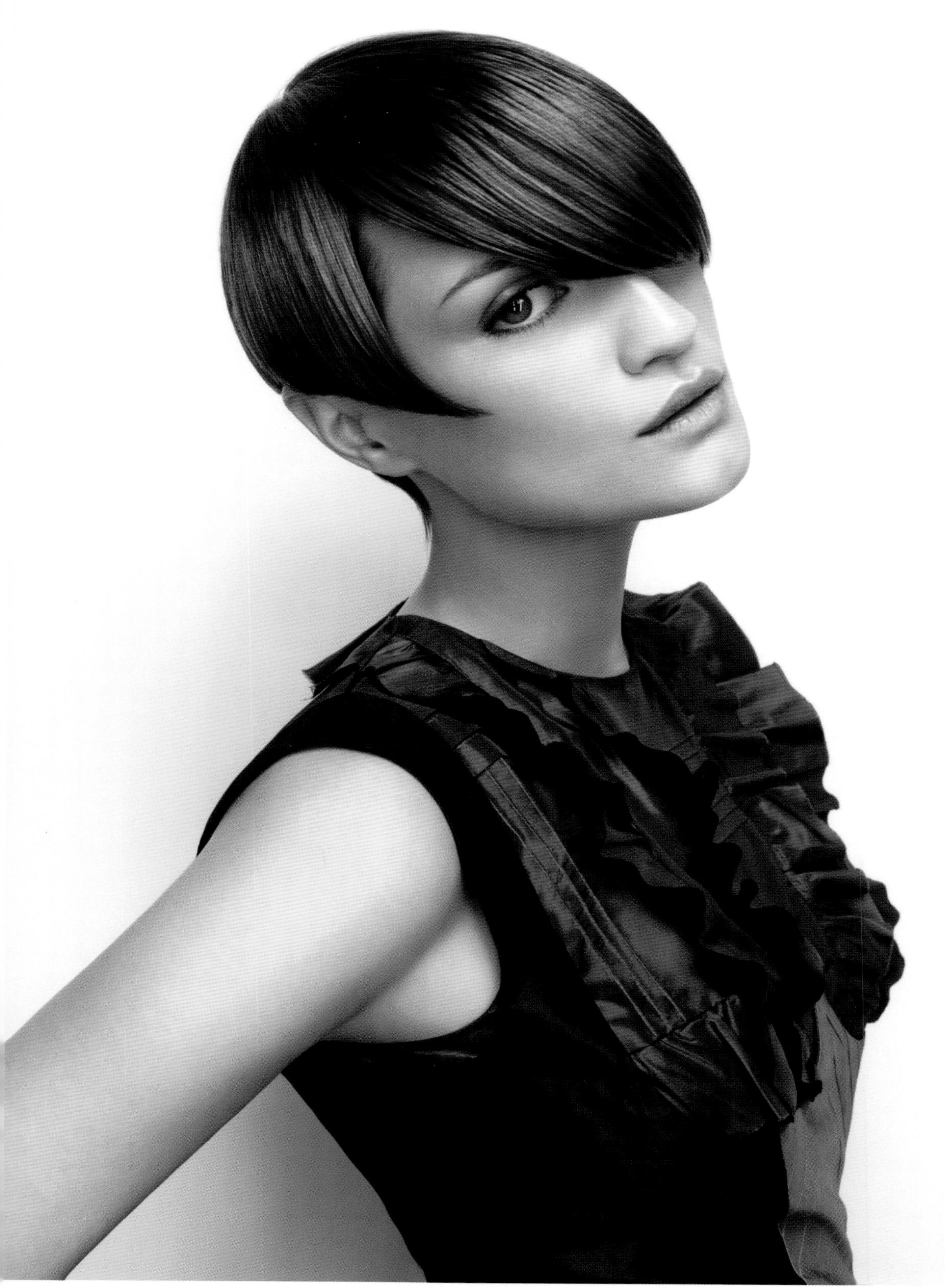

Hair by TONI&GUY, modelled by Miriam de Laco (FM/Elite), 2000s, photographed by Troyt Coburn

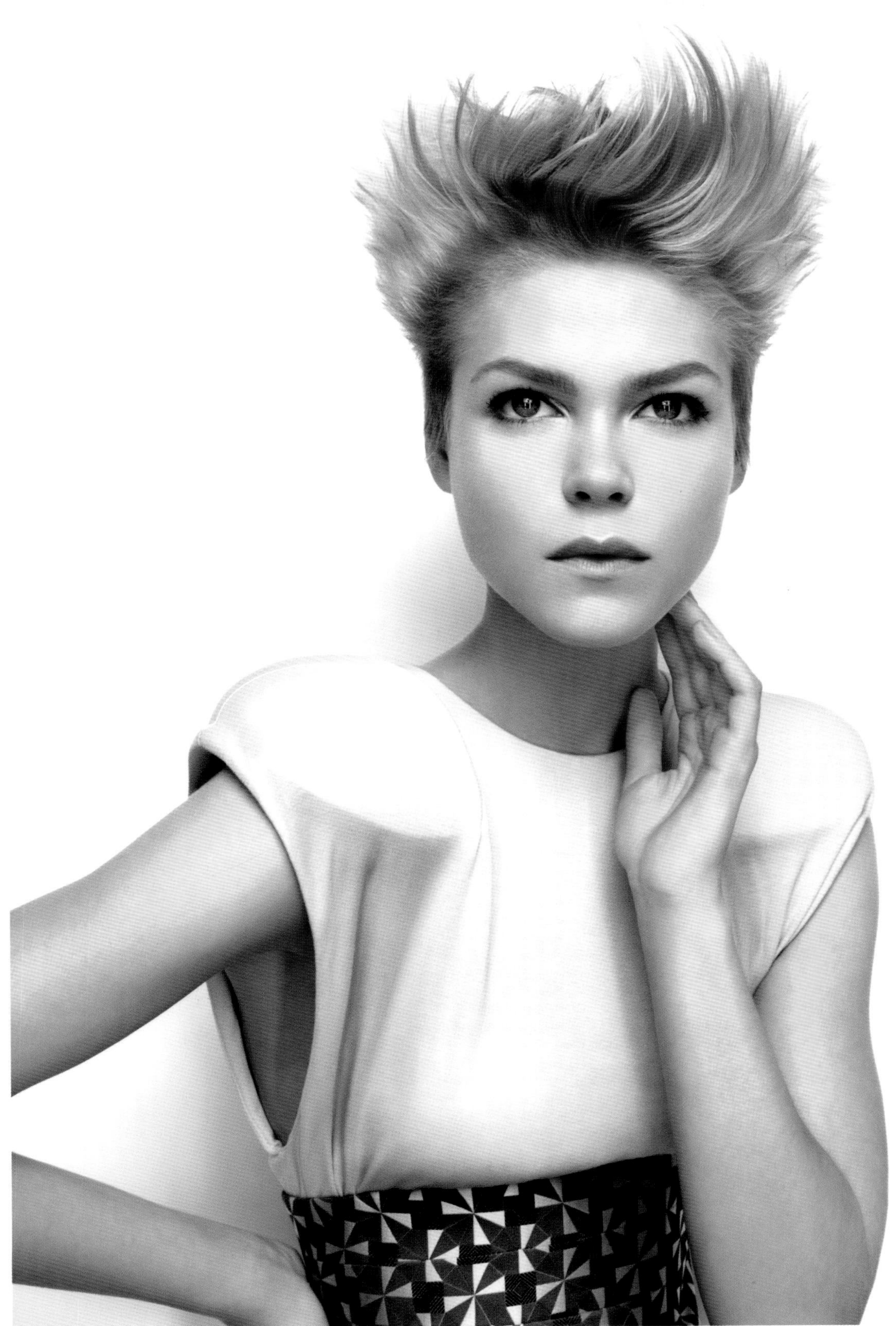

Hair by Richard Mannah and Lynsey Ashton for TONI&GUY, modelled by Marianne (Select) 2000s, photographed by Troyt Coburn

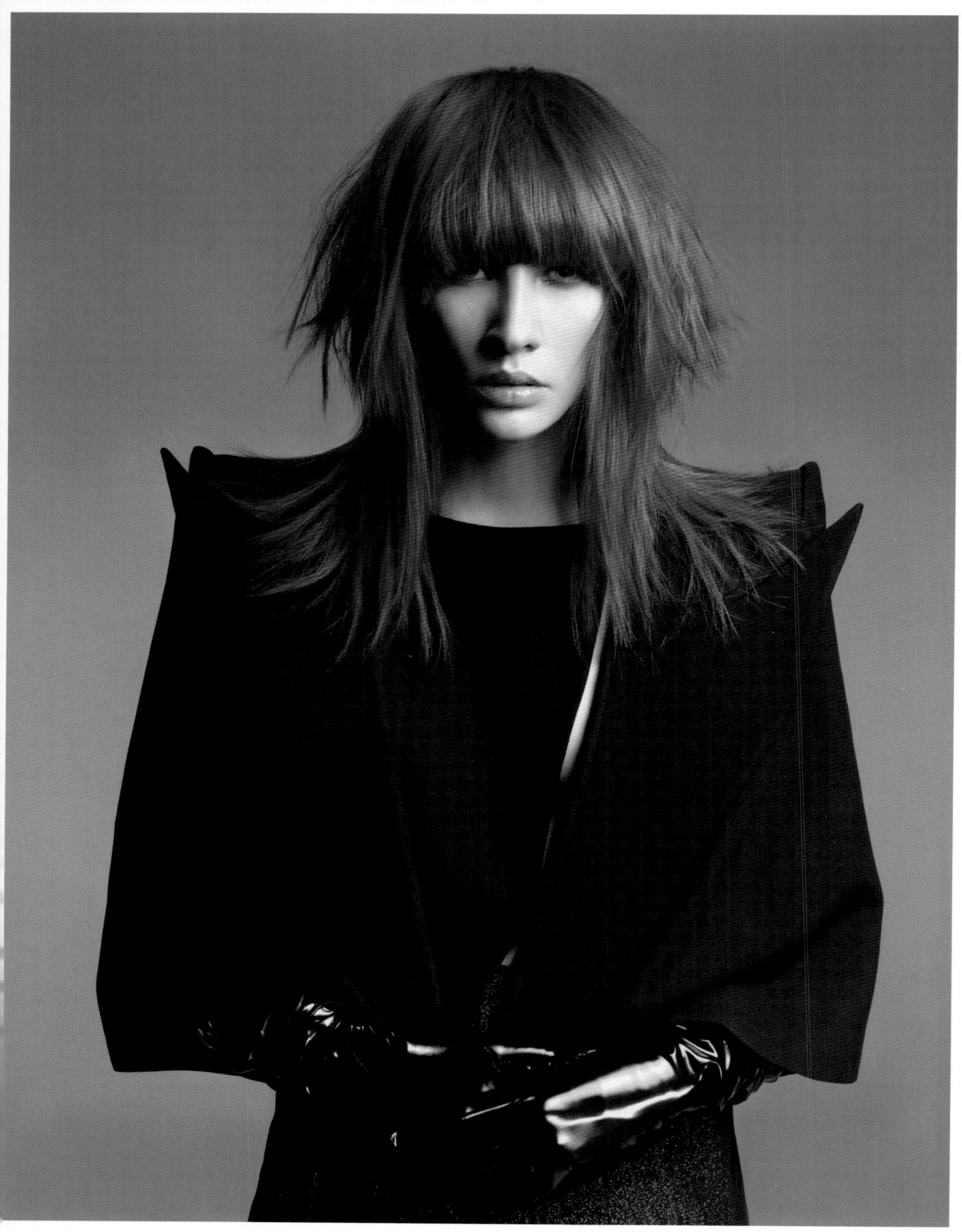

Hair by Hide Saiga for TONI&GUY, modelled by Lena (Profile), 2000s, photographed by Troyt Coburn

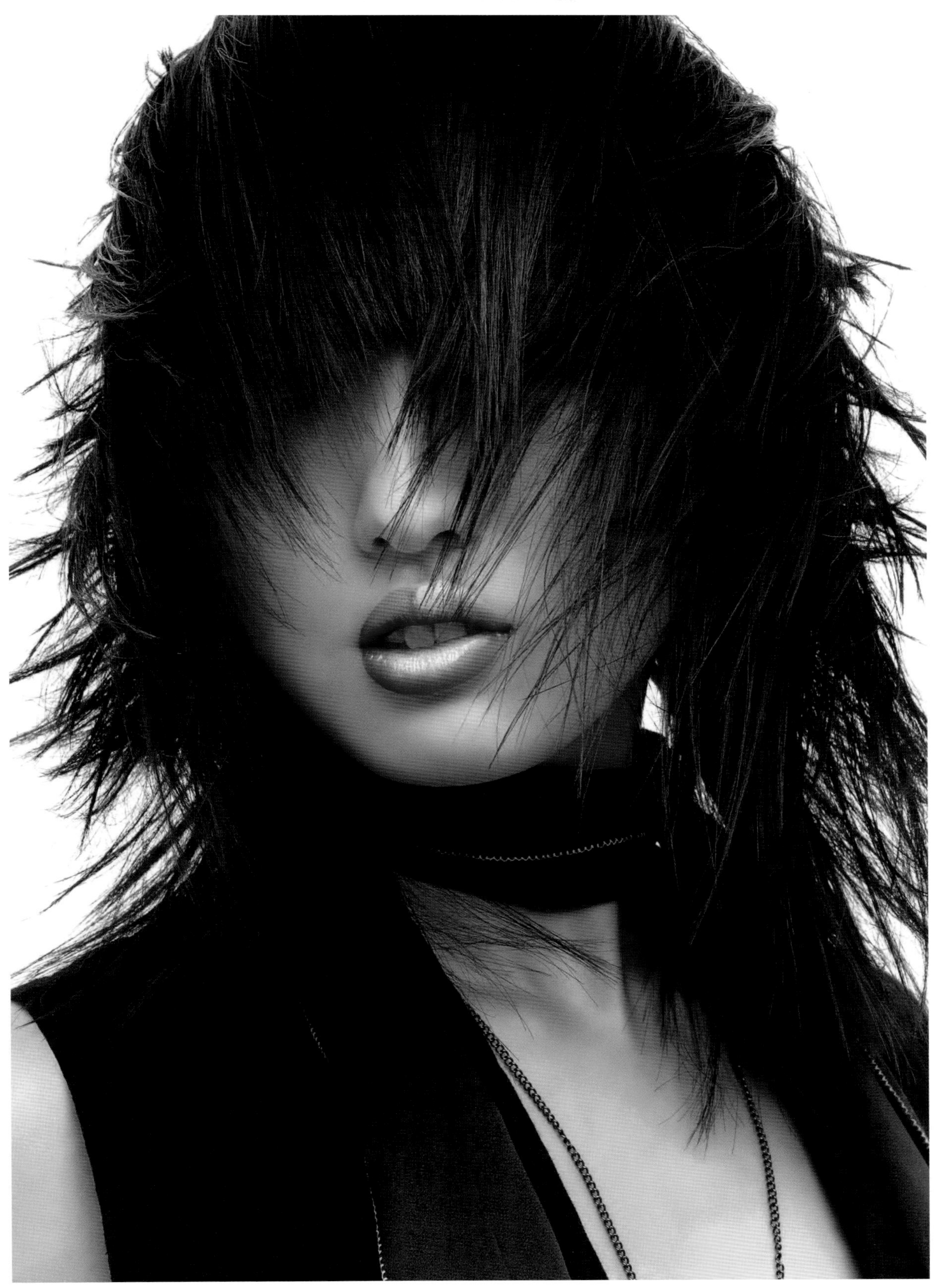

Hair by Simon Raby for TONI&GUY, 2000s

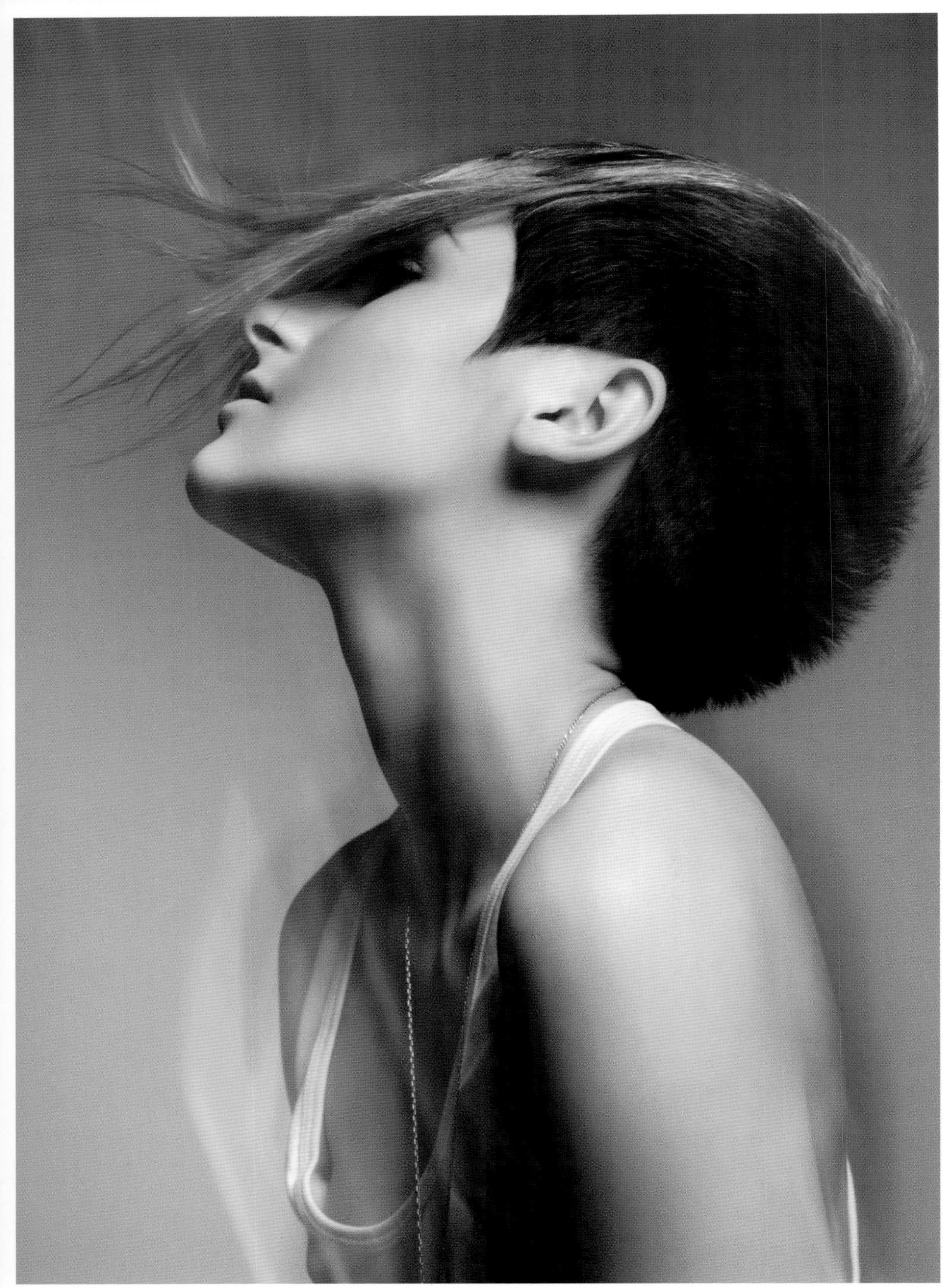

Hair by Grant Norton for TONI&GUY Australia, 2000s, photographed by Andrew O'Toole

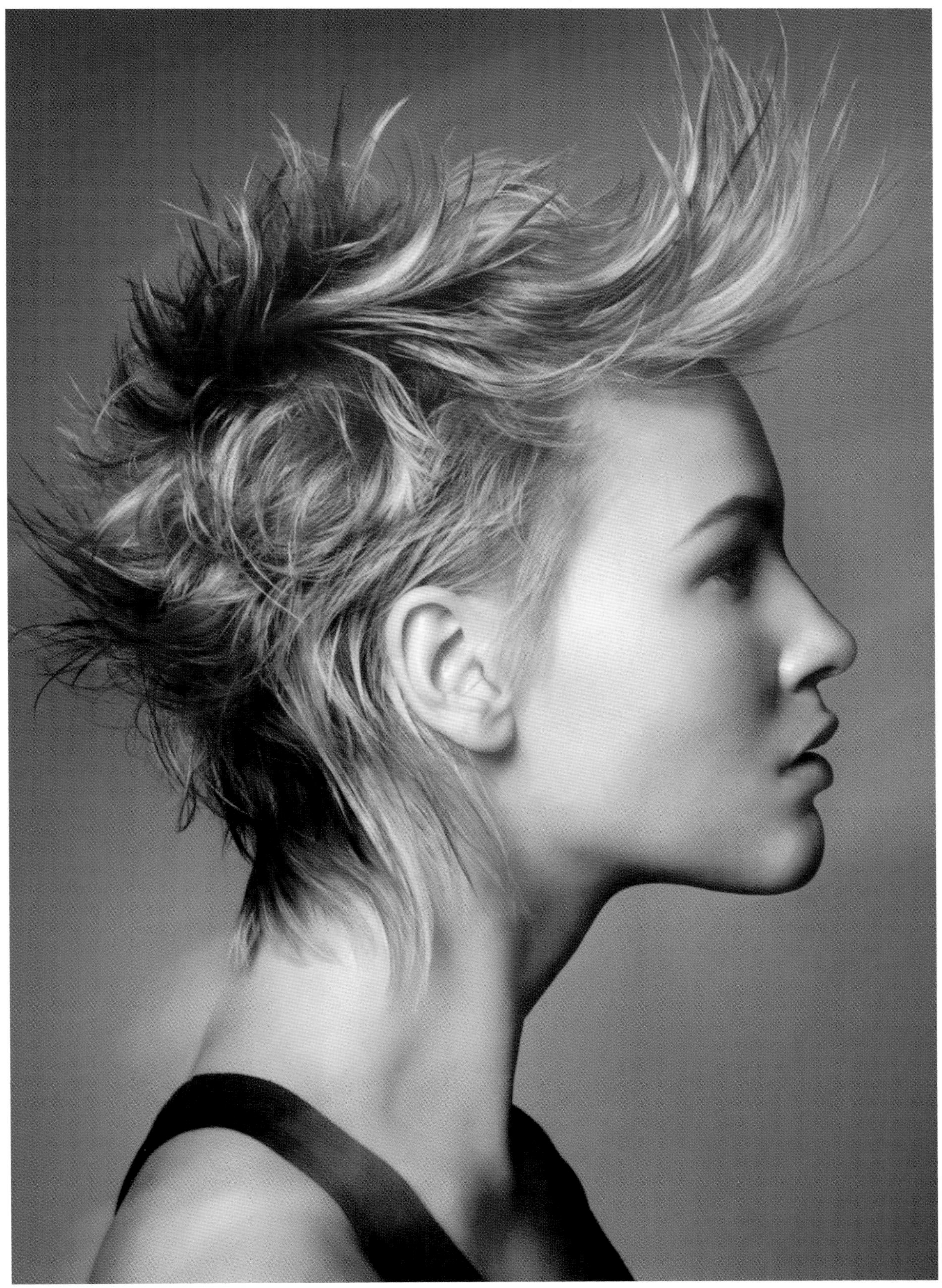

Hair by Grant Norton for TONI&GUY Australia, 2000s, photographed by Andrew O'Toole

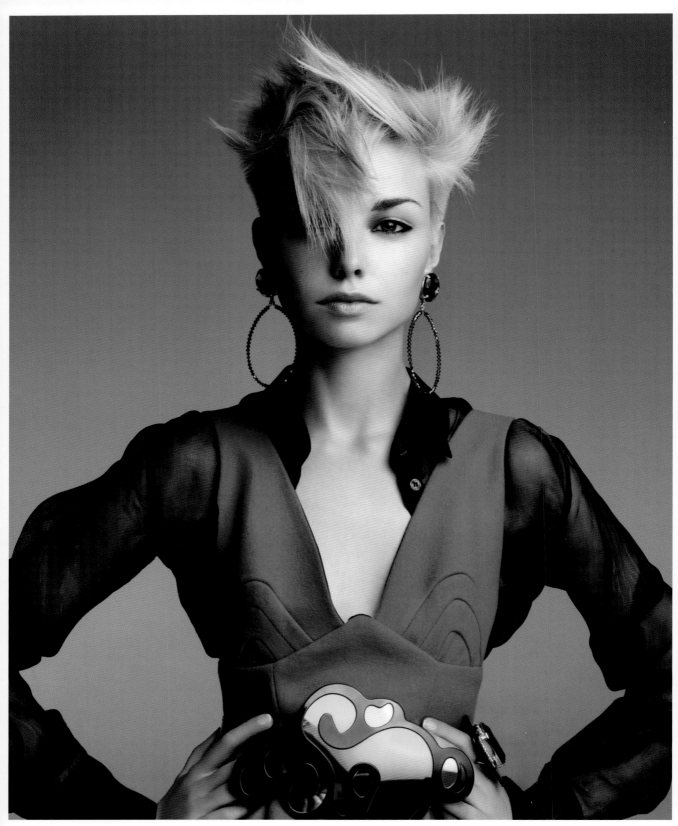

Hair by Cos Sakkas for TONI&GUY Covent Garden, modelled by Egle (Bookings), 2000s, photographed by Troyt Coburn

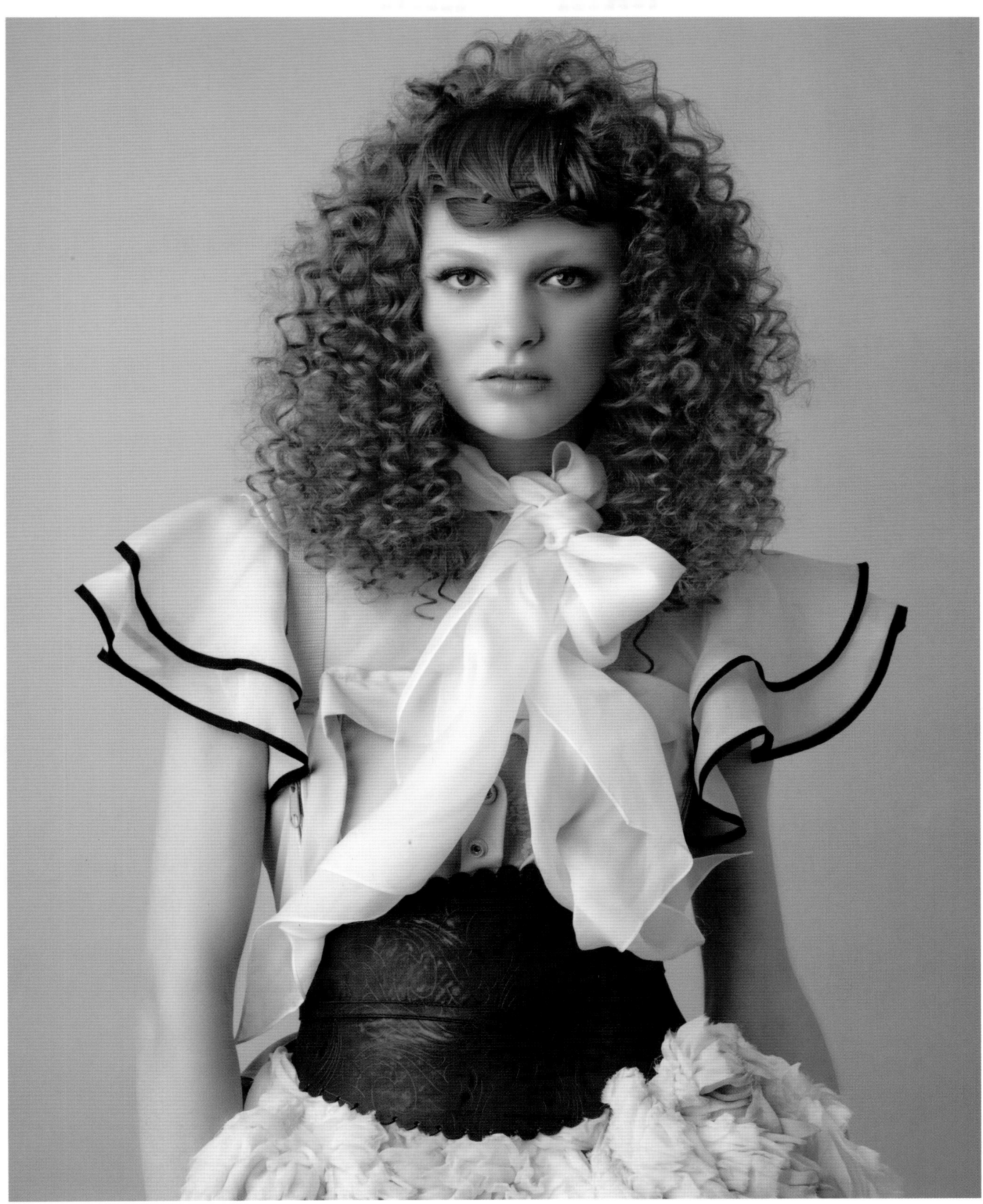

Hair by Jan Deighton at TONI&GUY Sunderland, 2000s, photographed by Wolfgang Mustain

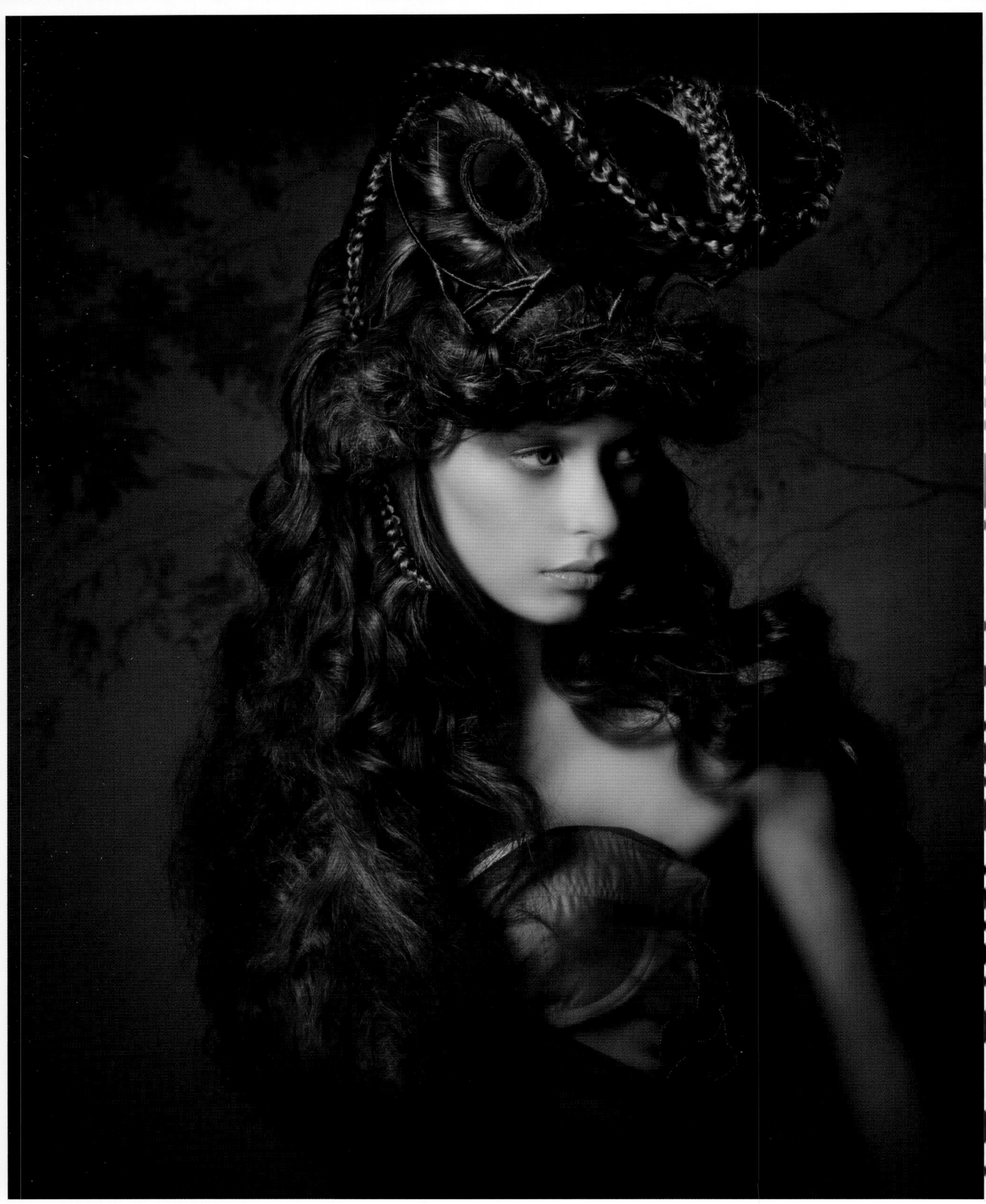

Hair by Indira Schauwecker for TONI&GUY Covent Garden, 2000s, photographed by Gitte Meldgaard Fritz

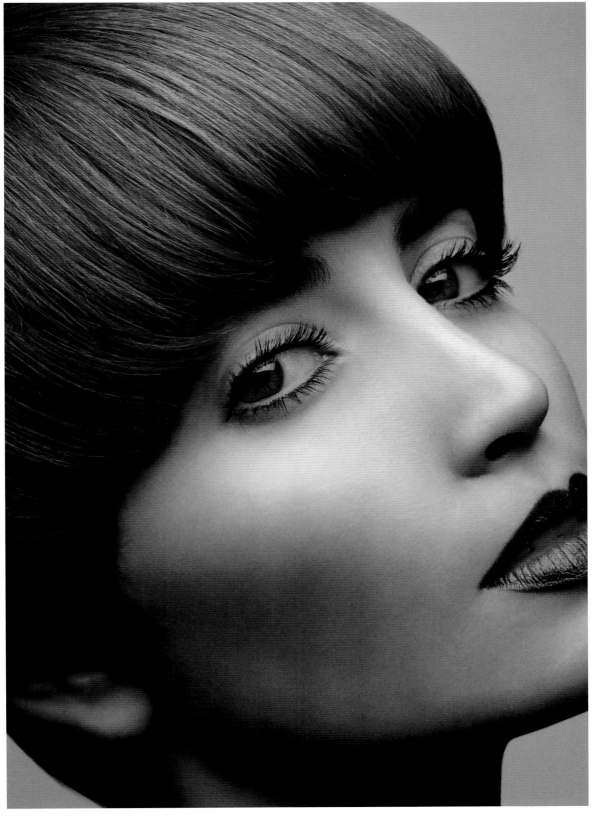

Hair by Jacen Ward for TONI&GUY Australia, 2000s, photographed by Andrew O'Toole

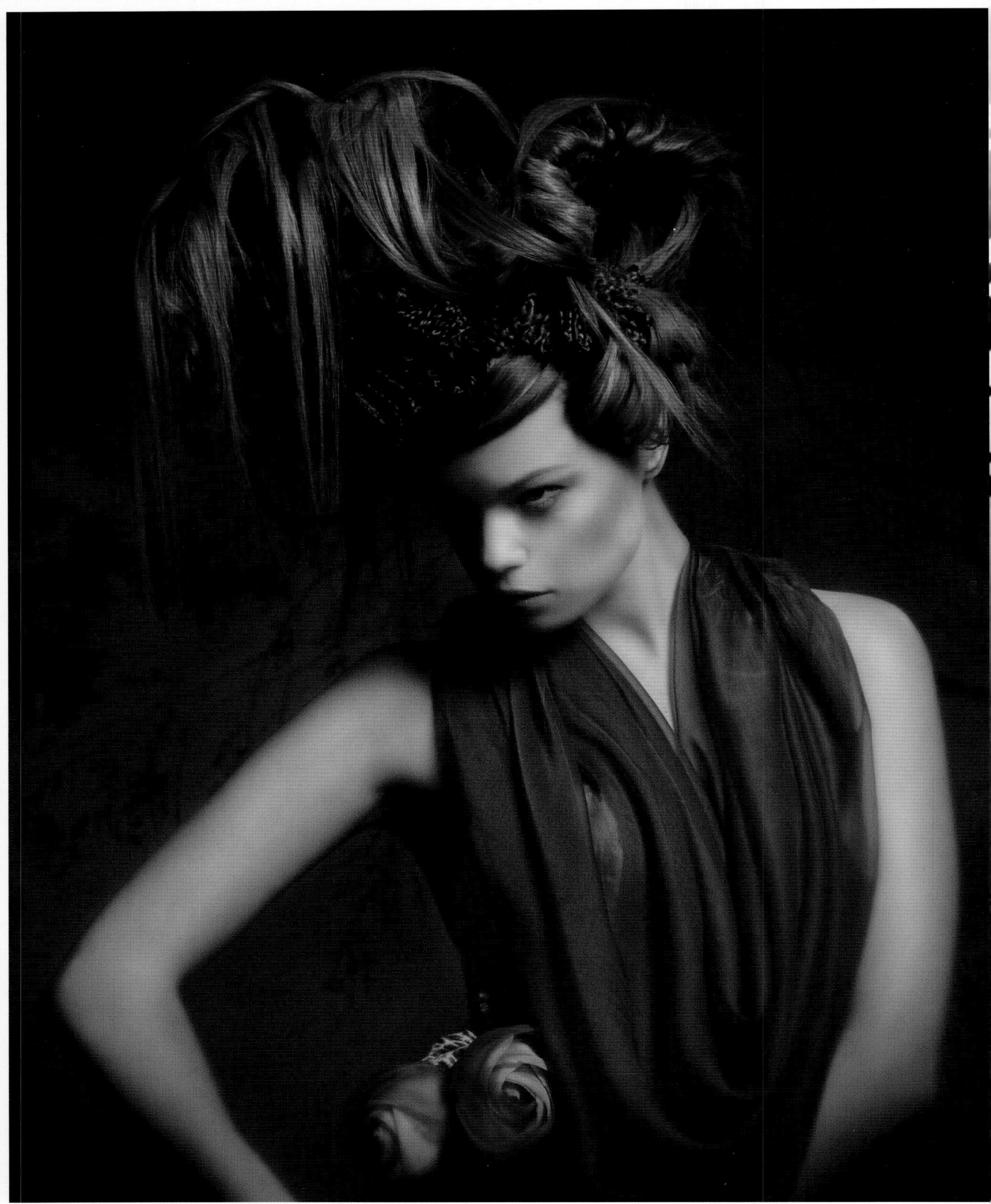

Hair by Indira Schauwecker for TONI&GUY Covent Garden, 2000s, photographed by Gitte Meldgaard Fritz

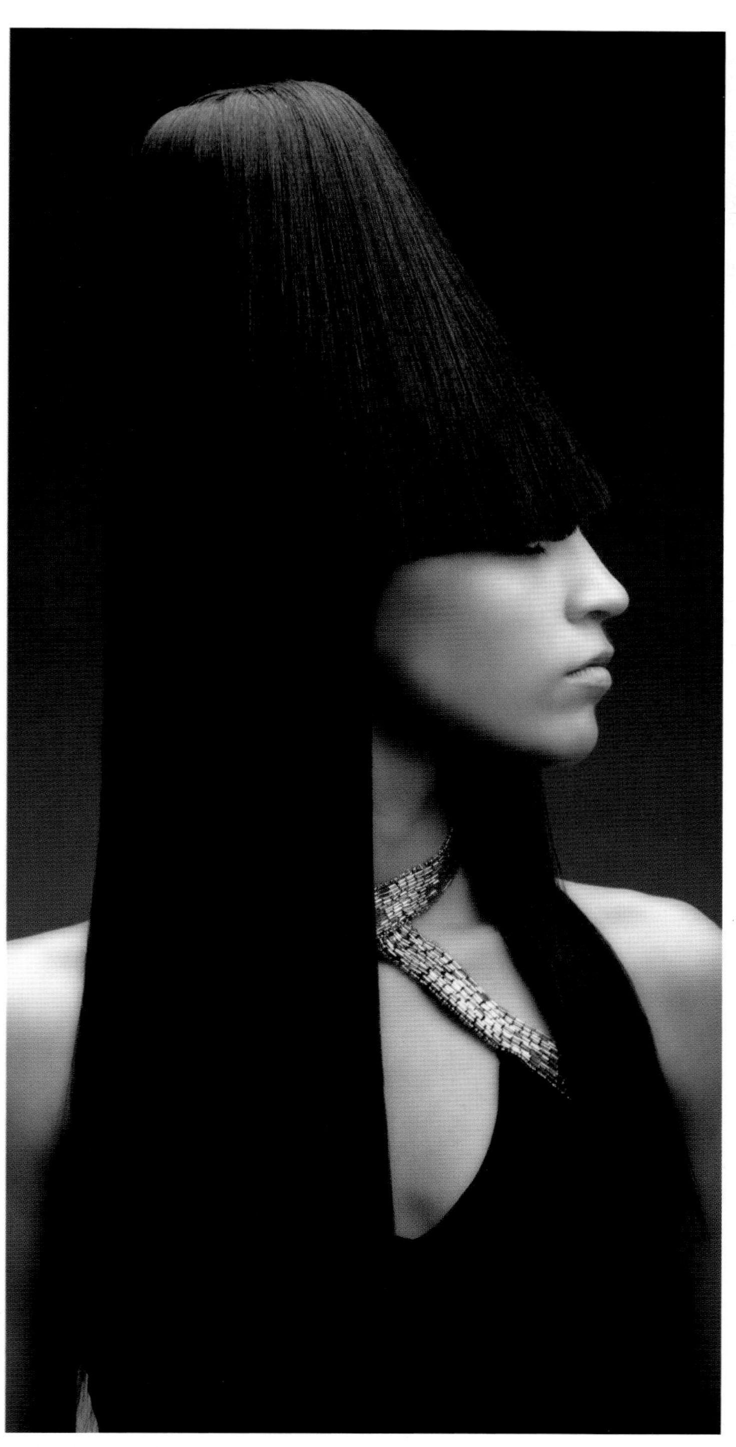

Hair by Philippe Gentner for TONI&GUY Paris, 2000s, photographed by Edward Deblay

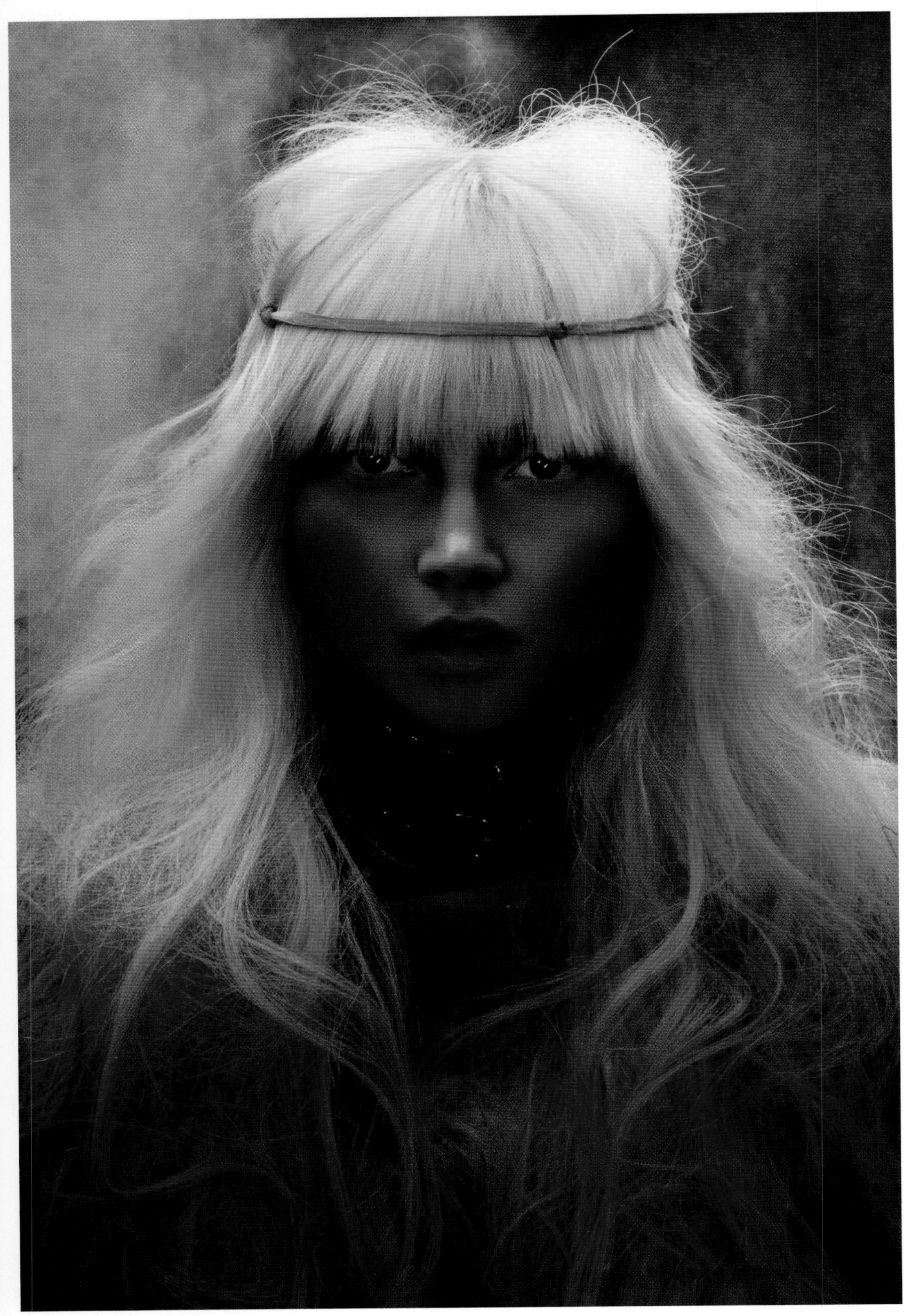

Hair by Matthew Webb for TONI&GUY Australia, 2000s, photographed by Andrew O'Toole

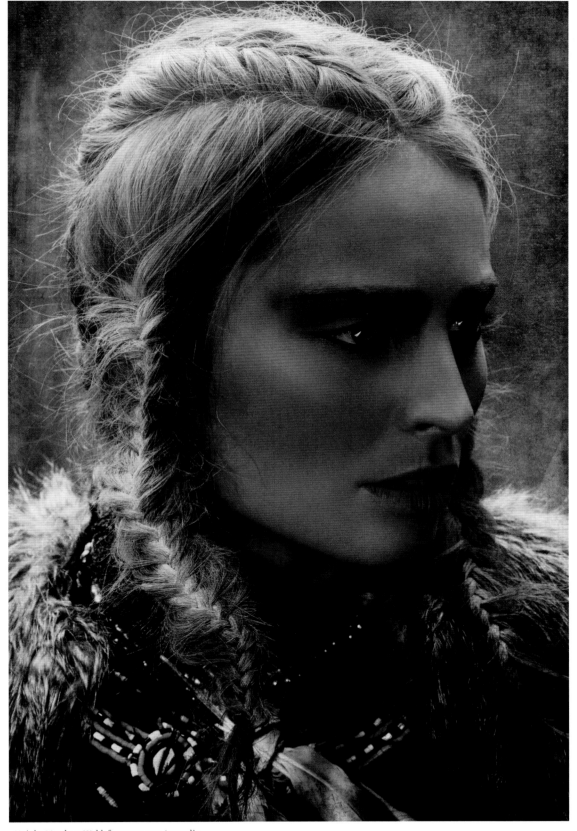

Hair by Matthew Webb for TONI&GUY Australia, 2000s, photographed by Andrew O'Toole

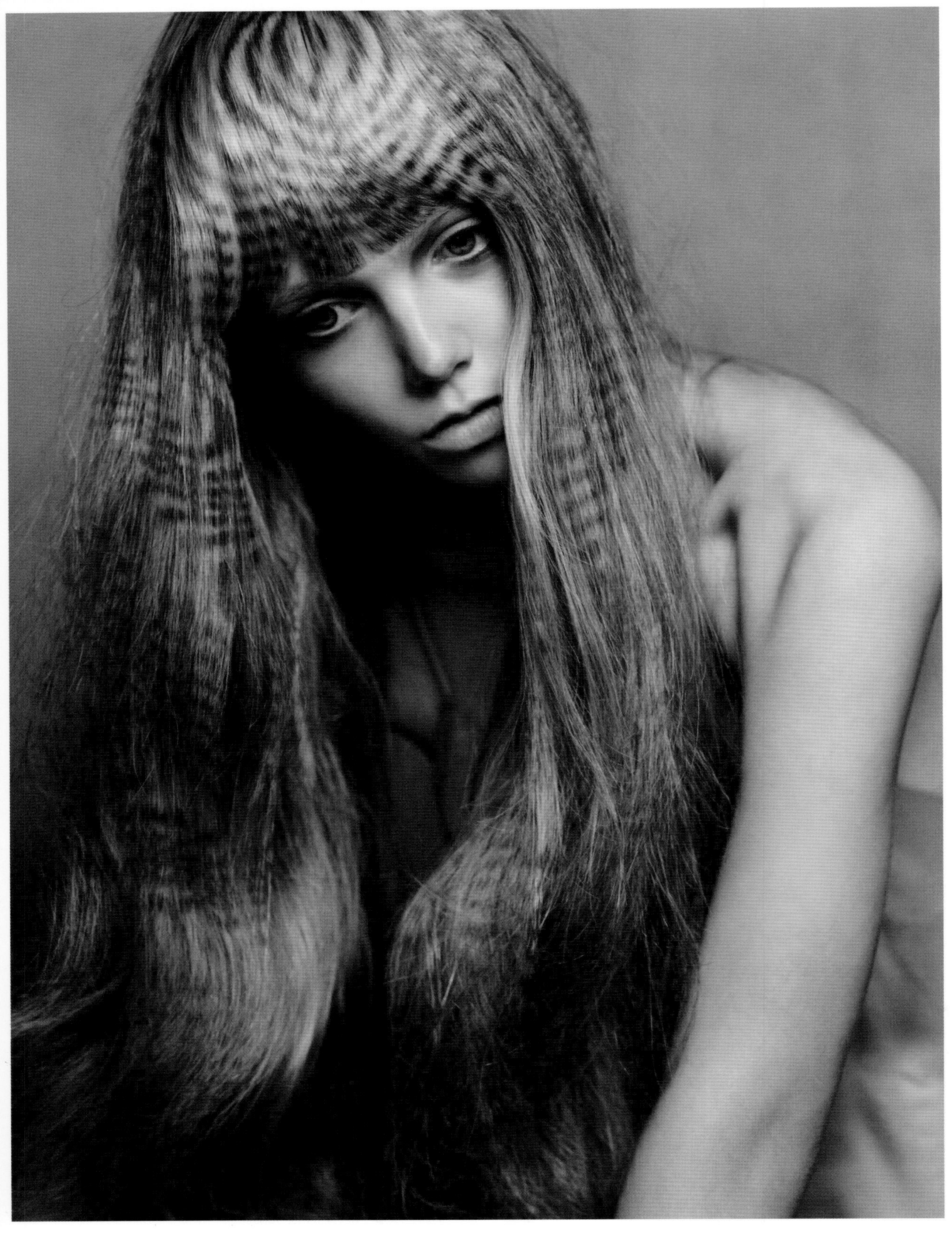

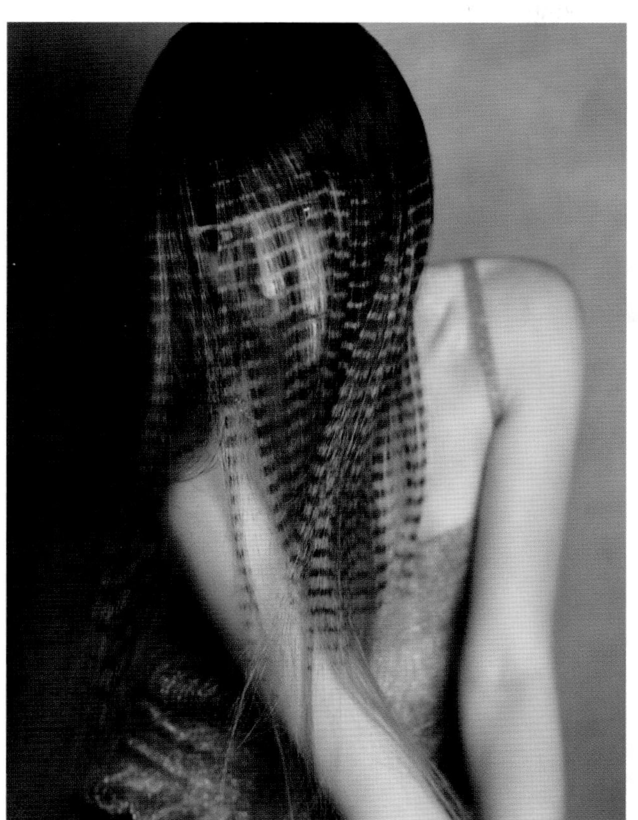

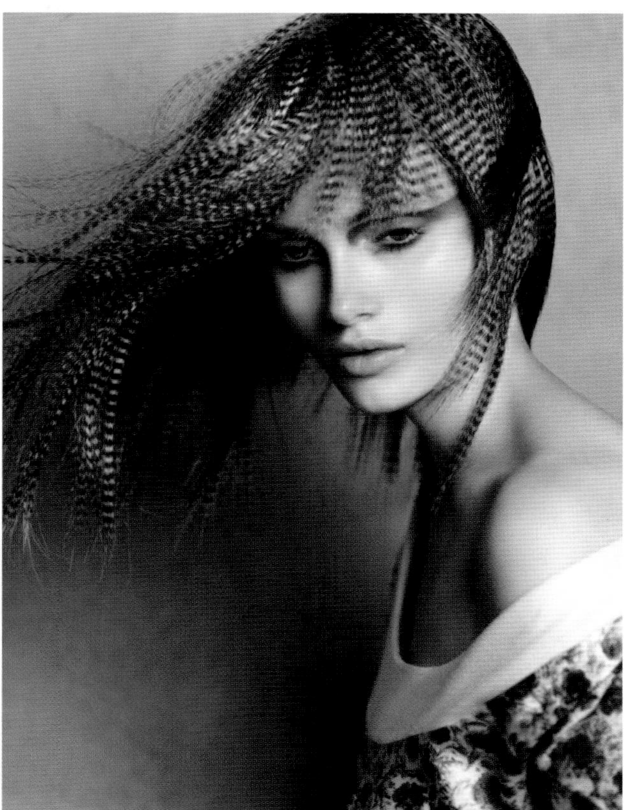

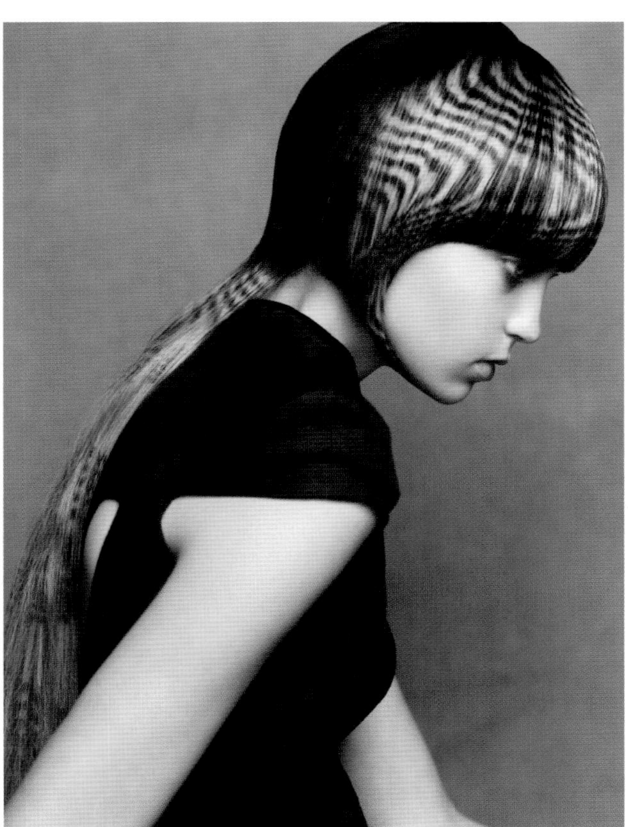

Hairstyles from Game Collection
for the British Hairdressing Awards
by Angelo Seminara (International
Creative Director, Trevor Sorbie), 2009

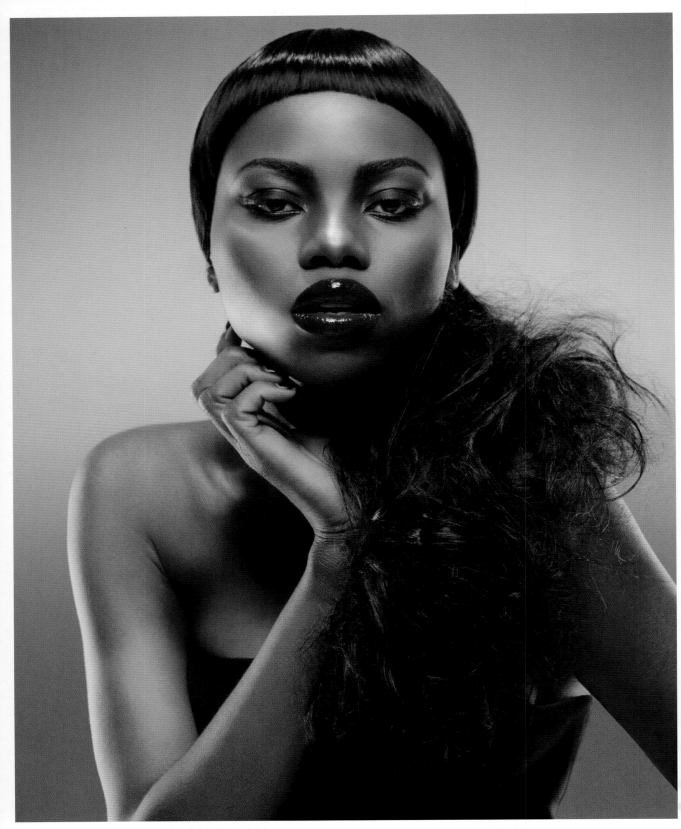

Black Beauty/Wahl Award winning hairstyle from the Definitive Power Collection by Michelle Thompson (Francesco Group), modelled by Syncha, 2009

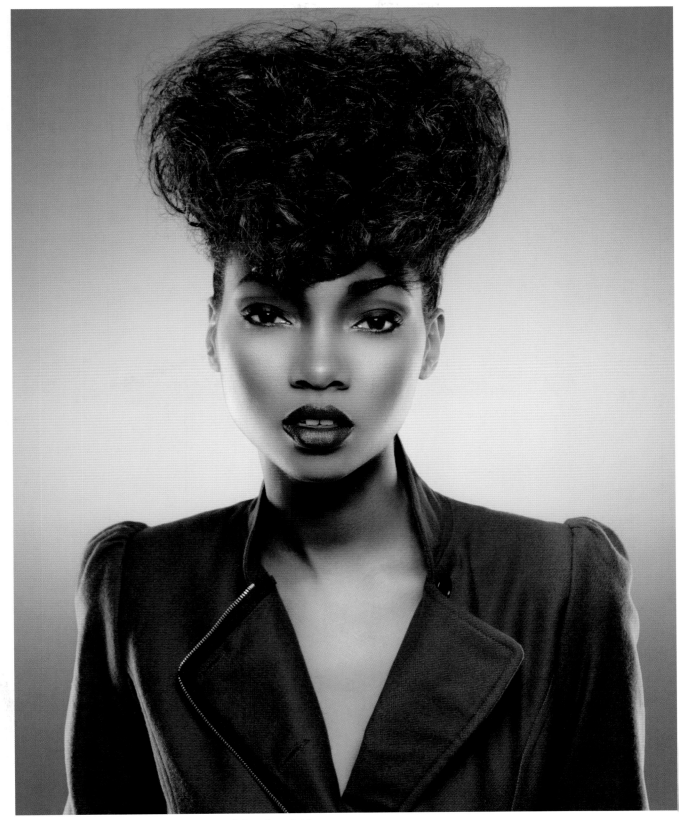

Black Beauty/Wahl Award winning Neo-1980s hairstyle from the Definitive Power Collection by Michelle Thompson (Francesco Group), modelled by Sylvie (Elite), 2009

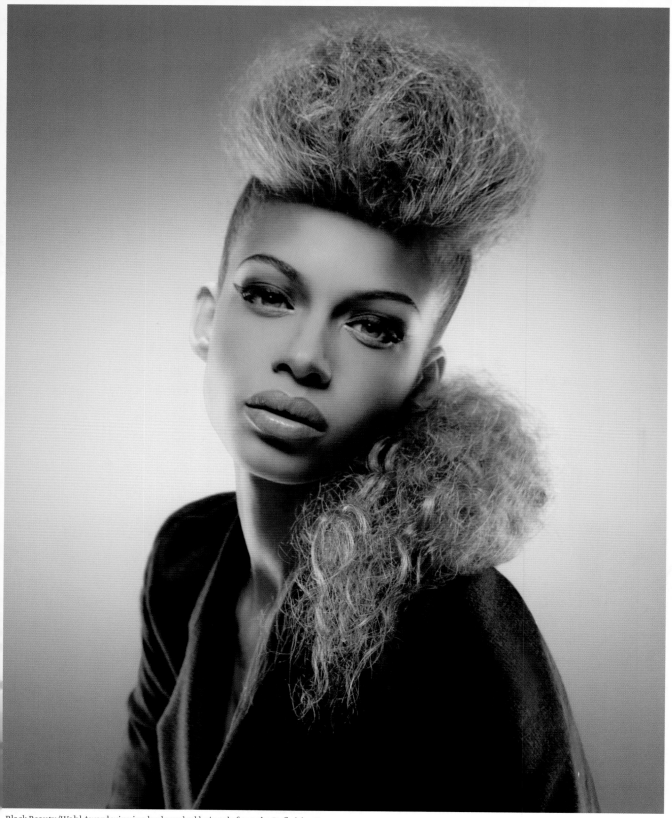

Black Beauty/Wahl Award winning backcombed hairstyle from the Definitive Power Collection by Michelle Thompson (Francesco Group), modelled by Annisa, 2009

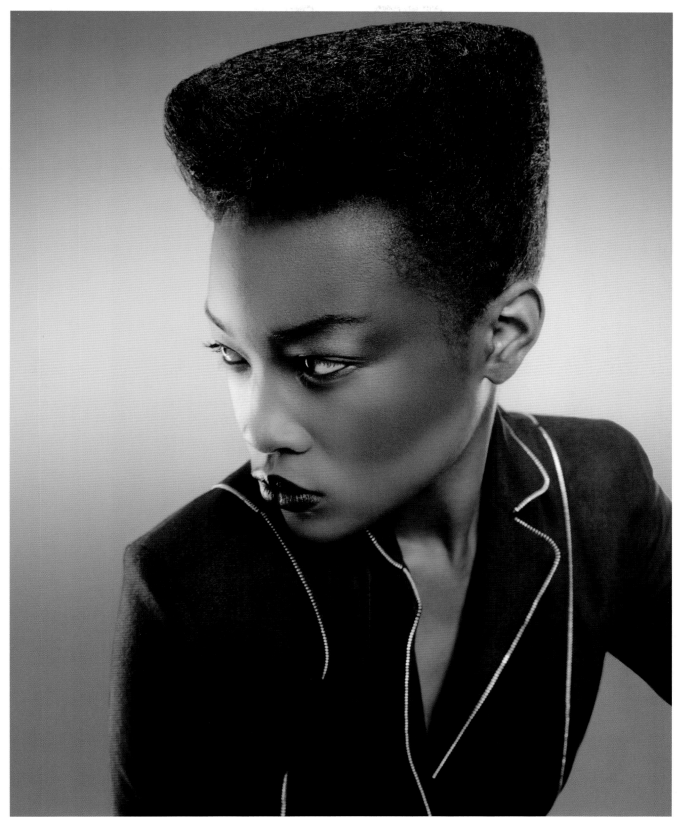

Black Beauty/Wahl Award winning geometric flat-top hairstyle from the Definitive Power Collection by Michelle Thompson (Francesco Group), modelled by Betty (Models 1), 2009

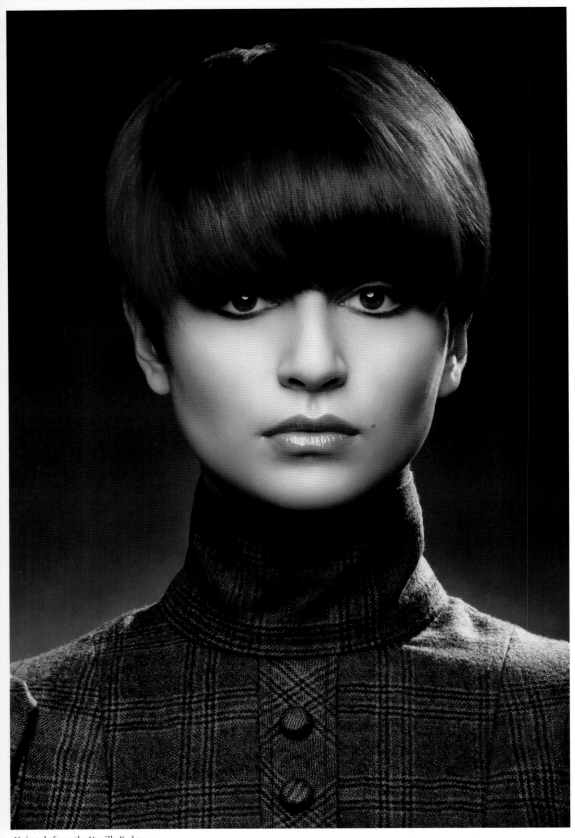

Hairstyle from the Vanilla Fudge
Collection by Anne Veck, 2009

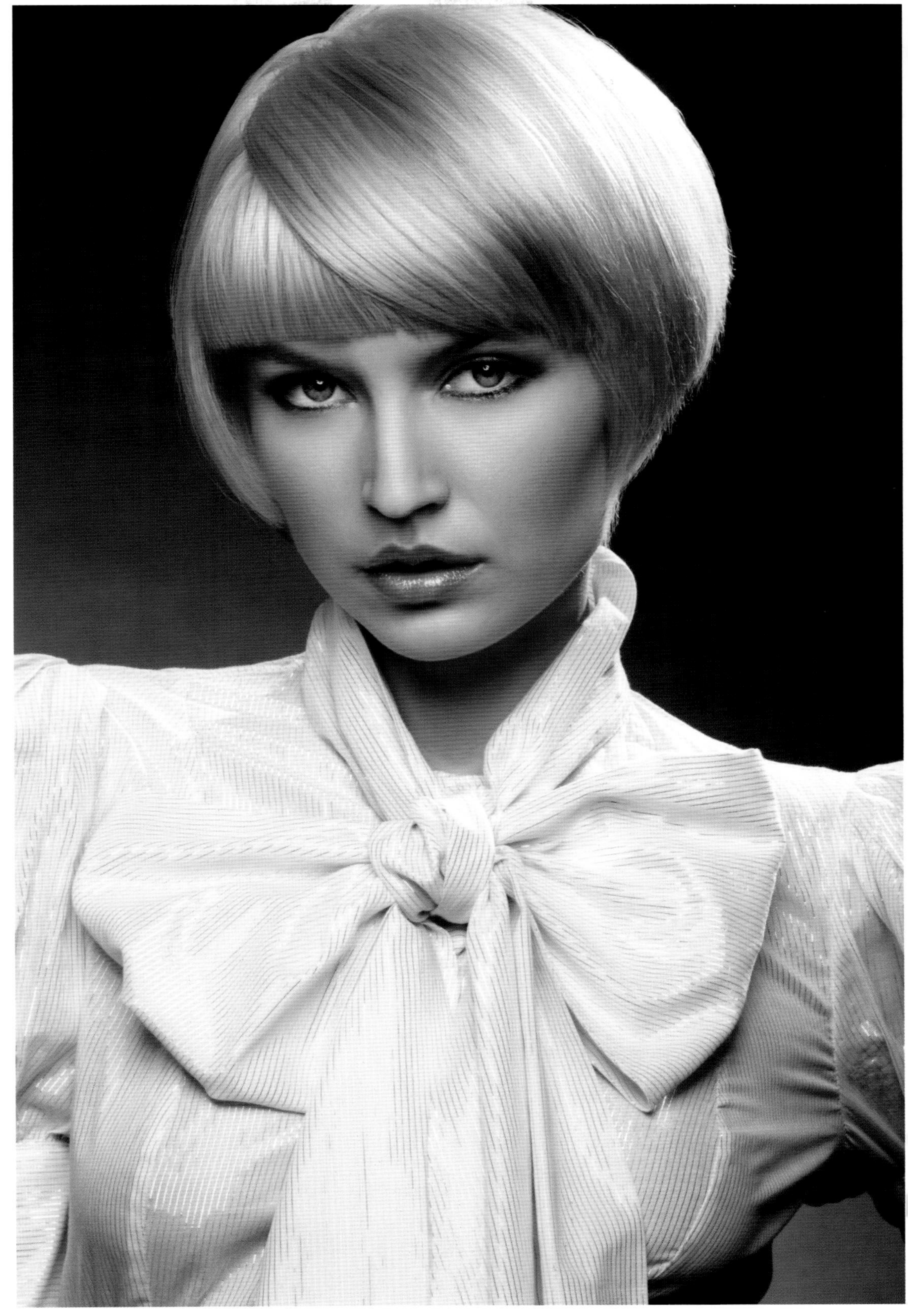

Hairstyle from the Vanilla Fudge
Collection by Anne Veck, 2009

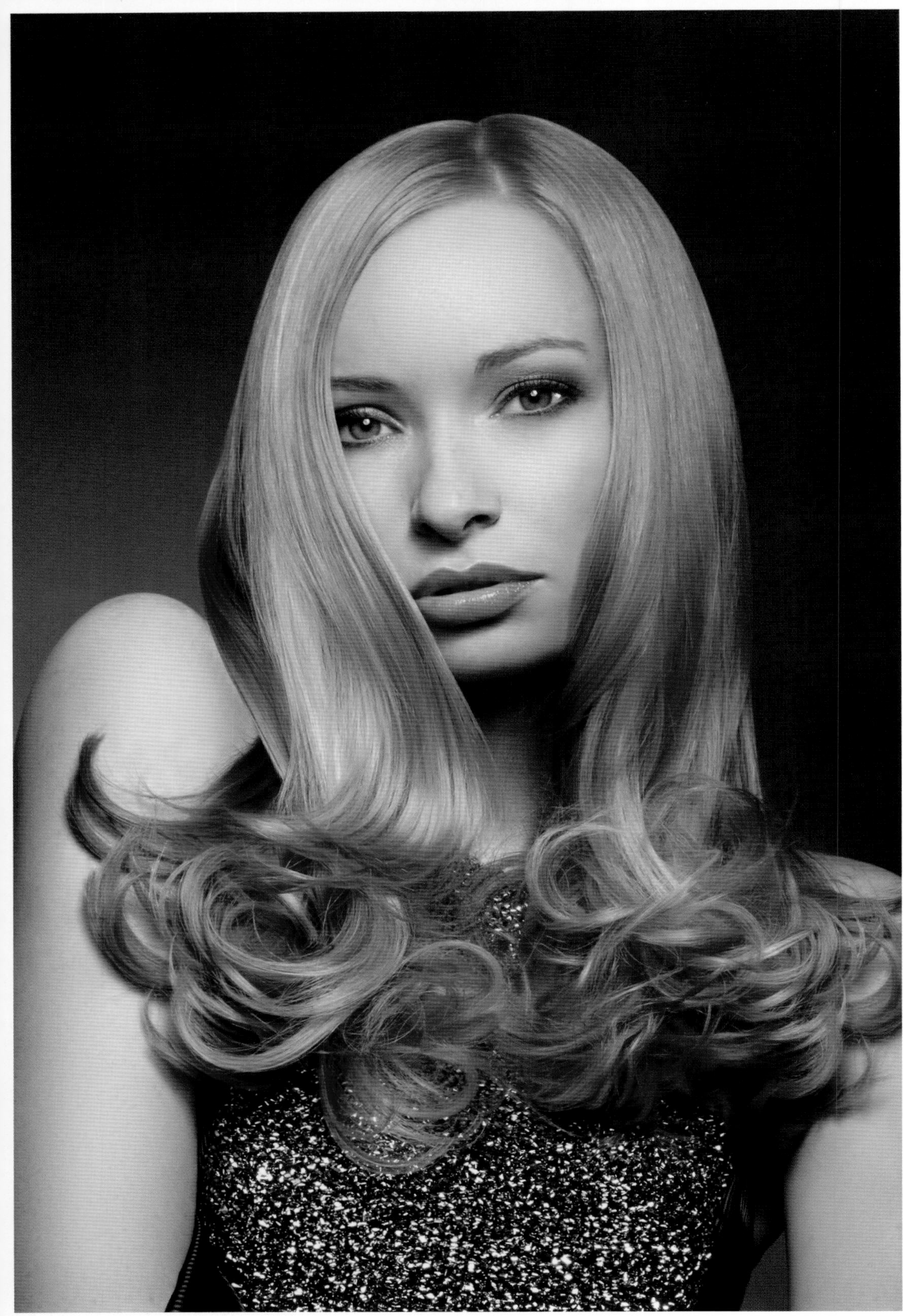

Hairstyle from the Vanilla Fudge
Collection by Anne Veck, 2009

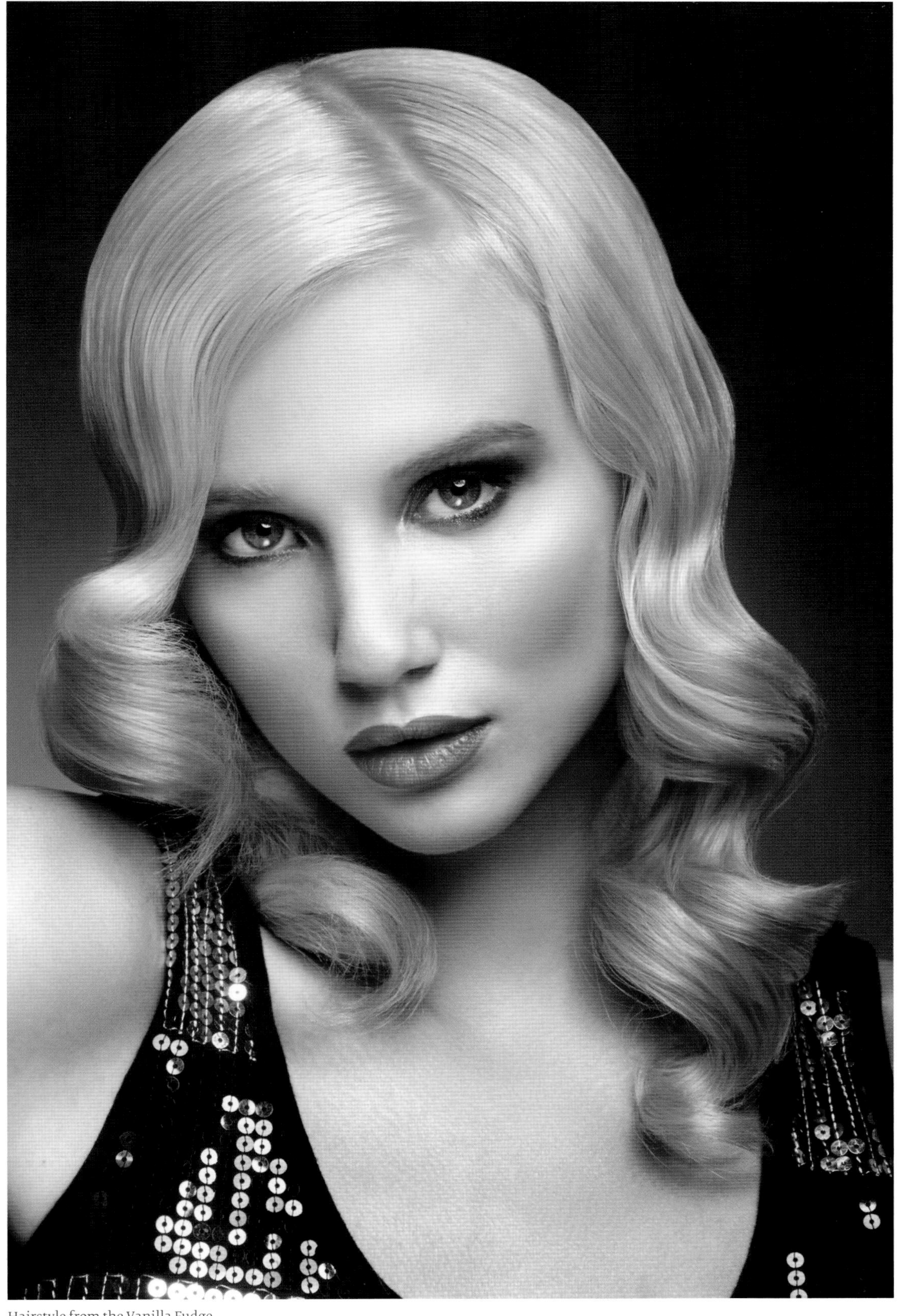

Hairstyle from the Vanilla Fudge
Collection by Anne Veck, 2009

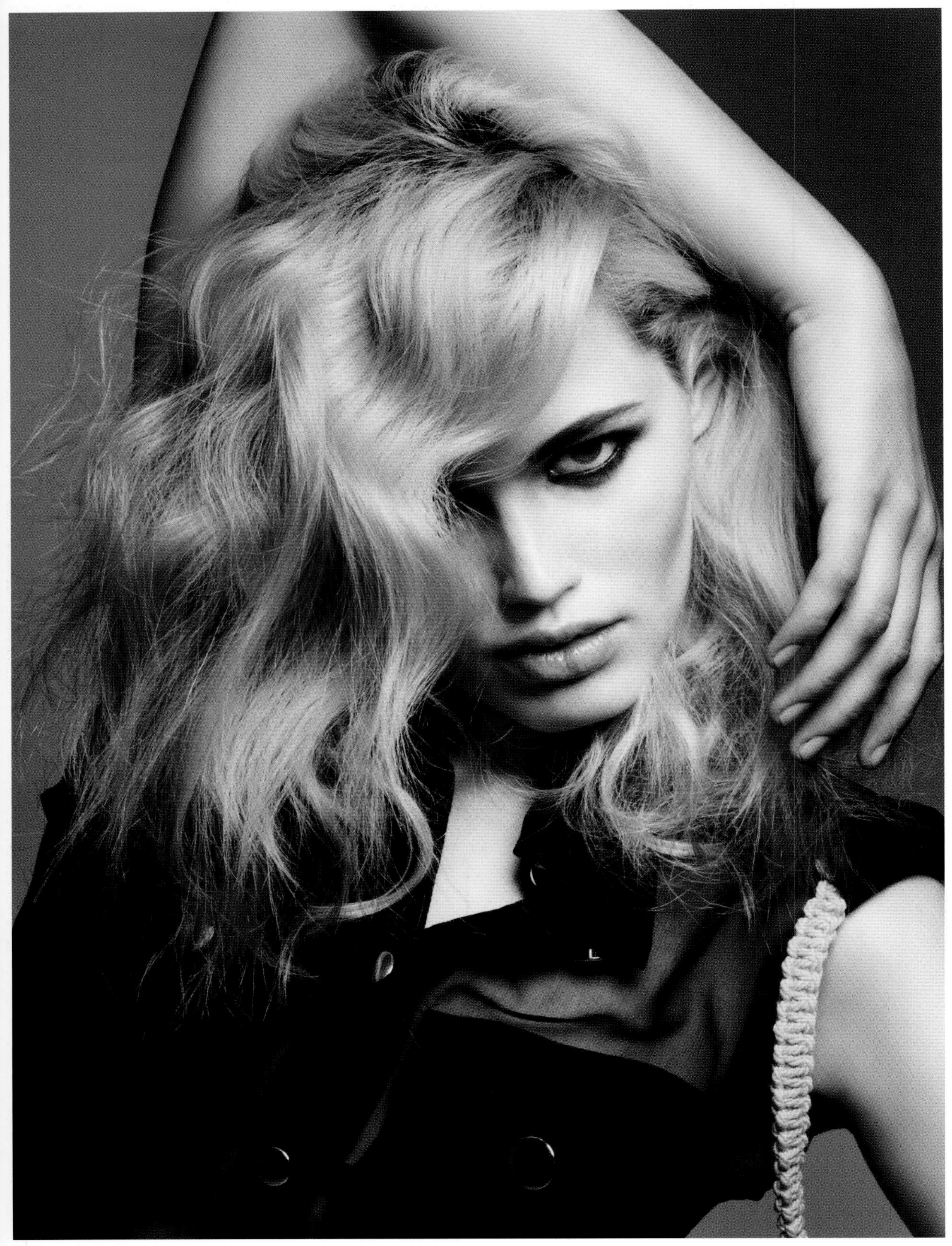

'Pink' hairstyle from the Glamazons
Collection by Lisa Shepherd, 2009

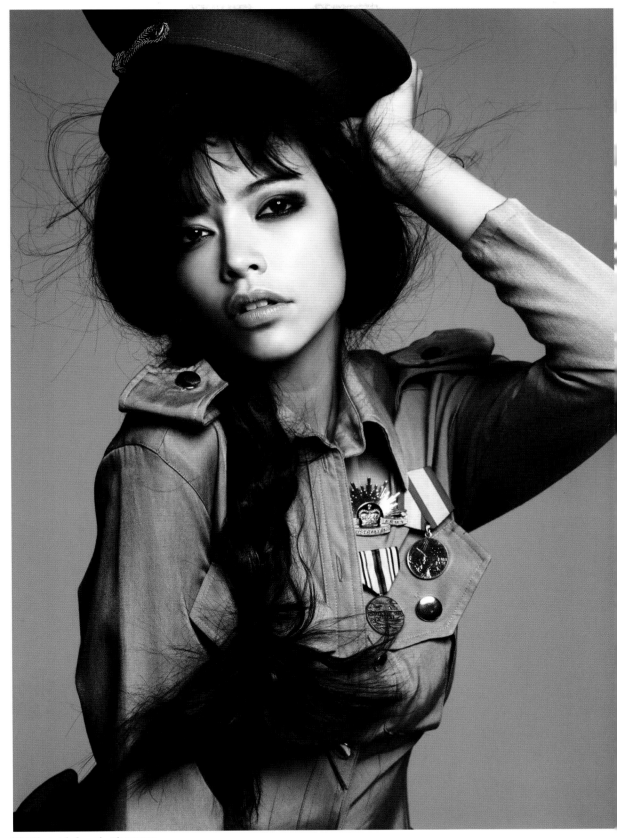

‘Plait’ hairstyle from the Glamazons Collection by Lisa Shepherd, 2009

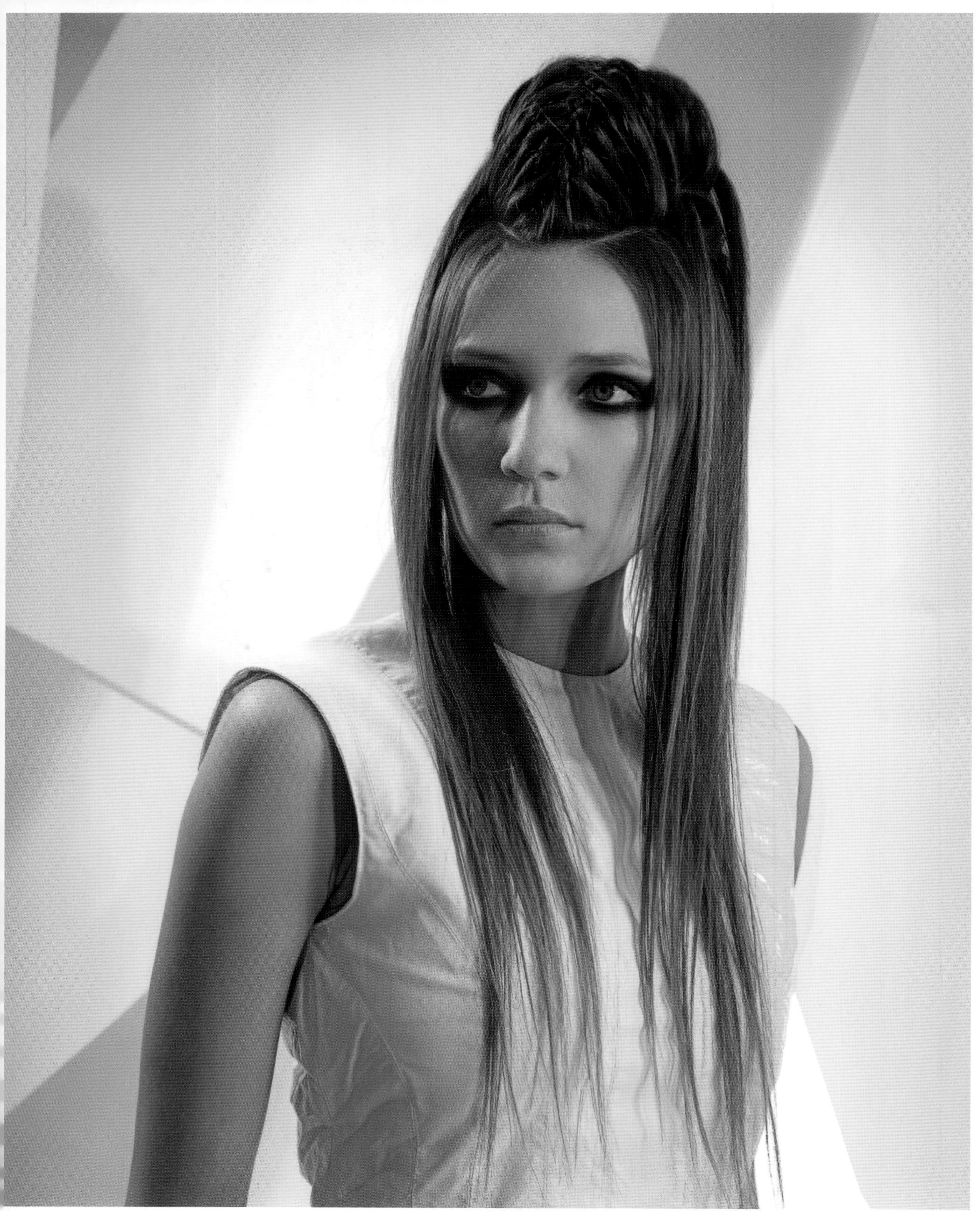

Hairstyle by Metropolis Artistic Team, 2009, photographed by Paul Godfrey

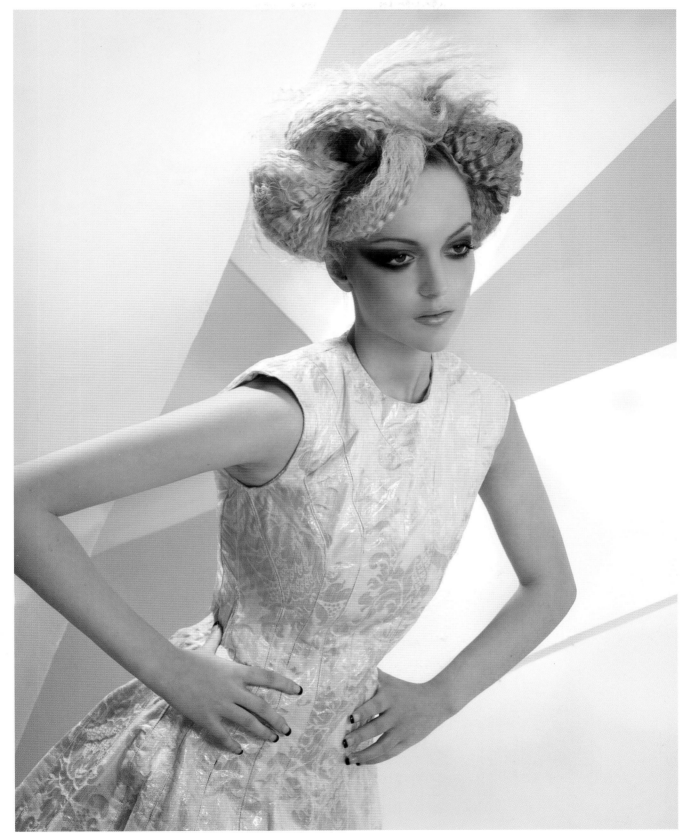

Hairstyle by Metropolis Artistic Team, 2009, photographed by Paul Godfrey

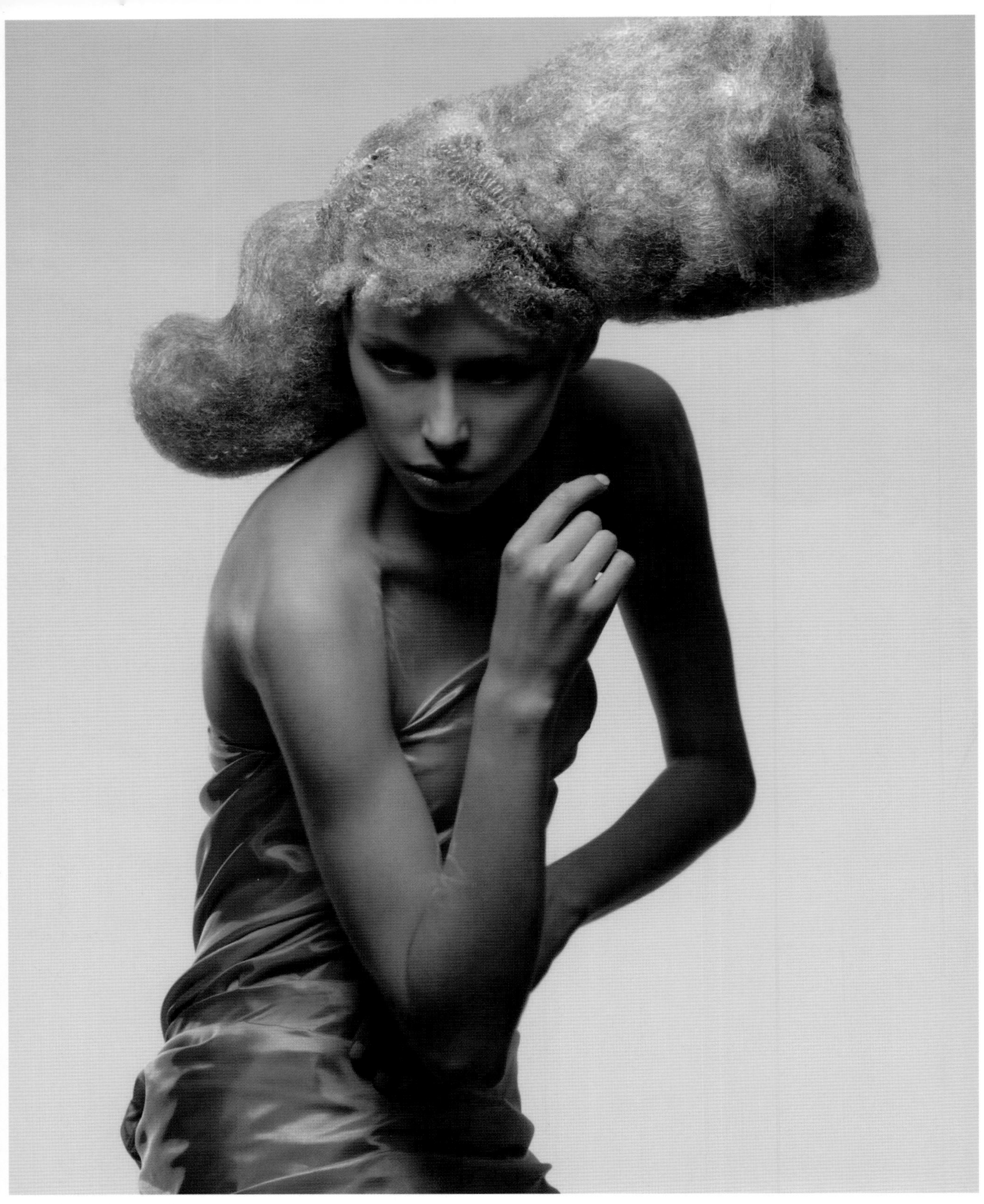

Hairstyle from the Magnolia
Collection by Anne Veck, 2010

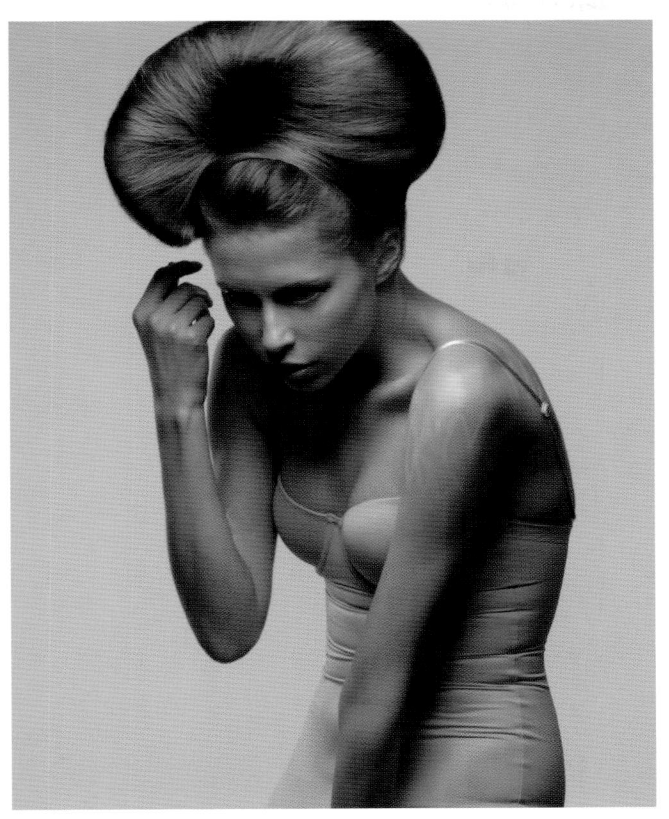
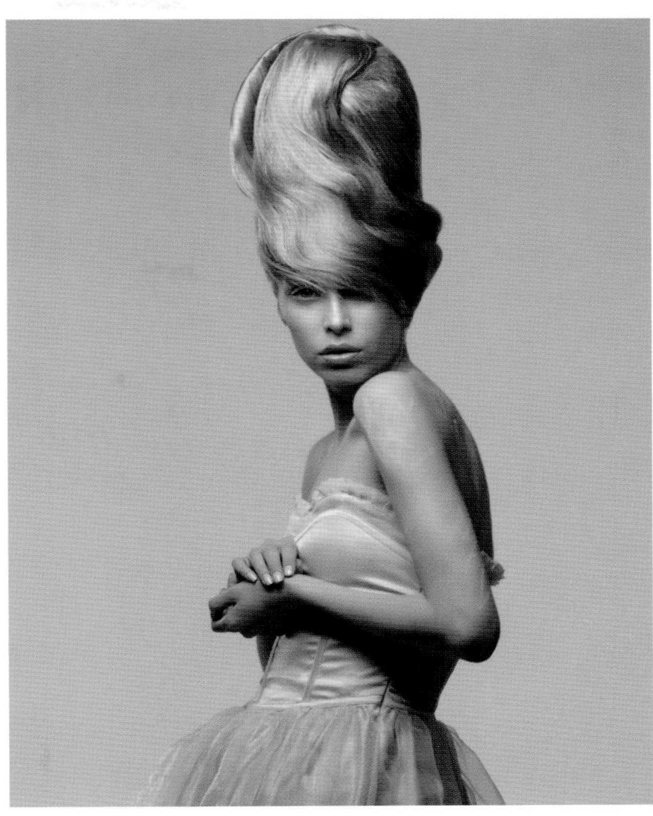
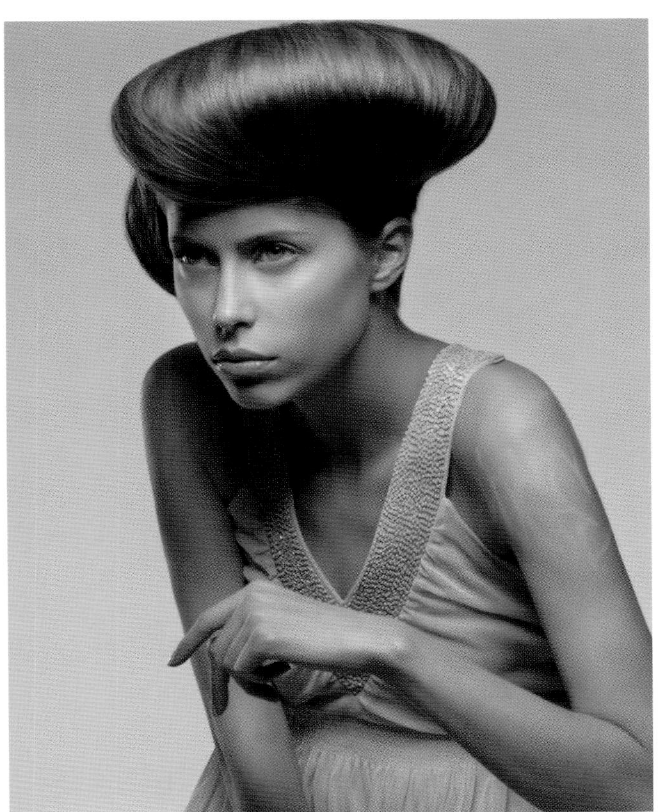
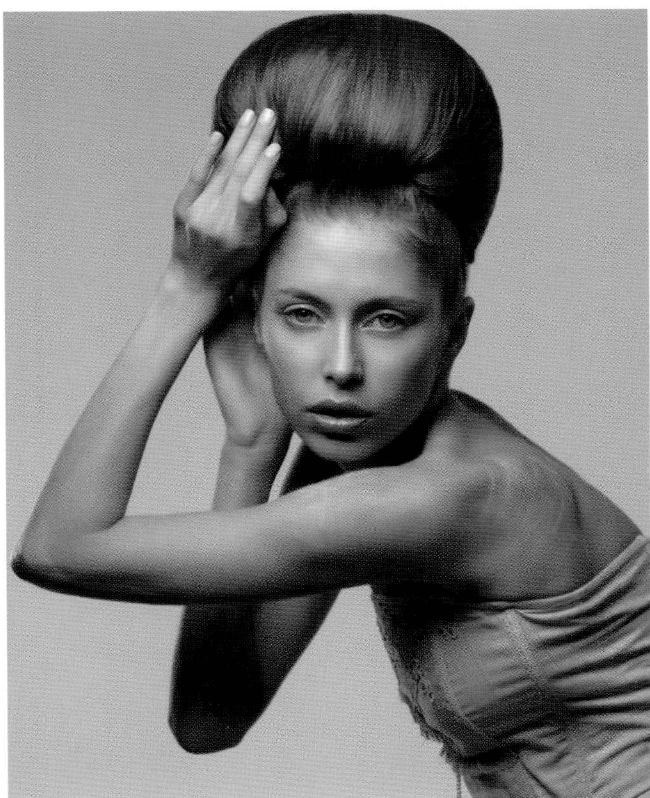

Hairstyles from the Magnolia Collection by Anne Veck, 2010

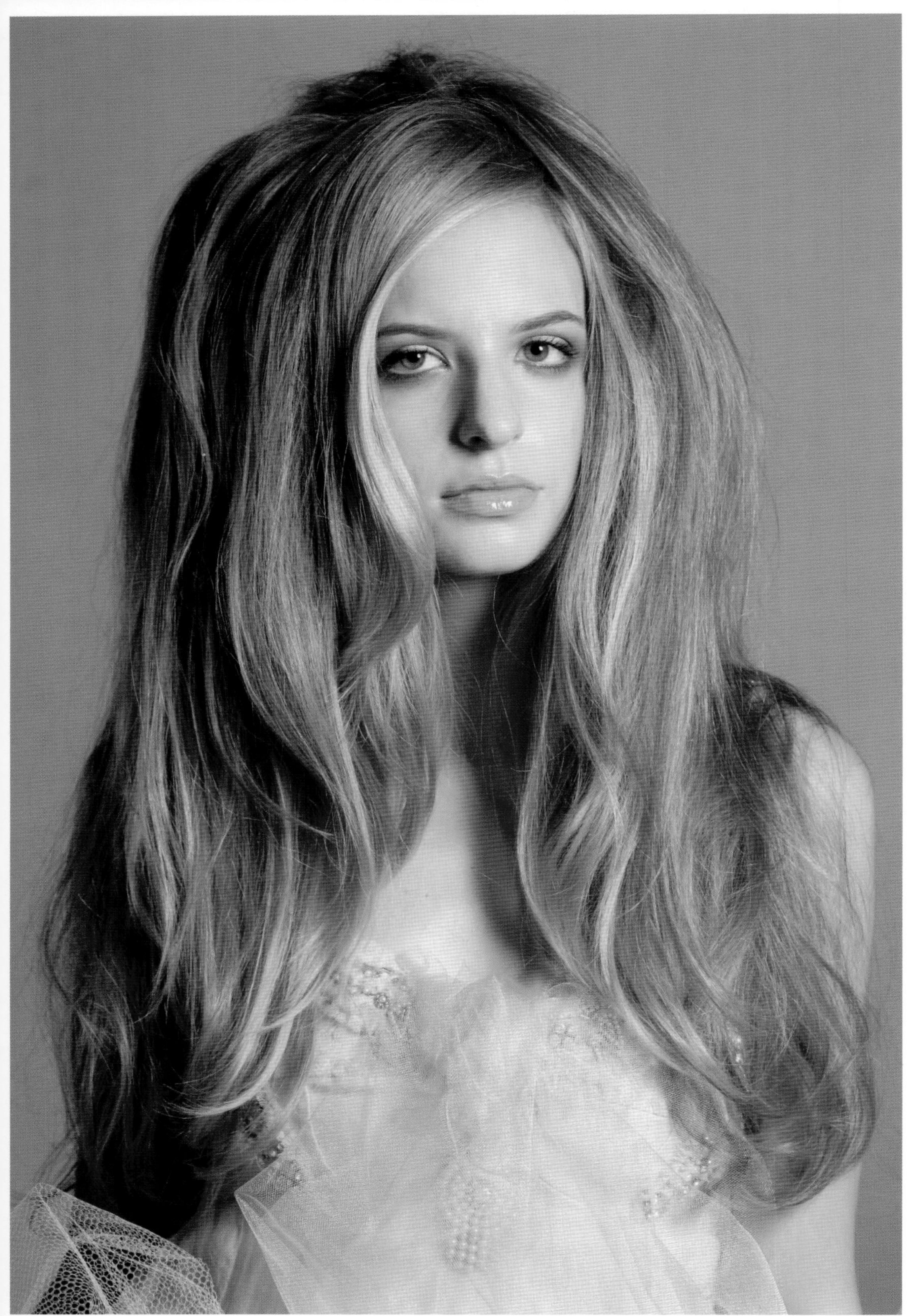

Elina O'Connor with the 'Princess Tease' hairstyle
by Luke & Rona O'Connor, 2010

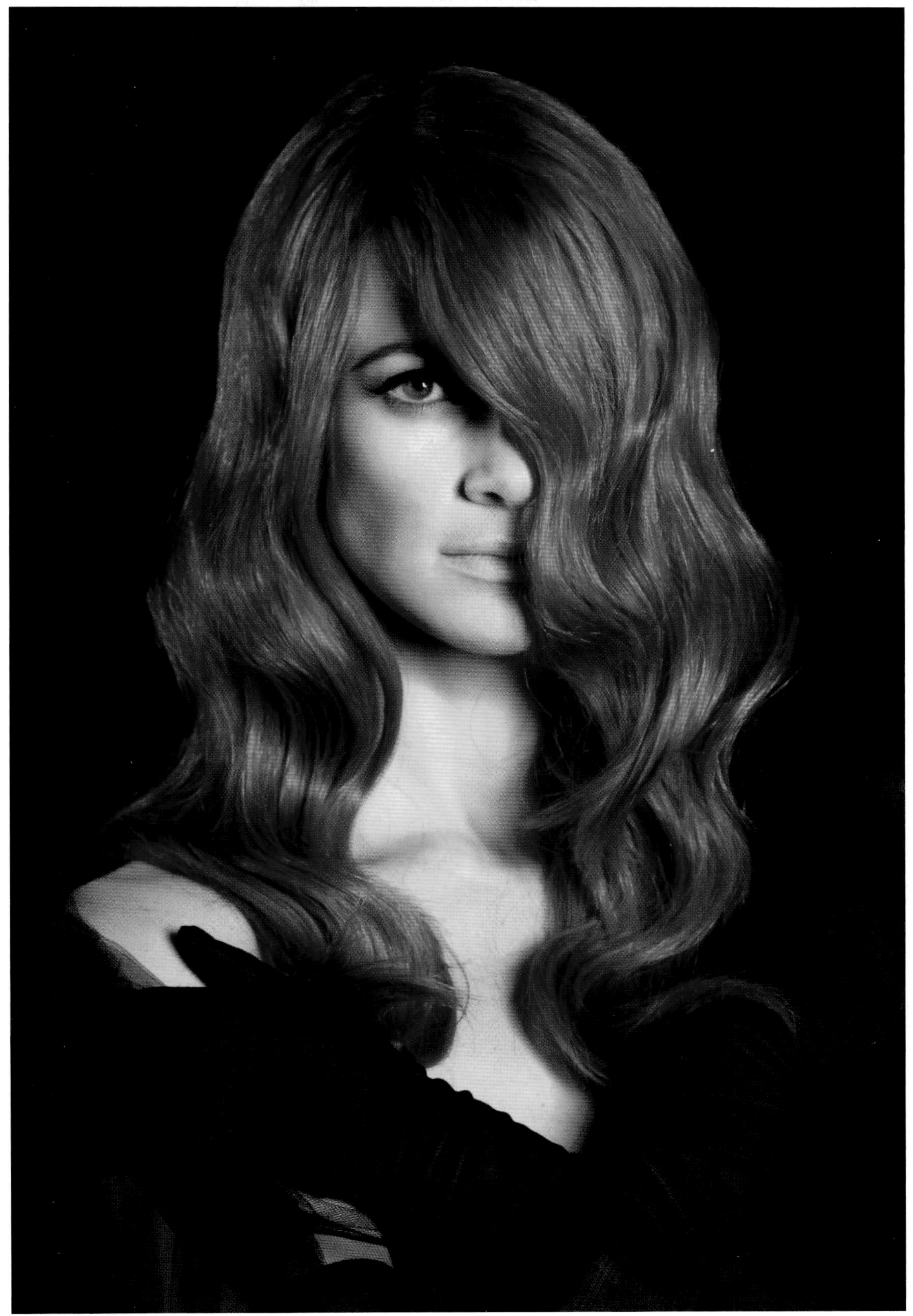

Kendra Andrews with the 'Liquid Ruby Red' hairstyle (in the 'Peek-a-boo' style made famous by 1940s Hollywood star, Veronica Lake) by Luke & Rona O'Connor, 2010

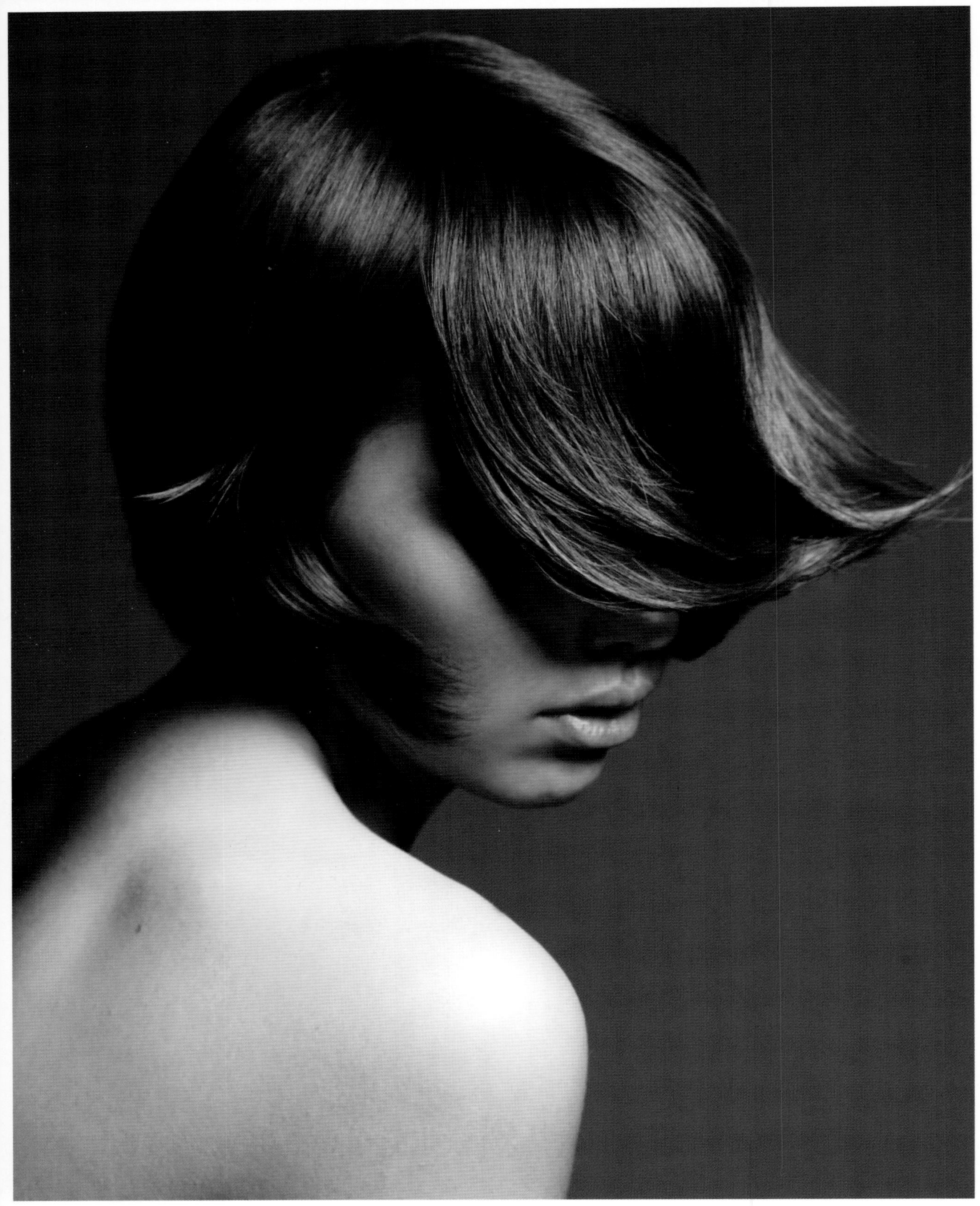

Hairstyle by Louis Byrne for Easton
Regal Hairdressing, 2010

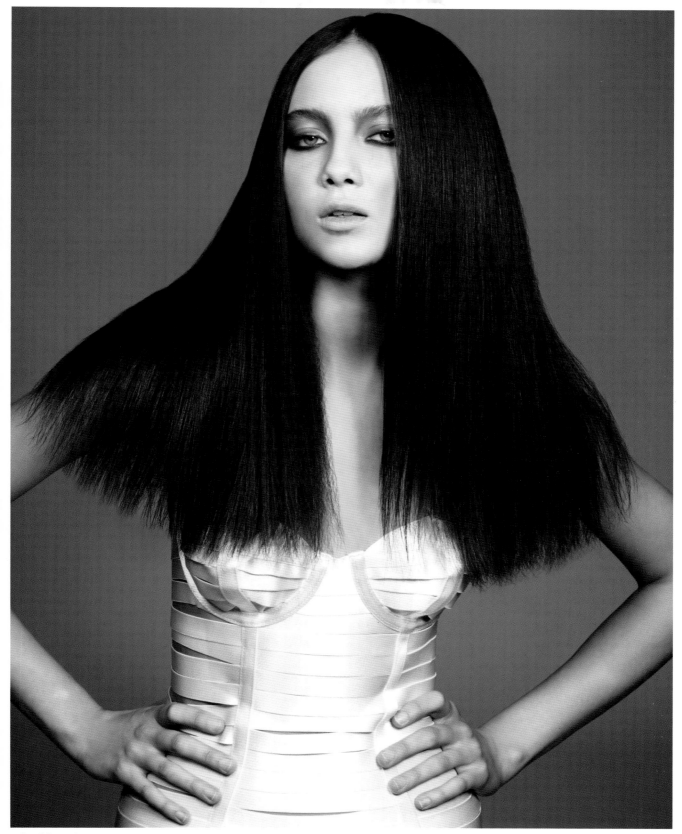

Hairstyle by Louis Byrne, 2000s

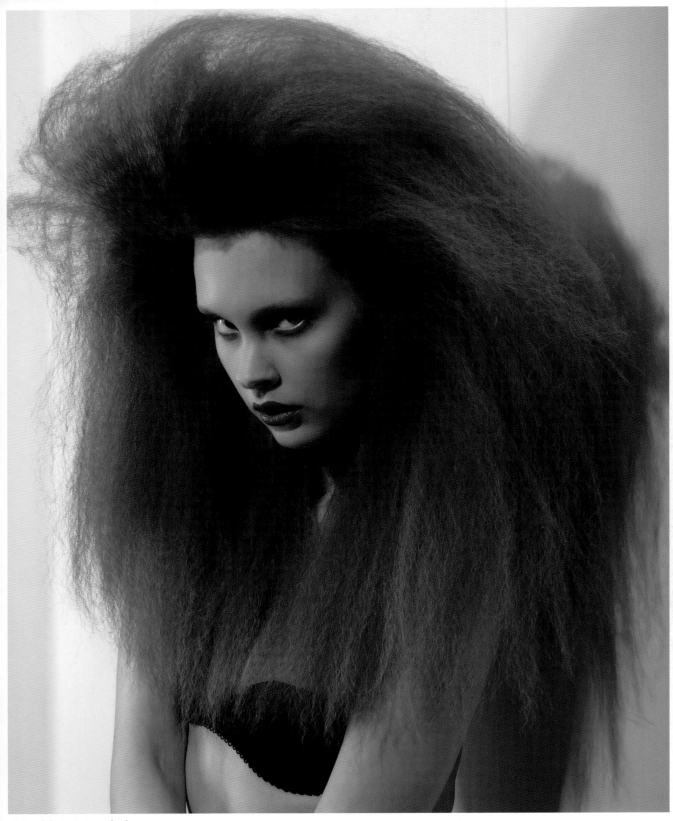

Hairstyle by Louis Byrne for the
British Hairdressing Awards, 2010

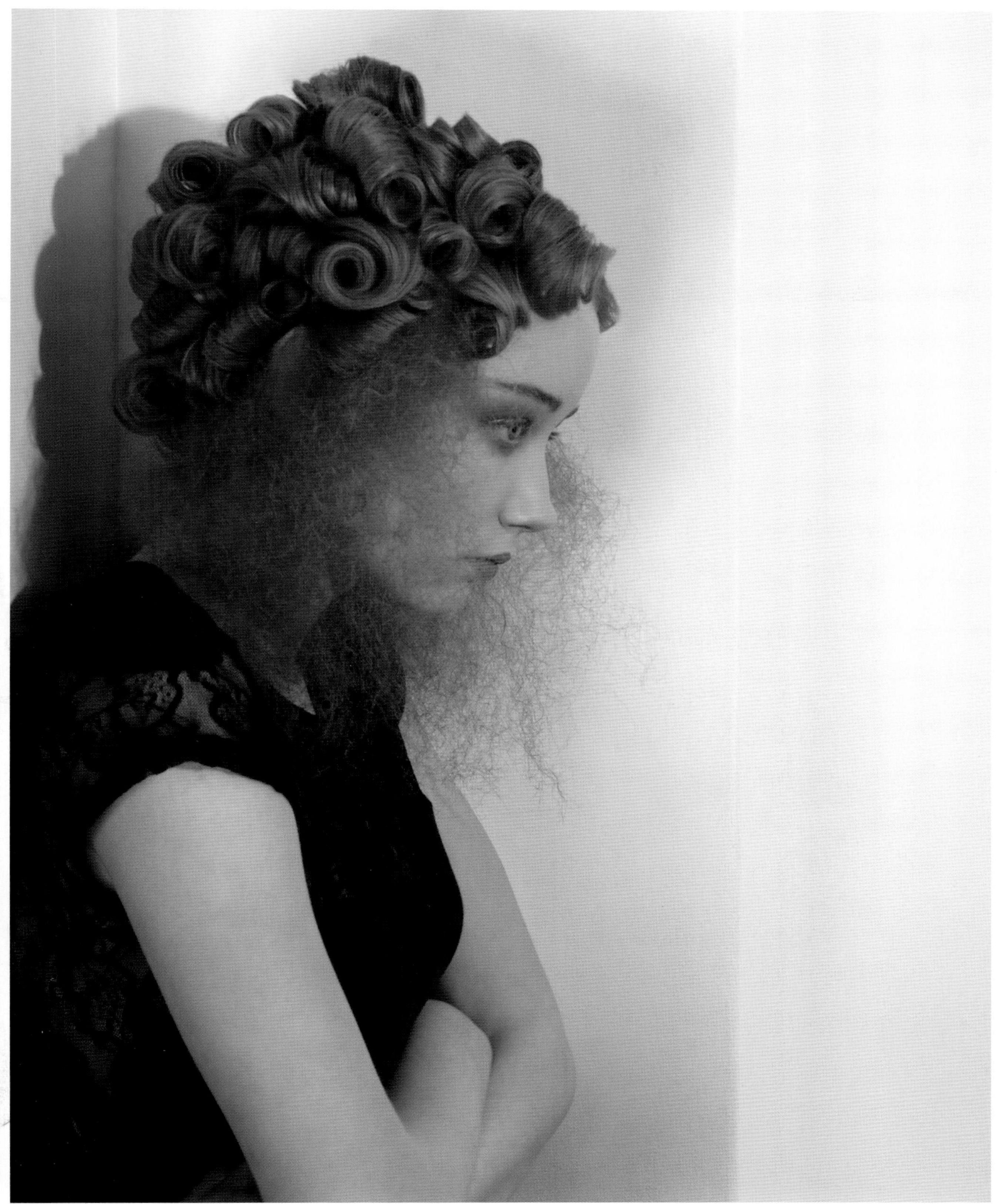

Hairstyle by Louis Byrne for the
British Hairdressing Awards, 2010

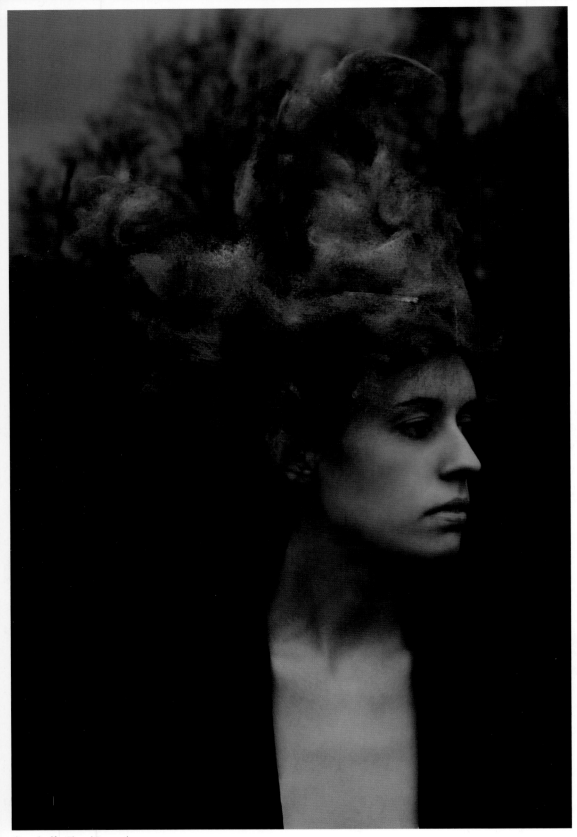

'Jazmine' by Gianni Scumaci,
photographer Colin Roy, 2010

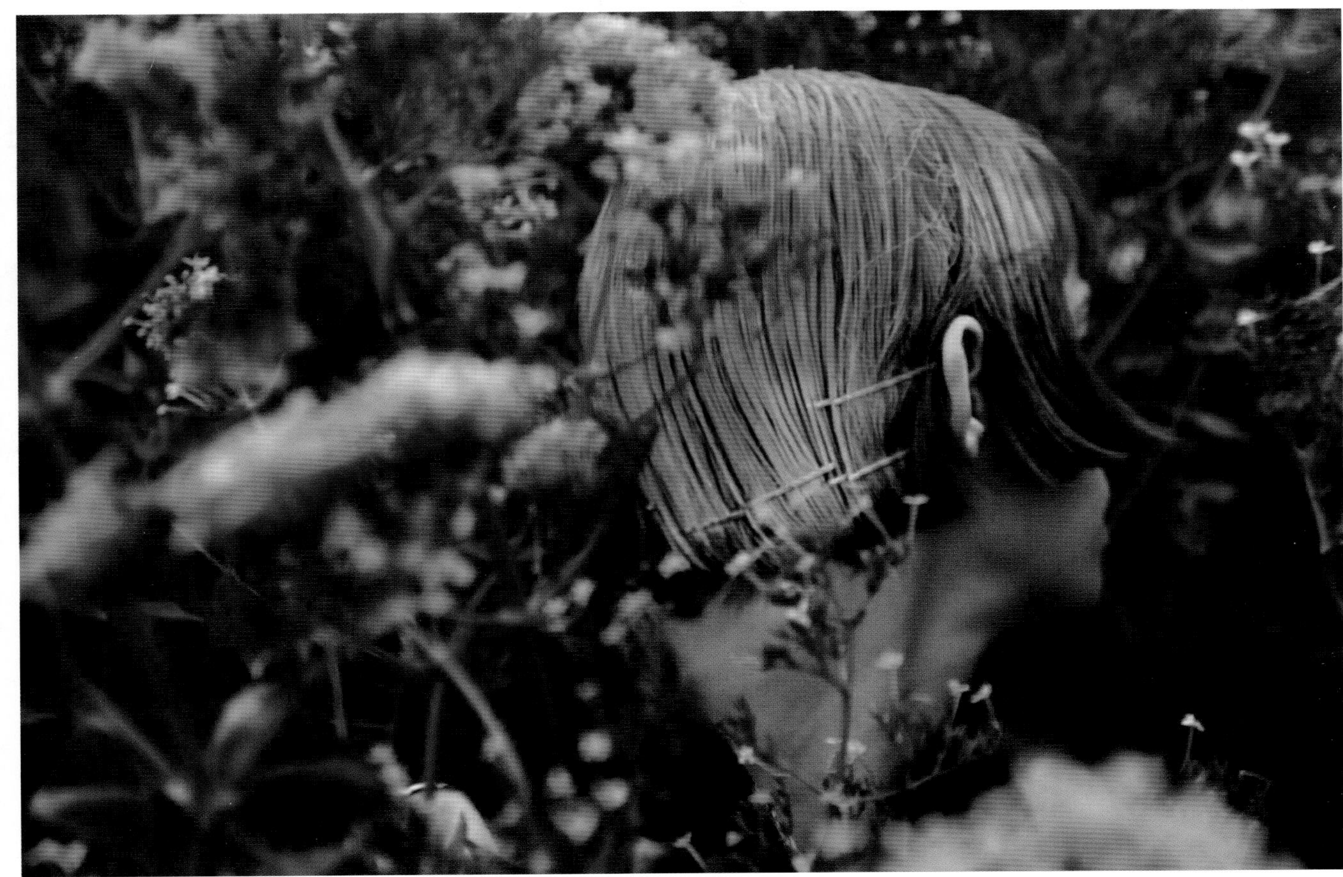

'Jazmine' by Gianni Scumaci,
photographer Colin Roy, 2010

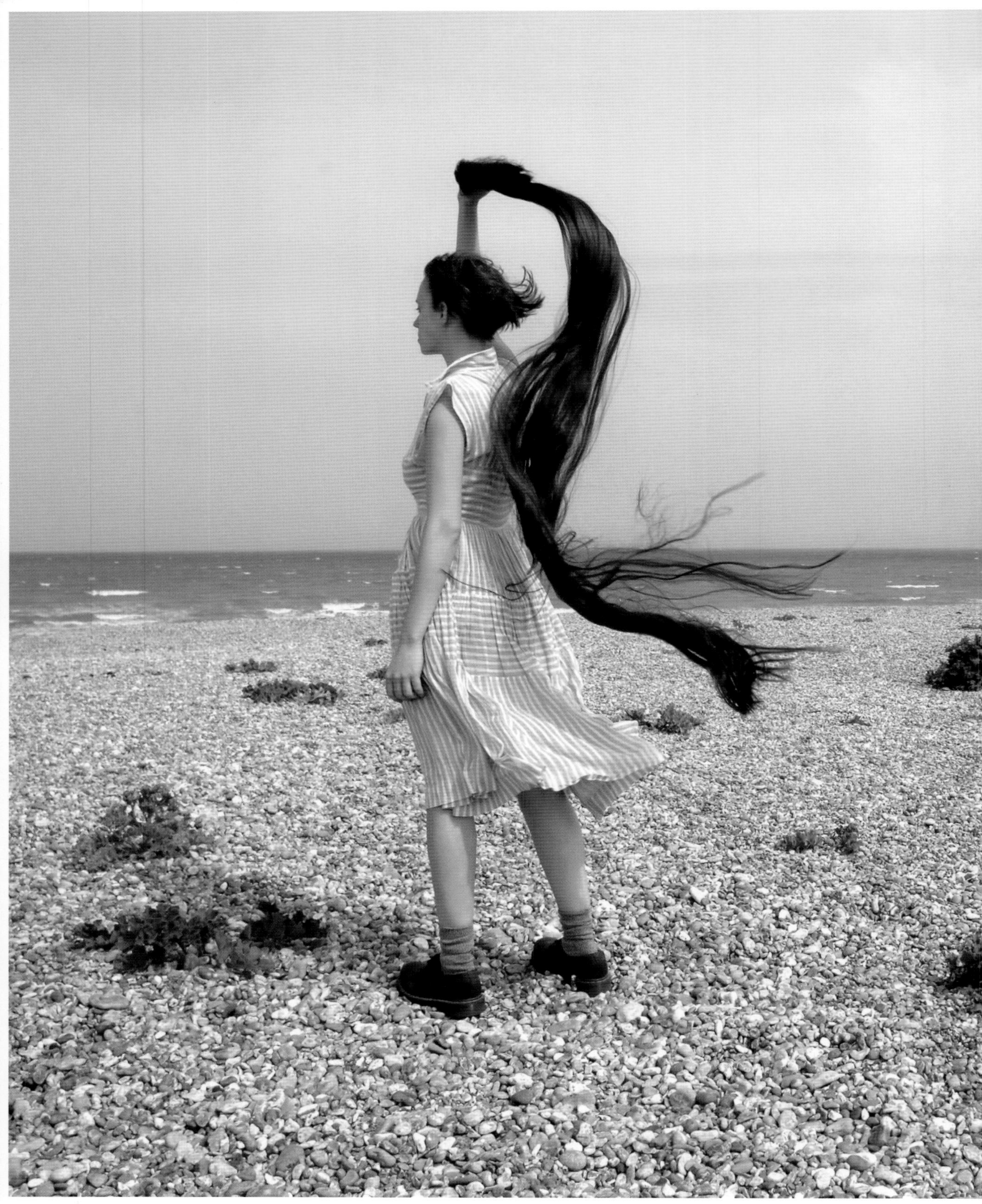

‘Jazmine’ by Gianni Scumaci,
photographer Colin Roy, 2010

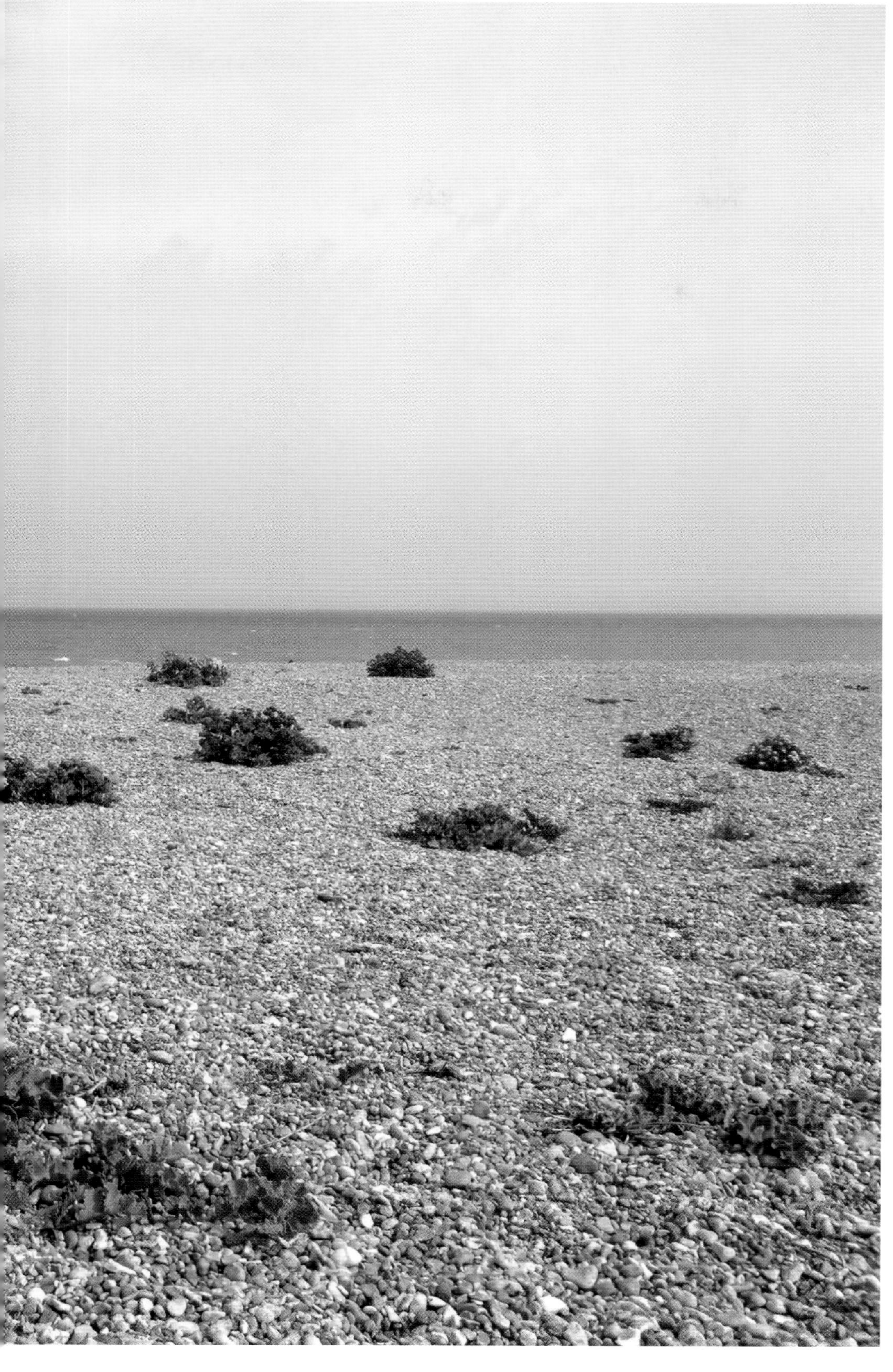

Bibliography

Asser, Joyce, *Historic Hairdressing*, Pitman, London, 1966

Bysterveld, Henri de, *Album de Coiffures Historiques*, Paris, 1863

Foan, Gilbert A., *The Art and Craft of Hairdressing*, The New Era Publishing Co. Ltd., London, 1936

Gordon, Michael, *Hair Heroes*, Bumble and bumble, USA, 2002

Jones, Dylan, *Haircults: Fifty Years of Styles and Cuts*, Thames and Hudson, London, 1990

Lewis, Leonard, *Leonard of Mayfair*, Hutchinson, London, 2000

Mallemont, A., *L'Art de la Coiffure Française*, E. Robinet, Paris, 1900

Moritz, Heinrich, *Album Historischer und Phantasie-Frisuren*, J.W. Zimmer, Frankfurt, 1900

Racinet, Auguste, *Le Costume Historique*, Firmin Didot, Paris, 1888

Rambaud, René, *Précis d'Histoire de la Coiffure Féminine à Travers les Ages*, Paris, 1937

Serventi, Henry, *Album of Period Coiffures, Historical and Modern*: (A.D. 1400 – A.D. 1927) from Medieval Times to the Present Day, London, c.1927

Sherrow, Victoria, *Encyclopaedia of Hair: A Cultural History*, Greenwood Press, USA, 2006

Smith, William, *Dictionary of Greek and Roman Antiquities*, John Murray, London, 1875

Stevens Cox, James, *An Illustrated Dictionary of Hairdressing and Wigmaking*, B. T. Batsford Ltd., London, 1966

Stewart, James, *Plocacosmos or, The whole art of hair dressing*, London, 1782

Zdatny, Steven, *Hairstyles and Fashion: A Hairdresser's History of Paris, 1910–1920*, Berg, Oxford International Publishers Ltd., Oxford/New York, 1999

Articles

Bicknell, J. P. C., *Hairdressing – and All That*, Progress Summer Issue, Lever Brothers & Unilever Limited, August 1938

Burnley, Florence and Schlesinger, Kathleen, *The Magic of Hairdressing in the 19th Century*, The Strand Magazine, George Newnes Ltd., London, 1900

Long, Carola, *Bob's your haircut*, The Independent, London, 10th of January 2009

Uzanne, Octave, *Weapons and Ornaments of Woman, Hairdressing and Head Coverings*, Cosmopolitan, August 1906

·

We are immensely grateful to those individuals, companies, picture libraries and institutions that have kindly allowed us to reproduce their images. We regret that in some cases it has not been possible to trace the original copyright holders of photographs from earlier publications or of early publicity images. The publisher has endeavoured to respect the rights of third parties and if any such rights have been overlooked in individual cases, the mistake will be correspondingly amended where possible. The majority of historic images included in this book are from the Fiell Archive.

Picture Credits

© Michael Barnes: photographs Chris Timtheou: 394 (all images), 395, 400, 401 (all images); photographs Rick Bonds: 408/409 (all images); photographs David Hindley: 410 (all images), 411, 412; photographs Marc Waller: 418 (all images), 419 (all images); 424, 425; photographs Kyoko Homma, courtesy of Goldwell: 452 (all images), 453 (all images), 458, 459; photographs Kyoko Homma: 462, 463, 468, 469

© Antoinette Beenders Archive Collection: 426, 427, 444 (both images), 445

© Brooks&Brooks: photographs Jenny Hands: 434 (all images), 435, 442, 443

© Louis Byrne: title page image (2), 454 (all images), 455, 466, 467; courtesy of Easton Regal Hairdressing: 502, 503, 504, 505

© Andrew Collinge: photographs Bill Ling: 342, 343 (left); photograph Mike Balfre: 343 (right); photographs Craig Johnston: 370, 371; photographs John Swannell: 450, 451

© Warren du Preez & Nick Thornton Jones: courtesy of Eugene Souleiman: 446/447, 448, 449

© Julien d'Ys: 413 (both images)

© Paul Edmonds: 367, 389, 390, 391, 402, 403, 420

Fiell Images/Fiell Publishing Limited, London: © Fiell Image Archive: 6, 13, 14, 15, 16, 17 (all images), 18, 19, 20, 21, 23, 24, 26 (all images), 27, 28, 29, 30 (all images), 31, 34, 35, 38 (all images), 39, 42, 43, 44, 45, 48, 49, 50, 51, 52, 53, 54, 55, 56, 57, 58, 60, (both images), 61, 62, 63 (all images), 64 (all images), 65, 66 (all images), 67, 68, 69, 70, 71, 72, 73, 74, 75, 76, 77, 78, 79, 80, 81, 82, 83, 84, 85 (all images), 86, 87, 88, 89, 90, 91, 92, 93, 94 (all images), 95, 96, 98 (both images), 99, 100, 101, 102 (all images), 103, 104, 105, 106, 107, 108, 109, 110, 111, 112 (all images), 113, 114, 115, 116, 117, 118, 119, 120, 121, 122, 123, 124, 125, 126 (both images), 127 (all images), 128, 129 (all images), 130, 131, 132, 133, 134, 135, 136, 138 (both images),

139, 140, 141, 142, 143, 144, 145, 146, 147, 148, 149, 150, 151, 152, 153, 154, 155, 156, 157, 158/159, 160, 161, 162, 163, 164, 165, 166/167, 168, 169, 170, 171, 172, 173, 176, 177 (both images), 178, 179, 180, 181, 182, 183, 184, 185, 186, 187, 188, 189, 190, 191, 192, 193, 194, 196, 198, 199, 200, 201, 202, 203, 204, 205, 206, 207, 208, 209, 210, 211, 212, 213, 214, 215, 216, 217, 218, 219, 220, 221, 222 (both images), 223, 224, 226 (all images), 227, 228, 229, 230, 232 (all images), 233, 234, 235, 236 (all images), 237 (all images), 238, 239, 240, 241, 242, 243, 244 (all images), 245 (all images), 246 (all images), 247, 248 (all images), 249, 250, 252, 253, 254, 255, 256 (both images), 257, 258, 259, 260, 261, 262, 263, 264 (all images), 265, 266, 267, 268 (all images), 269, 270, 271 (both images), 272 (both images), 273 (both images), 274, 275, 276, 277, 278 (all images), 279, 280, 281, 287, 290, 291 (all images), 292 (all images), 293, 294 (both images), 295, 296, 298 (both images), 299, 300, 301, 302 (both images), 303, 304, 305, 308, 309 (all images), 314, 318, 319, 320, 321, 322, 323, 324, 325, 326, 327, 330, 331, 332, 333, 350, 351, 354, 356

© Simon Forbes for Antenna: 352, 358, 359, 373, 376, 377, 378, 379, 382, 383, 384, 385

© Francesco Group, courtesy of Michelle Thompson: 460, 461; photographs Alessandro Cecchini: 486, 487, 488, 489

Getty Images: © Ronald Dumont/Express/Getty Images: 284; © Hulton Archive/Getty Images: 197, 286; © Eugene Robert Richee/Hulton Archive/Getty Images: 174, 386; Getty Images/Bridgeman Art Library: 46

© Barry Lategan: 285, 288 (courtesy of Twiggy), 289 (courtesy of Twiggy), 306

© Lukaro, courtesy of Luke & Rona O'Connor: photographs Tim Fielding: 398, 500, 501; photograph Ken Pivak: 399

© Metropolis: courtesy of Robert Masciave/Catalyst Consultancy: photographs Paul Godfrey: 496, 497

© Tomoko Nagakawa, 2000: 416

National Gallery, London: 37

© Ted Reynell: 355

© Colin Roy: courtesy of Gianni Scumaci: back cover image, 506, 507, 508/509

Scala Archives/Photo Scala, Florence: Scala Archives/Photo Scala, Florence © 2010 – courtesy of the Ministero Beni e Att. Culturali: 10; Photo Scala, Florence/Fotografica Foglia © 2010 – courtesy of the Ministero Beni e Att. Culturali: 22; Photo Scala, Florence © 2010: 32, 36; White Images/Scala, Florence © 2010: 40/41

© scpr, on behalf and courtesy of © Trevor Sorbie: 328 (both images), 349

© Angelo Seminara, courtesy of © Trevor Sorbie: photographs Andrew O'Toole: 484, 485 (all images)

© Lisa Shepherd: 421, 422, 423, 436, 437, 494, 495

© Smile, courtesy of Leslie Russell and Keith Wainwright: 8/9, 334; © Smile, photograph Tim Street-Porter: 335 (both images); © Smile, photograph James Wedge: 315; © Smile, photographs Steve Hiatt: 310, 311, 312 (both images), 313 (both images), 316, 317, 329, 338 (both images), 339, 340, 341, 362, 363, 369

© The Terence Donovan Archive: 282, 283

© TIGI: courtesy of Anthony Mascolo: 417, 428/429, 430, 431, 432, 433, 440, 441, 456, 457, 464, 465

© TONI&GUY: courtesy of Anthony Mascolo: front cover (photograph Pete Underwood), 336, 337, 344, 345, 346/347, 348, 357, 360, 361, 364, 365, 366, 368, 372, 374, 375, 380, 381, 388, 392, 393, 396, 397, 404, 405, 406, 407; photographs Troyt Coburn: 470, 471, 472, 473, 476; photographs Andrew O'Toole: 474, 475, 479, 482, 483; photograph Wolfgang Mustain: 477; photographs Gitte Meldgaard Fritz: 478, 480; photograph Edward Deblay: 481

© Anne Veck: photographs Charlotte Kibbles: 490, 491, 492, 493; photographs Barry Jeffery: 498, 499 (all images)

© Tim Walker: courtesy of Sasha Pivovarova/img Models: 414; courtesy of Coco Rocha/Storm: 438; courtesy of Stella Tennant/Select: 439

© Joanna Wilkinson: 297

Acknowledgements

This book is dedicated to Pat & Anthony Mascolo, whose groundbreaking hair creations inspired this project.

As with any publication of this nature, a great many people have been involved in this book's realisation and I would like to offer my immense gratitude to Isabel Wilkinson for her exceptional researching and picture sourcing skills, Mark Thomson and Rob Payne for their superb graphic design and painstaking execution of the layout, Rosanna Negrotti for her exacting copy-editing and proofing, and, of course, my husband, Peter for his enduring support and infective enthusiasm. I would also like to thank all the models, photographers and picture libraries that have allowed us to use their beautiful images. And lastly, but by no means least, I would like to offer up my immense gratitude to all the people involved in the hair industry who have kindly helped us with research and picture sourcing... this book is about you and as such you made this book happen – a big thank you!

Special thanks to:

Myles Ashby of Art + Commerce
Valentina Bandelloni of Scala Archives
Michael Barnes
Alex Barron-Hough of TIGI
Antoinette Beenders
Cliff Borress
Fanni Bostrom
Marilyn Braiterman
Sally & Jamie Brooks
Louis Byrne
Gosia Charles of Streeters Holdings Ltd.
Kelly Chin of Catalyst consultancy
Troyt Coburn
Andrew Collinge
Siobhan Cait Farrar of Streeters London
Diana Donovan
Warren Du Preez
Julien d'Ys
Easton Regal Hairdressing
Paul Edmonds
Simon Forbes of Antenna
Francesco Group
Kathy Griffin
Karen Harper of TONI&GUY
Katie Helman of Store PR
Elaine Hendrix
Daniel Hersheson
Milla Jovovich
Sophie Knight of Babel Fish PR
Barry Lategan
Marine Le Joncour
Leonard Lewis
Dominic Lewis
Lucy Liu
Bobby Loosmore of TONI&GUY
Soo Lucas, aka Soo Catwoman
Tristan Lund of the Michael Hoppen Gallery
Robert Masciave
Anthony & Pat Mascolo of TIGI
Jazmine Miles-Long
Calvin Morris at Storm
Sacha Mascolo-Tarbuck of TONI&GUY
Sarah McIntosh of the Terence Donovan Archive
Keith Mellen and Anne Veck
Metropolis Artistic Team
Tomoko Nagakawa
Tito Nath
Hayley Newman of Getty Images
Elina O'Connor
Luke and Rona O'Connor
Andrew O'Toole
Johnny Paterson of Catalyst consultancy
Maria Pitillo
Sasha Pivovarova
Coco Rocha
Colin Roy
Vidal Sassoon
Gianni Scumaci
Angelo Seminara of Trevor Sorbie
Tanya Shaw of SCPR
Lisa Shepherd
Ruth Sherlock of Andrew Collinge
Trevor Sorbie
Eugene Souleiman
John Swannell
Stella Tennant
Louise Thomas of SCPR
Michelle Thompson
Nick Thornton Jones
Lindsey Thurlow of Artist Representation/Management
Twiggy
Jacki Wadeson of JWPR
Keith Wainwright & Leslie Russell of Smile
Tim Walker and his assistant Polly Penrose
Vivienne Westwood
Anna Wintour